OXFORD CLINICAL NEPHROLOGY SERIES

Cardiovascular Disease in End-stage Renal Failure

Oxford Clinical Nephrology Series

Analgesic and NSAID-induced kidney disease
Edited by J.H. Stewart

Dialysis amyloid
Edited by Charles van Ypersele and Tilman B. Drüeke

Infections of the kidney and urinary tract
Edited by W.R. Cattell

Polycystic kidney disease
Edited by Michael L. Watson and Vicente E. Torres

Treatment of primary glomerulonephritis
Edited by Claudio Ponticelli and Richard J. Glassock

Inherited disorders of the kidney
Edited by Stephen H. Morgan and Jean-Pierre Grünfeld

Complications of long-term dialysis
Edited by Edwina A. Brown and Patrick S. Parfrey

Lupus nephritis
Edited by E. Lewis, M. Schwartz, and S. Korbet

Nephropathy in type 2 diabetes
Edited by Eberhard Ritz and Ivan Rychlík

Hemodialysis vascular access
Edited by Peter J. Conlon, Michael Nicholson and Steve Schwab

Mechanisms and clinical management of chronic renal failure (Second edition; formerly *Prevention of progressive chronic renal failure*)
Edited by A. Meguid El Nahas with Kevin Harris and Sharon Anderson

Cardiovascular disease in end-stage renal failure
Edited by Joseph Loscalzo and Gérard M. London

Cardiovascular Disease in End-stage Renal Failure

Edited by

JOSEPH LOSCALZO

Wade Professor and Chairman, Department of Medicine, and Director, Whitaker Cardiovascular Institute, Boston University School of Medicine, USA

and

GÉRARD M. LONDON

Chief of the Division of Nephrology, Mahnès Hospital, Fleury-Mérogis, France

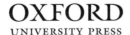

OXFORD

UNIVERSITY PRESS

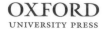

OXFORD
UNIVERSITY PRESS

Great Clarendon Street, Oxford OX2 6DP

Oxford Uninversity Press is a department of the University of Oxford.
It furthers the University's objective of excellence in research, scholarship,
and education by publishing worldwide in

Oxford New York

Athens Auckland Bangkok Bogotá Buenos Aires Calcutta
Cape Town Chennai Dar es Salaam Delhi Florence Hong Kong Istanbul
Karachi Kuala Lumpur Madrid Melbourne Mexico City Mumbai
Nairobi Paris São Paulo Singapore Taipei Tokyo Toronto Warsaw

with associated companies in Berlin Ibadan

Oxford is a registered trade mark of Oxford University Press
in the UK and in certain other countries

Published in the United States
by Oxford University Press Inc., New York

© Joseph Loscalzo and Gérard M. London 2000

The moral rights of the author have been asserted
Database right Oxford University Press (maker)

First published 2000

A catalogue record for this book is available from The British Library
Library of Congress Cataloging in Publication Data
(Data available)

ISBN 019 262 987 5

Typeset by EXPO Holdings, Malaysia

Printed and bound in Great Britain by
Biddles Ltd. Guildford & King's Lynn

PREFACE

A better understanding of the pathophysiology of renal failure, coupled with technological advances in dialysis techniques and renal transplantation, has greatly improved the prognosis and survival for patients with end-stage renal failure. Unfortunately, the advances and success of treatment are limited by a number of extrarenal complications that can cause significant morbidity and mortality. Of these, cardiovascular abnormalities are the most common, with cardiac complications alone accounting for more than 40 per cent of deaths in international registries. The importance of cardiovascular complications has become even more apparent in recent years with the increased prevalence of diabetes mellitus and vascular nephropathy and with the general aging of patients with end-stage renal failure.

The past decade has witnessed enormous advances in understanding the causes and pathophysiology of cardiovascular disease, and its diagnosis, treatment, and prevention. It is, therefore, of importance for physicians caring for patients with end-stage renal failure to understand the pathogenesis of cardiovascular complications, to become familiar with modern diagnostic tools and techniques, and to recognize and treat these complications. The goal of this text is to provide a comprehensive review of the pathophysiology and clinical manifestations of the principal cardiovascular complications in patients with chronic renal failure. This text is intended to assist nephrologists, cardiologists, and internists who care for these patients.

The book comprises 19 chapters and is organized into three parts. The first part comprises three chapters dealing with the epidemiology of cardiovascular disease in patients with end-stage renal failure. In the second part, eight chapters cover the basic pathophysiology and pathobiology of cardiovascular disease in the setting of end-stage renal failure. The final part comprises eight chapters focusing on the clinical manifestations, diagnosis, and management of cardiovascular disease in patients with end-stage renal failure.

Joseph Loscalzo
Gérard M. London

ACKNOWLEDGEMENTS

We thank Stephanie Tribuna for her assistance throughout the many phases of the development of this text, and Jalna Ross for her assistance in reference verification.

To our wives, Anita and Alena, and to our children, Julia and Alex Loscalzo, and Thomas and Marc London

CONTENTS

CONTRIBUTORS

Kerstin Amann, Department of Pathology, University of Heidelberg, 69120 Heidelberg, Germany

Thomas C. Andrews, Department of Internal Medicine, Cardiology Division, The University of Texas Southwestern Medical Center at Dallas, 5323 Harry Hines Boulevard, Dallas, TX 75235-9047, USA

Angel Argiles, Department of Medicine and Nephrology, University Hospital, 34295 Montpellier, France

Colin Baigent, Clinical Trial Service Unit and Epidemiological Studies Unit, University of Oxford, UK

George L. Bakris, Rush University Hypertension Center, Department of Preventive Medicine, Rush Presbyterian/St Luke's Medical Center, Chicago, IL 60612, USA

Benoît Barrou, Division of Renal Transplantation, CHU Pitié-Salpétrière, Paris, France

Marc-Olivier Bitker, Division of Renal Transplantation, CHU Pitié-Salpétrière, Paris, France

Andrew G. Bostom, Memorial Hospital of Rhode Island, Pawtucket, RI 02860, USA

M. Elizabeth Brickner, The University of Texas Southwestern Medical Center at Dallas, Department of Internal Medicine, Cardiology Division, 5323 Harry Hines Boulevard, Dallas, TX 75235–9047, USA

Liam F. Casserly, Nephrology Section, Department of Medicine, Boston Medical Center, Boston University School of Medicine, Boston, MA, USA

Alistair M.S. Chesser, Anthony Raine Research Laboratories, St Bartholomew's Hospital, London, UK

Philippe Cluzel, Division of Vascular Radiology, CHU Pitié-Salpétrière, Paris, France

Bruce F. Culleton, National Heart, Lung, and Blood Institute's Framingham Heart Study, Framingham, MA, USA

Gilbert Deray, Division of Nephrology, CHU Pitié-Salpétrière, Paris, France

Béatrice Descamps-Latscha, INSERM U507, Necker Hospital, 75743 Paris Cedex 15, France

Tilman L. B. Drüeke, INSERM U507, Necker Hospital, 75743 Paris Cedex 15, France

Robert N. Foley, The Divisions of Nephrology and Clinical Epidemiology, Memorial University of Newfoundland, The Health Sciences Centre, St. John's, Newfoundland, Canada A1B 3V6

Michael M. Givertz, Cardiovascular Section, Department of Medicine, Boston Medical Center, Boston, MA 02118, USA

Helene L. Glassberg, Cardiovascular Section, Department of Medicine, Boston University School of Medicine, Boston, MA 02118, USA

Alain P. Guérin, Nephrology Department, Manhès Hospital, Fleury-Mérogis, France

Kunitoshi Iseki, Dialysis Unit and Third Department of Internal Medicine, University of The Ryukyus, Okinawa, Japan

Bertram L. Kasiske, Division of Nephrology, Department of Medicine, Hennepin County Medical Center, University of Minnesota Medical School, Minneapolis, Minnesota, USA

Khoa T. N., INSERM U507, Necker Hospital, 75743 Paris Cedex 15, France

Edouard Kieffer, Division of Vascular Surgery, CHU Pitié-Salpétrière, Paris, France

J.P. Kooman, Department of Internal Medicine, University Hospital Maastricht, The Netherlands

Fabien Koskas, Division of Vascular Surgery, CHU Pitié-Salpétrière, Paris, France

Florian Kronenberg, Institute of Medical Biology and Human Genetics, Schöpfstrasse 41, Innsbruck A-6020, Austria

Eduardo K. Lacson, Renal Division, Department of Medicine, Brigham and Women's Hospital, Harvard Medical School, Boston, MA, USA

K.M. L. Leunissen, Department of Internal Medicine, University Hospital Maastricht, The Netherlands

Gérard M. London, Nephrology Department, Manhès Hospital, Fleury-Mérogis, France

Joseph Loscalzo, Department of Medicine and Whitaker Cardiovascular Institute, Boston University School of Medicine, Boston, MA 02118, USA

Sylvain J. Marchais, Nephrology Department, Manhès Hospital, Fleury-Mérogis, France

Ziad A. Massy, Division of Nephrology, C.H. Beauvais, and INSERM U507, Necker Hospital, Paris, France

Fabien Métivier, Nephrology Department, Manhès Hospital, Fleury-Mérogis, France

Albert Mimran, Department of Medicine and Nephrology, University Hospital, 34295 Montpellier, France

Georges Mourad, Department of Medicine and Nephrology, University Hospital, 34295 Montpellier, France

William F. Owen, Institute for Renal Outcomes Research & Health Policy, Duke Clinical Research Institute, Duke University School of Medicine, Durham, NC, USA

Patrick S. Parfrey, The Divisions of Nephrology and Clinical Epidemiology, Memorial University of Newfoundland, The Health Sciences Centre, St. John's, Newfoundland, Canada A1B 3V6

Thierry Petitclerc, Division of Nephrology, CHU Pitié-Salpétrière, Paris, France

Jean Ribstein, Department of Medicine and Nephrology, University Hospital, 34295 Montpellier, France

Claudio Rigatto, Divisions of Nephrology and Clinical Epidemiology, The Health Sciences Centre, Memorial University, St. John's, Newfoundland, Canada

Eberhard Ritz, Department of Nephrology, University of Heidelberg, 69115 Heidelberg, Germany

John D. Rutherford, The University of Texas Southwestern Medical Center at Dallas, Department of Internal Medicine, Cardiology Division, 5323 Harry Hines Boulevard, Dallas, TX 75235–9047, USA

Tessa Savage, Anthony Raine Research Laboratories, St Bartholomew's Hospital, London, UK

F.M. van der Sande, Department of Internal Medicine, University Hospital Maastricht, The Netherlands

David C. Wheeler, Department of Nephrology, University Hospital NHS Trust, Queen Elizabeth Hospital, Edgbaston, Birmingham B15 2TH, UK

Véronique Witko-Sarsat, INSERM U507, Necker Hospital, 75743 Paris Cedex 15, France

Jong-Yoon Yi, Rush University Hypertension Center, Department of Preventive Medicine, Rush Presbyterian/St Luke's Medical Center, Chicago, IL 60612, USA

PART I
Epidemiology

1

Cardiovascular risk factors in chronic renal failure

David C. Wheeler and Colin Baigent

Introduction

Prevalence of cardiovascular disease in chronic renal failure

Cardiovascular disease is now the leading cause of mortality among patients with chronic renal failure in Europe, the United States, and other developed countries. Approximately 60% of deaths among US dialysis patients can be attributed collectively to myocardial infarction, cardiac arrest, stroke, and 'other cardiac causes' (Table 1.1).[1] Some international variation may exist, although qualitatively similar patterns have been reported in Europe.[2] At all ages, the absolute mortality rates among dialysis patients are substantially higher than in the general population (Fig. 1.1).[3] Overall, such patients are at 10- to 20-fold increased risk of death from a cardiovascular cause, which in the US corresponds to an absolute cardiovascular mortality rate of about 9% per annum.[4] The relative risk is highest in younger patients and declines with age, suggesting that cardiovascular disease develops prematurely. As shown in Fig. 1.1, a dialysis patient aged 25–44 is at similar absolute risk of death from car-

Table 1.1 Adjusted[a] cause-specific annual percentage death rates for US never-transplanted dialysis patients, by age, sex, and diabetic status, 1991–1993 (modified from reference 1: USRDS 1996 Annual Data Report)

Cause of death	Total	Male	Female	Aged 20–64	Aged 65 or over	Diabetic	Non-diabetic
Acute MI	2.6	2.8	2.3	1.8	3.5	3.5	2.1
Cardiac arrest	4.3	4.5	4.2	2.9	6.1	6.1	3.6
Other cardiac[b]	4.1	4.4	3.7	2.4	6.0	5.0	3.6
Stroke	1.4	1.2	1.6	0.9	2.0	1.9	1.2
Total vascular	**12.4**	**12.9**	**11.8**	**8.0**	**17.6**	**16.5**	**10.4**
Infection	3.2	3.1	3.4	2.3	4.5	4.3	2.7
Cancer	0.9	1.1	0.7	0.6	1.4	0.6	1.1
Other (specified)	4.6	4.5	4.7	3.2	6.1	5.1	4.3
Total non-vascular	**8.7**	**8.7**	**8.8**	**6.0**	**12.0**	**9.9**	**8.1**
Unknown or missing[c]	4.3	4.6	4.0	2.7	6.2	5.4	3.8
All-cause mortality	**25.4**	**26.2**	**24.6**	**16.7**	**35.8**	**31.8**	**22.3**

[a]Data adjusted for sex, age (5-year categories), race, treatment modality, and diabetic status.
[b]Approximately two-thirds of other cardiac deaths were attributed to cardiac arrhythmia.
[c]Cause of death data were unavailable for approximately 10% of dialysis deaths.

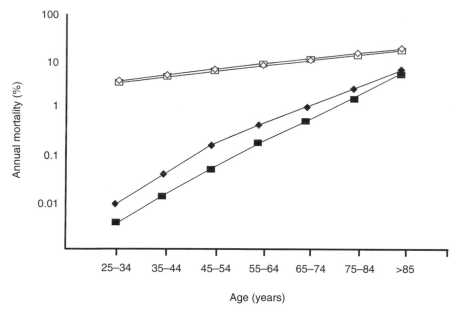

Fig. 1.1 Cardiovascular mortality (defined as death due to arrhythmias, cardiomyopathy, cardiac arrest, myocardial infarction, atherosclerotic heart disease and pulmonary edema) in patients with chronic renal failure. General population: ◆, male; ■, female. Dialysis: ◇, male; □, female. (From reference 4 with permission.)

diovascular disease as an individual without renal disease aged over 75 years. Furthermore, cardiovascular mortality in patients with diabetic nephropathy is around three times as high as in those with renal failure attributable to other causes, so the risk among young diabetics is especially high.[5]

Patients awaiting a renal allograft are usually selected for the absence of co-morbid conditions, so their absolute risk of cardiovascular disease will tend to be lower when compared with dialysis patients considered unsuitable for transplant listing. However, following successful renal transplantation, immunosuppressive drugs such as corticosteroids and cyclosporin may have an adverse impact on metabolic factors and blood pressure. Although this may complicate the identification of risk factors for cardiovascular disease among renal transplant recipients, it has been established that such individuals are about three to five times more likely to suffer a myocardial infarction than age- and sex-matched controls from the general population (Fig. 1.2).[6,7]

Temporal association between cardiovascular disease and chronic renal failure

Most data on cardiovascular disease complicating chronic renal failure have been derived from registries of patients receiving renal replacement therapy. However, observational studies in the general population suggest that even mild renal impairment, which may be more common, is associated with increased risk. In the British Regional Heart Study, for example, elevation of serum creatinine to around 150–200 μmol/l (1.7–2.3 mg/dl) was associated with a two- to fourfold excess of cardiovascular disease among unselected men.[8] Similar associations between renal impairment and increased risk of cardiovascular disease

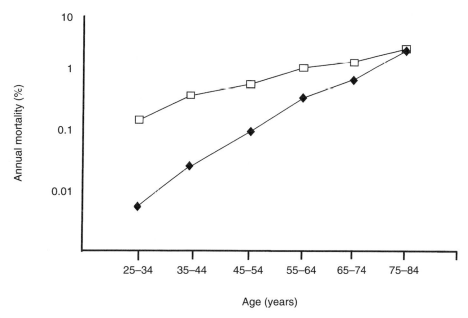

Fig. 1.2 Cardiovascular mortality (defined as death due to arrhythmias, cardiomyopathy, cardiac arrest, myocardial infarction, atherosclerotic heart disease and pulmonary edema) in renal transplant recipients. ◆, General population (all); □, renal transplants. (From reference 4 with permission.)

have been noted in individuals with diabetes and hypertension[9,10] and in those who have survived a myocardial infarction or stroke.[11,12] These observations might suggest that cardiovascular disease develops early in the course of chronic renal failure and that patients are exposed to cardiovascular risk factors such as hypertension for many years by the time they commence renal replacement therapy. Indeed, certain risk factors such as diabetes mellitus and hypertension may contribute to the development of both renal and cardiovascular disease, as is best illustrated in patients with atherosclerotic renal artery stenosis.[13–16] Furthermore, progression of renal failure may exacerbate pre-existing risk factors such as high blood pressure.[17] Thus, the likelihood of developing a myocardial infarction or congestive heart failure might increase in conjunction with deteriorating renal function. Unfortunately, owing to the lack of prospective studies, there is little detailed information about the temporal relationship between the progression of cardiovascular disease and renal dysfunction. However, these observations suggest that patients with moderate renal impairment could benefit from treatments known to prevent cardiovascular disease. Unfortunately, such patients have not been studied systematically because renal impairment is usually considered to be an exclusion criterion in randomized trials among patients at high risk of cardiovascular disease.

Features of cardiovascular disease in chronic renal failure

The high cardiovascular mortality rate among young dialysis patients was first reported in 1974 and was attributed to accelerated development of atherosclerotic lesions.[18] These early studies not only indicated an increased prevalence of ischaemic heart disease, which was reported in approximately 40% of dialysis patients, but also noted a high frequency of other complications attributed to arterial occlusion, including stroke and peripheral arterial embolization.[19] Atherosclerotic lesions in patients with chronic renal failure appear morphologically similar to those observed in individuals without renal disease, although they may be modified by medial degeneration, extensive calcification, and fibrous change.[19–21] In addition, the aorta and major arteries exhibit reduced compliance as a result of fibrous or fibro-elastic thickening.[21]

It has been recognized for many years that angina pectoris can develop in uraemic patients with angiographically normal coronary arteries.[22,23] Such observations imply a mismatch between oxygen demand and supply, probably caused by left ventricular hypertrophy in the presence of anaemia, thus highlighting the importance of structural myocardial disease in chronic renal failure (see Chapters 7 and 13). Changes in left ventricular geometry, including concentric wall thickening and increases in cavity volume, are frequently detected by echocardiography and may be associated with functional abnormalities.[24] For example, in one study, increased left ventricular mass was present in 74% of patients commencing a dialysis programme.[25] Other manifestations of the uraemic cardiomyopathy include left ventricular dilatation and systolic dysfunction, which may be detected by echocardiography at an early stage of renal failure, long before the initiation of dialysis treatment.[25,26] Ultrastructural changes to the heart include interstitial myocardial fibrosis and abnormalities of the microcirculation with a reduction in capillary density.[27]

Thus, cardiovascular pathology in patients with chronic renal failure is characterized by a combination of atheromatous narrowing of major arteries and structural changes to the heart and vessel walls. The pathogenesis of these abnormalities may be interrelated, since reduced arterial compliance may exacerbate the deleterious effects of hypertension and anaemia on cardiac workload and thereby contribute to myocardial disease.[27,28] Thus while one-fifth of cardiovascular deaths in dialysis patients can be attributed to acute myocardial infarction (resulting predominantly from atherosclerosis), two-thirds are caused by arrhythmias and cardiac arrest, possibly reflecting the high prevalence of left ventricular disease (Table 1.1).[1,24]

The importance of cardiovascular risk factors

Among healthy middle-aged individuals, several risk factors are known to be associated with an increased risk of ischaemic heart disease, congestive heart failure, or both.[29] Exposure to some of these risk factors may be increased among patients with impaired renal function, and may help to explain the high prevalence of cardiovascular disease that has been observed in those individuals who progress to end-stage renal failure and require dialysis.[13,30,31] However, reliable quantitative assessments of epidemiological associations between particular risk factors and cardiovascular events can only be provided by large longitudinal epidemiological studies or by randomized trials that reverse exposure to a particular risk factor (e.g. cholesterol-lowering treatment). Unfortunately, such data are lacking in patients with chronic renal failure, and in their absence nephrologists have been obliged to extrapolate guidelines for risk factor management in these individuals from studies in non-uraemic populations.[32]

The identification of risk factors for cardiovascular disease among patients with chronic renal failure may allow stratification of patients into levels of risk and help to target intervention at those most likely to benefit. If groups at high absolute risk of ischaemic or structural heart disease can be identified reliably, then treatments designed to prevent the development of these conditions could be tested in randomized trials. Such trials are essential because although the absolute benefits of treatments could be large, there might also be major predictable or unanticipated hazards. Drug toxicity, for example, might arise due to reduced renal drug clearance, or patients might be intolerant of treatment. As has been noted in a recent survey of the available evidence,[33] there is a lack of reliable randomized trials of this nature involving individuals with chronic renal disease, so that treatment decisions are currently difficult.

This chapter describes how the development of chronic renal failure changes cardiovascular risk factors in patients with kidney disease and assesses the possible aetiological importance of these factors in the development of occlusive and structural cardiovascular complications. Since the main aim is to assess epidemiological relationships between particular risk factors and cardiovascular diseases, it is first necessary to characterize such relationships *before* they become distorted by biases and the effects of treatment. Hence, the chapter is focused on pre-dialysis and dialysis patients, rather than on renal transplant recipients.

Hypertension

Elevated blood pressure is a common complication of renal parenchymal disease and occurs in patients with mildly impaired renal function, even before plasma creatinine concentration rises.[34] The prevalence of hypertension (usually defined as >150/90 mmHg) is higher in Blacks than Whites and in patients with glomerular as opposed to tubulointerstitial disease. Its prevalence increases as renal failure progresses, being present in 80–90% of patients commencing dialysis.[35] Furthermore, hypertensive patients with renal failure more often develop systolic hypertension compared with hypertensive patients without renal failure, perhaps reflecting reduced vascular compliance.[36] The pathophysiology of high blood pressure complicating chronic renal disease is complex and will be discussed in detail in Chapter 12. Contributory factors include volume expansion, sodium retention, overactivity of both the sympathetic nervous system and the renin–angiotensin–aldosterone axis, and accumulation of circulating endogenous vasoactive substances.[35,37,38] The net result is an increased cardiac output with an inappropriately high peripheral vascular resistance.[39] Hypertension is a persistent problem following renal transplantation with a prevalence of 70–85%.[17] Vasoconstriction in response to immunosuppressive agents such as cyclosporin and activation of the renin–angiotensin system in the graft or native kidney may be important in its pathogenesis.[40,41]

Management of hypertension includes dietary sodium restriction, as high salt intakes sustain extracellular volume expansion and limit the efficacy of antihypertensive medications.[42] All classes of antihypertensive drug can be used in chronic renal failure, although once renal function deteriorates significantly, failure of tubular concentrating function reduces the efficacy of diuretics.[43] Once dialysis has been initiated, control can be improved by careful attention to fluid balance, and sustained control of blood pressure within a range comparable to non-uraemic patients has been reported to be achievable with rigorous dialysis regimens.[44] In practice, however, even with the use of antihypertensive drugs, only about 50% of patients in most dialysis units have a blood pressure of 140/90 mmHg or lower.[45]

Epidemiological associations

Prospective observational studies in individuals without pre-existing cardiovascular disease have demonstrated that for each increment of 5–6 mmHg in 'usual' diastolic or 10 mmHg of systolic blood pressure, there is a 20–25% greater risk of ischaemic heart disease, 35–40%

greater risk of stroke, and 50% greater risk of congestive cardiac failure.[46,47] Furthermore, hypertension increases the risk of left ventricular hypertrophy, which, once established, is associated with a twofold increased risk of congestive cardiac failure and a 50% increased risk of ischaemic heart disease that is independent of blood pressure.[48] Left ventricular hypertrophy is also associated with a four- to ninefold increase in the risk of serious ventricular arrhythmias.[49] Similar associations between blood pressure and coronary artery disease have been observed among individuals at higher risk of cardiovascular disease, including those with diabetes[50] or a preceding history of myocardial infarction.[51]

However, analogous prospective studies in dialysis and renal transplant populations have been inconsistent and several have shown that lower blood pressure is associated with excess mortality.[52–56] One possible explanation for this inconsistency is the high prevalence of congestive cardiac failure and of co-morbid conditions such as malnutrition, diabetes, and infection, particularly in the dialysis population. As in other chronically ill populations, such as the very elderly, blood pressure may fall as a consequence of ischaemic or structural changes to the heart, or as an adaptation to serious disease, producing a U-shaped or even negative association between blood pressure and mortality.[57] A recent prospective study showed that the apparent association between low pre-dialysis blood pressure and an increased risk of mortality among 4499 haemodialysis patients was strongest among individuals known to have heart failure—as might be expected—but the association was also evident among individuals without such a history.[58] Pre-dialysis hypotension was associated with an increased risk of death from ischaemic heart disease, heart failure, and non-vascular causes. Therefore, this study suggests that chronic, non-vascular conditions that contribute to increased mortality may play a role in reducing blood pressure through mechanisms that are poorly understood.

A particular difficulty in assessing epidemiological associations between blood pressure and cardiovascular disease in haemodialysis populations is that large fluctuations in blood pressure occur, partly as a result of fluid accumulations between dialysis sessions, and partly because ultrafiltration during dialysis lowers both systolic and diastolic pressure.[17] Many dialysis units recommend that patients avoid their antihypertensive medications on treatment days in an effort to avoid intradialytic hypotension. Owing to the effects of 'regression dilution',[46] the combination of systematic and random errors in blood pressure measurement among dialysis patients may lead to substantial underestimation of the true strength of epidemiological associations between blood pressure and cardiovascular outcomes. Ambulatory blood pressure monitoring suggests that pre-dialysis recordings are higher than average blood pressure, and that the mean of pre-dialysis and postdialysis readings is usually a reliable estimate of the mean interdialytic pressure.[17] Future prospective studies need to correct for the effects of 'regression dilution' by ensuring that repeated assessments of blood pressure are obtained at regular intervals throughout the follow-up period.

Thus, several important biases must be taken into account before it is possible to assess the quantitative importance of hypertension as a risk factor in patients with chronic renal failure. Failure to do so might lead to underestimation of the benefits of antihypertensive therapy in these individuals. This is particularly important among pre-dialysis patients, when blood pressure may be substantially elevated but relatively easy to control. In diabetics without renal failure, another group at high risk of cardiovascular disease but with substantially less co-morbid illness, reductions in blood pressure produce large absolute reductions in the risk of cardiovascular disease.[59,60]

Regression of left ventricular hypertrophy has been reported in dialysis patients following control of blood pressure, suggesting the potential to reverse end-organ damage.[61,62]

Similarly, progressive left ventricular wall thickening in renal transplant recipients can be prevented by antihypertensive therapy.[63] However, given that large volume changes during haemodialysis treatments may result in severe hypotension, the safety of intensive blood pressure control in this population has been questioned.[64] Large-scale randomized trials comparing different levels of blood pressure control would help to resolve several current clinical uncertainties, the most important of which are: (i) how low is it safe to reduce blood pressure in dialysis patients; and (ii) does more aggressive blood pressure reduction during the period of chronic renal failure prior to dialysis help prevent cardiovascular disease once such patients commence renal replacement therapy? Such randomized trials would also help to assess the aetiological importance of hypertension in the development of the cardiovascular complications of chronic renal disease, the study of which is made particularly difficult by the various inherent methodological limitations of non-randomized observational studies among this population.

Anaemia

Anaemia resulting from a deficiency of erythropoietin is present in the majority of patients with advanced chronic renal failure and leads to structural and functional changes to the cardiovascular system.[65] Physiological responses include increased stroke volume and heart rate, reduced peripheral vascular resistance, and sympathetic overactivity. The net result is an increase in both venous return and cardiac output. In the longer term, these changes, along with hypertension, are thought to contribute to left ventricular hypertrophy. Correction of anaemia with recombinant human erythropoietin therapy is now established practice in the management of patients with end-stage renal failure.[66]

Epidemiological associations

The cardiovascular consequences of chronic anaemia are not well understood owing to a lack of prospective studies. Information from dialysis registries suggests that a low haemoglobin is associated with increased all-cause mortality,[66] but in the only such study to examine causes of death, there was no clear association between a low haemoglobin and a higher risk of fatal cardiovascular events.[67] In another study, 432 dialysis patients with a mean haemoglobin concentration of 8.9 (±1.5) g/dl were followed for an average of 41 months. A 1 g/dl lower mean haemoglobin was associated with a significant 42% increased risk of new left ventricular dilatation and a 28% greater risk of new congestive cardiac failure.[68] However, it remains unclear whether low haemoglobin is the cause of increased mortality or a physiological consequence of other co-morbid conditions that contribute to heart failure and to death among dialysis patients.

Correction of anaemia with erythropoietin has been shown to reduce left ventricular muscle mass and to correct ventricular dysfunction despite associated increases in blood pressure.[61,69–71] However, the effects of such an intervention on serious vascular events are unclear. In the only published randomized trial to have addressed this issue, 1233 dialysis patients with a history of cardiovascular disease were assigned to normal or low haematocrit groups (targets of 42% and 30% respectively).[72] Following concerns about safety, the trial was terminated after 14 months of the planned 3-year follow-up period. During this time only 237 cardiovascular deaths (125/618 normal vs. 112/615 low haemoglobin) and 33 non-fatal myocardial infarctions (19/618 vs. 14/615) had occurred, with no significant differences between the two groups. This study cannot therefore exclude moderate benefits or hazards associated with increasing haematocrit. Two other unpublished randomized studies, conducted in Canada and Scandinavia, were too small when combined to provide much additional information on major cardiovascular outcomes.[73] Because structural cardiac abnormalities develop early in the course of chronic renal failure, correcting anaemia in the pre-dialysis stages may be necessary to prevent the development of left ventricular disease. Further large-scale, long-term, randomized trials are, therefore, required to establish whether correction of anaemia produces worthwhile reductions in cardiovascular events.

Dyslipidaemia

Lipoprotein metabolism in chronic renal failure

Chronic renal failure leads to a complex disturbance of lipoprotein metabolism, the precise manifestations of which may be influenced by other factors such as nutritional state, diabetes, and the presence of proteinuria.[74–76] In general, the characteristic pattern is the accumulation of apo-B-containing triglyceride-rich particles of the very low-density lipoprotein (VLDL) and intermediate-density lipoprotein (IDL) classes, leading to hypertriglyceridaemia.[77,78] High-density lipoprotein (HDL)-cholesterol levels are low and while low-density lipoprotein (LDL)-cholesterol is normal, there is a preponderance of small, dense LDL particles.[79–81] Apolipoprotein (apo) metabolism is also disturbed, leading to an increase in apo B and C-III and a decrease in apo A-I and A-II. The resultant decrease in the apo A-I:C-III ratio is characteristic of the uraemic dyslipidaemia and is the earliest detectable abnormality of lipoprotein metabolism in these individuals.[77]

The pathophysiology of uraemic dyslipidaemia is not fully understood, although impaired activity of lipoprotein lipase may in part explain the accumulation of triglyceride-rich particles.[82] Abnormalities of lipoprotein metabolism develop early in the course of renal failure and tend to progress as renal function declines.[83] Pooling data from multiple studies, the prevalence of hypertriglyceridaemia (defined as plasma triglyceride >2.2 mmol/l, or equivalently >200 mg/dl) among patients with mild to moderate renal insufficiency has been estimated to be approximately 40%, with 35% having a low HDL-cholesterol level (defined as <0.9 mmol/l, or equivalently <35 mg/dl).[84] Patients with heavy proteinuria are more likely to develop hypercholesterolaemia (plasma cholesterol >6.2 mmol/l or >240 mg/dl) reflecting accumulation of LDL particles, with a prevalence of around 90% compared with 30% in patients with non-proteinuric uraemia.[84] Diabetes tends to accentuate the changes in these lipid fractions, so that diabetic patients with renal failure have somewhat higher triglyceride and lower HDL-cholesterol levels.[84] In patients who become malnourished, cholesterol levels may fall owing to a compensatory reduction in hepatic cholesterol synthesis.[85]

The initiation of dialysis therapy has little impact on lipid abnormalities associated with uraemia. In comparison with haemodialysis patients, a higher proportion of continuous ambulatory peritoneal dialysis (CAPD) patients have elevated LDL-cholesterol and decreased HDL-cholesterol levels.[84] Lipid abnormalities are modified by successful renal transplantation, following which triglyceride levels tend to fall and HDL-cholesterol rises with correction of uraemia. However, approximately 60% of patients develop hypercholesterolaemia, reflecting an increase in LDL-cholesterol.[84,86] Immunosuppressive drugs, particularly steroids and cyclosporin, may contribute to the pathogenesis of dyslipidemia following renal transplantation, although the mechanisms have not been fully elucidated.[87] For example, in a randomized trial of steroid withdrawal among transplant patients,[88] there was a significant reduction of about 1 mmol/l in serum cholesterol, suggesting that steroids on their own may produce substantial increases in the risk of ischaemic heart disease. In general, when compared with patients receiving prednisolone and azathioprine, cyclosporin-based immunosuppressive regimens have been associated with higher triglyceride and cholesterol levels.[89] Conversion from cyclosporin to tacrolimus may lead to a fall in both total and LDL-cholesterol.[90]

Lipid abnormalities in patients with chronic renal failure can be partially corrected by modification of diet and, if appropriate, control of diabetes.[91] However, such measures usually produce only modest proportional reductions in cholesterol (e.g. 5–10%), and pharmacological interventions are required to achieve the levels of reduction (e.g. 30–40%) that have been shown to prevent cardiovascular events in other high-risk populations. The 3-hydroxy-3-methylglutaryl CoA reductase inhibitors ('statins') effectively reduce total and LDL-cholesterol concentrations in patients with renal failure.[87,91] Fibric acid derivatives lower both triglyceride and cholesterol while correcting HDL levels, but tend to accumulate when renal function is impaired. Similarly, blood levels of certain statins may increase in combination with cyclosporin, enhancing the risk of myotoxicity. Hence, if either drug is to be used in transplant patients, then it may be appropriate to reduce doses to minimize risks of muscle injury.[91,92] A large number of predominantly short-term studies have examined the effects of these lipid-lowering therapies in patients with chronic renal disease, although even when combined, they have been too small to determine reliably whether any such treatments result in a reduction in the risk of serious cardiovascular events.[91]

Lipoprotein (a)

Lipoprotein (a) (Lp(a)) is composed of an LDL like particle covalently linked to a polymorphic apoprotein, apo(a). Apo(a) has over 30 isoforms of varying size determined by the number of repeats of a single kringle domain.[93] In healthy individuals, plasma Lp(a) concentrations are primarily determined by genotype and not influenced by external factors. Lp(a) levels are increased among uraemic patients, an abnormality that is detectable early in the course of progressive renal failure.[94] When renal function is normal, high Lp(a) concentrations are associated with a predominance of low-molecular-weight apo(a) isoforms, whereas when renal function is abnormal, most individuals with raised Lp(a) levels exhibit a predominance of high-molecular-weight isoforms.[95] Protein wasting states, such as the nephrotic syndrome, and treatment with peritoneal dialysis, as well as conditions that produce an acute phase reaction, all lead to elevated Lp(a) concentrations.[96–98] Increased concentrations of high-molecular-weight apo(a) isoforms are reversed following successful renal transplantation,[99] suggesting that isoform concentrations are strongly influenced by renal function in patients with kidney disease. Although the precise mechanisms remain uncertain, experimental studies indicate that Lp(a) is extracted from the circulation by the normal kidney.[100] Thus, loss of renal function may impair the metabolism of this lipoprotein, leading to elevated plasma levels.

Lipid peroxidation

Oxidation of LDL or other lipoproteins may play a fundamental role in the development of atherosclerotic lesions.[101] The susceptibility of these particles to oxidative modification may, therefore, reflect their atherogenic potential. Small LDL subclasses are more prone to oxidation than larger ones, so the pattern of lipoprotein abnormality associated with chronic renal failure might be expected to accelerate vascular injury. In addition, a deficiency of natural antioxidants including vitamin C and glutathione peroxidase has been described in patients with pre-dialysis renal failure.[102] However, levels of vitamin E (α-tocopherol), the principal lipid-soluble antioxidant associated with the LDL particle, are not reduced.[103] The dialysis process itself may promote lipid peroxidation and further deplete antioxidant defences.[104,105] Studies in haemodialysis patients have confirmed that LDL particles are more susceptible to copper-induced oxidative damage *in vitro* compared with particles from matched non-uraemic controls.[103] In addition, haemodialysis patients were shown to have higher levels of autoantibodies to oxidized lipoproteins.[106] Similar abnormalities have been reported in stable renal transplant recipients.[107]

Epidemiological associations

Hypercholesterolaemia   Observational studies among healthy individuals have shown that the relationship between the risk of ischaemic heart disease and serum cholesterol is positively 'log-linear', with no evidence of a 'threshold' below which a lower cholesterol is not associated with a lower risk.[108] Associations between the risk of ischaemic heart disease and serum cholesterol appear to show a similar log-linear relationship in a wide range of populations at somewhat higher risk, including those with established cardiovascular disease[109] and diabetes mellitus.[110]

Unfortunately, our understanding of the relationship between lipid abnormalities and cardiovascular disease in patients with chronic renal failure is limited by a lack of available data. One observational study, based on data from a registry of around 12 000 haemodialysis patients treated in the US during 1988, showed that there was an *inverse* association between total cholesterol and all-cause mortality.[111] A similar (but much smaller) study showed an analogous relationship between low cholesterol and cardiovascular deaths,[112] which is the opposite of what might have been expected. Furthermore, in renal transplant recipients, who are more likely to develop hypercholesterolaemia, positive associations between total cholesterol levels and cardiovascular complications have not been found consistently.[6,54]

These inconsistencies might be partly explained by the following points. First, it is unclear what proportion of cardiovascular mortality is attributable directly to atheromatous cardiac disease (i.e. ischaemic heart disease) as opposed to structural myocardial disease (i.e. left ventricular hypertrophy), and real associations between cholesterol and ischaemic heart disease may be substantially diluted by cardiac deaths that are unrelated to atherosclerotic narrowing of coronary arteries (and hence the level of serum cholesterol). More importantly, in contrast to studies among patients with diabetes or a previous history of cardiovascular disease, dialysis registries include patients with severe co-morbid conditions, such as malnutrition and infection, that themselves cause reductions in hepatic cholesterol synthesis.[85] As in other populations with substantial levels of co-morbid illness, such as the very elderly,[113] the importance of blood cholesterol level may not become clear until adjustments have been made for co-morbidity and pre-existing disease.[114] Given such difficulties, the aetiological relevance of cholesterol to the development of cardiovascular disease in patients with chronic renal disease may be underestimated in observational studies that do not adequately adjust for co-morbidity.

Randomized trials of statins have shown that proportional reductions in cardiovascular disease produced by a fixed statin dose are smaller among populations with low baseline-cholesterol levels, such as those found in patients with chronic renal failure.[108] Thus, for a given statin dose, the proportional effects of lipid-lowering therapy on cardiovascular events are uncertain. In particular, if reducing cholesterol does not lower the risk of congestive cardiac failure or arrhythmias, which account for two-thirds of cardiovascular mortality among dialysis patients (Table 1.1), then the overall proportional effect of intervention on cardiac mortality may be diluted. However, the absolute effects on atherosclerotic coronary artery disease may still be worthwhile in some high risk patients.

Thus, the strength of any association between serum cholesterol and cardiovascular events may only be established by large, randomized, placebo-controlled trials of lipid-lowering drugs. Two such trials are currently in progress. In the 4D (Die Deutsche Diabetes Dialyse Studie), it is planned to randomize a total of 1200 dialysis patients with type II diabetes to either atorvastatin (20 mg daily) or matching placebo.[115] In the second study, the ALERT (Assessment of Lescol in Renal Transplantation), around 2000 transplant recipients have been randomized to either fluvastatin, 40 mg daily, or placebo medication. Further studies are likely to be required to provide reliable information about the effects of reducing cholesterol among the large majority of patients with chronic renal failure who do not meet the eligibility criteria of either of these trials.

Hypertriglyceridaemia, low HDL-cholesterol, and small LDL particles   Plasma triglyceride is a marker for hepatic production of triglyceride-rich lipoproteins, although the aetiological relationship between triglyceride levels and ischaemic heart disease is unclear from studies to date. This is due to measurement variability, intra-individual variability, and the close association between raised triglyceride, low HDL-cholesterol levels, and reductions in LDL particle size.[116–118]

A meta-analysis of 17 population-based studies showed a weak association between triglyceride levels and cardiovascular risk, but this was substantially attenuated after correcting for HDL-cholesterol.[117] However, in an overview of observational studies in non-renal populations, each 0.1 mmol/l (3.9 mg/dl) lower HDL-cholesterol was associated with a 10% increased risk of cardiovascular disease, independent of other factors.[119] These data suggest that the combination of raised triglyceride, low HDL-cholesterol, and small dense LDL may contribute to an increased risk of cardiovascular disease among patients with renal failure, although it is not possible at present to identify any aetiologically distinct component of this metabolic cluster. Thus, although measurement of total blood triglyceride among patients with chronic renal failure may identify patients at high risk, at present it remains unclear whether reducing triglycerides will prevent cardiovascular events.

Raised lipoprotein (a)   Prospective studies in non-uraemic populations suggest that elevated Lp(a) may be an independent risk factor for ischaemic heart disease.[120] Longitudinal studies in pre-dialysis patients[121] and in patients on haemodialysis[122] have also suggested that elevated levels of this lipoprotein are associated with an increased risk of a variety of vascular outcomes. However, Lp(a) levels correlate with markers of the acute phase response in these individuals,[96] so it remains unclear whether elevated levels are a cause of cardiovascular disease or a consequence of other co-morbid conditions that contribute to increased mortality among dialysis patients. Thus, further studies are required to clarify the importance of Lp(a) as a cardiovascular risk factor, both in the general population and in patients with chronic renal failure. Even if Lp(a) does turn out to be important in the pathogenesis of ischaemic heart disease, it is likely to be of value mainly as an indicator of cardiovascular risk rather than as a target for modification, as there are currently no widely practicable methods for reducing the plasma levels of this lipoprotein.

Lipid peroxidation   Some observational studies have shown that dietary antioxidant intake and plasma antioxidant levels are inversely associated with the risk of ischaemic heart disease.[123] In addition, plasma levels of autoantibodies to oxidized LDL and the degree of susceptibility of this lipoprotein to oxidative damage were associated with atherosclerosis.[128,129] To date, there are few reliable data concerning the effects of dietary supplementation with antioxidant vitamins. In the only large randomized trial of α-tocopherol, 6 years of a low dose (50 mg daily) did not prevent ischaemic heart disease.[129] The risk of non-fatal myocardial infarction was reported to be reduced in a relatively small trial of about 18 months of 400–800 IU daily of α-tocopherol, but there was no effect on cardiac mortality, and there were too few cardiovascular events for this study to be reliable.[130] There are currently no randomized studies designed to examine the effects of antioxidant vitamin supplementation among patients with chronic renal disease.

Diabetes mellitus and insulin resistance

Diabetes is the primary cause of renal failure in 15–30% of patients requiring dialysis, with equal proportions having type I and type II disease.[131] However, even among patients with chronic renal failure who are not diabetic, some degree of insulin resistance may develop.[132] These abnormalities are usually detectable well before there have been appreciable reductions in renal function, but do not usually lead to overt glucose intolerance.[133] The mechanisms that contribute to impaired insulin action in uraemia are not fully understood. Binding of insulin to muscle and adipose tissue is normal, suggesting that there is a post-receptor defect.[132] In severe renal impairment, this may be exacerbated by reduced insulin secretion, possibly due to secondary hyperparathyroidism.[132,134] Insulin sensitivity may improve following initiation of dialysis.[135] Hyperinsulinaemia and insulin resistance are thought to play an important aetiological role in the development of post-transplant diabetes which occurs *de novo* in approximately 10% of patients.[136,137]

The management of diabetes and insulin resistance in patients with chronic renal failure is based on the same principles as in diabetic individuals with normal renal function. Thus, weight-reducing diets and lifestyle changes which increase physical activity should be encouraged.[138] A number of medications commonly used in the treatment of renal disease and its complications exacerbate abnormalities of glucose metabolism. These include thiazide diuretics, which induce glucose intolerance in many non-diabetic patients.[139] In renal transplant recipients, administration of corticosteroids impairs glucose uptake and promotes insulin resistance, whilst both cyclosporin and tacrolimus are diabetogenic, possibly due to a direct toxic effect on pancreatic beta cells.[140,141] For type II diabetic patients with renal failure who do not respond to diet and lifestyle changes, oral hypoglycaemic drugs must be used with caution. First-generation sulphonylureas such as chlorpropamide are excreted by the kidney and are best avoided. Second-generation drugs in this class undergo hepatic metabolism making gliclazide and glipizide safer options. Biguanides, including metformin, accumulate in patients with renal insufficiency, thereby increasing the risk of lactic acidosis, and are contraindicated.[142] When attempting to achieve tight control in type I and type II diabetic patients, it must be remembered that the half-life of insulin is prolonged in renal failure, thus increasing the risk of hypoglycaemia. In addition, lack of awareness of low blood sugar levels may be more common.[135,138]

Epidemiological associations

Diabetes Complications of diabetes mellitus include macrovascular disease, microvascular disease, and diabetic cardiomyopathy.[131] Observational studies suggest that the overall risk of death resulting from myocardial infarction is about three times higher in diabetic patients than in those without diabetes, with younger individuals being at even higher relative risk.[143] Diabetic patients are also at a similarly increased risk of congestive cardiac failure.[144] The development of nephropathy, a manifestation of diabetic microvascular disease, may enhance the likelihood of macrovascular complications. For example, during 14-year follow-up of 3234 type II diabetic patients, after correction for confounding factors, the presence of heavy proteinuria was associated with not only a 13-fold increased risk of renal failure but also a 2.5-fold increased risk of cardiovascular mortality.[145] A high prevalence of ischaemic heart disease in diabetic patients with renal failure has been observed among those screened for their suitability for renal transplantation.[146,147] In one study, coronary angiography showed that over half had at least one atheromatous lesion causing greater than 50% stenosis.[148]

Randomized trials have indicated that strict glycaemic control reduces the risk of microvascular complications of diabetes, although patients with nephropathy have generally been excluded.[149,150] In a *post hoc* analysis of the largest study of intensive control in type I diabetes published to date, which was not designed to examine cardiovascular endpoints and included relatively few patients with renal disease, intensive glycaemic control produced a non-significant 41% reduction in macrovascular events.[151] Patients with tighter control, however, had an increased frequency of hypoglycaemic events, although there did not appear to be any adverse effect on cognitive function.[150] In the UK prospective diabetes study, intensive control in type II diabetic patients, either with hypoglycaemic drugs or insulin, did not conclusively reduce the risk of myocardial infarction.[149] However, like the Diabetes Control and Complications Trial, the benefits of intensive treatment were clearly justified by the reduction in microvascular complications.

Thus the available data suggest that intensive diabetic control is appropriate in diabetic patients without nephropathy in order to prevent microvascular complications, although it remains uncertain whether such treatment also reduces the risk of cardiovascular events. Although reductions in microvascular disease might outweigh the hazards of hypoglycaemia, in diabetic patients with adequate renal function. The balance of benefit to risk may be less favourable in patients with nephropathy, who are more likely to develop hypoglycaemia.[138] Thus, randomized trials among patients with diabetes and renal disease are required in order to determine whether tight glycaemic control prevents vascular events in this very high risk group.

Insulin resistance Insulin resistance produces hypertriglyceridaemia, low HDL-cholesterol, and an increase in small dense LDL particles.[152] This metabolic abnormality may therefore explain, at least in part, the analogous changes in lipid profile observed in uraemic patients. Such abnormalities, which are also associated with increased activity of the sympathetic nervous system and hypertension, may contribute to an increased risk of cardiovascular disease in patients with insulin resistance.[152]

Some prospective studies have demonstrated positive correlations between insulin levels and cardiovascular risk whilst others have found J- or U-shaped relationships.[153] At the present time, it is not clear whether insulin resistance is a risk factor for cardiovascular disease in patients with chronic renal failure.

Hyperhomocysteinaemia

Homocysteine is a non-essential sulphur-containing amino acid formed as an intermediate during the metabolism of methionine (see Chapter 9). Patients with an inherited deficiency of the enzyme cystathionine β-synthetase develop elevated plasma homocysteine levels of up to 400 μmol/l and vascular disease in early adulthood. This observation led to the original hypothesis that more moderate degrees of hyperhomocysteinaemia may be a risk factor for atherosclerosis.[154] Normal plasma homocysteine concentrations are between 5 and 15 μmol/l, approximately 80% of which is protein bound.[155] Pathways of homocysteine metabolism involve either remethylation or transulphuration. Remethylation of the amino acid requires a methyl group donated by methyltetrahydrofolate, a metabolite of folic acid, in a reaction dependent on vitamin B_{12}. Alternatively, during transulphuration, homocysteine is converted to cystathionine by the action of a pyridoxine-dependent enzyme, cystathionine β-synthetase.[156] Homocysteine levels may be elevated as a result of deficiency of folic acid, vitamin B_{12}, or vitamin B_6, and they may be lowered pharmacologically by oral folate or B vitamin supplementation.[157] Experimental studies have shown that homocysteine may induce oxidative damage to endothelial cells and smooth muscle cell proliferation, suggesting possible mechanisms of vascular injury.[158]

Homocysteine levels may be increased up to fourfold in dialysis patients, while in those with pre-dialysis chronic renal failure, each increment of 100 μmol/l (1.1 mg/dl) in serum creatinine is associated with around a 2 μmol/l increase in plasma homocysteine levels.[159] Furthermore, in individuals with milder renal disease and with normal serum creatinine concentrations, there is an inverse linear relationship between glomerular filtration rate (as assessed by iohexol clearance) and plasma homocysteine concentrations.[160] Such observations suggest that moderate hyperhomocysteinaemia is present at a very early stage in the natural history of chronic renal disease. The mechanisms that result in elevated homocysteine levels in uraemia are not fully understood (see Chapter 9). Possible contributory factors include altered amino acid metabolism, reduced enzyme activity, and, in dialysis patients, losses of water-soluble B group vitamins. Homocysteine levels fall, but do to not return to normal, following successful renal transplantation.[161]

Epidemiological associations

In a meta-analysis of prospective observational studies in the general population, a 5 μmol/l increment in plasma homocysteine corresponded to a 30% greater risk of vascular disease.[162] In patients with chronic renal failure, both retrospective and prospective studies have demonstrated associations between elevated homocysteine levels and the risk of vascular events.[163–166] Randomized trials in patients without chronic renal impairment suggest that dietary supplementation with micronutrients reduces plasma homocysteine levels. A meta-analysis of these trials showed that 0.5–5.0 mg folic acid and 0.5 mg vitamin B_{12} reduced homocysteine levels by between a quarter and a third.[167] For dialysis patients already taking a standard regimen of 1 mg folic acid, 10 mg vitamin B_6, and 12 μg vitamin B_{12}, the addition of 15 mg folic acid, 100 mg vitamin B_6, and 1 mg vitamin B_{12} produced a 30% reduction in homocysteine levels.[168] Hence, higher doses of micronutrients may be appropriate among patients with chronic renal failure in order to produce the maximum possible reduction in homocysteine levels.

At the present time there are no completed trials, either in uraemic or non–uraemic populations, examining whether lowering plasma homocysteine levels reduces the risk of serious cardiovascular events. Since levels of this amino acid are particularly high in patients with chronic renal failure, as is the absolute risk of cardiovascular disease, an appropriate micronutrient regimen might well result in large absolute benefits.

Smoking

The few published studies of smoking prevalence in patients with chronic renal failure suggest that the proportion reporting regular cigarette smoking is somewhat lower than among their healthy counterparts in the general population.[169,170] A larger proportion had smoked before the onset of renal failure, perhaps suggesting that chronic illness may have caused a few sick patients to stop.[171] Among patients with chronic renal failure, therefore, smoking is unlikely to account for much of the proportional increase in the risk of cardiovascular disease compared with the general population.

Epidemiological associations

In non–uraemic populations, cigarette smoking causes around a fourfold increase in the risk of non-fatal myocardial infarction,[172] with the risk somewhat higher among younger individuals. Although there is some direct evidence of the hazards of smoking in patients with chronic renal failure, these studies are too small to be reliable.[31,173] In the general population, cessation of smoking leads to a reversal of this excess risk within 2 to 5 years.[174] Thus, encouraging patients with chronic renal failure to stop smoking may produce large absolute benefits and all efforts should be made to assist them to do so. Nicotine accumulates in chronic renal failure and although replacement therapy is generally safe, it may exacerbate hypertension.[175]

Acute phase responses

Acute phase responses, which result from acute or chronic inflammatory processes, lead to characteristic changes in the concentrations of certain plasma proteins. By definition, an 'acute phase reactant' is a protein that either increases or decreases in concentration by at least 25% under such conditions. Such responses are thought to result from cytokine-mediated modulation of hepatic protein production.[176] Typical examples of acute phase reactants are fibrinogen and C-reactive protein (which increase) and albumin (which decreases during an inflammatory process). Changes in the levels of these plasma constituents have been shown to be associated with moderate increases in cardiovascular disease risk in the general population.[177]

Fibrinogen

Fibrinogen is required for platelet aggregation and is the major determinant of both plasma and blood viscosity.[178] Clinical studies have shown that hyperfibrinogenaemia in chronic renal failure is part of an acute-phase reaction that also produces reductions in plasma albumin in association with increased interleukin-6 levels.[179] Mean plasma fibrinogen levels are also increased in patients with large protein losses such as those with nephrotic syndrome or those treated with peritoneal dialysis.[177,179]

Epidemiological associations

A meta-analysis of prospective studies in non–uraemic populations suggested that a differ-ence of around 3 μmol/l (0.1 g/dl) in mean 'usual' fibrinogen concentration was associated with around an 80% increase in the risk of cardiovascular disease.[177] Hence, prolonged ele-vation of fibrinogen levels in patients with chronic renal disease might predispose to occlu-sive vascular events. To date, at least one study has indicated that raised fibrinogen concentrations are associated with an increased risk of death in diabetic patients with end-stage renal failure.[180]

Serum albumin

Approximately 40% of total body albumin circulates in the intravascular compartment trans-porting molecules such as fatty acids, hormones, and drugs. In healthy individuals, plasma albumin concentrations are held fairly constant at 35–45 g/l by equilibration with the extravascular space.[181] Even in the absence of proteinuria, plasma albumin levels fall in chronic renal disease, as in other serious illness, particularly if patients develop protein-calorie malnutrition as renal function declines.[182]

Epidemiological associations

A 4 g/l difference in mean 'usual' serum albumin concentration is associated with about a 50% increased risk of ischaemic heart disease in healthy populations.[177] Similar associations have been observed between albumin and the risk of other diseases, such as cancer.[183] To date, no single aetiological mechanism has been established linking hypoalbuminaemia with such disparate disease processes. In dialysis patients, observational studies suggest that a low serum albumin is a good predictor of short-term mortality.[184,185] However, as in patients with other severe illnesses, the largest falls in serum albumin tend to occur in those patients who are most seriously ill and who are also those most likely to die.[183] Thus, it remains unclear whether serum albumin is a cause of increased cardiovascular disease risk in patients with chronic renal disease or merely a marker of ill health among those at high risk of dying.

C-reactive protein (CRP)

CRP increases up to 1000-fold in acute inflammation and elevated levels are a common finding in individuals with chronic renal failure. In one study, 35% of 1054 haemodialysis patients had a raised CRP, which was associated with a low plasma albumin, suggesting that increased concentrations of this acute phase reactant were associated with malnutrition.[186]

Epidemiological associations

A meta-analysis of prospective studies in non–uraemic populations has indicated that patients with a CRP in the top third of the baseline measurement were 1.7 times more likely to die from ischaemic heart disease, or suffer a non-fatal myocardial infarction, compared with those in the bottom third.[177] A prospective study among haemodialysis patients did not find any association between CRP levels and an increased risk of death.[186] As with other acute phase reactants, this may be because in chronic renal disease, multiple determinants of patient outcome (including infection, nutritional state, and co-morbid illness such as dia-betes) may also directly influence the level of CRP, thus confounding any true association between CRP and the risk of cardiovascular disease. Prospective studies among individuals with various degrees of renal impairment are required to assess the possible aetiological relevance of acute phase reactants to cardiovascular disease in chronic renal impairment.

Conclusions

Pathological and functional studies suggest that atherosclerosis, in combination with structural changes to the heart and arterial wall, contributes to the clinical manifestations of cardiovascular disease in chronic renal failure. Since these diseases are rare in middle-aged individuals in the general population, but occur in young dialysis patients, they must develop prematurely. Renal impairment causes substantial changes to several known (and possible) risk factors for atherosclerotic and structural heart disease. Many of these disturbances are present very early in the natural history of renal failure when renal function is only mildly abnormal. Moreover, certain causes of chronic renal failure (e.g. diabetes and hypertension) also contribute to the development of cardiovascular diseases. However, the precise quantitative relationship between risk factors and cardiovascular disease in chronic renal failure is complex, and may be substantially modified by the nature of the primary renal disease, nutritional status, age, and pre-existing co-morbidity.

Existing epidemiological studies of cardiovascular diseases in patients with chronic renal failure have been based largely on data obtained from dialysis registries. These may give a misleading picture of the true relevance of known risk factors to the development of specific cardiovascular diseases because epidemiological relationships can become distorted in populations with a high prevalence of co-morbid illness. Such distortions have been observed in the study of relationships between cholesterol and cardiovascular disease among individuals aged 80 or more.[114] In uraemic patients, the levels of co-morbidity (and mortality) are similar to those found in very elderly people. Although statistical correction can be made, registry data do not generally allow confounding variables to be measured accurately enough to determine associations reliably. This methodological difficulty might be circumvented by long-term prospective observational studies of individuals with initially minor degrees of renal dysfunction, among whom the distortions produced by the effects of renal disease or co-morbid illnesses on risk factors might be minimized. Alternatively, when particular risk factors can be modified by intervention, randomized trials comparing intervention versus placebo might avoid such confounding. Unconfounded estimates of the importance of cholesterol in promoting cardiovascular disease among dialysis patients could, for example, be produced by trials of cholesterol-lowering drugs in pre-dialysis populations.

This chapter has highlighted how little is known about the causes of cardiovascular morbidity and mortality among patients with chronic renal failure. As noted in a recent report from the US National Kidney Foundation,[32] there is a pressing need for well-designed prospective observational studies and randomized trials to gain a better understanding of the causes of cardiovascular disease in chronic renal failure. If collaborative studies can be undertaken in future years then it might be possible to reduce the high morbidity and mortality resulting from cardiovascular disease in patients with chronic renal failure, thereby increasing both the quantity and quality of their lives.

Acknowledgments

Dr Baigent is a career track scientist with the UK Medical Research Council. The authors are grateful to Kate Burbury for help in preparation of the manuscript and to Jan Palfrey for bibliographic assistance.

References

1. *USRDS 1996 Annual Data Report*, National Institutes of Health, National Institute of Diabetes and Digestive and Kidney Diseases, Bethesda, MD, April 1996.
2. Raine AE, Margreiter R, Brunner FP, Ehrich JH, Geerlings W, Landais P *et al.* Report on the management of renal failure in Europe, XXII, 1991. *Nephrol Dial Transplant* 1992;7 Suppl 2:7–35.
3. Sarnak MJ, Levey AS. Cardiovascular mortality in ESRD compared to the general population. *J Am Soc Nephrol* 1998;9:160A (abstract).
4. Foley RN, Parfrey PS, Sarnak MJ. Clinical epidemiology of cardiovascular disease in chronic renal disease. *Am J Kidney Dis* 1998;32 Suppl 3:S112–19.
5. Held PJ, Levin NW, Port FK. Cardiac disease in chronic uremia: an overview. In: Parfrey PS, Harnett JD, editors. Cardiac dysfunction in chronic uremia. Boston: Kluwer, 1991:3–17.
6. Kasiske BL. Risk factors for accelerated atherosclerosis in renal transplant recipients. *Am J Med* 1988;84:985–92.
7. Lindholm A, Albrechtsen D, Frödin L, Tufveson G, Persson NH, Lundgren G. Ischemic heart disease—major cause of death and graft loss after renal transplantation in Scandinavia. *Transplantation* 1995;60:451–7.
8. Wannamethee SG, Shaper AG, Perry IJ. Serum creatinine concentration and risk of cardiovascular disease. A possible marker for increased risk of stroke. *Stroke* 1997;28:557–63.
9. Shulman NB, Ford CE, Hall WD, Blaufox MD, Simon D, Langford HG *et al.* on behalf of the Hypertension Detection and Follow-up Program Cooperative Group. Prognostic value of serum creatinine and effect of treatment of hypertension on renal function. Results from the hypertension detection and follow-up program. *Hypertension* 1989;13 Suppl I:I-80–93.
10. Aronow WS. Usefulness of serum creatinine as a marker for coronary events in elderly patients with either systemic hypertension or diabetes mellitus. *Am J Cardiol* 1991;68:678–9.
11. Friedman PJ. Serum creatinine: an independent predictor of survival after stroke. *J Intern Med* 1991;229:175–9.
12. Matts JP, Karnegis JN, Campos CT, Fitch LL, Johnson JW, Buchwald H and the POSCH group. Serum creatinine as an independent predictor of coronary heart disease mortality in normotensive survivors of myocardial infarction. *J Fam Pract* 1993;36:497–503.
13. Ma KW, Greene EL, Raij L. Cardiovascular risk factors in chronic renal failure and hemodialysis populations. *Am J Kidney Dis* 1992;19:505–13.
14. Rimmer JM, Gennari FJ. Atherosclerotic renovascular disease and progressive renal failure. *Ann Intern Med* 1993;118:712–19.
15. Klag MJ, Whelton PK, Randall BL, Neaton JD, Brancati FL, Ford CE *et al.* Blood pressure and end-stage renal disease in men. *New Engl J Med* 1996;334:13–18.
16. Brancati FL, Whelton PK, Randall BL, Neaton JD, Stamler J, Klag MJ. Risk of end-stage renal disease in diabetes mellitus. A prospective cohort study of men screened for MRFIT. *JAMA* 1997;278:2069–74.
17. Mailloux LU, Levey AS. Hypertension in patients with chronic renal disease. *Am J Kidney Dis* 1998;32 Suppl 3:S120–41.
18. Lindner A, Charra B, Sherrard DJ, Scribner BH. Accelerated atherosclerosis in prolonged maintenance hemodialysis. *New Engl J Med* 1974;290:697–701.
19. Ibels LS, Stewart JH, Mahony JF, Neale FC, Sheil AG. Occlusive arterial disease in uraemic and haemodialysis patients and renal transplant recipients. A study of the incidence of arterial disease and of the prevalence of risk factors implicated in the pathogenesis of arteriosclerosis. *Quart J Med* 1977;46:197–214.
20. Vincenti F, Amend WJ, Abele J, Feduska NJ, Salvatierra O. The role of hypertension in hemodialysis-associated atherosclerosis. *Am J Med* 1980;68:363–9.
21. London GM, Marchais SJ, Guerin AP, Métivier F, Pannier B. Cardiac hypertrophy and arterial alterations in end-stage renal disease: hemodynamic factors. *Kidney Int* 1993;43 Suppl 41:S42–9.

22. Roig E, Betriu A, Castañer A, Magriña J, Sanz G, Navarro-Lopez F. Disabling angina pectoris with normal coronary arteries in patients undergoing long-term hemodialysis. *Am J Med* 1981;71:431–4.

23. Rostand SG, Kirk KA, Rutsky EA. Dialysis-associated ischemic heart disease: insights from coronary angiography. *Kidney Int* 1984;25:653–9.

24. Hutchins GM. Cardiac pathology in chronic renal failure. In: Parfrey PS, Harnett JD, editors. Cardiac dysfunction in chronic uremia. Boston: Kluwer, 1991:85–115.

25. Foley RN, Parfrey PS, Harnett JD, Kent GM, Martin CJ, Murray DC *et al.* Clinical and echocardiographic disease in patients starting end-stage renal disease therapy. *Kidney Int* 1995;47:186–92.

26. Stefanski A, Schmidt KG, Waldherr R, Ritz E. Early increase in blood pressure and diastolic left ventricular malfunction in patients with glomerulonephritis. *Kidney Int* 1996;50:1321–6.

27. Amann K, Ritz E. Cardiac structure and function in renal disease. *Current Opin Nephrol Hypertens* 1996;5:102–6.

28. Ritz E, Koch M. Morbidity and mortality due to hypertension in patients with renal failure. *Am J Kidney Dis* 1993;21 Suppl 2:113–18.

29. Wilson PW, Culleton BF. Epidemiology of cardiovascular disease in the United States. *Am J Kidney Dis* 1998;32 Suppl 3:S56–65.

30. Rostand SG, Kirk KA, Rutsky EA. Relationship of coronary risk factors to hemodialysis associated ischemic heart disease. *Kidney Int* 1982;22:304–8.

31. Lameire N, Bernaert P, Lambert M-C, Vijt D. Cardiovascular risk factors and their management in patients on continuous ambulatory peritoneal dialysis. *Kidney Int* 1994;46 Suppl 48:S31–8.

32. Levey AS, Beto JA, Coronado BE, Eknoyan G, Foley RN, Kasiske BL *et al.* Controlling the epidemic of cardiovascular disease in chronic renal disease: What do we know? What do we need to learn? Where do we go from here? *Am J Kidney Dis* 1998;32:853–906.

33. Levey AS. Controlling the epidemic of cardiovascular disease in chronic renal disease: where do we start? *Am J Kidney Dis* 1998;32 Suppl 3:S5–13.

34. Acosta JH. Hypertension in chronic renal disease. *Kidney Int* 1982;22:702–12.

35. Mailloux LU, Haley WE. Hypertension in the ESRD patient: pathophysiology, therapy, outcomes, and future directions. *Am J Kidney Dis* 1998;32:705–19.

36. London G, Guerin A, Pannier B, Marchais S, Benetos A, Safar M. Increased systolic pressure in chronic uremia. Role of arterial wave reflections. *Hypertension* 1992;20:10–19.

37. Shichiri M, Hirata Y, Ando K, Emori T, Ohta K, Kimoto S *et al.* Plasma endothelin levels in hypertension and chronic renal failure. *Hypertension* 1990;15:493–6.

38. Glatter KA, Graves SW, Hollenberg NK, Soszynski PA, Tao QF, Frem GJ *et al.* Sustained volume expansion and (Na–K) ATPase inhibition in chronic renal failure. *Am J Hypertens* 1994;7:1016–25.

39. Smith MC, Dunn MJ. Hypertension in renal parenchymal disease. In: Laragh JH, Brenner BM, editors. *Hypertension: pathophysiology, diagnosis and management.* New York: Raven, 1990:1583–99.

40. Luke RG. Mechanisms of cyclosporin-induced hypertension. *Am J Hypertens* 1991;4:468–71.

41. Curtis JJ. Hypertension following kidney transplantation. *Am J Kidney Dis* 1994;23:471–5.

42. Bauer JM, Reams GP. Antihypertensive drugs. In: Brenner BM, editor. *The kidney.* 5th ed. Philadelphia: Saunders, 1996:2299–330.

43. Suki WN. Use of diuretics in chronic renal failure. *Kidney Int* 1997;51 Suppl 59:S33–5.

44. Charra B, Calemard E, Ruffet M, Chazot C, Terrat J-C, Vanel T *et al.* Survival as an index of adequacy of dialysis. *Kidney Int* 1992;41:1286–91.

45. Buckalew VM, Berg RL, Wang S-R, Porush JG, Rauch S, Schulman G and the Modification of Diet in Renal Disease Study Group. Prevalence of hypertension in 1,795 subjects with chronic renal disease: The Modification of Diet in Renal Disease Study Baseline Cohort. *Am J Kidney Dis* 1996;28:811–21.

46. MacMahon S, Peto R, Cutler J, Collins R, Sorlie P, Neaton J *et al.* Blood pressure, stroke and coronary heart disease. Part I. Prolonged differences in blood pressure: prospective observational studies corrected for the regression dilution bias. *Lancet* 1990;335:765–74.

47. Levy D, Larson MG, Vasan RS, Kannel WB, Ho KK. The progression from hypertension to congestive heart failure. *JAMA* 1996;275:1557–62.

48. Levy D, Garrison RJ, Savage DD, Kannel WB, Castelli WP. Prognostic implications of echocardiographically determined left ventricular mass in the Framingham Heart Study. *New Engl J Med* 1990;322:1561–6.

49. Levy D, Anderson KM, Savage DD, Balkus SA, Kannel WB, Castelli WP. Risk of ventricular arrhythmias in left ventricular hypertrophy: The Framingham Heart Study. *Am J Cardiol* 1987;60:560–5.

50. Turner RC, Millns H, Neil HA, Stratton IM, Manley SE, Matthew DR *et al.* for the United Kingdom Prospective Diabetes Study Group. Risk factors for coronary artery disease in non-insulin dependent diabetes mellitus: United Kingdom Prospective Diabetes Study (UKPDS:23). *BMJ* 1998;316:823–8.

51. Wong ND, Cupples LA, Ostfeld AM, Levy D, Kannel WB. Risk factors for long-term coronary prognosis after initial myocardial infarction: The Framingham Study. *Am J Epidemiol* 1989;130;469–80.

52. Abdulmassih Z, Chevalier A, Bader C, Drüeke TB, Kreis H, Lacour B. Role of lipid disturbances in the atherosclerosis of renal transplant patients. *Clin Transplant* 1992;6:106–13.

53. Ponticelli C, Montagnino G, Tarantino A, Aroldi A, Banfi G, Campise MR. Hypertension in renal transplantation. *Contrib Nephrol* 1994;106:190–2.

54. Kasiske BL, Guijarro C, Massy ZA, Wiederkehr MR, Ma JZ. Cardiovascular disease after renal transplantation. *J Am Soc Nephrol* 1996;7:158–65.

55. Iseki K, Miyasato F, Tokuyama K, Nishime K, Uehara H, Shiohira Y *et al.* Low diastolic blood pressure, hypoalbuminemia, and risk of death in a cohort of chronic hemodialysis patients. *Kidney Int* 1997;51:1212–17.

56. Zager PG, Nikolic J, Brown RH, Campbell MA, Hunt WC, Peterson D *et al.* for the Medical Directors of Dialysis Clinic, Inc. 'U' curve association of blood pressure and mortality in hemodialysis patients. *Kidney Int* 1998:54:561–9.

57. Mattila K, Haavisto M, Rajala S, Heikinheimo R. Blood pressure and five year survival in the very old. *BMJ* 1988;296:887–9.

58. Port FK, Hulbert-Shearon TE, Wolfe RA, Bloembergen WE, Golper TA, Agodoa LYC *et al.* Predialysis blood pressure and mortality risk in a national sample of maintenance hemodialysis patients. *Am J Kidney Dis* 1999;33:507–17.

59. MacMahon S, Rodgers A, Neal B, Chalmers J. Blood pressure lowering for the secondary prevention of myocardial infarction and stroke. *Hypertension* 1997;29:537–8.

60. UK Prospective Diabetes Study Group. Tight blood pressure control and risk of macrovascular and microvascular complications in type 2 diabetes: UKPDS 38. *BMJ* 1998;317:703–13.

61. Cannella G, Paoletti E, Delfino R, Peloso G, Molinari S, Traverso GB. Regression of left ventricular hypertrophy in hypertensive dialyzed uremic patients on long-term antihypertensive therapy. *Kidney Int* 1993;44:881–6.

62. Schmieder RE, Martus P, Klingbeil A. Reversal of left ventricular hypertrophy in essential hypertension. A meta-analysis of randomized double-blind studies. *JAMA* 1996;275:1507–13.

63. Rockstroh JK, Schobel HP, Vogt-Ladner G, Hauser I, Neumayer HH, Schmieder RE. Blood pressure independent effects of nitrendipine on cardiac structure in patients after renal transplantation. *Nephrol Dial Transplant* 1997;12:1441–7.

64. Robson R, Collins J, Johnson R, Kitching R, Searle M, Walker R *et al.* on behalf of the PERFECT study collaborative group. Effects of simvastatin and enalapril on serum lipoprotein concentrations and left ventricular mass in patients on dialysis. *J Nephrol* 1997;10:33–40.

65. Silberberg JS, Rahal DP, Patton DR, Sniderman AD. Role of anemia in the pathogenesis of left ventricular hypertrophy in end-stage renal disease. *Am J Cardiol* 1989;64:222–4.

66. National Kidney Foundation–Dialysis Outcomes Quality Initiative. NKF-DOQI clinical practice guidelines for the treatment of anemia of chronic renal failure. *Am J Kidney Dis* 1997;30 Suppl 3:S192–240.

67. Locatelli F, Conte F, Marcelli D. The impact of haematocrit levels and erythropoietin treatment on overall and cardiovascular mortality and morbidity—the experience of the Lombardy Dialysis Registry. *Nephrol Dial Transplant* 1998;13:1642–4.

68. Foley RN, Parfrey PS, Harnett JD, Kent GM, Marray DC, Barré PE. The impact of anemia on cardiomyopathy, morbidity, and mortality in end-stage renal disease. *Am J Kidney Dis* 1996;28:53–61.

69. Pascaul J, Teruel JL, Moya JL, Liaño F, Jiménez-Mena M, Ortuño J. Regression of left ventricular hypertrophy after partial correction of anemia with erythropoietin in patients on hemodialysis: a prospective study. *Clin Nephrol* 1991;35:280–7.

70. Raine AE, Roger SD. Effects of erythropoietin on blood pressure. *Am J Kidney Dis* 1991;18:76–83.

71. Fellner SK, Lang RM, Neumann A, Korcarz C, Borow KM. Cardiovascular consequences of correction of the anemia of renal failure with erythropoietin. *Kidney Int* 1993;44:1309–15.

72. Besarab A, Bolton WK, Browne JK, Egrie JC, Nissenson AR, Okamoto DM *et al.* The effects of normal as compared with low hematocrit values in patients with cardiac disease who are receiving hemodialysis and epoetin. *New Engl J Med* 1998;339:584–90.

73. Jacobs C. Normalization of haemoglobin: why not? *Nephrol Dial Transplant* 1999;14 Suppl 2:75–9.

74. Avram MM, Goldwasser P, Burrell DE, Antignani A, Fein PA, Mittman N. The uremic dyslipidemia: a cross-sectional and longitudinal study. *Am J Kidney Dis* 1992;20:324–35.

75. Attman P-O, Nyberg G, William-Olsson T, Knight-Gibson C, Alaupovic P. Dyslipoproteinemia in diabetic renal failure. *Kidney Int* 1992;42:1381–9.

76. Wheeler DC, Bernard DB. Lipid abnormalities in the nephrotic syndrome: causes, consequences and treatment. *Am J Kidney Dis* 1994;23:331–46.

77. Attman P-O, Samuelsson O, Alaupovic P. Lipoprotein metabolism and renal failure. *Am J Kidney Dis* 1993;21:573–92.

78. Oda H, Keane WF. Lipid abnormalities in end stage renal disease. *Nephrol Dial Transplant* 1998;13 Suppl 1:45–9.

79. Shoji T, Nishizawa Y, Nishitani H, Yamakawa M, Morii H. Impaired metabolism of high density lipoprotein in uremic patients. *Kidney Int* 1992;41:1653–61.

80. O'Neal D, Lee P, Murphy B, Best J. Low-density lipoprotein particle size distribution in end-stage renal disease treated with hemodialysis or peritoneal dialysis. *Am J Kidney Dis* 1996;27:84–91.

81. Rajman I, Harper L, McPake D, Kendall MJ, Wheeler DC. Low-density lipoprotein subfraction profiles in chronic renal failure. *Nephrol Dial Transplant* 1998;13:2281–7.

82. Joven J, Vilella E, Ahmad S, Cheung MC, Brunzell JD. Lipoprotein heterogeneity in end-stage renal disease. *Kidney Int* 1993;43:410–18.

83. Grützmacher P, März W, Peschke B, Gross W, Schoeppe W. Lipoproteins and apolipoproteins during the progression of chronic renal disease. *Nephron* 1988;50:103–11.

84. Kasiske BL. Hyperlipidemia in patients with chronic renal disease. *Am J Kidney Dis* 1998;32 Suppl 3:S142–56.

85. Bologa RM, Levine DM, Parker TS, Cheigh JS, Serur D, Stenzel KH *et al.* Interleukin-6 predicts hypoalbuminemia, hypocholesterolemia, and mortality in hemodialysis patients. *Am J Kidney Dis* 1998;32:107–14.

86. Kasisike BL, Umen AJ. Persistent hyperlipidemia in renal transplant patients. *Medicine* 1987;66:309–16.

87. Arnadottir M, Berg A-L. Treatment of hyperlipidemia in renal transplant recipients. *Transplantation* 1997;63:339–45.
88. Ratcliffe PJ, Dudley CR, Higgins RM, Firth JD, Smith B, Morris PJ. Randomised controlled trial of steroid withdrawal in renal transplant recipients receiving triple immunosuppression. *Lancet* 1996;348:643–8.
89. Kasiske BL, Tortorice KL, Heim-Duthoy KL, Awni WM, Rao KV. The adverse impact of cyclosporin on serum lipids in renal transplant recipients. *Am J Kidney Dis* 1991;17:700–7.
90. McCune TR, Thacker LR, Peters TG, Mulloy L, Rohr MS, Adams PA *et al.* Effects of tacrolimus on hyperlipidemia after successful renal transplantation. A Southeastern Organ Procurement Foundation Multicenter Clinical Study. *Transplantation* 1998;65:87–92.
91. Massy ZA, Ma JZ, Louis TA, Kasiske BL. Lipid-lowering therapy in patients with renal disease. *Kidney Int* 1995;48:188–98.
92. Regazzi MB, Iacona I, Campana C, Raddato V, Lesi C, Perani G *et al.* Altered disposition of pravastatin following concomitant drug therapy with cyclosporin A in transplant recipients. *Transplant Proc* 1993;25:2732–4.
93. Fortmann SP, Marcovina SM. Lipoprotein (a), a clinically elusive lipoprotein particle. *Circulation* 1997;95:295–6.
94. Sechi LA, Zingaro L, De Carli S, Sechi G, Catena C, Falleti E *et al.* Increased serum lipoprotein (a) levels in patients with early renal failure. *Ann Intern Med* 1998;129:457–61.
95. Dieplinger H, Lackner C, Kronenberg F, Sandholzer C, Lhotta K, Hoppichler F *et al.* Elevated plasma concentrations of lipoprotein (a) in patients with end-stage renal disease are not related to the size polymorphism of apolipoprotein (a). *J Clin Invest* 1993;91:397–401.
96. Wanner C, Rader D, Bartens W, Krämer J, Brewer HB, Schollmeyer P *et al.* Elevated plasma lipoprotein (a) in patients with the nephrotic syndrome. *Ann Intern Med* 1993;119:263–9.
97. Levine DM, Gordon BR. Lipoprotein (a) levels in patients receiving renal replacement therapy: methodologic issues and clinical implications. *Am J Kidney Dis* 1995;26:162–9.
98. Maeda S, Abe A, Seishima M, Makino K, Noma A, Kawade M. Transient changes of serum lipoprotein (a) as an acute phase protein. *Atherosclerosis* 1989;78:145–50.
99. Kronenberg F, König P, Lhotta K, Öfner D, Sandholzer C, Margreiter R *et al.* Apolipoprotein (a) phenotype-associated decrease in lipoprotein (a) plasma concentrations after renal transplantation. *Arterioscler Thromb* 1994;14:1399–1404.
100. Kronenberg F, Trenkwalder E, Lingenhel A, Friedrich G, Lhotta K, Schober M *et al.* Renovascular arteriovenous differences in Lp(a) plasma concentrations suggest removal of Lp(a) from the renal circulation. *J Lipid Res* 1997;38:1755–63.
101. Steinberg D, Parthasarathy S, Carew TE, Khoo JC, Witztum JL. Beyond cholesterol. Modifications of low-density lipoprotein that increase its atherogenicity. *New Engl J Med* 1989;320:915–24.
102. Richard MJ, Arnaud J, Jurkovitz C, Hachache T, Meftahi H, Laporte F *et al.* Trace elements and lipid peroxidation abnormalities in patients with chronic renal failure. *Nephron* 1991;57:10–15.
103. Maggi E, Bellazzi R, Falaschi F, Frattoni A, Perani G, Finardi G *et al.* Enhanced LDL oxidation in uremic patients: an additional mechanism for accelerated atherosclerosis? *Kidney Int* 1994;45:876–83.
104. Toborek M, Wasik T, Drózdz M, Klin M, Magner-Wróbel K, Kopieczna-Grzebieniak E. Effect of hemodialysis on lipid peroxidation and antioxidant system in patients with chronic renal failure. *Metabolism* 1992;41:1229–32.
105. Jackson P, Loughrey CM, Lightbody JH, McNamee PT, Young IS. Effect of hemodialysis on total antioxidant capacity and serum antioxidants in patients with chronic renal failure. *Clin Chem* 1995;41:1135–8.
106. Maggi E, Bellazzi R, Gazo A, Seccia M, Bellomo G. Autoantibodies against oxidatively-modified LDL in uremic patients undergoing dialysis. *Kidney Int* 1994;46:869–76.

107. Ghanem H, van den Dorpel MA, Weimar W, Man in 't Veld AJ, El-Kannishy MH, Jansen H. Increased low density lipoprotein oxidation in stable kidney transplant recipients. *Kidney Int* 1996;49:488–93.

108. Baigent C, Armitage J. Cholesterol reduction among patients at increased risk of coronary heart disease. *Proc R Coll Physicians Edin* 1999;29 Suppl 5:10–15.

109. Pekkanen J, Linn S, Heiss G, Suchindran CM, Leon A, Rifkind BM *et al.* Ten-year mortality from cardiovascular disease in relation to cholesterol level among men with and without preexisting cardiovascular disease. *New Engl J Med* 1990;322:1700–7.

110. Stamler J, Vaccaro O, Neaton JD, Wentworth D for the Multiple Risk Factors Intervention Trial Research Group. Diabetes, other risk factors, and 12-year cardiovascular mortality for men screened in the Multiple Risk Factor Intervention Trial. *Diabetes Care* 1993;16;434–44.

111. Lowrie EG, Lew NL. Death risk in hemodialysis patients: the predictive value of commonly measured variables and an evaluation of death rate differences between facilities. *Am J Kidney Dis* 1990;15:458–82.

112. Degoulet P, Legrain M, Réach I, Aimé F, Devriès C, Rojas P *et al.* Mortality risk factors in patients treated by chronic hemodialysis. Report of the Diaphane Collaborative Study. *Nephron* 1982;31:103–10.

113. Weverling-Rijnsburger AW, Blauw GJ, Lagaay AM, Knook DL, Meinders AE, Westendorp RG. Total cholesterol and risk of mortality in the oldest old. *Lancet* 1997;350:1119–23.

114. Corti M-C, Guralnik JM, Salive ME, Harris T, Ferrucci L, Glynn RJ *et al.* Clarifying the direct relation between total cholesterol levels and death from coronary heart disease in older persons *Ann Intern Med* 1997;126:753–60.

115. Wanner C, Krane V, Ruf G, März W, Ritz E fordie Deutsche Diabetes Dialyse Studie investigators. Rationale and design of a trial improving outcome of type 2 diabetics on hemodialysis. *Kidney Int* 1999;56 Suppl 71:S-222–6.

116. Gardner CD, Fortmann SP, Krauss RM. Association of small low-density lipoprotein particles with the incidence of coronary artery disease in men and women. *JAMA* 1996;276:875–81.

117. Hokanson JE, Austin MA. Plasma triglyceride level is a risk factor for cardiovascular disease independent of high-density lipoprotein cholesterol level: a meta-analysis of population-based prospective studies. *J Cardiovasc Risk* 1996;3:213–19.

118. Stampfer MJ, Krauss RM, Ma J, Blanche PJ, Holl LG, Sacks FM *et al.* A prospective study of triglyceride level, low-density lipoprotein particle diameter, and risk of myocardial infarction. *JAMA* 1996;276:882–8

119. Gordon DJ, Probstfield JL, Garrison RJ, Neaton JD, Castelli WP, Knoke JD *et al.* High-density lipoprotein cholesterol and cardiovascular disease. Four prospective American studies. *Circulation* 1989;79:8–15.

120. Nguyen TT, Ellefson RD, Hodge DO, Bailey KR, Kottke TE, Abu-Lebdeh HS. Predictive value of electrophoretically detected lipoprotein(a) for coronary heart disease and cerebrovascular disease in a community-based cohort of 9936 men and women. *Circulation* 1997;96:1390–7.

121. Jungers P, Massy ZA, Nguyen Khoa T, Fumeron C, Labrunie M, Lacour B *et al.* Incidence and risk factors of atherosclerotic cardiovascular accidents in predialysis chronic renal failure patients: a prospective study. *Nephrol Dial Transplant* 1997;12:2597–602.

122. Cressman MD, Heyka RJ, Paganini EP, O'Neil J, Skibinski CI, Hoff HF. Lipoprotein (a) is an independent risk factor for cardiovascular disease in hemodialysis patients. *Circulation* 1992;86:475–82.

123. Gey KF, Puska P, Jordan P, Moser UK. Inverse correlation between plasma vitamin E and mortality from ischemic heart disease in cross-cultural epidemiology. *Am J Clin Nutr* 1991;53:326S–34S.

124. Riemersma RA, Wood DA, Macintyre CC, Elton RA, Gey KF, Oliver MF. Risk of angina pectoris and plasma concentrations of vitamins A, C, and E and carotene. *Lancet* 1991;337:1–5.

125. Gaziano JM, Manson JE, Branch LG, LaMotte F, Colditz GA, Buring JE *et al.* Dietary beta carotene and decreased cardiovascular mortality in an elderly cohort. *J Am Coll Cardiol* 1992;19 Suppl A:377A (abstract).

126. Rimm EB, Stampfer MJ, Ascherio A, Giovannucci E, Colditz GA, Willett WC. Vitamin E consumption and the risk of coronary heart disease in men. *New Engl J Med* 1993;328:1450–6.
127. Stampfer MJ, Hennekens CH, Manson JE, Colditz GA, Rosner B, Willett WC. Vitamin E consumption and the risk of coronary disease in women. *New Engl J Med* 1993;328:1444–9.
128. Salonen JT, Salonen R, Penttilä I, Herranen J, Jauhiainen M, Kantola M *et al.* Serum fatty acids, apolipoproteins, selenium and vitamin antioxidants and the risk of death from coronary artery disease. *Am J Cardiol* 1985;56:226–31.
129. Rapola JM, Virtamo J, Ripatti S, Huttunen JK, Albanes O, Taylor PR *et al.* Randomised trial of α-tocopherol and β-carotene supplements on incidence of major coronary events in men with previous myocardial infarction. *Lancet* 1997; 349:1715–20.
130. Stephens NG, Parsons A, Schofield PM, Kelly F, Cheeseman K, Mitchinson MJ *et al.* Randomised controlled trial of vitamin E in patients with coronary disease: Cambridge Heart Antioxidant Study (CHAOS). *Lancet* 1996;347:781–6.
131. Clark CM, Lee DA. Prevention and treatment of the complications of diabetes mellitus. *New Engl J Med* 1995;332:1210–17.
132. Hager SR. Insulin resistance in uremia. *Am J Kidney Dis* 1989;14:272–6.
133. Fliser D, Pacini G, Engelleiter R, Kautzky-Willer A, Prager R, Franek E *et al.* Insulin resistance and hyperinsulinemia are already present in patients with incipient renal disease. *Kidney Int* 1998;53:1343–7.
134. Akmal M, Massry SG, Goldstein DA, Fanti P, Weisz A, DeFronzo RA. Role of parathyroid hormone in the glucose intolerance of chronic renal failure. *J Clin Invest* 1985;75:1037–44.
135. DeFronzo RA, Smith JD. Is glucose intolerance harmful for the uremic patient? *Kidney Int* 1985;28 Suppl 17:S88–97.
136. Sumrani NB, Delaney V, Ding Z, Davis R, Daskalakis P, Friedman EA *et al.* Diabetes mellitus after renal transplantation in the cyclosporin era—an analysis of risk factors. *Transplantation* 1991;51:343–7.
137. Ekstrand AV, Eriksson JG, Grönhagen-Riska C, Ahonen PJ, Groop LC. Insulin resistance and insulin deficiency in the pathogenesis of posttransplantation diabetes in man. *Transplantation* 1992;53:563–9.
138. Manske CL. Hyperglycemia and intensive glycemic control in diabetic patients with chronic renal disease. *Am J Kidney Dis* 1998;32 Suppl 3:S157–71.
139. Breckenridge A, Welborn TA, Dollery CT, Fraser R. Glucose tolerance in hypertensive patients on long-term diuretic therapy. *Lancet* 1967;i:61–4.
140. Pagano G, Cavallo-Perin P, Cassader M, Bruno A, Ozzello A, Masciola P *et al.* An *in vivo* and *in vitro* study of the mechanism of prednisone-induced insulin resistance in healthy subjects. *J Clin Invest* 1983;72:1814–20.
141. Danovitch GM. Immunosuppressive medications and protocols for renal transplantation. In: Danovitch GM, editor. *Handbook of kidney transplantation.* 1st ed. Boston: Little Brown, 1996:67–103.
142. Bailey CJ, Turner RC. Metformin. *New Engl J Med* 1996;334:574–9.
143. Kannel WB. Lipids, diabetes, and coronary heart disease: insights from the Framingham Study. *Am Heart J* 1985;110:1100–7.
144. Wilson PW. An epidemiologic perspective of systemic hypertension, ischemic heart disease, and heart failure. *Am J Cardiol* 1997;80 Suppl 9B:3J–8J.
145. Stephenson JM, Kenny S, Stevens LK, Fuller JH, Lee E and the WHO Multinational Study Group. Proteinuria and mortality in diabetes: the WHO Multinational Study of Vascular Disease in Diabetes. *Diabetic Medicine* 1995;12:149–55.
146. Rimmer JM, Sussman M, Foster R, Gennari FJ. Renal transplantation in diabetes mellitus. Influence of preexisting vascular disease on outcome. *Nephron* 1986;42:304–10.
147. Lemmers MJ, Barry JM. Major role for arterial disease in morbidity and mortality after kidney transplantation in diabetic recipients. *Diabetes Care* 1991;14:296–301.

148. Manske CL, Wilson RF, Wang Y, Thomas W. Atherosclerotic vascular complications in diabetic transplant candidates. *Am J Kidney Dis* 1997;29:601–7.

149. UK Prospective Diabetes Study (UKPDS) Group. Intensive blood-glucose control with sulphonylureas or insulin compared with conventional treatment and risk of complications in patients with type 2 diabetes (UKPDS 33). *Lancet* 1998;352:837–53.

150. The Diabetes Control and Complications Trial Research Group. The effect of intensive treatment of diabetes on the development and progression of long-term complications in insulin-dependent diabetes mellitus. *New Engl J Med* 1993;329:977–86.

151. The Diabetes Control and Complications Trial (DCCT) Research Group. Effect of intensive diabetes management on macrovascular events and risk factors in the Diabetes Control and Complications Trial. *Am J Cardiol* 1995;75:894–903.

152. Reaven GM, Lithell H, Landsberg L. Hypertension and associated metabolic abnormalities—the role of insulin resistance and the sympathoadrenal system. *New Engl J Med* 1996;334:374–81.

153. Ruige JB, Assendelft WJ, Dekker JM, Kostense PJ, Heine RJ, Bouter LM. Insulin and risk of cardiovascular disease. A meta-analysis. *Circulation* 1998;97:996–1001.

154. McKully KS. Vascular pathology of homocysteinaemia: implications for the pathogenesis of arteriosclerosis. *Am J Pathol* 1969;56:111–28.

155. Ueland PM, Refsum H, Stabler SP, Malinow MR, Andersson A, Allen RH. Total homocysteine in plasma or serum: methods and clinical applications. *Clinical Chem* 1993;39:1764–79.

156. Mayer EL, Jacobsen DW, Robinson K. Homocysteine and coronary atherosclerosis. *J Am Coll Cardiol* 1996;27:517–27.

157. Omenn GS, Beresford SA, Motulsky AG. Preventing coronary heart disease. B vitamins and homocysteine. *Circulation* 1998;97:421–4.

158. Welch GN, Loscalzo J. Homocysteine and atherothrombosis. *New Engl J Med* 1998;338;1042–50.

159. Chauveau P, Chadefaux B, Coudé M, Aupetit J, Hannedouche T, Kamoun P *et al.* Hyperhomocysteinemia, a risk factor for atherosclerosis in chronic uremic patients. *Kidney Int* 1993;43 Suppl 41:S72–7.

160. Arnadottir M, Hultberg B, Nilsson-Ehle P, Thysell H. The effect of reduced glomerular filtration rate on plasma total homocysteine concentration. *Scand J Clin Lab Invest* 1996;56:41–6.

161. Bostom AG, Gohh RY, Beaulieu AJ, Nadeau MR, Hume AL, Jacques PF *et al.* Treatment of hyperhomocysteinemia in renal transplant recipients. A randomized, placebo-controlled trial. *Ann Intern Med* 1997;127:1089–92.

162. Danesh J, Lewington S. Plasma homocysteine and coronary heart disease: systematic review of published epidemiological studies. *J Cardiovasc Risk* 1998;5:229–32.

163. Bostom AG, Shemin D, Lapane KL, Miller JW, Sutherland P, Nadeau MR *et al.* Hyperhomocysteinemia and traditional cardiovascular disease risk factors in end-stage renal disease patients on dialysis: a case-control study. *Atherosclerosis* 1995;114:93–103.

164. Bostom AG, Shemin D, Lapane KL, Sutherland P, Nadeau MR, Wilson PW *et al.* Hyperhomocysteinemia, hyperfibrinogenemia, and lipoprotein (a) excess in maintenance dialysis patients: a matched case-control study. *Atherosclerosis* 1996;125:91–101.

165. Bostom AG, Shemin D, Verhoef P, Nadeau MR, Jacques PF, Selhub J *et al.* Elevated fasting total plasma homocysteine levels and cardiovascular disease outcomes in maintenance dialysis patients. A prospective study. *Arterioscler Thromb Vasc Biol* 1997;17:2554–8.

166. Moustapha A, Naso A, Nahlawi M, Gupta A, Arheart KL, Jacobsen DW *et al.* Prospective study of hyperhomocysteinemia as an adverse cardiovascular risk factor in end-stage renal disease. *Circulation* 1998;97:138–41.

167. Homocysteine Lowering Trialists' Collaboration. Lowering blood homocysteine with folic acid based supplements: meta-analysis of randomised trials. *BMJ* 1998;316:894–8.

168. Bostom AG, Shemin D, Lapane KL, Hume AL, Yoburn D, Nadeau MR *et al.* High dose B-vitamin treatment of hyperhomocysteinemia in dialysis patients. *Kidney Int* 1996;49: 147–52.

169. Anonymous. Comorbid conditions and correlations with mortality risk among 3,399 incident haemodialysis patients. *Am J Kidney Dis* 1992;20 (5 suppl 2):32–8.
170. Rubin HR, Jenckes M, Fink NE, Meyer K, Wu AW, Bass EB *et al.* for the CHOICE study. Patient's view of dialysis care: development of a taxonomy and rating of importance of different aspects of care. *Am J Kidney Dis* 1997;30:793–801.
171. Beto JA, Bansal VK. Interventions for other risk factors: tobacco use, physical inactivity, menopause, and homocysteine. *Am J Kidney Dis* 1998;32 Suppl 3:S172–84.
172. Parish S, Collins R, Peto R, Youngman L, Barton J, Jayne K *et al.* for the International Studies of Infarct Survival (ISIS) Collaborators. Cigarette smoking, tar yields, and non-fatal myocardial infarction: 14000 cases and 32000 controls in the United Kingdom. *BMJ* 1995;311:471–7.
173. Haire HM, Sherrard DJ, Scardapane D, Curtis FK, Brunzell JD. Smoking, hypertension and mortality in a maintenance dialysis population. *Cardiovasc Med* 1978;3:1163–8.
174. Doll R, Peto R, Wheatley K, Gray R, Sutherland I. Mortality in relation to smoking: 40 years' observations on male British doctors. *BMJ* 1994;309:901–11.
175. Orth SR, Ritz E, Schrier RW. The renal risks of smoking. *Kidney Int* 1997;51:1669–77.
176. Gabay C, Kushner I. Acute-phase proteins and other systemic responses to inflammation. *New Engl J Med* 1999;340,448–54.
177. Danesh J, Collins R, Appleby P, Peto R. Association of fibrinogen, C-reactive protein, albumin, or leukocyte count with coronary heart disease. Meta-analyses of prospective studies. *JAMA* 1998;279:1477–82.
178. Meade TW. Fibrinogen in ischaemic heart disease. *Europ Heart J* 1995;16 Suppl A:31–5.
179. Irish A. Cardiovascular disease, fibrinogen and the acute phase response associations with lipids and blood pressure in patients with chronic renal disease. *Atherosclerosis*: 1998;137:133–9.
180. Koch M, Kutkuhn B, Grabensee B, Ritz E. Apolipoprotein A, fibrinogen, age, and history of stroke are predictors of death in dialysed diabetic patients: a prospective study in 412 subjects. *Nephrol Dial Transplant* 1997;12:2603–11.
181. Doweiko JP, Nompleggi DJ. Role of albumin in human physiology and pathophysiology. *J Parenter Enter Nutr* 1991;15:207–11.
182. Kaysen GA, Stevenson FT, Depner TA. Determinants of albumin concentration in hemodialysis patients. *Am J Kidney Dis* 1997;29:658–68.
183. Goldwasser P, Feldman J. Association of serum albumin and mortality risk. *J Clin Epidemiol* 1997;50:693–703.
184. Owen WF, Lew NL, Liu Y, Lowrie EG, Lazarus JM. The urea reduction ratio and serum albumin concentration as predictors of mortality in patients undergoing hemodialysis. *New Engl J Med* 1993;329:1001–6.
185. Foley RN, Parfrey PS, Harnett JD, Kent GM, Murray DC, Barré PE. Hypoalbuminaemia, cardiac morbidity, and mortality in end-stage renal disease. *J Am Soc Nephrol* 1996;7:728–36.
186. Owen WF, Lowrie EG. C-reactive protein as an outcome predictor for maintenance hemodialysis patients. *Kidney Int* 1998;54:627–36.

2

Mortality and cardiovascular risk factors influencing survival in end-stage renal failure

Robert N. Foley and Patrick S. Parfrey

Clinical epidemiology of cardiovascular disease in end-stage renal failure (ESRF)

Pericarditis and pericardial effusion were common manifestations of terminal uremia before renal replacement therapies became available. The availability of chronic hemodialysis led to an almost miraculous change in that the inexorable progression to death associated with the uremic syndrome was stalled. It became rapidly apparent, however, that the reprieve was temporary, and that the survival of dialysis patients was still at least an order of magnitude shorter than in a general population sample of similar age.[1] During this time it became evident that cardiovascular disease was the attributed cause of death in an unexpectedly large proportion of patients.[2-4] This was unexpected because limited availability meant that patients were selected for dialysis based on younger age and absence of other major co-morbid illnesses. In 1974, Doctors Lindner, Charra, Sherrard, and Scribner blew the whistle alerting the nephrology community of this epidemic. In the Seattle experience, 60% of deaths in their dialysis patients were due to cardiovascular disease. It was suggested that accelerated atherosclerosis was responsible for this premature cardiovascular demise.[5] This notion has become very widespread, although it is far from universally accepted. It is probably fair to comment that attention to the muscular or pump function of the cardiovascular system has received inadequate attention until more recently.

It has been consistently observed that approximately half of all deaths in dialysis patients are attributed to cardiovascular disease.[6,7] This observation is consistent over time, in populations with very different practices of renal replacement therapy and very different underlying rates of cardiovascular disease in the general population. These observations suggest a strong connection between uremia and cardiovascular disease. It is equally plausible that cardiovascular disease leads to uremia and that uremia leads to cardiovascular disease.

Mortality from cardiovascular disease is orders of magnitude higher in dialysis patients, while transplant patients appear to have rates that are intermediate (see Figs 1.1 and 1.2), though still excessive.[8]

Most clinical studies aimed at identifying reversible cardiovascular risk factors have used death as outcome measure. Applying a Framingham type approach late in the natural history of cardiovascular disorders is fraught with potential pitfalls, especially because many patients have already developed clinical or silent versions of the disease destined to kill them. Using death alone as an outcome in natural history studies can lead to tenuous conclusions for many reasons. Cause-specific mortality, for example using cardiac death as an outcome to identify treatable cardiac risk factors, is somewhat of a house of cards, because the validity of how physicians assign cause of death is questionable. For example, Perneger *et al.*[9]

compared dialysis registry reporting forms from 335 ESRF patients to cause of death from death certificates. Agreement on cause of death in these dialysis patients was only 31%. Using death as an outcome parameter to pick out reversible risk factors can also lead to major problems. The level of a risk factor may change dramatically before and after developing the condition that leads to death. By analogy, we would not examine blood pressure or cholesterol levels from patients in coronary artery units to determine the influence of these parameters on death from coronary artery disease in the general population. The ideal epidemiological study should identify a population demonstrably free of cardiac disease, and should include the morbid events that subsequently cause death as study outcomes, in addition to using death as an end-point.

The incidence rates of coronary artery disease and cardiac failure are very high in dialysis patients. For example, in the Canadian Hemodialysis Morbidity Study admission rates for ischemic heart disease and cardiac failure were 10% per year for each condition.[10] Most patients beginning dialysis therapy can be considered to have cardiac disease. For example, in the ongoing, prospective, US Renal Data System (USRDS) Wave 2 study 40% of patients starting dialysis therapy have had antecedent ischemic heart disease and 40% have had cardiac failure.[11] We performed a 10-year study from the inception of dialysis therapy in 433 ESRF patients. Subclinical cardiac disease was the rule at the time of first dialysis: 74% had left ventricular hypertrophy, 32% had left ventricular dilatation, and 15% had systolic dysfunction.[12] Several echocardiographic studies have had similar findings. It is implausible that the huge burden of cardiac disease already present in patients starting dialysis therapy can fully explain the very high subsequent incidence rates. In our study, over a mean follow-up on dialysis therapy of 28 months, 12% of patients went on to develop their first episode of ischemic heart disease,[13] while 25% went on to develop their first episode of cardiac failure.[14] Expressed in another way, among patients without clinical manifestations of these diseases starting dialysis, the incidence rates of new ischemic heart disease and new cardiac failure were 5% and 11% respectively per year of follow-up.

As defined by clinical criteria, cardiovascular disease is clearly associated with short survival in ESRF patients. Cardiac failure has been consistently associated with dialysis mortality. The association has been neither as consistent nor as strong for ischemic heart disease. This is particularly true when the possibility of concomitant cardiac failure is taken into account in survival analyses. One of the larger studies, from the USRDS, suggested that both ischemic heart disease and cardiac failure were independently associated with death in dialysis patients.[15] We found that patients with ischemic heart disease starting dialysis therapy had shorter survival than those that did not. However, multivariate models suggested that much of the latter mortality effect appeared through cardiac failure. The impact of ischemic heart disease was not independent of cardiac failure.[16] The presence of both conditions was especially lethal (Fig. 2.1).

With regard to left ventricular (LV) disorders present on echocardiography, we found a hierarchy of risk as follows: normal LV, concentric LV hypertrophy, LV dilatation, and systolic dysfunction. This risk grading strongly predicted the development of ischemic heart disease, cardiac failure, and death. It was noteworthy, as shown in Fig. 2.2, that the relationship between echocardiographic abnormalities and death came into effect after a lag phase of 2 years, which suggests a window of opportunity, with an ideal time for intervention prior to this.[16,17] Silberberg *et al.*[18] have also shown an association between LV hypertrophy and mortality in patients starting dialysis therapy. In a recent analysis, we found that regression of LV hypertrophy and systolic dysfunction between baseline and 1 year of dialysis was

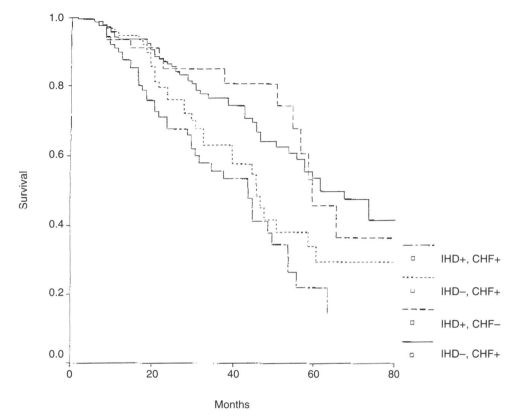

Fig. 2.1 Mortality, adjusted for age and diabetes mellitus, according to the presence or absence of ischemic heart disease (IHD) and congestive heart failure (CHF) at inception of dialysis therapy. (Primary data taken from references 13 and 14.)

associated with a lower risk of new-onset cardiac failure. This effect was independent of, and additive to, baseline echocardiographic parameters.[19]

One of the major problems hindering advance in determining the clinical epidemiology of coronary artery disease in ESRF is the lack of an easy-to-apply quantitative and accurate diagnostic test. Most epidemiological studies have used various permutations of angina pectoris, myocardial infarction, and a prior history of coronary revascularization procedure as a surrogate marker for the presence of coronary artery disease. However, silent coronary artery disease and angina with normal coronary arteries are both common in dialysis patients. Dahan *et al.*[20] recently published a very interesting study in which thallium imaging and coronary angiography were both performed in 60 asymptomatic hemodialysis patients who were followed prospectively for 2.8 years. The prevalence of asymptomatic coronary artery disease was 21%. Thallium testing, using a combination of dipyridamole and exercise as a stressor, was a highly accurate diagnostic test with sensitivity, specificity, positive, and negative predictive values of 92, 89, 71, 98, and 90%, respectively. The odds of remaining free of coronary events was 9.2-fold lower in patients with normal thallium uptake than in those with abnormal thallium ($p <$ 0.005), even after adjustment for several risk factors including left ventricular mass index and systolic function.[20] Validation of these results in a larger group of ESRF patients would

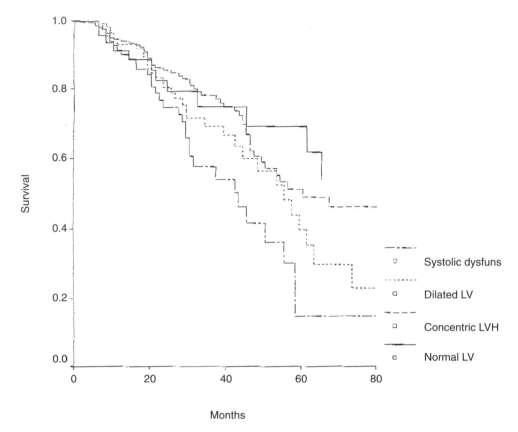

Fig. 2.2 Mortality, adjusted for age and diabetes mellitus, according to left ventricular (LV) echocardiographic morphology at inception of dialysis therapy. (Primary data taken from references 12 and 16.)

provide us with a useful tool for the study of coronary artery disease in ESRF patients. Electron-beam computed tomography[21,22] has many attractive features for non-invasively and directly imaging the coronary arterial tree, but has yet to be evaluated in ESRF patients.

Although the clinical epidemiology of cardiovascular disease in chronic renal failure has received much attention in recent years, there are still glaring gaps in our knowledge. Intuitively, it seems that early intervention will be the way forward. Unfortunately, our information on the incidence and risk factors of cardiovascular disease in those with predialysis chronic renal insufficiency, including renal transplant recipients, is quite rudimentary. Intervention trials are urgently needed to lessen the burden of cardiovascular disease in chronic renal failure. To do this sensibly, we need accurate information about cardiovascular event rates and reversible risk factors from large-scale prospective studies, in all categories of patients with renal dysfunction.

Risk factors

Should we intervene in classical cardiovascular risk factors in ESRF patients?

The decade of the 1990s has been memorable for the profusion of large trials that have shown that intervention in risk factors derived from observational studies translates into clinical benefit. Thus, in general population medicine, very few physicians doubt that we should intervene in hypertension or hypercholesterolemia. What has been equally impressive is that those already at higher risk gain relatively more from a given intervention. For example, the benefits of controlling blood pressure are very clear in older subjects.[23–25] Similarly, aggressive lipid strategies are clearly beneficial in survivors of myocardial infarction,[26–29] while aspirin therapy is most clearly indicated in those with coronary artery disease[30–34] or in older diabetic patients.[35] It is clear that these results are difficult to ignore and that the interventions employed are easily applicable to ESRF patients. It is equally clear that classic cardiovascular risk factors such as hypertension, hypercholesterolemia, and hyperglycemia are common, and often severe in chronic renal failure patients. However, these patients also have risk factors unique to uremia and its therapies that could overshadow the impact of classical risk factors. It is the opinion of these authors that these intervention trials in classic cardiovascular risk factors need to be repeated in ESRF patients if logical treatment algorithms are to be developed. Because therapeutic uncertainty is so pervasive, it would appear that ESRF patients are an ideal group in which to perform these trials.[36]

Smoking

Smoking is known to double the risk of cardiovascular disease in the general population. It is also known that smoking is even riskier in subjects with otherwise greater risks of cardiovascular disease.[37] Smoking is rarely considered when trying to identify reversible mortality risk factors in ESRF patients. Little has been written about the impact of smoking in ESRF patients. In the USRDS Special Study of Case Mix Severity smoking increased mortality by 26% in hemodialysis patients.[18] In another study it was associated with a doubling of mortality rates in diabetic ESRF patients.[38]

Hypertension

Hypertension is very common in ESRF populations. Hypertension is clearly implicated in the pathogenesis of cardiovascular disease in the general population and the progression of chronic renal disease.

Clinical trials in the general population have demonstrated repeatedly that lowering blood pressure in hypertensive individuals lowers cardiovascular risk.[23–25] However, it remains to be determined how low our blood pressure targets should be. Some observational studies have suggested a 'U' or 'J' curve relationship between diastolic blood pressure and cardiovascular risk in this population, in which risk increases as diastolic blood pressure falls below 85 mmHg and rises above 90 mmHg.[39,40] It is plausible that these findings may reflect the danger of reducing perfusion pressure in vascular beds with fixed stenoses. The Hypertension Optimal Trial was designed to address this contentious issue. 18 790 hypertensive patients aged 50 to 80 years were randomly assigned to target diastolic blood pressures of ≤90 or ≤85 or ≤80 mmHg using felodipine as principal antihypertensive therapy. Overall, there were no differences in cardiovascular outcome according to assigned target blood pressure. Diabetic patients (who might be expected to be more prone to undiagnosed fixed vascular stenoses) appeared to be different, as those in the ≤80 mmHg target had a cardiovascular event rate half that of the >90 mmHg. A major problem with this study was the failure to adequately separate blood pressure levels in the three patient groups. A *post hoc* analysis, ignoring random group assignment, suggested a threshold diastolic blood pressure level of 82.6 mmHg for major cardiovascular events, and 86.5 mmHg for cardiovascular events.[35] Thus, the 'J/U' curve controversy rages on.

The debate regarding cardiovascular risk and target blood pressure in ESRF has become an even more contentious issue than in essential hypertension. Until recently, nephrologists 'knew', by intuition, that hypertension is a major reversible cardiac risk factor in dialysis patients. Recent observational data to support this intuition have been anything but consistent. For example, in the study of Charra *et al.*[41] patients received long-duration hemodialysis with exceptionally high urea clearance (a universally accepted measure of how dialysis cleans the uremic internal milieu). Five-year survival rates were extremely good. Of these patients, 98% had 'normal' blood pressure levels, without recourse to antihypertensive medications. Even within this relatively normotensive range, higher blood pressure levels were directly associated with mortality.[41] On the other hand, several observational studies have reported that low blood pressure is independently associated with mortality in ESRF.[9,42] Others have reported no relationship between blood pressure and mortality in adequately hemodialyzed patients.[10,43,44] If a true cause–effect relationship is present, these results suggest that high blood pressure is protective. In patients with progressive renal disease, it is hard to conceptualize (and even harder to explain to patients) how blood pressure levels could suddenly switch from being harmful immediately before, to beneficial immediately after, starting dialysis therapy. A recent study by Zager *et al.*[45] suggested that pre-dialysis blood pressure was unrelated to cardiovascular mortality. A U-curve association between post-dialysis blood pressure and mortality was seen, with systolic blood pressures greater than 180 mmHg, diastolic blood pressure greater than 90 mmHg, and systolic blood pressure less than 110 mmHg associated with increased cardiovascular mortality.[45] In our study,[46] mean arterial blood pressure levels were 101 mmHg. An inverse relationship between blood pressure levels and mortality was seen. Mortality increased by 22% for each 10 mmHg decrease in the time-averaged mean arterial blood pressure. High blood pressure, however, was independently associated with an increase in LV mass index and cavity volume on follow-up, as well as with new-onset ischemic heart disease and cardiac failure. These data produce conclusions that appear to be internally incongruous: high blood pressure may have caused the conditions that killed these patients, while lower average blood pressure was associated with shorter survival. It is worth highlighting several results from our study: (1) admission for cardiac failure predated most deaths; (2) high blood pressure was very strongly predictive of the development of cardiac failure; (3) blood pressures fell following the development of cardiac failure; (4) low blood pressure strongly predicted mortality after the development of cardiac failure.[46] Even if interpreted in a very conservative way, these data suggest, at least, that high blood pressure is not good for dialysis patients without pre-established cardiac disease. The huge prevalence of hypertension in ESRF populations and the lack of uniformity in the blood pressure–mortality relationship indicates the necessity for a large randomized trial in dialysis patients. There are very few randomized trials to guide antihypertensive therapy in ESRF patients. London *et al.*[47] randomly assigned 24 hypertensive dialysis patients with LV hypertrophy to either the ACE-inhibitor perindopril or the calcium channel blocker nitrendipine. The blood pressure reductions seen were similar in both groups. However, there was a greater reduction in LV mass index in those assigned ACE-inhibitors. This study suggests that blood pressure reduction is beneficial and that ACE-inhibitors may have an impact that is independent of their blood pressure lowering effect.[47]

It is clear that large randomized controlled trials in ESRF are needed to determine the ideal target blood pressure and the optimum way to reduce blood pressure in ESRF patients.

Lipid abnormalities

High triglyceride levels, decreased high-density lipoprotein (HDL) and high lipoprotein (a) (Lp(a)) levels are frequently observed in both hemodialysis and peritoneal dialysis, while peritoneal dialysis patients also have higher low-density lipoprotein (LDL) levels.[48-56] The associations between quantitative lipid abnormalities and outcome in ESRF are not as consistent as seen in the general population. For example, Lowrie and Lew[42] found an inverse association between cholesterol levels and mortality, possibly because low cholesterol reflects malnutrition. Some studies, however, have reported that dyslipidemia may be associated with cardiac mortality in diabetic hemodialysis patients[57] and that Lp(a) levels are associated with cardiovascular disease in a mixed population of hemodialysis patients.[58] A recent cross-sectional study reported that apoB levels, low-molecular-weight apo(a) phenotype and low HDL levels were independently associated with the presence of coronary artery disease.[59] Yet again, there is a clear need to perform randomized clinical trials to determine whether aggressive therapy of hypercholesterolemia has a beneficial impact on patient outcome in ESRF.

Hyperhomocysteinemia

Hyperhomocysteinemia is a potent cardiovascular risk factor in the general population.[60] Very high homocysteine levels are found in ESRF patients.[61]

Several studies have reported that high homocysteine levels may lead to vascular disease in uremic patients.[62-68] This risk factor may be amenable to intervention with high dose B-vitamin therapy, even in renal patients. Bostom and colleagues performed a randomized trial in renal transplant patients demonstrating that vitamin B_6 and a combination of folic acid plus vitamin B_{12} have additive effects in reducing homocysteine levels.[69] Perna *et al.* gave 14 hemodialysis patients 2 months of therapy with oral methyltetrahydrofolate at a dose of 15 mg per day.[69a] Homocysteine levels fell dramatically. The cardiovascular benefit of interventions like this has yet to be established.

Anemia

Anemia has been shown consistently to be a risk factor for the cardiac abnormalities seen in ESRF. In our study, which reflected clinical practice in the 1980s, hemoglobin levels averaged 8.8 g/dl. Anemia, over time, was independently associated with progressive LV dilatation on echocardiography, the development of *de novo* cardiac failure, and overall mortality.[70] Several observational studies have suggested that anemia leads to LV dilatation and/or hypertrophy.[71,72] More recently, a number of large dialysis databases have shown associations between anemia and mortality, with the mortality risk increasing as hematocrit falls below 33%.[73-75] This paradigm, whereby anemia and decreased peripheral oxygen delivery cause harm exclusively via central hemodynamic and cardiac maladaptation, may be overly simplistic. For example, an extensive body of evidence suggests that the beneficial effect of red blood cell transfusions in hypovolemic patients with traumatic injuries may be predominantly related to restoration of the peripheral blood volume as opposed to the central blood volume.[76]

Many studies have examined the effect of partial correction of anemia with epoetin on echocardiographic abnormalities. These have shown that partial correction of anemia partially reverses hypoxic vasodilatation, increases peripheral resistance, reduces cardiac output, and partially reverses LV dilatation and hypertrophy.[77–86] The consistency of these data lead naturally to several questions: what if anemia was never allowed to develop in the ESRF spectrum, especially in those without established cardiomyopathy? What is the impact of normalization of anemia in patients allowed to develop both sustained anemia and cardiomyopathy? Several observational studies of patients with advancing chronic renal failure show that cardiac enlargement progresses rapidly as glomerular filtration rate falls; nascent renal anemia has been associated with this cardiac enlargement in the studies reported thus far.[87,88] We have recently examined the annual evolution of cardiomyopathy in a group of dialysis patients with serial echocardiograms from baseline to 3 years on dialysis therapy.[89] LV dilatation with compensatory LV wall thickening occurred over time. The greatest degree of cardiac enlargement took place in the first year. Risk factors (anemia and hemodialysis compared to peritoneal dialysis) could only be identified in the first year. The cardiac enlargement after this was autonomous of several standard risk factors.[89] These data suggest that earlier intervention to prevent anemia might be superior to late intervention.

Three randomized clinical trials comparing partial to complete correction of anemia have recently been completed. In the US trial 1233 patients (56% of whom were diabetic, with a mean duration dialysis duration of 3.2 years) were randomly assigned to target hematocrits of 30% or 42%. The presence of congestive heart failure or ischemic heart disease was a prerequisite for inclusion in the trial. The primary end-point was the combined outcome of death or a first nonfatal myocardial infarction. After an average of 2.4 years of follow-up, there were 183 deaths and 19 first nonfatal myocardial infarctions among the patients in the high-hematocrit group and 150 deaths and 14 nonfatal myocardial infarctions among those in the low-hematocrit group (risk ratio for the normal-hematocrit group compared with the low-hematocrit group, 1.3; 95% confidence interval, 0.9–1.9). The patients in the normal-hematocrit group had a decline in the adequacy of dialysis and received intravenous iron dextran more often than those in the low-hematocrit group. In particular, there was an excess of vascular access thrombosis, with rates of thrombosis of 39% vs. 29% respectively,[90] translating into an increase of relative risk of approximately one-third. Thus, in target hemodialysis patients with advanced cardiac disease, the conservative target hematocrit appears warranted. We have recently completed a Canadian multicenter trial in hemodialysis patients without symptoms of cardiac disease. The principal objectives were to compare target hemoglobin levels of 100 and 135 g/l with respect to regression of concentric LV hypertrophy and LV dilatation. The results of this trial are being analysed at the time of writing. A Swedish trial has also finished recently, in which partial versus complete correction of renal anemia are compared in patients with advancing chronic renal failure, dialysis patients, and renal transplant recipients. These trials should help us to select appropriate target hemoglobin levels in hemodialysis patients.

Abnormal calcium-phosphate homeostasis

We found that chronic hypocalcemia in dialysis patients was strongly associated with ischemic heart disease and death. The association was seen in both peritoneal dialysis patients and hemodialysis patients, and was only partly explained by the relationship between mean serum calcium and time spent on dialysis therapy.[91] Hypocalcemia induces hyperparathyroidism, which may lead to intracellular calcium overload, altered myocardial bioenergetics, and myocardial ischemia.[92] Hyperparathyroidism has been associated with LV abnormalities and arterial thickening in dialysis patients.[93,94] A recent study from the USRDS showed that phosphorus levels above 6.5 mg/dl and hyperparathyroidism were both associated with mortality in hemodialysis patients.[95] Should it transpire that hyperparathyroidism is truly a major vascular risk factor, we may need to change our approach to the treatment of hyperparathyroidism to one which considers both its bony and cardiovascular effects. Once again, this is a question that can be addressed with a clinical trial.

Hypoalbuminemia

Hypoalbuminemia and dialysis intensity are among the more dominant outcome predictors in ESRF.[96-98] The contribution of acute phase reaction and actual malnutrition to the hypoalbuminemia of ESRF is not fully known. Regardless of causation, the relationship between hypoalbuminemia and mortality is strong; the consistent observation that cardiovascular disease far outpaces any other cause of death in ESRF suggests that hypoalbuminemia and cardiac disease in dialysis patients are inter-related. In our prospective cohort study falling mean serum albumin levels were strongly associated with the development of *de novo* and recurrent cardiac failure, *de novo* and recurrent ischemic heart disease, cardiac mortality, and overall mortality in hemodialysis patients. Among peritoneal dialysis patients hypoalbuminemia was independently associated with progressive LV dilatation on serial echocardiograms, *de novo* cardiac failure, and overall mortality. It is worth reiterating that low serum albumin levels came before these clinical events.[99]

The mechanisms connecting hypoalbuminemia to coronary artery disease and cardiomyopathy in dialysis patients are not known. Several are theoretically possible, including hypercoagulability, as in the nephrotic syndrome, direct effects related to inadequate protein stores, and as a surrogate marker for the pathogenic effects of a chronic inflammatory state.

Uremia

Animal studies show that uremia leads to deposition of interstitial ground substance, followed by collagen deposition, and a reduction in capillary surface density.[100,101] Uremic serum directly depresses myocardial contractility.[102] Uremia has been shown to cause chronic activation of the vascular endothelium.[103]

The evidence that uremia leads to clinical cardiovascular disease in human ESRF is indirect. For example, in the National Co-operative Dialysis Study there were more cardiac events in patients who received less intensive dialysis therapy.[104] Renal transplantation leads to an improvement in many of the echocardiographic abnormalities seen in dialysis patients.[105] The ongoing Hemodialysis (HEMO) study should shed considerable light on this issue. The latter is a very large multicenter trial sponsored by the National Institutes of Health whose objective is to test the effects of dialysis dosage and membrane flux on morbidity and mortality.

Conclusion

The clinical epidemiology of cardiac disease in chronic uremia is a rapidly evolving field. The traditional cardiac risk factors are common and modifiable, but need to be rigorously tested for clinical benefit in uremic populations. Many modifiable factors that are related to the uremic state may lead to cardiac morbidity and mortality. High-quality prospective epidemiological data, as well as randomized controlled clinical trials, are needed in ESRF.

References

1. Drukker, W. Haemodialysis: a historical review. In: Maher JF, editor. *Replacement of renal function by dialysis.* 3rd ed. Boston: Kluwer Academic, 1989.
2. Drukker W, Alberts C, Ode A, Roosedall KJ, Wilmink JM. Report on regular dialysis treatment in Europe. *Proceedings of the European Dialysis Transplantation Association* 1966;3:90.
3. Brunner FP, Garland HJ, Harlen H, Scharer K, Parsons FM. Combined report on regular dialysis and transplantation in Europe. *Proceedings of the European Dialysis Transplantation Association* 1966;3:90.
4. Bryan F Jr. National Dialysis Registry Report. *Proc 6th Annu Contractors Conf, Artif Kidney Program*, NIAMDD, DHEW Publ No NIH 74. 1973;248:201.
5. Lindner A, Charra B, Sherrard DJ, Scribner BH. Accelerated atherosclerosis in prolonged maintenance hemodialysis. *New England Journal of Medicine* 1974;290:697–701.
6. *US Renal Data System (USRDS) Annual Report*, 1997.
7. Fenton S, Desmeules M, Copleston P, Arbus G, Froment D, Jeffery J *et al*. Renal replacement therapy in Canada: a report from the Canadian Organ Replacement Register. *American Journal of Kidney Diseases* 1995;25:134–150.
8. Foley RN, Parfrey PS, Sarnak MJ. Clinical epidemiology of cardiovascular disease in chronic renal disease. *American Journal of Kidney Diseases* 1998;32:S112–S119.
9. Perneger TV, Klag MJ, Whelton PK. Cause of death in patients with end-stage renal disease: death certificates vs registry reports. *American Journal of Kidney Diseases* 1993;83:1735–1738
10. Churchill DN, Taylor DW, Cook RJ, LaPlante P, Barre P, Cartier P *et al*. Canadian Hemodialysis Morbidity Study. *American Journal of Kidney Diseases* 1992;19:214–234.
11. The USRDS Dialysis Morbidity and Mortality Study: Wave 2. United States Renal Data System. *American Journal of Kidney Diseases* 1997;30(2 Suppl 1):S67–S85.
12. Foley RN, Parfrey PS, Harnett JD, Kent GM, Martin CJ, Murray DC *et al*. Clinical and echocardiographic disease in patients starting end-stage renal disease therapy. *Kidney International* 1995;47:186–192.
13. Parfrey PS, Foley RN, Harnett JD, Kent GM, Martin CJ, Murray DC *et al*. Outcome and risk factors of ischemic heart disease in chronic uremia. *Kidney International* 1996;49:1428–1434.
14. Harnett JD, Foley RN, Kent GM, Barre P, Murray DC, Parfrey PS. Congestive heart failure in dialysis patients: prevalence, incidence, prognosis and risk factors. *Kidney International* 1995;47:884–890.
15. US Renal Data System 1992 Annual Report. IV. Comorbid conditions and correlations with mortality risk among 3,399 incident hemodialysis patients. *American Journal of Kidney Diseases* 1992;20(Suppl 2):32–38.
16. Foley RN, Parfrey PS, Harnett JD, Kent GM, Murray DC, Barre PE. The prognostic importance of left ventricular geometry in uremic cardiomyopathy. *Journal of the American Society of Nephrology* 1995;5:2024–2031.
17. Parfrey PS, Foley RN, Harnett JD, Kent GM, Murray DC, Barre PE. Outcome and risk factors for left ventricular disorders in chronic uremia. *Nephrology, Dialysis and Transplantation* 1996;11:1277–1285.

18. Silberberg JS, Barre P, Prichard S, Sniderman AD. Impact of left ventricular hypertrophy on survival in end-stage renal disease. *Kidney International* 1989;36:286–290.

19. Foley RN, Parfrey PS, Kent GM, Harnett JD, Murray DC, Barre PE. Serial change in echocardiographic parameters and cardiac outcome in ESRD. *Journal of the American Society of Nephrology* 1998;9:249A.

20. Dahan M, Viron BM, Faraggi M, Himbert DL, Lagallicier BJ *et al.* Diagnostic accuracy and prognostic value of combined dipyridamole–exercise thallium imaging in hemodialysis patients. *Kidney International* 1998;54:255–262.

21. Achenbach S, Moshage W, Ropers D, Nossen J, Daniel W. Value of electron-beam computed tomography for the noninvasive detection of high-grade coronary artery stenoses and occlusions. *New England Journal of Medicine* 1998;339:1964–1971.

22. Callister TQ, Raggi P, Cooil B, Lippolis NJ, Russo DJ. Effect of HMG-CoA reductase inhibitors on coronary artery disease as assessed by electron-beam computed tomography. *New England Journal of Medicine* 1998;339:1972–1978.

23. MacMahon S, Rodgers A. The effects of blood pressure reduction in older patients: an overview of five randomized controlled trials in elderly hypertensives. *Clinical Experiments in Hypertension* 1998;15:967–978.

24. MRC Working Party. Medical Research Council trial of blood pressure reduction in older patients: principal results. *British Medical Journal* 1992;304:405–412.

25. Staessen JA, Fagard R, Thijs L, Arabidze GG, Birkenhager WH, Bulpitt CJ *et al.* Randomised double-blind comparison of placebo and active treatment for older patients with isolated hypertension. The Systolic Hypertension in Europe (Syst-Eur) Trial Investigators. *Lancet* 1997;350:757–764.

26. Scandanavian Simvastatin Survival (4S) Study Group. A randomized trial of cholesterol lowering in 4444 patients with coronary heart disease. *Lancet* 1994;344:1383–1389.

27. Sacks FM, Pfeffer MA, Moye LA, Rouleau JL, Rutherford JD, Cole TG *et al.* The effect of pravastatin on coronary events after myocardial infarction in patients with average cholesterol levels. Cholesterol and Recurrent Events Trial. *New England Journal of Medicine* 1996;335:101–109.

28. Prevention of cardiovascular events and death with pravastatin in patients with coronary heart disease and a broad range of initial cholesterol levels. The Long-Term Intervention with Pravastatin in Ischaemic Disease (LIPID) Study Group. *New England Journal of Medicine* 1998;339:1349–1357.

29. Ross SD, Allen IE, Connelly JE, Korenblat BM, Smith ME, Bishop D, Luo D. Clinical outcomes in statin treatment trials: a meta-analysis. *Arch Intern Med* 1999;159:1793–1802

30. ISIS-2 (Second International study of Infarct Survival) Collaborative Group. Randomized trial of intravenous streptokinase, oral aspirin, both, or neither among 17,187 cases of suspected acute myocardial infarction. *Lancet* 1988;2:349–360.

31. RISC Group. Risk of myocardial infarction and death during treatment with low-dose aspirin and intravenous heparin in men with unstable coronary artery disease. *Lancet* 1990;3:827–830.

32. Theroux P, Ouimet H, McCans J, Latour JG, Joly P, Levy G *et al.* Aspirin, heparin, or both to treat unstable angina. *New England Journal of Medicine* 1988;319:1105–1111.

33. Elwood PC, Cochrane AL, Burr ML, Sweetnam PM, Williams G, Wilsby E *et al.* A randomized controlled trial of acetylsalicylic acid in the prevention of mortality from myocardial infarction. *British Medical Journal* 1974;1:436–440.

34. Anand SS, Yusuf S. Oral anticoagulant therapy in patients with coronary artery disease: a meta-analysis. *Journal of the American Medical Association* 1999;282:2058–2067

35. Hanssen L, Zanchetti A, Carruthers SG, Dahlof B, Elmfeldt D, Julius S *et al.* Effects of intensive blood-pressure lowering and low-dose aspirin in patients with hypertension: principal results of the Hypertension Optimal Treatment (HOT) trial. HOT Study Group. *Lancet* 1998;351:1755–1762.

36. Baigent C. The need for large-scale randomized evidence. *British Journal of Clinical Pharmacology* 1997;43:349–353.

37. Kannel WB. Update on the role of cigarette smoking in coronary artery disease. *American Heart Journal* 1981;101:319–328.

38. McMillan MA, Briggs JD, Junor BJ. Outcome of renal replacement therapy in patients with diabetes mellitus. *British Medical Journal* 1990;301:540–544.

39. Cruickshank JM, Thorp JM, Zacharias FJ. Benefits and potential harm of lowering high blood pressure. *Lancet* 1987;1:581–584.

40. D'Agostino RB, Belanger AJ, Kannel WB, Cruickshank JM. Relation of low blood pressure to coronary artery disease in presence of myocardial infarction: the Framingham Study. *British Medical Journal* 1991;303:385–389.

41. Charra B, Calemard E, Ruffet M, Chazot C, Terrat JC, Vanel T *et al.* Survival as an index of adequacy of dialysis. *Kidney International* 1992;41:1286–1291.

42. Lowrie EG, Lew NL. Death risk in hemodialysis patients: the predictive value of commonly measured variables and an evaluation of death rate differences between facilities. *American Journal of Kidney Diseases* 1990;15:458–482.

43. Duranti E, Imperiali P, Sasdelli M. Is hypertension a mortality factor in dialysis? *Kidney International* 1996;55:S173–174.

44. Salem MM, Bower J. Hypertension in the hemodialysis population: any relation to one-year survival? *American Journal of Kidney Diseases* 1996;28:737–740.

45. Zager PG, Nikolic J, Brown RH, Campbell MA, Hunt WC, Peteson D *et al.* 'U' curve association of blood pressure and mortality in hemodialysis patients. Medical Directors of Dialysis, Inc. *Kidney International* 1998;54:561–569.

46. Foley RN, Parfrey PS, Harnett JD, Kent GM, Murray DC, Barre PE. Impact of hypertension on cardiomyopathy, morbidity and mortality in end-stage renal disease. *Kidney International* 1996;49:1379–1385.

47. London GM, Pannier B, Guerin AP, Marchais SJ, Safar ME, Cuche JL. Cardiac hypertrophy, aortic compliance, peripheral resistance and wave reflection in end-stage renal disease. Comparative effects of ACE-inhibition and calcium channel blockade. *Circulation* 1996;90:2786–2796.

48. Shapiro J. Atherogenesis in chronic renal failure. In: Parfrey PS, Harnett JD, editors. *Cardiac dysfunction in chronic uremia*. Boston: Kluwer Academic, 1992;187–204.

49. Toto RD, Lena Vega GL, Grundy SM. Mechanisms and treatment of dyslipidemia of renal diseases. *Current Opinion in Nephrology and Hypertension* 1993;2:784–790.

50. Parra HJ, Mezdour H, Cachera C, Dracon M, Tacquet A, Fruchart JC. Lp(a) lipoprotein in patients with chronic renal failure treated by hemodialysis. *Clinical Chemistry* 1987;33:721.

51. Murphy BG, McNamee P, Duly E, Henry W, Archbold P, Trinick T. Increased serum apolipoprotein(a) in patients with chronic renal failure treated with continuous ambulatory peritoneal dialysis. *Atherosclerosis* 1992;93:53–57.

52. Hirata K, Kikuchi S, Saku K, Jimi S, Zhang B, Naito S *et al.* Apolipoprotein(a) phenotypes and serum lipoprotein(a) levels in hemodialysis patients with/without diabetes mellitus. *Kidney International* 1993;44:1062–1070.

53. Okura Y, Saku K, Hirata K, Zhang B, Liu R, Ogahara S *et al.* Serum lipoprotein(a) levels in maintenance hemodialysis patients. *Nephron* 1993;65:46–50.

54. Auguet T, Senti M, Rubies-Prat J, Pelegri A, Pedro-Botet J, Nogues X. Serum lipoprotein(a) concentrations in patients with chronic renal failure receiving hemodialysis: influence of apolipoprotein(a) genetic polymorphism. *Nephrology, Dialysis and Transplantation* 1993;8:1099–1103.

55. Webb AT, Reaveley DA, O'Donnell M, Seed M, Brown EA. Lipoprotein(a) in patients on maintenance hemodialysis and continuous ambulatory peritoneal dialysis. *Nephrology, Dialysis and Transplantation* 1993;8:609–613.

56. Thillet J, Faucher C, Issad B, Allouche M, Chapman A, Jacobs C. Lipoprotein(a) in patients treated by continuous ambulatory peritoneal dialysis. *American Journal of Kidney Diseases* 1993;22:226–232.

57. Tschope W, Koch M, Thomas B, Ritz E. Serum lipids predict cardiac death in diabetic patients on maintenance hemodialysis. Results of a prospective study. The German Study Group Diabetes and Uremia. *Nephron* 1993;64:354–358.

58. Cressman MD, Heyka RJ, Paganini FP, O'Neil J, Skibinski CI, Hoff HF. Lipoprotein(a) is an independent risk factor for cardiovascular disease in hemodialysis patients. *Circulation* 1992;86:475–482.

59. Koch M, Kutkuhn B, Trenkwalder E, Bach D, Grabensee B, Dieplinger H *et al.* Apolipoprotein B, fibrinogen, HDL cholesterol, and apolipoprotein(a) phenotypes predict coronary artery disease in hemodialysis patients. *Journal of the American Society of Nephrology* 1997;8:1889–1898.

60. Clarke R, Daly L, Robinson K, Naughten E, Cahalane S, Fowler B *et al.* Hyperhomcysteinemia: an independent risk factor for vascular disease. *New England Journal of Medicine* 1991;324:1149–1155.

61. Wilcken DEL, Gupta VJ, Reddy SG. Accumulation of sulfur-containing amino acids including cysteine-homocysteine in patients on maintenance hemodialysis. *Clinical Science* 1980;58:427–430.

62. Chauveau P, Chadefaux B, Coude M, Aupetit J, Hannedouche T, Kamoun D *et al.* Hyperhomocysteinemia, a risk factor for atherosclerosis in chronic uremic patients. *Kidney International* 1993;(Suppl) 41:S72–S77.

63. Bachmann J, Tepel M, Raidt H, Reizler R, Graefe U, Langer K. Hyperhomocysteinemia and the risk for vascular disease in hemodialysis patients. *Journal of the American Society of Nephrology* 1995;6:121–125.

64. Robinson K, Gupta A, Dennis V, Arheart K, Chaudhary D, Green R *et al.* Hyperhomocysteinemia confers an independent increased risk of atherosclerosis in end-stage renal disease and is closely linked to plasma folate and pyridoxine concentrations. *Circulation* 1996;94:2743–2748.

65. Jungers P, Chauveau P, Bandin O, Chadefaux B, Aupetit J, Labrunie M *et al.* Hyperhomocysteinemia is associated with atherosclerotic occlusive arterial accidents in predialysis chronic renal failure patients. *Mineral and Electrolyte Metabolism* 1997;23:170–173.

66. Bostom AG, Shemin D, Verhoef P, Nadeau MR, Jacques PF, Selhub J *et al.* Elevated fasting total plasma homocysteine levels and cardiovascular disease outcome in maintenance dialysis patients. A prospective study. *Arteriosclerosis, Thrombosis, and Vascular Biology* 1997;17:2554–2558.

67. Moustapha A, Naso, Nahlawi M, Gupta A, Arheart KL, Jacobsen DW *et al.* Prospective study of hyperhomocysteinemia as an adverse risk factor in end-stage renal disease. *Circulation* 1998;97:138–141.

68. Ducloux D, Fournier V, Rebibou JM, Bresson-Vautrin C, Gibey R, Chalopin JM. Hyperhomocyst(e) inemia in renal transplant recipients with and without cyclosporin. *Clinical Nephrology* 1998;49:232–235.

69. Bostom AG, Gohh RY, Beaulieu AJ, Nadeau MR, Hume AL, Jacques PF *et al.* Treatment of hyperhomocysteinemia in renal transplant recipients. A randomized, placebo-controlled trial. *Annals of Internal Medicine* 1997;127:1089–1092.

69a. Perna AF, Ingrosso D, De Santo NG, Galletti P, Brunone M, Zappia V. Metabolic consequences of folate-induced reduction of hyperhomocysteinemia in uremia. *Journal of the American Society of Nephrology* 1997; 8:1899–1905.

70. Foley RN, Parfrey PS, Harnett JD, Kent GM, Murray DC, Barre PE. The impact of anemia on cardiomyopathy, morbidity, and mortality in end-stage renal disease. *American Journal of Kidney Diseases* 1996;28:53–61.

71. Hutting J, Kramer W, Schutterle G, Wizemann V. Analysis of left ventricular changes associated with chronic hemodialysis: a non-invasive follow-up study. *Nephron* 1988;49:284–290.

72. Huting J, Kramer W, Reitinger J, Kuln K, Wizemann V, Schutterle G. Cardiac structure and function in continuous ambulatory dialysis: influence of blood purification and hypercirculation. *American Heart Journal* 1990;119:244–352.

73. Madore F, Lowrie EG, Brugnara C, Lew NL, Lazarus JM *et al.* Anemia in hemodialysis patients: variables affecting this outcome predictor. *Journal of the American Society of Nephrology* 1997;8:1921–1929.
74. Locatelli F, Conte F, Marcelli D. The impact of haematocrit levels and erythropoietin treatment on overall and cardiovascular mortality and morbidity—the experience of the Lombardy Dialysis Registry. *Nephrology, Dialysis and Transplantation* 1999;13:1642–1644.
75. Collins A, Ma J, Ebben J. Patient survival is associated with hematocrit level. Journal of the American Society of Nephrology 1997;8:190A.
76. Valeri CR, Crowley JP, Loscalzo J. The red cell transfusion trigger: has a sin of commission now become a sin of omission? *Transfusion* 1998;38:602–610.
77. London GM, Zins B, Pannier B, Naret C, Berthelot JM, Jacquot C *et al.* Vascular changes in hemodialysis patients in response to recombinant human erythropoietin. *Kidney International* 1989;36:878–882.
78. Low I, Grutzmacher P, Bergmann M, Schoeppe W. Echocardiographic findings in patients on maintenance hemodialysis substituted with recombinant human erythropoietin. *Clinical Nephrology* 1989;31:26–30.
79. Macdougall IC, Lewis NP, Saunders MJ, Cochlin DL, Davies ME, Hutton RD *et al.* Long-term cardiorespiratory effect of amelioration of renal anaemia by erythropoietin. *Lancet* 1990;335:489–493.
80. Cannlla G, LaCanna G, Sandrini M, Gaggiotti M, Nardio G, Movilli E *et al.* Renormalization of high cardiac output and left ventricular size following long-term recombinant human erythropoietin treatment of anemia in dialyzed uremic patients. *Clinical Nephrology* 1990;34:272–278.
81. Silberberg J, Racine N, Barre PE, Sniderman AD. Regression of left ventricular hypertrophy in dialysis patients following correction of anemia with recombinant human erythropoietin. *Canadian Journal of Cardiology* 1990;6:1–4.
82. Pascual J, Teruel JL, Moya JL, Liano F, Jimenez-Mena M, Ortuno J. Regression of left ventricular hypertrophy after partial correction of anaemia with erythropoietin in patients on hemodialysis: a prospective study. *Clinical Nephrology* 1991;35:280–287.
83. Tagawa H, Nagano M, Saito H, Umezu M, Yamakado M. Echocardiographic findings in hemodialysis patients treated with recombinant human erythropoietin: proposal for a hematocrit most beneficial to hemodynamics. *Clinical Nephrology* 1991;35:35–38.
84. Goldberg N, Lundin AP, Delano B, Friedman JA, Stein RA. Changes in left ventricular size, wall thickness, and function in anemic patients treated with recombinant human erythropoietin. *American Heart Journal* 1992;124:424–427.
85. Martinez-Vea A, Bardaji A, Garcia C, Ridao C, Richart C, Oliver JA. Long-term myocardial effects of correction of anemia with recombinant human erythropoietin in aged patients on hemodialysis. *American Journal of Kidney Diseases* 1992;19:353–357.
86. Fellner SK, Lang RM, Neumann A, Korcarz C, Borow KM. Cardiovascular consequences of the correction of the anemia of renal failure with erythropoietin. *Kidney International* 1993;44:1309–1315.
87. Levin A, Singer J, Thompson CR, Ross H, Lewis M. Prevalent left ventricular hypertrophy in the predialysis population: identifying opportunities for intervention. *American Journal of Kidney Diseases* 1996;27:347–354.
88. Tucker B, Fabbian F, Giles M, Thuraisingham RC, Raine AE, Baker LR. Left ventricular hypertrophy and ambulatory blood pressure monitoring in chronic renal failure. *Nephrology, Dialysis and Transplantation* 1997;12:724–728.
89. Foley RN, Parfrey PS, Kent GM, Harnett JD, Murray DC, Barre PE. Long-term evolution of cardiomyopathy in dialysis patients. *Kidney International* 1998;54:1720–1725.
90. Besarab A, Bolton WK, Browne JK, Egrie JC, Nissenson AR, Okamoto DM *et al.* The effects of normal as compared with low hematocrit values in patients with cardiac disease who are receiving hemodialysis and epoetin. *New England Journal of Medicine* 1998;339:584–590.

91. Foley RN, Parfrey PS, Harnett JD, Kent GM, Murray DC, Barre PE. Hypocalcemia, morbidity and mortality in end-stage renal disease. *American Journal of Nephrology* 1996;16:386–393.

92. Massry SG, Smogorzweski M. Mechanisms through which parathyroid hormone mediates its deleterious effects on organ function in uremia. Seminars in Nephrology 1994;14:219–231.

93. London GM, Fabiani F, Marchais SJ, de Vernejoul MC, Guerin AP, Safar ME *et al.* Uremic cardiomyopathy: an inadequate left ventricular hypertrophy. *Kidney International* 1987;31:973–980.

94. Kawagishi T, Nishizawa Y, Konishi T, Kawasaki K, Emoto M, Shoji T *et al.* High-resolution B-mode ultrasonography in evaluation of atherosclerosis in uremia. *Kidney International* 1995;48:820–826.

95. Block GA, Hulbert-Shearon TE, Levin NW, Port FK. Association of serum phosphorus and calcium × phosphate product with mortality risk in chronic hemodialysis patients: a national study. *American Journal of Kidney Diseases* 1998;31:607–617.

96. Canada–USA (CANUSA) Peritoneal Dialysis Study Group. Adequacy of dialysis and nutrition in continuous peritoneal dialysis: association with clinical outcome. *Journal of the American Society of Nephrology* 1996;7:1998–2007.

97. Owen WF Jr, Lew NL, Yan Liu SM, Lowrie EG, Lazarus JM. The urea reduction ratio and serum albumin concentrations as predictors of mortality in patients undergoing hemodialysis. *New England Journal of Medicine* 1993;329:1001–1006.

98. Held PJ, Levin NW, Bovbjerg RR, Panly MV, Diamond LH. Mortality and duration of hemodialysis treatment. Journal of the American Medical Association 1991;265:871–875.

99. Foley RN, Parfrey PS, Harnett JD, Kent GM, Murray DC, Barre PE. Hypoalbuminemia, cardiac morbidity, and mortality in end-stage renal disease. *Journal of the American Society of Nephrology* 1996;7:728–736.

100. Mall G, Rambausek, Neumeister A, Kollmar S, Vetterlein F, Ritz E. Myocardial interstitial fibrosis in experimental uremia–implications for cardiac compliance. *Kidney International* 1988;33:804–811.

101. Amann K, Wiest G, Zimmer G, Gretz N, Ritz E, Mall G. Reduced capillary density in the myocardium of uremic rats–a stereological study. *Kidney International* 1992;42:1079–1085.

102. Penpargkul S, Scheuer J. Effect of uremia upon the performance of the rat heart. *Cardiovascular Research* 1978;6:702–708.

103. Gris J-C, Branger B, Vecina F, al Sabadini BA, Fourcade J, Schved J-F. Increased cardiovascular risk factors and features of cardiovascular activation and dysfunction in dialyzed uremic patients. Kidney International 1994;46:807–813.

104. Lowrie EG, Laird NM, Parker TF, Sargeant JA. Effect of the hemodialysis prescription on patient morbidity. Report from the National Co-operative Dialysis Study. *New England Journal of Medicine* 1981;305:1176–1181.

105. Parfrey PS, Harnett JD, Foley RN, Kent GM, Murray DC, Barre PE *et al.* Impact of renal transplantation on uremic cardiomyopathy. *Transplantation* 1995;60:908–914.

3

Ischemic heart disease in end-stage renal failure

Thomas C. Andrews, M. Elizabeth Brickner, and John D. Rutherford

Introduction

The prevalence of end-stage renal failure (ESRF) in the United States is growing at the rate of 7 to 9% per year, and by the year 2010 an estimated 350 000 patients will be afflicted.[1] Diabetes mellitus is the cause of 35% of new cases of ESRF and hypertension accounts for an additional 30% of new cases. Therefore, since ESRF is an end-stage manifestation of two conditions that increase the risk of atherosclerosis, it is not surprising that cardiovascular disease is the leading cause of death in this patient population. As coronary revascularization carries much greater mortality and morbidity in hemodialysis patients,[2,3] emphasis must be placed on prevention of atherosclerosis. In this chapter, we discuss the epidemiology, natural history, pathophysiology, and mechanisms of ischemic heart disease in ESRF with a focus on potentially modifiable risk factors.

Epidemiology and natural history

There are two hypotheses to explain the high incidence of coronary artery disease in patients with ESRF. First, dialysis therapy may accelerate atherogenesis as suggested in the original report of Lindner and colleagues in 1974.[4] Second, the development of coronary artery disease may precede the initiation of dialysis, and may be due primarily to coexistent conditions that are associated with coronary artery disease.[5] To further study this issue, investigators from Japan performed coronary angiography within 1 month of initiation of dialysis on 24 unselected ESRF patients aged 40 to 80 years. The incidence of both cigarette smoking and diabetes mellitus was greater than 60%. The mean age was 64 years and 67% were male. Almost half of the patients had a history of angina and resting electrocardiography demonstrated ischemic changes in two-thirds. Fifteen of the 24 patients (63%) demonstrated coronary disease on angiography ($\geq$75% stenosis), and of these 11 had multivessel disease. The prevalence of coronary artery disease was 73% in those with angina pectoris and 54% of patients without such symptoms. Thus, in this small series of patients with many risk factors for coronary disease, there was a high prevalence of coronary artery disease in both symptomatic and asymptomatic subjects.[6] In a prospective cohort study of 147 pre-dialysis renal failure patients, Jungers and colleagues found a three times higher rate of cardiac events compared with matched controls without renal disease. In multivariate analysis, cigarette smoking, systolic blood pressure, HDL-cholesterol, and fibrinogen were all independent risk factors for developing cardiovascular events. These data suggest that dialysis therapy is not associated with cardiac events, but rather patients who initiate dialysis suffer from coexistent coronary artery disease.[7]

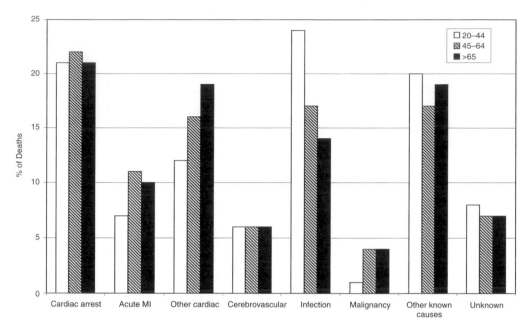

Fig. 3.1 Causes of death for all dialysis patients by age (in years), 1994–1996. (Data from reference 8.)

According to the US Renal Data Systems 1998 Annual Data Report, cardiovascular disease accounts for almost half of the overall mortality in patients with ESRF on chronic dialysis therapy (Fig. 3.1) and 18–37% of the mortality of the transplant population (Fig. 3.2). In general, cardiovascular risk is higher in diabetics, those undergoing peritoneal vs. hemodialysis, and patients of older age.[8] The influence of race and gender on life expectancy differs in patients with ESRF compared with the general US population. In the US population without ESRF, the life expectancy is greater for Whites than Blacks regardless of gender through age 85. In the population with ESRF (including transplant patients) expected lifespan is 19–47% of an age–sex–race-matched US population, and after the age of 35 years Blacks have a longer life expectancy than Whites.[8] In dialysis patients, Whites have a 29% higher risk of death than Blacks due to acute myocardial infarction, other cardiac causes, dialysis withdrawal, and infection, and males have a 22% higher risk of death than females due to acute myocardial infarction, other cardiac causes, and malignancy.[9]

Several large, prospective studies have described correlates of overall mortality in patients with ESRF. For example, Foley *et al.*[10] followed 433 Canadian ESRF patients from initiation of dialysis for a mean of 41 months. Mean age at baseline was 51 years and two-thirds were male. In contrast to the US ESRF population, glomerulonephritis was the most common etiology of renal disease (31%), followed by diabetic nephropathy (20%). All patients underwent baseline echocardiography, which was abnormal in most patients: 15% demonstrated systolic dysfunction and 32% left ventricular dilatation. Although blood pressure was reasonably well controlled (mean 151/83 mmHg) and only 29% had long-standing hypertension (defined as >10 years), 74% demonstrated left ventricular hypertrophy. Overall median survival was 50 months. Independent correlates of death included age, diabetes mellitus, cardiac failure, peripheral vascular disease, and left ventricular systolic dysfunction. In

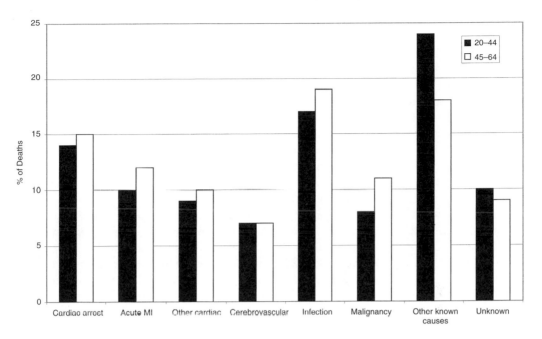

Fig. 3.2 Causes of death for all transplant patients by age (in years), 1994–1996. (Data from reference 8.)

patients with cardiac failure at baseline, coronary artery disease was associated with a worse prognosis.[10] Specific correlates of cardiovascular morbidity and mortality were determined in a prospective French study of 147 ESRF patients.[7] In multivariate analysis, cigarette smoking, systolic blood pressure, HDL-cholesterol, and fibrinogen were all independent risk factors for developing a cardiovascular or cerebrovascular event.[7] As in patients without ESRF, cardiovascular morbidity and mortality are also related to left ventricular systolic dysfunction and the extent of coronary artery disease.

Characterization of the natural history of coronary artery disease in this population is confounded by a high rate of angiographically normal coronary arteries in ESRF patients with angina pectoris. Rostand and colleagues reviewed the records of 44 ESRF patients with a clinical diagnosis of angina pectoris. Only 53% of those patients demonstrated obstructive coronary disease on angiography. In this series, all patients with obstructive coronary disease were White, and most were older males.[11] Angina in the presence of normal coronary arteries was found more commonly in females, Blacks, and those with hypertension and left ventricular hypertrophy.[12] Explanations for anginal symptoms with normal coronary arteries include subendocardial ischemia due to severe left ventricular hypertrophy, microvascular dysfunction with impaired vasodilator reserve, and/or severe limitations of oxygen delivery. Some have suggested that coronary angiography should be performed routinely in patients with uremia because of the high incidence of coronary disease in asymptomatic patients and the moderate incidence of normal coronary angiograms in dialysis patients with angina.[6]

ESRF patients who sustain a myocardial infarction demonstrate very poor long-term survival due to subsequent cardiac events. Herzog and colleagues studied the outcome of 34 189 dialysis patients hospitalized between 1977 and 1995 for a first acute myocardial infarction. More than half of the infarctions occurred in the first 2 years after initiation of dialysis. The overall mortality was 59% at 1 year, 73% at 2 years, and 90% at 5 years, with two-thirds of the deaths due to cardiac causes. Mortality was highest in older patients and in those who suffered from diabetes mellitus. Although the crude 1-, 3-, and 5-year survival after myocardial infarction showed no improvement on comparing the outcomes of myocardial infarction occurring in 1977–1984 with those occurring in 1990–1995, after adjusting for co-morbidity a recent small improvement in survival was evident. Large reductions in cardiac mortality were evident in ESRF patients who underwent renal transplantation. For example, the 2-year mortality rate from cardiac causes was 11% in transplant recipients compared with 52% in the dialysis patients. After adjusting for demographic characteristics, etiology and duration of renal failure, and co-morbidity, the relative risk of cardiac death was 4.45 (95% confidence interval 4.01–4.94) for dialysis patients compared with transplant recipients. Because of the poor long-term survival, the authors suggest a more aggressive strategy for the detection and treatment of coronary artery disease in this patient population.[13]

Patients with ESRF who undergo revascularization with coronary artery bypass surgery (CABG) or percutaneous transluminal coronary angioplasty (PTCA) also have a poor long-term prognosis. In a retrospective study, Rinehart and colleagues studied 84 chronic dialysis patients with symptomatic coronary disease. Twenty-four underwent PTCA and 60 received CABG. Mean age was 62–64 years, 71% were male and 83% Caucasian. The cause of ESRF was diabetes in 35% and hypertension in 23%. Procedural mortality was 3.3% for CABG and 5% for PTCA, and the incidence of procedure-related myocardial infarction was 7% and 5% respectively. Patients were followed for an average of 20 months in the PTCA group and 31 months in the CABG group. Despite the relatively low rate of procedural complications, the 2- and 5-year survival rates were 66% and 40% respectively for the CABG group and 51% and 14% respectively for the PTCA group (p = NS comparing PTCA and CABG). Patients undergoing PTCA were more likely to have recurrence of angina.[14] Younger patients may fare somewhat better. In a cohort of diabetic patients undergoing CABG prior to renal transplantation (mean age 45), the 2- and 4-year survival was 73% and 66% respectively with a 3% operative mortality.[15]

Thallium scintigraphy has been used to identify high and low risk subgroups of ESRF patients. Le and co-workers developed a cardiac risk assessment algorithm in 189 patients referred for renal transplant evaluation. Low risk patients less than age 50, without angina, diabetes, congestive heart failure, and with a normal electrocardiogram had only a 1% cardiac mortality at 4 years. Those with one or more of these five clinical risk factors were further stratified with thallium scanning into those without reversible defects at low risk (5% 4-year mortality) and those with reversible defects at high risk (23% 4-year mortality).[16]

Pathophysiology and mechanisms

Much of the cardiovascular morbidity and mortality associated with ESRF can be ascribed to a high prevalence of risk factors for atherosclerosis. In this population, diabetes mellitus is a particularly strong risk factor for coronary artery disease, while hypertension and hypercholesterolemia are less important. Several recently described 'new risk factors' for coronary disease are perhaps of relative greater importance (or at least more prevalent) in ESRF patients compared to the general population, including elevations in lipoprotein(a) and homocysteine, and a disordered balance of hemostasis, thrombosis, and fibrinolysis. Disordered calcium and phosphate metabolism with secondary hyperparathyroidism may be an important contributor to the accelerated atherothrombosis of ESRF. Sympathetic overactivity is common in ESRF patients and may accelerate atherosclerosis directly or worsen hypertension. Finally, the anemia associated with renal failure is an important and potentially reversible risk factor for cardiovascular disease in this population.

Diabetes mellitus

The presence of diabetes mellitus is an important marker of increased cardiovascular risk in the ESRF population. The rate of death is significantly higher in dialysis patients with diabetes mellitus compared with such patients without diabetes (202 vs. 135 deaths per 1000 patient years), and in renal transplant recipients, patients with diabetes are much more likely to die of myocardial infarction than non-diabetic patients (Fig. 3.3). It has been postulated that high levels of advanced glycation end-products (AGEs) may account for some of the cardiac morbidity of diabetes and ESRF, since very high levels of AGEs accumulate in patients with both disorders.[17] Injected into animal models, these substances induce a vasculopathy and activate mononuclear cells, and perhaps accelerate atherogenesis in humans.[18] Braun and colleagues performed coronary angiography on 100 diabetic patients with ESRF and found 25 with significant disease (greater than 70% stenosis of one major epicardial coronary artery). During follow-up, myocardial infarction occurred in 52% of patients with significant disease and 11% of those without significant stenoses.[19] Koch *et al.*[20] performed angiography on 105 diabetics under consideration for transplantation, and found significant coronary disease in 36%. There were no differences in other atherosclerosis risk factors in patients with and without coronary disease, which led the authors to suggest that all diabetics should undergo catheterization prior to renal transplantation.[20]

Intravenous dipyridamole thallium imaging can be used to determine cardiac risk in patients with diabetes under evaluation for renal transplantation. Camp and colleagues

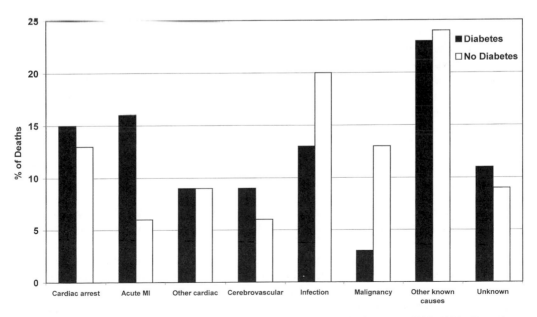

Fig. 3.3 Causes of death for transplant patients aged 20–44 by diabetic status, 1994–1996. (Data from reference 8.)

studied 40 such patients, and nine demonstrated reversible defects on thallium scanning. Six of nine subjects with reversible defects suffered cardiac events (three preoperative events and three postoperative events). There were no cardiac events in patients with normal scans ($n =$ 23) or fixed defects only ($n = 8$).[21] Manske and colleagues[15] developed a risk stratification strategy using clinical and coronary angiographic data from 141 asymptomatic Caucasian patients with ESRF and type I diabetes mellitus. In patients of at least 45 years, 88% demonstrated significant coronary artery disease. In those under 45 years, 42% had at least one 50% stenosis. Most patients with significant coronary disease in the under-45 group had at least one of three predictors: smoking, ST–T wave changes on resting EKG, or diabetes longer than 25 years.

Hypertension

The prevalence of hypertension is higher in Blacks than Whites in the United States, and, when present, hypertension is also more severe.[22] In 1987 in Jefferson County, Alabama, ESRF due to hypertension occurred at a rate of 9.6 per 100 000 in Blacks and 0.62 per 100 000 Whites.[23] Fifty percent of diabetics with ESRF also suffer from hypertension, compared with 28% of non-diabetic ESRF patients.[24] In the United States, hypertension remains undertreated in more than half of patients undergoing dialysis, defined by systolic blood pressure greater than 150 mmHg before dialysis.[1] The most common causes of hypertension in this group are fluid overload and pre-existing essential hypertension. Other less common causes of high blood pressure in ESRF patients include increased sympathetic activity, elevated plasma renin activity, hypercalcemia, elevated plasma levels of endothelin-1, and derangements of the L-arginine–nitric oxide pathway.[25] In addition to contributing to atherogenesis, hypertension has a number of deleterious effects on cardiac function, causing left ventricular hypertrophy with associated abnormalities of diastolic function, left ventricular systolic dysfunction (when chronically undertreated), reduced coronary artery vasodilator reserve, and myocardial ischemia (even in the absence of coronary stenoses).[26]

Dyslipidemia

Overt hypercholesterolemia is relatively uncommon in the ESRF population. For example, in one study the average total serum cholesterol level was 178 mg/dl, LDL-cholesterol 104 mg/dl, HDL-cholesterol 35 mg/dl, and triglycerides 187 mg/dl.[27] The most common lipid abnormality is hypertriglyceridemia due to reduced chylomicron clearance.[28] However, levels of lipoprotein(a) (Lp(a)) are markedly elevated in hemodialysis patients.[29] This cholesterol-rich lipoprotein is structurally similar to LDL-cholesterol but contains apolipoprotein(a) which shares sequence homology with plasminogen. Lp(a) has been implicated as a risk factor for myocardial infarction and stroke, perhaps by interfering with fibrinolysis as well as accelerating atherogenesis by incorporation into the atherosclerotic plaque. In a prospective cohort study of 129 dialysis patients, median Lp(a) levels were 38.4 mg/dl compared with 8 mg/dl in similar unselected, White non-dialysis patients and 16.9 mg/dl in coronary patients. Twenty-six patients suffered a cardiac event over the 48-month follow-up period. The mean Lp(a) level was significantly higher in patients with an event compared with those without an event (78.9 vs. 35.4 mg/dl), and stepwise logistic regression analysis indicated that Lp(a) was a strong predictor of cardiovascular events in the follow-up period.[27] Levels of intermediate-density lipoprotein cholesterol (IDL-cholesterol) are often elevated in patients with chronic renal failure[30,31] and correlate with non-invasive measures of aortic atherosclerosis as assessed by aortic pulse wave velocity.[32] Finally, levels of oxidized LDL-particles are elevated in ESRF patients, and this lipoprotein is highly atherogenic.[33] After renal transplantation additional patients develop dyslipidemia due to treatment with corticosteroids and cyclosporin. In a study of 500 transplantation patients treated with cyclosporin, overt dyslipidemia developed in 37%, usually within 6 months of transplantation. In this study, cardiovascular or cerebrovascular events were three times more likely in transplant patients with dyslipidemia (15 vs. 5%, $p < 0.001$).[34]

Homocysteinemia

Levels of homocysteine are elevated in dialysis patients, and a markedly high level is an independent risk factor for cardiovascular events in this population.[29,35] Treatment with high dose-B-vitamins is effective in lowering the levels of plasma homocysteine in dialysis patients[36] and in transplant recipients.[37] This topic is reviewed extensively in Chapter 9.

Hyperparathyroidism

Disordered calcium–phosphate metabolism and secondary hyperparathyroidism have been suggested as potential contributors to atherogenesis in patients with ESRF. Rostand and colleagues first studied the relationship between myocardial calcium content and left ventricular ejection fraction in uremic patients undergoing dialysis. There was a significant inverse relationship between left ventricular systolic function and both myocardial calcium content and serum parathyroid hormone levels.[38] Using electron beam computed tomography, a European group found a very high incidence of coronary artery calcification in ESRF patients. Compared with age-matched, non-ESRF patients with documented coronary artery disease, the coronary total calcium score was three to four times higher in ESRF patients in all age groups. In addition, dialysis patients aged 40 to 60 demonstrated a 25% worsening of coronary calcium score on a second measurement within 1 year of baseline testing. There was no correlation between calcium, phosphate, or parathyroid hormone values and coronary calcium scores.[39] Kawagishi and colleagues used high-resolution B-mode ultrasonography to determine the intima–media thickness of the carotid and femoral arteries in dialysis patients and age-matched controls. They found that intima–media thickness values were higher in the dialysis patients, and, using multiple regression analysis found independent correlates of intima–media thickness of the femoral artery to be age, cigarette smoking, and serum parathyroid hormone level.[40] Both hypocalcemia and hyperparathyroidism suppress hepatic triglyceride lipase and thus contribute to the high levels of intermediate density-lipoprotein and low levels of high density-lipoprotein levels of uremia. As discussed above, these lipoprotein abnormalities are associated with functional abnormalities of the vasculature[32] and the development of coronary artery disease.[31]

Abnormalities of hemostasis and fibrinolysis

Levels of several proteins important for hemostasis and fibrinolysis are abnormal in ESRF. Using a case-control design, Bostom and colleagues found 50% higher levels of fibrinogen in 71 dialysis patients compared with 71 controls.[29] Gris and co-workers studied 22 French patients on maintenance hemodialysis after excluding those with clinical cardiovascular disease, diabetes, vasculitis, or systemic lupus erythematosus. Levels of fibrinogen, factor VII, and type-1 tissue plasminogen activator inhibitor (PAI-1) were higher in ESRF patients compared with controls. When desmopressin was administered intravenously, ESRF patients had less release of tissue-type plasminogen activator (t-PA) than controls. The investigators concluded that all measured hemostatic and fibrinolytic cardiovascular risk factors were abnormal in ESRF patients, predisposing these patients to arterial thrombotic events.[41]

Sympathetic overactivity

Converse and colleagues studied sympathetic nerve discharge to skeletal muscle blood vessels in 23 dialysis patients and 11 normal controls using peroneal nerve microneurography. Sympathetic activity was similar in the five dialysis patients who had also undergone bilateral nephrectomy compared with normal controls. However, in the 18 dialysis patients who had not undergone nephrectomy, sympathetic nerve discharge was 2.5 times that of controls or dialysis patients with nephrectomy. Moreover, in dialysis patients without nephrectomy, both mean arterial pressure and calf vascular resistance was higher than in dialysis patients with nephrectomy. The authors concluded that chronic renal failure is associated with reversible sympathetic overactivity caused by an afferent signal from the failing kidneys.[42] It is possible that sympathetic overactivity may accelerate atherosclerosis directly or contribute to coronary artery disease by worsening systemic hypertension.

Anemia

In addition to hypertension, the anemia associated with renal disease increases cardiac workload and contributes to the development of left ventricular hypertrophy, which is an independent risk factor for cardiovascular death in patients with ESRF.[43,44] A recent survey demonstrated that 69% of dialysis patients had hematocrits between 27 and 33%, and 15% had values less than 27%.[45] The anemia associated with ESRF is primarily from deficient erythropoietin production. Most studies suggest that increasing hematocrit above 30% in patients with ESRF improves quality of life, reduces transfusion need, reduces left ventricular hypertrophy, improves exercise capacity, improves sleep and, perhaps, cognitive function. However, blood pressure is also increased in a minority of patients with erythropoietin therapy. Besarab and colleagues[45] conducted a large-scale randomized trial examining the effects of normalization of hematocrit values with recombinant human erythropoietin on death or myocardial infarction in patients with cardiac disease undergoing hemodialysis. The hypothesis of the study was supported by previous observations that correction of anemia reduces exercise-induced myocardial ischemia and leads to regression of left ventricular hypertrophy in ESRF patients treated with erythropoietin.[46,47] In this trial, 1233 ESRF patients with clinical evidence of coronary artery disease or congestive heart failure were randomized to receive escalating doses of erythropoietin to achieve and maintain a hematocrit value of at least 42% ('normal-hematocrit' group) or 30% ('low-hematocrit' group) for the duration of the study period. The study was halted after 29 months because of an excess number of deaths and nonfatal myocardial infarctions in the 'normal-hematocrit' group (risk ratio 1.3, 95% confidence interval 0.9–1.9). The investigators suggested that inadequate dialysis and increased treatment with iron-dextran therapy might have led to the increased mortality observed in the normal hematocrit group.

Importantly, both groups of patients demonstrated decreasing mortality rates with increasing hematocrit, and the calculated magnitude of the benefit was a 30% decrease in the risk of death or myocardial infarction per 10% increase in hematocrit for all patients. While there are no data to support normalization of the hematocrit in patients with cardiovascular disease undergoing hemodialysis, maintenance of the hematocrit around 30–35% seems to be advantageous.[45]

Usefulness of risk factors in predicting coronary artery disease

Some have suggested that the prevalence of conventional cardiovascular risk factors may not be highly useful in predicting the presence of coronary artery disease in ESRF patients. Rostand and co-workers examined the records of 320 dialysis patients at risk for developing ischemic heart disease. They found that older patients and those with chronic pyelonephritis as an etiology of renal failure were at higher risk for ischemic heart disease. On univariate analysis, blood pressure, smoking status, serum triglycerides, race, and gender did not correlate with the presence of ischemic heart disease.[48] In a more recent study, Koch and colleagues[20] studied 105 consecutive diabetic patients with coronary arteriography in the first 6 months after initiation of dialysis therapy. They found significant coronary disease in 36% of patients, and 29% of these coronary artery disease patients underwent some form of revascularization therapy. Risk factors for atherosclerosis, including hypertension, cigarette use, dyslipidemia, and levels of lipoprotein(a) and fibrinogen, were similar in patients with and without coronary artery disease. In addition, the presence of peripheral vascular disease did not correlate with the presence of angiographically significant coronary artery disease. Based on these data, the authors recommended coronary angiography for all diabetic patients in whom renal transplantation is contemplated.[20] Joki and colleagues reported similar findings in a small group of 25 patients who underwent coronary angiography within 1 month of dialysis initiation.[6] In a second study, Koch and colleagues[49] collected data from 607 hemodialysis patients (33% diabetics) to determine predictors of coronary disease defined as previous infarction by history and ECG criteria and/or significant stenosis by coronary arteriography. Seven independent predictors for coronary artery disease were identified, including level of apolipoprotein B, apo(a) phenotype, male gender, age, fibrinogen level, diabetes mellitus, and HDL-cholesterol level. Of these seven predictors, only two were associated with odds ratios of greater than 2: apo(a) phenotype (OR = 2.11, 95% CI 1.34–3.31) and sex (OR = 2.09, 95% CI 1.34–3.27). Thus, given the lack of either strong positive or negative predictors for coronary artery disease, it is difficult to predict with a high degree of certainty which patients are so afflicted without further testing.[49]

Summary and conclusions

There is a high prevalence of ischemic heart disease in patients with ESRF, primarily owing to a high prevalence of cardiovascular risk factors. Many of these risk factors are readily identifiable and treatable. Greater efforts at atherosclerosis prevention may prevent or delay the cardiovascular mortality and morbidity associated with ESRF, although clinical trials are needed to determine which therapies are most effective from a clinical and cost standpoint.

References

1. Pastan, S. and Bailey, J. (1998). Dialysis therapy. *New England Journal of Medicine*, **338**, 1428–1437.
2. Deutsch, E., Bernstein, R., Addonizio, V., and Kussmaul, W. (1989). Coronary artery bypass surgery in patients on chronic hemodialysis. *Annals of Internal Medicine*, **110**, 369–372.
3. Rostand, S., Kirk, K., Rutsky, E., and Pacifico, A. (1988). Results of coronary artery bypass grafting in end-stage renal disease. *American Journal of Kidney Diseases*, **12**, 266–270.
4. Lindner, A., Charra, B., Sherrard, D., and Scribner, B. (1974). Accelerated atherosclerosis in prolonged maintenance hemodialysis. *New England Journal of Medicine*, **290**, 697–701.
5. Nicholls, A., Catto, G., Edward, N., Engeset, J., and Macleod, M. Accelerated atherosclerosis in long-term dialysis and renal-transplant patients: fact or fiction? *Lancet*, **1**, 276–278.
6. Joki, N., Hase, H., Nakamura, R., and Yamaguchi, T. (1997). Onset of coronary artery disease prior to initiation of haemodialysis in patients with end-stage renal disease. *Nephrology Dialysis Transplantation*, **12**, 718–723.
7. Jungers, P., Massy, Z., Khoa, T., Fumeron, C., Labrunie, M., Lacour, B., *et al.* (1997). Incidence and risk factors of atherosclerotic cardiovascular accidents in predialysis chronic renal failure patients: a prospective study. *Nephrology Dialysis Transplantation*, **12**, 2597–2602.
8. Renal Data Systems. (1998). USRDS 1998 Annual Data Report. National Institute of Diabetes and Digestive and Kidney Diseases: Bethesda, MD.
9. Bloembergen, W., Port, F., Mauger, E., and Wolfe, R. (1994). Causes of death in dialysis patients. Racial and gender differences. *Journal of the American Society of Nephrology*, **5**, 1231–1242.
10. Foley, R., Parfrey, P., Harnett, J., Kent, G., Martin, C., Murray, D., *et al.* (1995). Clinical and echocardiographic disease in patients starting end-stage renal disease therapy. *Kidney International*, **47**, 186–192.
11. Rostand, S., Kirk, K., and Rutsky, E. (1984). Dialysis-associated ischemic heart disease: insights from coronary angiography. *Kidney International*, **25**, 653–659.
12. Rostand, S., Kirk, K.A., and Rutsky, E.A. (1986). The epidemiology of coronary artery disease in patients on maintenance hemodialysis: implications for management. *Contributions to Nephrology*, **52**, 34–41.
13. Herzog, C., Ma, J., and Collins, A. (1998). Poor long-term survival after acute myocardial infarction among patients on long-term dialysis. *New England Journal of Medicine*, **339**, 799–805.
14. Rinehart, A., Herzog, C., Collins, A., Flack, J., Ma, J., and Opsahl, J. (1995). A comparison of coronary angioplasty and coronary artery bypass grafting outcomes in chronic dialysis patients. *American Journal of Kidney Disease*, **25**, 281–290.
15. Manske, C., Nelluri, G., Thomas, W., and Shumway, S. (1998). Outcome of coronary artery bypass surgery in diabetic transplant candidates. *Clinical Transplantation*, **12**, 73–79.
16. Le, A., Wilson, R., Douek, K., Pulliam, L., Tolzman, D., Norman, D., *et al.* (1994). Prospective risk stratification in renal transplant candidates for cardiac death. *American Journal of Kidney Disease*, **24**, 65–71.
17. Makita, Z., Bucala, R., Rayfield, E., Friedman, E., Kaufman, A.M., Korbet, S.M., *et al.* (1994). Reactive glycosylation endproducts in diabetic uremia and treatment of renal failure. *Lancet*, **343**, 1519–1522.
18. Schmidt, A., Yan, S., Brett, J., Mora, R., Nowygrod, R., and Stern, D.S. (1993). Regulation of human mononuclear phagocyte migration by cell surface binding protein for advanced glycation end products. *Journal of Clinical Investigation*, **91**, 2155–2168.
19. Braun, W., Phillips, D., Vidt, D., Novick, A., Nakamoto, S., Popowniak, K., *et al.* (1984). Coronary artery disease in 100 diabetics with end-stage renal failure. *Transplantation Proceedings*, **16**, 603–607.
20. Koch, M., Gradaus, F., Schoebel, F.-C., Leschke, M., and Grabensee, B. (1997). Relevance of conventional cardiovascular risk factors for the prediction of coronary artery disease in diabetic patients on renal replacement therapy. *Nephrology Dialysis Transplantation*, **12**, 1187–1191.

21. Camp, A., Garvin, P., Hoff, J., Marsh, J., Byers, S., and Chaitman, B. (1990). Prognostic value of intravenous dipyridamole thallium imaging in patients with diabetes mellitus considered for renal transplantation. *American Journal of Cardiology*, **65**, 1459–1463.

22. Dustan, II., Curtis, J., Luke, R., and Rostand, S. (1987). Systemic hypertension and the kidney in black patients. *American Journal of Cardiology*, **60**, 731–77I.

23. Qualheim, R., Rostand, S., Kirk, K., Rutsky, E., and Luke, R. (1991). Changing patterns of end-stage renal disease due to hypertension. *American Journal of Kidney Disease*, **18**, 336–343.

24. Weinrauch, L., D'Elia, J.A., Gleason, R.E., Hampton, L.A., Smith-Ossman, S., DeSilva, R.A., *et al.* (1992). Usefulness of left ventricular size and function in predicting survival in chronic dialysis patients with diabetes mellitus. *American Journal of Cardiology*, **70**, 300–303.

25. Ifudu, O. (1998). Care of patients undergoing hemodialysis. *New England Journal of Medicine*, **339**, 1054–1062.

26. Rostand, S., Brunzell, J., Cannon, R., and Victor, R. (1991). Cardiovascular complications in renal failure. *Journal of the American Society of Nephrology*, **2**, 1053–1062.

27. Cressman, M., Heyka, R., Paganini, F., O'Neil, J., Skibinski, C., and Hoff, H. (1992). Lipoprotein (a) is an independent risk factor for cardiovascular disease in hemodialysis patients. *Circulation*, **86**, 475–482.

28. Appel, G. (1991). Lipid abnormalities in renal disease. *Kidney International*, **39**, 169–183.

29. Bostom, A., Shemin, D., Lapane, K., Sutherland, P., Nadeau, M., Wilson, P., *et al.* (1996). Hyperhomocysteinemia, hyperfibrinogenemia, and lipoprotein(a) excess in maintenance dialysis patients: a matched case-control study. *Atherosclerosis*, **125**, 91–101.

30. Shoji, T., Nishizawa, Y., Kawagishi, T., Tanaka, M., Kawasaki, K., Tabata, T., *et al.* (1997). Atherogenic lipoprotein changes in the absence of hyperlipidemia in patients with chronic renal failure treated by hemodialysis. *Atherosclerosis*, **131**, 229–236.

31. Nishizawa, Y., Shoji, T., Kawagishi, T., and Morii, H. (1997). Atherosclerosis in uremia: possible roles of hyperparathyroidism and intermediate density lipoprotein accumulation. *Kidney International*, **62**, S90–S92.

32. Shoji, T., Nishizawa, Y., Kawagishi, T., Kawasaki, K., Taniwaki, H., Tabata, T., *et al.* (1998). Intermediate-density lipoprotein as an independent risk factor for aortic atherosclerosis in hemodialysis patients. *Journal of the American Society of Nephrology*, **9**, 1277–1284.

33. Becker, B., Himmelfarb, J., Henrich, W., and Hakim, R. (1997). Reassessing the cardiac risk profile in chronic hemodialysis patients: a hypothesis on the role of oxidant stress and other non-traditional cardiac risk factors. *Journal of the American Society of Nephrology*, **8**, 475–486.

34. Vathsala, A., Weinberg, R.B., Schoenberg, L, Greve, L.J., Goldstein, R.A., Van Buren, C.T., *et al.* (1989). Lipid abnormalities in cyclosporin-prednisone-treated renal transplant recipients. *Transplantation*, **48**, 37–43.

35. Bostom, A., Shemin, D., Verhoef, P., Nadeau, M., Jacques, P., Selhub, J., *et al.* (1997). Elevated fasting total plasma homocysteine levels and cardiovascular disease outcomes in maintenance dialysis patients. A prospective study. *Arteriosclerosis Thrombosis and Vascular Biology*, **17**, 2554–2558.

36. Bostom, A., Shemin, D., Lapane, K., Hume, A., Yoburn, D., Nadeau, M., *et al.* (1996). High dose-B-vitamin treatment of hyperhomocysteinemia in dialysis patients. *Kidney International*, **49**, 147–152.

37. Bostom, A., Gohh, R., Beaulieu, A., Nadeau, M., Hume, A., Jacques, P., *et al.* (1997). Treatment of hyperhomocysteinemia in renal transplant recipients. A randomized, placebo-controlled trial. *Annals of Internal Medicine*, **127**, 1089–1092.

38. Rostand, S., Sanders, C., Kirk, C., Rutsky, E., and Fraser, R. (1988). Myocardial calcification and cardiac dysfunction in chronic renal failure. *American Journal of Medicine*, **85**, 651–657.

39. Braun, J., Oldendorf, M., Moshage, W., Heidler, R., Zeitler, E., and Luft, F. (1996). Electron beam computed tomography in the evaluation of cardiac calcifications in chronic dialysis patients. *American Journal of Kidney Disease*, **27**, 394–401.

40. Kawagishi, T., Nishizawa, Y., Konishi, T., Kawasaki, K., Emoto, M., Shoji, T., *et al.* (1995). High-resolution B-mode ultrasonography in evaluation of atherosclerosis in uremia. *Kidney International*, **48**, 820–826.

41. Gris, J.-C., Branger, B., Vecina, F., al Sabadani, B., Fourcade, J., and Schved, J.-F. (1994). Increased cardiovascular risk factors and features of endothelial activation and dysfunction in dialyzed uremic patients. *Kidney International*, **46**, 807–813.

42. Converse, R.J., Jacobsen, T., Toto, R., Jost, C., Cosentino, F., Fouad-Tarazi, F., *et al.* (1992). Sympathetic overactivity in patients with chronic renal failure. *New England Journal of Medicine*, **327**, 1912–1918.

43. Silberberg, J., Barre, P., Prichard, S., and Sniderman, A. (1989). Impact of left ventricular hypertrophy on survival in end-stage renal disease. *Kidney International*, **36**, 286–290.

44. Venkatesan, J. and Henrich, W. (1997). Anemia, hypertension, and myocardial dysfunction in ESRD. *Seminars in Nephrology*, **17**, 257–269.

45. Besarab, A., Bolton, W., Browne, J., Egrie, J., Nissenson, A., Okamoto, D., *et al.* (1998). The effects of normal as compared with low hematocrit values in patients with cardiac disease who are receiving hemodialysis and epoetin. *New England Journal of Medicine*, **339**, 584–590.

46. Wizemann, V., Kaufmann, J., and Kramer, W. (1992). Effect of erythropoietin on ischemia tolerance in anemic hemodialysis patients with confirmed coronary artery disease. *Nephron*, **62**, 161–165.

47. Goldberg, N., Lundin, A., Delano, B., Friedman, E., and Stein, R. (1992). Changes in left ventricular size, wall thickness, and function in anemic patients treated with recombinant human erythropoietin. *American Heart Journal*, **124**, 424–427.

48. Rostand, S., Kirk, K., and Rutsky, E. (1982). Relationship of coronary risk factors to hemodialysis-associated ischemic heart disease. *Kidney International*, **22**, 304–308.

49. Koch, M., Kutkuhn, B., Trenkwalder, E., Bach, D., Grabensee, B., Dieplinger, H., *et al.* (1997). Apolipoprotein B, fibrinogen, HDL-cholesterol, and apolipoprotein (a) phenotypes predict coronary artery disease in hemodialysis patients. *Journal of the American Society of Nephrology*, **8**, 1889–1898.

PART II
Pathophysiology and pathobiology

4

Structural basis of cardiovascular dysfunction in uremia

Kerstin Amann and Eberhard Ritz

Introduction

As early as 1827 Richard Bright drew attention to the common presence of left ventricular hypertrophy and thickening of the aortic wall in patients with end-stage renal failure.[1] He postulated that the cause 'for the unusual efforts to which the heart has been impelled' were 'that it so affects the minute and capillary circulation, as to render greater action necessary to force the blood through the distant subdivisions of the vascular system.'

Today, cardiovascular complications are a major clinical problem in uremic patients. They account for 44% of all deaths in this population.[2] Death from cardiac causes is 10–20 times more common in patients with renal failure than in matched segments of the general population.[3,4] Recently, Herzog and co-workers[5] reported that the 1-year mortality rate in survivors of myocardial infarction was 59.3% in patients with renal failure. Mortality after myocardial infarction is 16–19 times higher than in the general population.

Several structural (Table 4.1) and non-structural alterations of the heart and the vasculature (Table 4.2) are present in uremic patients, and they presumably contribute to the increased cardiovascular risk in renal failure.

Recent clinical and experimental studies[6,7,20–25] clearly demonstrate that the pathogenesis of cardiovascular abnormalities in renal failure is much more complex than initially thought. Apart from elevated blood pressure, hypervolemia, and anemia, activation of local endocrine systems such as the renin–angiotensin system (RAS) and the endothelin (ET) system plays an important role.[26–29] Furthermore, it is widely acknowledged that parathyroid hormone (PTH) is a permissive factor for the development of cardiac and vascular alterations.[30,31] Whether

Table 4.1 Structural alterations of the heart and the vasculature in renal failure[6–9]

1. Heart	Left ventricular hypertrophy
	Hypertrophy of cardiomyocytes, alterations in myocyte number
	Intermyocytic fibrosis
	Coronary heart disease
	Microvascular disease
	Arteries
	Capillaries
2. Central elastic arteries	Wall thickening due to hyperplasia of vascular smooth muscle cells
	Changes of architecture and composition
	(abnormal embedding of fibres; reduction in elastin content;
	increase in extracellular matrix content)

Table 4.2   Functional changes in the heart and the vasculature in renal failure[10-20]

1. Heart	Reduction of insulin-mediated glucose uptake
	Reduction in the activity of the insulin-dependent glucose transporter (Glut 4)
	Reduced stability of energy-rich nucleotides
	Abnormal control of intracellular calcium in cardiomyocytes
	(impaired sarcoplasmic calcium uptake, increased cytosolic calcium
	concentrations during diastole)
	Reduction of the inotropic and chronotropic response to β-adrenergic stimulation
2. Central elastic arteries	
	Increased stiffness with reduced arterial compliance

atherogenesis is really accelerated in renal failure as initially postulated by Lindner *et al.*[32] remains controversial.

In the following we shall discuss the issues of left ventricular hypertrophy, coronary heart disease, microvascular disease, cardiac fibrosis, and changes of the structure of the central elastic arteries. All these structural abnormalities must compromise cardiovascular function. More importantly, they probably also contribute to the increase in cardiovascular mortality that is seen in the uremic patient.

Left ventricular hypertrophy (LVH)

In subtotally nephrectomized rats[33,34] as well as in uremic patients[35] an increase in left ventricular mass is seen very early in the course of renal failure. Stefanski and colleagues examined normotensive patients with biopsy-proven immunoglobulin A-nephritis and normal serum creatinine concentration; they exhibited an increase in septal wall thickness and a decrease in left ventricular compliance as reflected by a low E/A ratio.[35] Parfrey and co-workers[21] found that left ventricular disease was present in 85% of patients starting dialysis treatment. Sixteen percent of patients had systolic dysfunction, 41% concentric left ventricular hypertrophy, 28% left ventricular dilatation, and only 16% had normal cardiac findings on echocardiography. These cardiac abnormalities are closely correlated to the development of heart failure and reduced patient survival. Silberberg and colleagues noted significantly lower actuarial survival in patients whose left ventricular mass was elevated.[36] In a non-blinded study Canella and co-workers reported that left ventricular hypertrophy could be reversed by antihypertensive treatment using angiotensin-converting enzyme (ACE) inhibitors.[37] This was later on confirmed in a randomized and double-blind study by London and colleagues.[38] LVH was also found to be reversed by correction of anemia with human recombinant erythropoietin (rhEPO).[39,40]

In experimental renal failure LVH is associated with an increase in cardiomyocyte diameter and cardiomyocyte volume (Table 4.3).[41] These changes lead to an increase in oxygen diffusion distance and must impede diffusion of oxygen to the center of the cardiomyocyte.

Apart from cardiomyocyte hypertrophy there may also be changes in cardiomyocyte number possibly due to increased apoptosis of cardiomyocytes during the course of renal failure. Based on recent morphologic studies it is questionable whether myocytes are indeed postmitotic cells.[42-44] We noted that a certain number of cardiomyocytes in the left ventricle of uremic rats stained positive for the proliferation marker PCNA (proliferating nuclear

Table 4.3 Changes in cardiomyocyte geometry and number in experimental renal failure

Groups	Mean myocyte cross-sectional area (μm^2)	Mean myocyte volume (μm^3)	Total number of myocytes per heart ($\times 10^6$)	Myocyte number per volume myocardium ($\times 10^6$)
Sham-operated ($n = 11$)	545 ± 110	42396 ± 10869	23.64 ± 5.81	23.22 ± 4.66
Subtotal nephrectomy ($n = 9$)	682 ± 97.9	57522 ± 17778	18.54 ± 5.49	15.78 ± 4.52
t-test	$p < 0.05$	$p < 0.05$	$p < 0.05$	$p < 0.05$

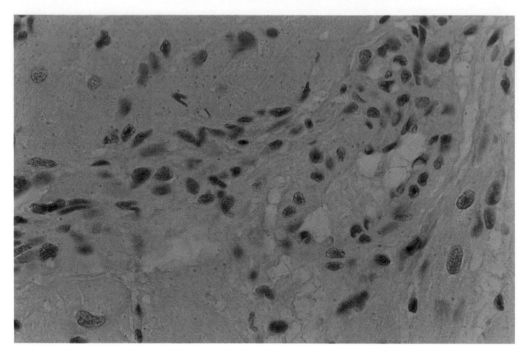

Fig. 4.1   Several PCNA (proliferating nuclear antigen) positive myocytes, interstitial cells, and vascular smooth muscle cells in the heart of a subtotally nephrectomized rat with renal failure of 8 weeks. Immunohistochemistry; original magnification ×240.

antigen) (Fig. 4.1) indicating myocyte activation and possible triggering of apoptosis.[45] Finally, a significant decrease in the number of cardiomyocytes was noted in subtotally nephrectomized rats compared to sham-operated controls (Table 4.3). In contrast, the volume density of myocytes, i.e. the fraction of myocytes per myocardial volume, was similar between both groups. Ultrastructural investigations documented hypertrophied cardiomyocytes without signs of cell damage or necrosis in the heart of subtotally nephrectomized rats.[30,33,46]

Rambausek and colleagues found differences in the relative proportion of isomyosins in the hearts of subtotally nephrectomized rats. In particular, they found an increased proportion of the fast contracting V1 fraction with high ATPase activity in contrast to what is seen in other forms of cardiac hypertrophy.[47]

Using polymerase chain reaction (PCR), *in situ* hybridization, and immunohistochemistry, increased mRNA and protein expression of endothelin 1 could be demonstrated in the heart of subtotally nephrectomized rats compared to controls.[48] Expression of endothelin 1 was also found in the heart of uremic patients using immunohistochemistry.[49] In addition, LVH was found to correlate closely with serum endothelin 1 concentrations.[50]

In experimental animals LVH could be demonstrated despite interventions to correct anemia and hypertension.[34] By contrast, LVH could be prevented by administration of ACE inhibitors, sympatholytic agents (Table 4.4), endothelin receptor blockers, and rhEPO.[8,48,51]

Table 4.4 Left ventricular hypertrophy in experimental renal failure—effect of antihypertensive treatment with angiotensin-converting enzyme (ACE) inhibitor, calcium channel blocker, and antisympatholytic agent[8]

Groups (n = 7–11 animals per group)	Left ventricular weight (g)	Left ventricular weight/ body weight ratio (mg/g)
Sham-operated controls	$1.053 \pm 0.10^{+}$	$1.89 \pm 0.16^{+}$
Untreated subtotal nephrectomy	$1.232 \pm 0.09^{*}$	$2.31 \pm 0.19^{*}$
Subtotal nephrectomy + ramipril	$0.758 \pm 0.08^{+}$	$1.79 \pm 0.13^{+}$
Subtotal nephrectomy + moxonidine	$0.895 \pm 0.04^{+}$	$2.15 \pm 0.52^{+}$
Subtotal nephrectomy + nifedipine	1.105 ± 0.19	$2.09 \pm 0.38^{*}$
Analysis of variance	$p < 0.05$	$p < 0.05$

$*p < 0.05$ vs. sham-operated controls.
$^{+}p < 0.05$ vs. untreated subtotal nephrectomy.

Coronary heart disease

Based on postmortem[52] and coronarography studies[53,54] it is well known that ischemic heart disease due to stenosis of coronary arteries is very common in patients with renal failure. Apart from sudden death, myocardial infarction is the most common cause of death in these patients. The prevalence of coronary artery stenosis varies from 24% in young non-diabetic hemodialysis patients[55,56] to 85% in elderly uremic patients (>45 years) with type I diabetes.[57]

Recent findings point to the importance of the morphology of the atherosclerotic plaque: it was shown that the plaque is not a static but rather a dynamic structure undergoing permanent remodeling. The balance between metalloproteinases and tissue inhibitors of metalloproteinases determines the stability of the fibrous cap. Plaques covered by a thick fibrous cap are stable lesions, i.e. the risk of rupture is relatively small. By contrast, lesions with a large lipid core are unstable and entail a high risk of rupture.[58–61] This concept of plaque stability may explain why only a loose correlation exists between coronary artery stenosis by angiography and cardiac events. It is of interest that in uremic patients atherosclerotic lesions are far more advanced, i.e. more calcified, than in non-renal control patients. Uremic patients also have a much higher risk of plaque rupture (Fig. 4.2) and this may be due to the high density of activated macrophages in the plaques.[7,62]

Microvascular disease

Intramyocardial arteries

Confirming previous observations of Roig and colleagues,[63] Rostand and co-workers noted that up to 50% of uremic patients with angina pectoris have patent coronary arteries on coronarography.[64–69] This finding is comparable to what was documented in hypertensive patients with so-called syndrome X;[70] such patients have microangiopathy of small intramyocardial arteries, i.e. wall thickening and reduced arteriolar lumen.[71,72]

In experimental renal failure (Table 4.5), as well as in uremic patients, wall thickening of intramyocardial arteries is also noted.[7,73] The functional consequences of increased arteriolar

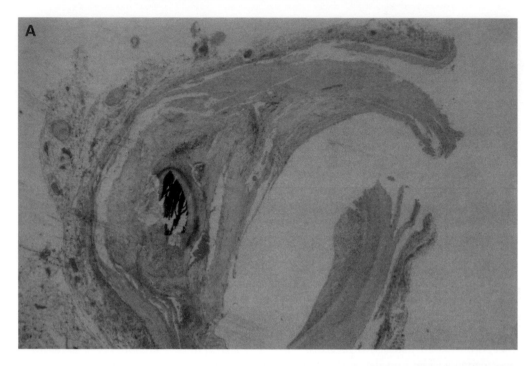

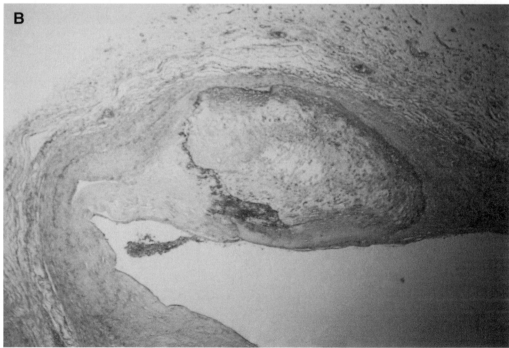

Fig. 4.2 Coronary atheroma of a uremic (A) and an age- and sex-matched non-renal control patient (B). Note severe plaque calcification in the uremic patient (A). Paraffin section; Kossa stain; original magnification ×60.

Table 4.5 Changes of intramyocardial arteries and of the aorta in experimental renal failure—effect of non-specific antihypertensive therapy[73]

Groups (n = 5–10 animals per group) (μm)	Intramyocardial arteries Wall thickness (μm)	Wall :lumen ratio (μm/μm)	Aorta Wall thickness
Untreated sham-operated controls	1.71 ± 0.27	0.055 ± 0.011	103 ± 14
Treated sham-operated controls	1.61 ± 0.13	0.052 ± 0.006	110 ± 1
Untreated subtotal nephrectomy	2.33 ± 0.35*	0.077 ± 0.011*	138 ± 29*
Treated subtotal nephrectomy	2.15 ± 0.19*	0.066 ± 0.007*	130 ± 19*
Analysis of variance	$p < 0.001$	$p < 0.001$	$p < 0.005$

*$p < 0.05$ vs. sham-operated controls.

Table 4.6 Hypertrophy of intramyocardial vascular smooth muscle cells in experimental renal failure[9]

Groups	Wall thickness (μm)	Mean nuclear volume (μm^3)	Mean cell volume (μm^3)
Sham-operated rats ($n = 10$)	4.42 ± 0.99	19.9 ± 2.2	430 ± 90
Subtotal nephrectomy ($n = 9$)	5.69 ± 1.11	26.0 ± 4.5	650 ± 230
Student's t-test	$p < 0.05$	$p < 0.01$	$p < 0.01$

wall thickness have not been defined. It may not necessarily lead to an increase in vascular resistance, but it could interfere with vasodilatation, i.e. with perfusion reserve.

Quantitative morphological studies, using unbiased stereological techniques and electron microscopy, demonstrated that the increase in wall thickness is due to an increase in intracellular actin filament content resulting in hypertrophy of arteriolar smooth muscle cells.[73,74] (Table 4.6). Immunohistochemical investigations showed increased expression of the vascular endothelial growth factor (VEGF, Fig. 4.3), the platelet-derived growth factor (PDGF-AB), collagen IV, actin, and integrin-beta 1 in the arteriolar wall of intramyocardial arteries in experimental renal failure.[45]

Experimental studies clearly demonstrated a permissive role for PTH in the genesis of wall thickening of intramyocardial arteries.[31] This observation is consistent with several clinical studies showing that PTH concentrations correlate with cardiac morbidity and cardiac death in dialysis patients.[75] Treatment with ACE inhibitors, endothelin receptor blockers, and calcium channel blockers prevented intramyocardial wall thickening after subtotal nephrectomy.[8,48,76] In contrast, non-specific antihypertensive treatment (dihydralazine and furosemide), sympatholytic agents, or correction of anemia with rhEPO did not prevent intramyocardial microarteriopathy (Table 4.4).[8,51]

Cardiac capillaries

In addition to arteriolar changes, changes in capillary density may further interfere with myocardial blood and oxygen supply.

In subtotally nephrectomized rats with moderate renal failure of short[8] and long duration,[46] cardiac capillary length density, i.e. the total length of all capillaries contained within a unit volume of myocardium, is reduced compared to controls (Fig. 4.4, Table 4.7). Such a

Table 4.7 Changes in cardiac capillarization in two models of left ventricular hypertrophy (experimental renal failure and genetic hypertension, see reference 46)

Groups ($n = 5$–8 animals per group)	Length density of intramyocardial capillaries (mm/mm^3)	Systolic blood pressure (mmHg)	Left ventricular weight (g)
Sham-operated controls	3329 ± 199	119 ± 6.61	1.10 ± 0.15
Subtotally nephrectomized rats (SNX)	2485 ± 264*	140 ± 20.3*	1.43 ± 0.32*
Spontaneously hypertensive rats (SHR-SP)	3800 ± 270	178 ± 16.2#	1.01 ± 0.22#
Normotensive controls (WKY)	3900 ± 440	128 ± 17.6	0.88 ± 0.07

*$p < 0.05$ vs. sham-operated controls.
#$p < 0.05$ vs. normotensive controls.

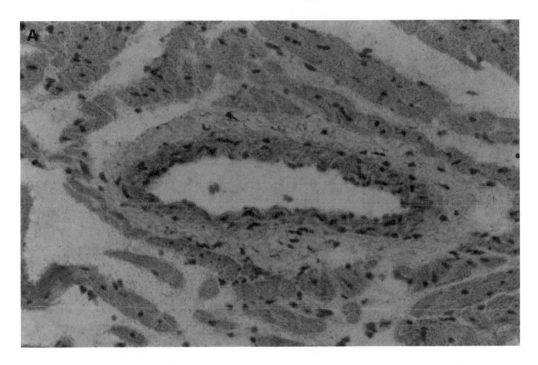

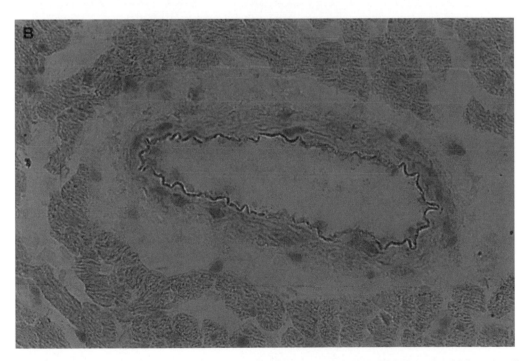

Fig. 4.3 Increased expression of the vascular endothelial growth factor (VEGF) in the thickened wall of an intramyocardial artery after subtotal nephrectomy (A) compared with no expression in a sham-operated control animal (B). Immunohistochemistry; original magnification ×150.

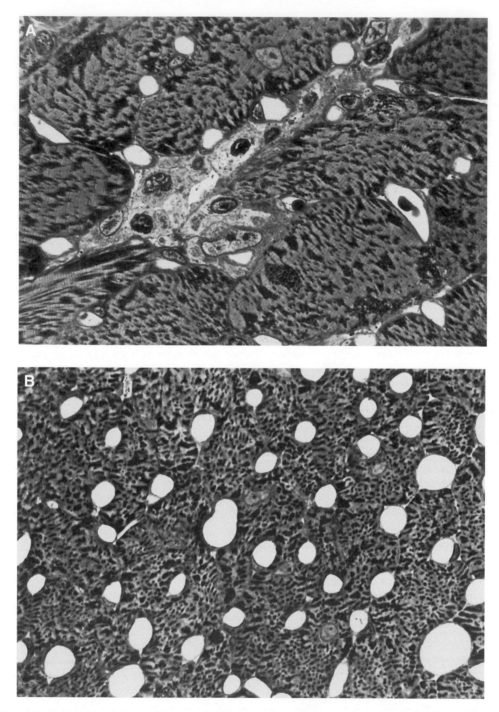

Fig. 4.4 Expansion of the cardiac interstitial tissue with activation of interstitial cells in a subtotally nephrectomized rat (A) compared with the normal myocardium in a sham-operated control rat (B). In addition, a markedly decreased number of capillary profiles per area of myocardium is seen after subtotal nephrectomy (A) compared with controls (B). Semi-thin section; original magnification ×600.

Table 4.8 Changes in cardiac capillarization, myocyte diameter, and interstitial tissue in patients with renal failure compared with patients with essential hypertension and normotensive control patients[77]

Groups (n = 9–10 per group)	Length density of myocardial capillaries (mm/mm³)	Myocyte diameter (μm)	Volume density of non-vascular interstitium (%)
Controls	2898 ± 456	13.8 ± 1.0	14.5 ± 2.2
Essential hypertension	$1872 \pm 243^*$	23.7 ± 2.2	16.7 ± 2.3
Uremia	$1483 \pm 283^{*+}$	$26.1 \pm 1.3^{*+++}$	$24.0 \pm 5.6^{*++}$
Analysis of variance	$p < 0.001$	$p < 0.001$	$p < 0.001$

$^*p < 0.001$ vs. controls.
$^+p < 0.05$ vs. essential hypertension.
$^{++}p < 0.01$ vs. essential hypertension.
$^{+++}p < 0.001$ vs. essential hypertension.

decrease in myocardial capillary supply was not noted in an experimental model of essential hypertension (SHR-SP). Capillary rarefaction is, therefore, specific for uremia and is not a non-specific consequence of hypertension or left ventricular hypertrophy. Such a decrease in capillary density leads to an increase in intercapillary distance.[8] Blood and oxygen supply of cardiomyocyte, therefore, will be diminished, making the myocardium more susceptible to ischemic injury.

Similar observations were made in uremic patients.[77] Reduced cardiac capillary length density was noted in the left ventricles of patients with renal failure compared with patients with essential hypertension and normotensive control patients (Table 4.8). This finding implies that in the hypertrophied left ventricle of uremic patients, capillary growth does not keep pace with cardiomyocyte growth, apparently because of some selective inhibition of capillary angiogenesis.[77] The finding of reduced capillary supply is specific for the heart since comparable changes could not be found in skeletal muscle, e.g. m. psoas.[78]

In experimental renal failure, the reduction in cardiac capillary supply could be prevented by the central sympatholytic agent moxonidine[8] and selective and non-selective endothelin receptor blockers.[27,48] In contrast, treatment with the calcium channel blocker nifedipine, the ACE inhibitor ramipril, and correction of anemia with rhEPO did not affect myocardial capillary density (Table 4.9a–c).[8,51]

Intermyocardiocyte fibrosis

A selective increase in intermyocytic fibrotic tissue was first described by Rössle and Pirani as early as the 1940s.[79,80] Using quantitative morphologic techniques the increase in cardiac interstitial fibrous tissue was later confirmed in short- and long-term experimental renal failure (Fig. 4.5a)[8,33] and also in uremic patients (Fig. 4.5b).[77] Ultrastructurally and morphometrically, a selective increase in cardiac interstitial cell and nuclear volume, but not in endothelial cell volume, was found with signs of cell activation (Fig. 4.5).[33] PTH was found to have a permissive effect on interstitial cell activation.[30] PTH also stimulates cardiac fibroblast proliferation *in vitro* (Fig. 4.6). Using immunohistochemistry, a significantly increased number of interstitial cells stained positive for the proliferation marker PCNA in

Table 4.9   Changes in myocardial capillaries in experimental renal failure

Groups (n = 7–11 animals per group)	Length density of myocardial capillaries (mm/mm^3)

(a) Effect of unspecific antihypertensive therapy, angiotensin-converting enzyme (ACE) inhibition, Ca-channel blockade, and sympathetic blockade[8]

Sham-operated controls	3915 ± 645[+]
Untreated subtotal nephrectomy	3036 ± 885*
Subtotal nephrectomy + ramipril	3452 ± 952
Subtotal nephrectomy + moxonidine	3729 ± 594[+]
Subtotal nephrectomy + nifedipine	3102 ± 575*
Analysis of variance	$p < 0.05$

(b) Effect of selective endothelin receptor A blocker (LU 135252) and ACE inhibitor (trandolapril)[48]

Sham-operated controls	3995 ± 471[+]
Sham-operated controls + LU 135252	3929 ± 558[+]
Untreated subtotal nephrectomy	3307 ± 535*
Subtotal nephrectomy + LU 135252	3800 ± 303[+]
Subtotal nephrectomy + trandolapril	3503 ± 533
Analysis of variance	$p < 0.05$

(c) Effect of correction of anemia by human recombinant erythropoietin (rhEPO)[51]

Sham-operated controls	4293 ± 501
Sham-operated controls + rhEPO	4124 ± 719
Sham-operated controls + rhEPO + antihypertensive treatment	4285 ± 796
Untreated subtotal nephrectomy	3237 ± 601*
Subtotal nephrectomy + rhEPO	3651 ± 576*
Subtotal nephrectomy + rhEPO + antihypertensive treatment	3620 ± 829*
Analysis of variance	$p < 0.05$

*$p < 0.05$ vs. sham-operated controls.
[+]$p < 0.05$ vs. untreated subtotal nephrectomy.

subtotally nephrectomized rats compared with controls (Fig. 4.1). In addition, increased expression of PDGF-AB, integrin-beta 1, and laminin were found in the cardiac interstitium (Fig. 4.7). Similar to what was noted with respect to the capillary changes, this increase was not seen in experimental models of genetic and renovascular hypertension or in patients with essential hypertension, respectively. Using non-radioactive *in situ* hybridization, increased cardiac renin mRNA expression was noted in the cardiac interstitium of subtotally nephrectomized rats compared with controls (Fig. 4.8).

Interstitial fibrosis presumably has important functional consequences. Interposition of collagen fibers between cardiomyocytes and capillaries may contribute to myocardial ischemia by causing displacement of capillaries, reduction of myocardial compliance, changes

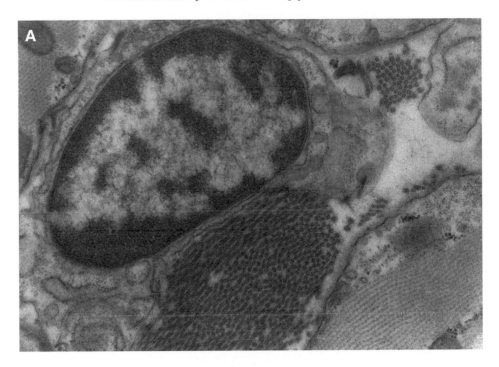

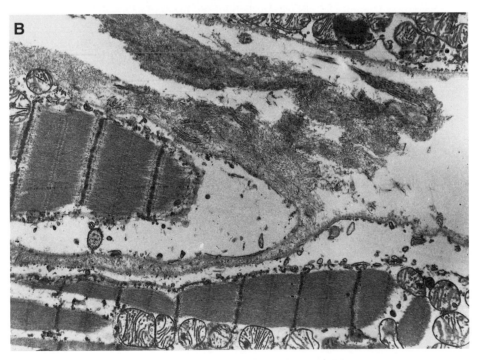

Fig. 4.5 Expansion of interstitial tissue with increased amounts of collagen fibers in the heart of a subtotally nephrectomized rat (A) and of a uremic patient (B). Electron microscopy; ultrathin section; original magnification ×10 000.

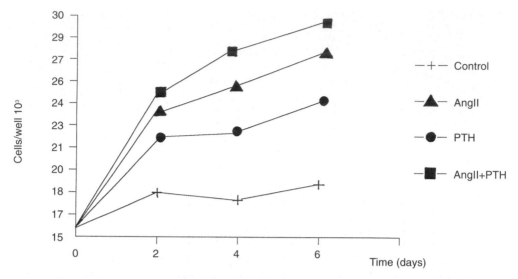

Fig. 4.6 Effects of angiotensin II (AngII) (10^{-7} M) and parathyroid hormone (PTH) (10^{-10} M) on proliferation of cardiac fibroblasts (passages 2–7). Cell number is higher in AngII- and PTH-stimulated fibroblasts compared with medium controls (0.8% fetal calf serum). Combined treatment with AngII + PTH leads to a further increase in cell number.

in the stress–strain relation and electrical instability by promoting re-entrant type of arrhythmias. The latter is thought to be due to fragmentation of the front of the action potential by interposed collagen fibers with dispersal of refractoriness. In patients with essential hypertension, cardiac fibrosis is known to be associated with an increased risk of cardiac death due to arrhythmias.[81]

Central elastic arteries

In experimental renal failure wall thickening is noted in elastic (aorta) and peripheral (mesenteric) arteries and veins. Wall thickening persists after blood pressure lowering with non-specific agents and is therefore partly independent of blood pressure.[73] It can be prevented, however, by ACE inhibitors, calcium channel blockers, sympatholytic agents, and, to some extent, also by endothelin receptor blockers.[8,76] Interpretation is somewhat difficult, however, as blood pressure was reduced to subnormal levels in these experiments.

Ultrastructural and stereological investigations demonstrated that the increase in aortic wall thickness is mainly due to vascular smooth muscle cell (VSMC) hyperplasia. Moderate hypertrophy of VSMCs and some increase in extracellular matrix further contribute to wall thickening. Elastic fiber content is decreased compared with controls and is accompanied by irregular 'embedding,' i.e. abnormal architectural arrangement of fibers in the three-dimensional space (Fig. 4.9, Table 4.10).[82,83]

In uremic patients wall thickening and reduced compliance of the carotid artery has been documented by ultrasonography and echotracers, respectively.[84] Those abnormalities were found to be closely correlated to serum endothelin levels.[50]

In addition, a decrease in aortic compliance was noted in uremic patients by London and co-workers.[24,25,85–89] This finding is comparable to what is found during aging. This observa-

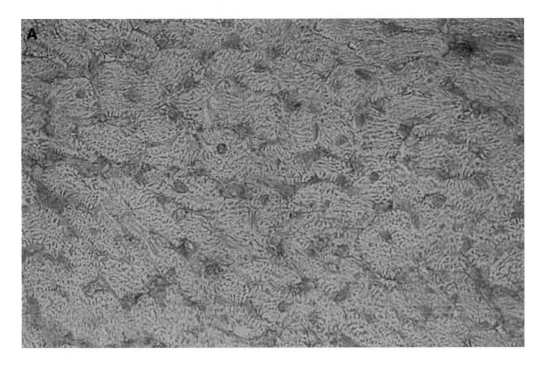

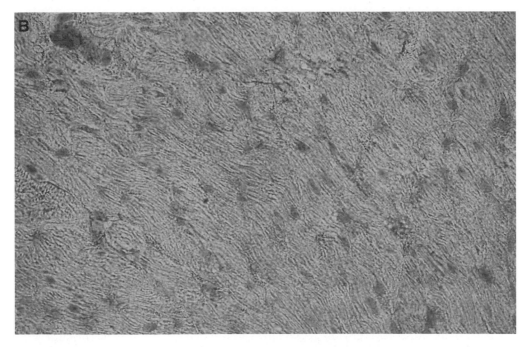

Fig. 4.7 Increased expression of platelet-derived growth factor (PDGF-AB) in the interstitium of a subtotally nephrectomized rat (A) compared with a sham-operated control rat (B). Paraffin section; immunohistochemistry; original magnification ×400.

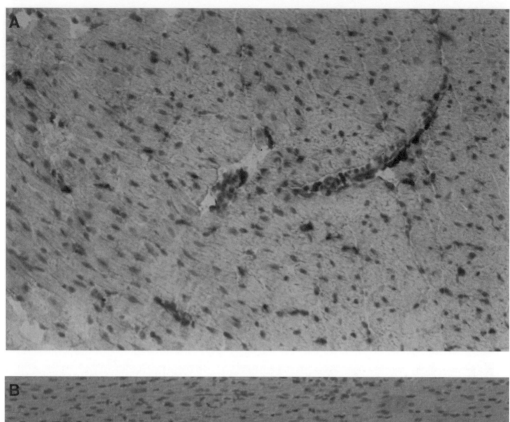

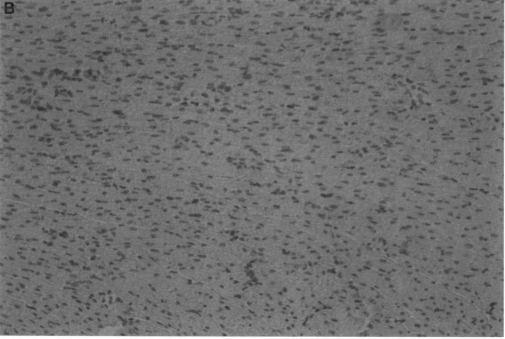

Fig. 4.8 Increased expression of cardiac renin mRNA by *in situ* hybridization in a subtotally nephrectomized rat (A) compared with a sham-operated control animal (B).

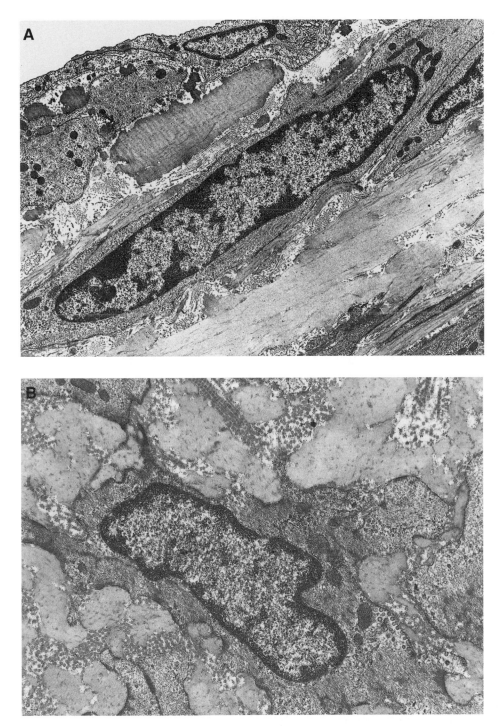

Fig. 4.9 Wall thickening of the aorta with disturbed aortic architecture (increase in cell number and extracellular matrix, reduced elastic fiber content). Comparison of subtotally nephrectomized rat (B) and sham–operated control rat (A).

Table 4.10 Formal pathogenesis of arteriolar and aortic wall thickening in experimental renal (hyperplasia *vs.* hypertrophy of vascular smooth muscle cells (VSMCs), see reference 83)

Groups (n = 8–10 animals per group)	Intramyocardial arteries		Aorta			
	Mean number of VSMCs ($\times 10^5$)	Mean volume of VSMCs (μm^3)	Mean nuclear volume (μm^3) segment	Mean number of VSMCs per 1 mm aortic	Mean volume of VSMCs (μm^3)	Mean nuclear volume (μm^3)
Sham-operated controls	10.4 ± 5.4	430 ± 90	19.9 ± 2.2	281 ± 60	85.5 ± 14.8	5.8 ± 3.0
Subtotal nephrectomy	10.7 ± 5.3	650 ± 230	26.0 ± 4.5	470 ± 110	97.7 ± 5.8	7.1 ± 2.3
Student's *t*-test	n.s.	$p < 0.01$	$p < 0.01$	$p < 0.05$	$p < 0.05$	n.s.

Table 4.11 Cardiac and aortic endothelin-1 (ET1) mRNA expression in short-term experimental renal failure—effect of angiotensin-converting enzyme (ACE) inhibitor (trandolapril) and angiotensin II (AngII) receptor blocker (losartan)

Groups	Cardiac ET1 mRNA (ratio to internal standard)	Aortic ET1 mRNA (ratio to internal standard)
Sham operated controls ($n = 8$)	2.12 ± 0.44	1.40 ± 0.36
Sham operated controls + AngII ($n = 10$)	2.86 ± 1.00	1.22 ± 0.30
Subtotal nephrectomy ($n = 10$)	2.86 ± 0.95	0.98 ± 0.11
Subtotal nephrectomy + trandolapril ($n = 9$)	2.34 ± 0.74	1.18 ± 0.33
Subtotal nephrectomy + losartan ($n = 9$)	2.71 ± 0.64	$1.21 \pm 0.37^+$
Analysis of variance	n.s.	n.s.

tion could be partly explained by an increase in aortic wall thickness, but is mainly due to alteration of the mechanical wall properties (per unit volume). Such increased stiffness has repercussions on the heart, as reduced aortic compliance leads to an increase of aortic pulse wave velocity and of the kinetic work load of the heart, thus affecting left ventricular hypertrophy and coronary perfusion.

Endothelin 1 mRNA in the heart is significantly increased after subtotal nephrectomy.[48] By contrast, it is somewhat lower in the aorta of subtotally nephrectomized rats and after angiotensin II (AngII) infusion (Table 4.11). This might explain why endothelin receptor blockers are less effective in the prevention of increased aortic wall thickness compared with ACE inhibitors.

Acknowledgments

This work was supported by the Deutsche Forschungsgemeinschaft (Am 93/2–2), the Faculty of Medicine, University of Heidelberg, and the Else-Kröner-Fresenius Stiftung. We thank Z. Antoni, H. Derks, G. Gorsberg, D. Lutz, P. Numrich, P. Rieger, S. Wessels, M. Weckbach, and H. Ziebart for technical assistance.

References

1. Bright, R. (1836) Cases and observations, illustrative of renal disease accompanied with the secretion of albuminous urine. *Guy's Hospital Reports* 1, 338–379.
2. US Renal Data System (1995) Causes of Death. *Annual Data Report* 14, pp. 79–90. Bethesda, MD. The National Institutes of Health, National Institute of Diabetes and Digestive and Kidney Disease.
3. Raine, A.E., McMahon, S., Selwood, N.H., Wing, A.J. and Brunner, F.P. (1991) Mortality from myocardial infarction in patients on renal replacement therapy in the UK. *Nephrology Dialysis and Transplantation* 6, 902 (Abstract).
4. Raine, A.E., Margreiter, R., Brunner, F.P., Ehrich, J.H., Geerlings, W., Landais, P., *et al.* (1992) Report on management in renal failure in Europe, XXII, 1991. *Nephrology Dialysis and Transplantation* 7 (Suppl. 2), 7–35.
5. Herzog, C., Ma, J.Z. and Colins, A.J. (1998) Poor long-term survival after acute myocardial infarction among patients on long-term dialysis. *New England Journal of Medicine* 339, 799–805.

6. Amann, K. and Ritz, E. (1997) Cardiac disease in chronic uremia: pathophysiology. *Advances in Renal Replacement Therapy* 4, 212–224.

7. Amann, K., Schwarz, U., Törnig, J., Stein, G. and Ritz, E. (1997) Some cardiac abnormalities in renal failure. In: Grünfeld, J.P., Bach, J.F. and Kreis, H. (eds). *Actualités néphrologiques Jean Hamburger*. Hôpital Necker 1997, pp. 1–15. Paris: Médecine-Sciences Flammarion.

8. Törnig, J., Amann, K., Ritz, E., Nichols, C., Zeier, M. and Mall, G. (1996) Arteriolar wall thickening, capillary rarefaction and interstitial fibrosis in the heart of rats with renal failure: the effect of ramipril, nifedipine and moxonidine. *Journal of the American Society of Nephrology* 7, 667–675.

9. Törnig, J., Gross, M.L., Simonaviciene, A., Mall, G., Ritz, E. and Amann, K. (1999) Hypertrophy of intramyocardial arteriolar smooth muscle cells in experimental renal failure. *Journal of the American Society of Nephrology* 10, 77–83.

10. Mann, J.F., Hausen, M., Jacobs, K.H., Kutter, A., Nagel, W., Rascher, W., *et al.* (1984) Adrenergic responsiveness in experimental uremia. *Contributions to Nephrology* 41, 108–112.

11. Mann, J.F., Jakobs, K., Riedel, J. and Ritz, E. (1986) Reduced chronotropic responsiveness of the heart in experimental uremia. *American Journal of Physiology* 250, H846–852.

12. Kreusser, W., Mann, J.F., Rambausek, M., Klooker, P., Mehls, O. and Ritz, E. (1983) Cardiac function in experimental uremia. *Kidney International* (Suppl. 15), S83–88.

13. Kuczera, M., Hilgers, K., Lisson, C., Ganten, D., Hilgenfeldt, U., Ritz, E., *et al.* (1991) Local angiotensin formation in hindlimbs of uremic hypertensive and renovascular hypertensive rats. *Journal of Hypertension* 9, 41–48.

14. Raine, A.E., Seymour, A.M., Roberts, A.F., Radda, G.K. and Ledingham, J.G. (1993) Impairment of cardiac function and energetics in experimental renal failure. *Journal of Clinical Investigation* 92, 2934–2940.

15. McMahon, A.C., Naqvi, R.U., Hurst, M.J., MacLeod, K.T. and Raine, A.E. (1995) Raised intracellular calcium in isolated single ventricular myocytes in experimental uremia. *Journal of the American Society of Nephrology* 6, 1023 (Abstract).

16. McMahon, A.C., Naqvi, R.U., Hurst, M.J. and Raine, A.E. (1995) Na/Ca exchange in isolated ventricular myocytes in experimental renal failure. *Journal of the American Society of Nephrology* 6, 1024 (Abstract).

17. Ronen, S.M., Seymour, A.-M. and Raine, A.E. (1996) Impaired phosphocreatinine (PCR) recovery after ischemia in the uraemic heart. *Nephrology Dialysis and Transplantation* 11, 1440–1441 (Abstract).

18. Matthias, S., Hönack, C., Rösen, P., Zebe, H. and Ritz, E. (1995) Glucose uptake and expression of glucose transporters in the heart of uremic rats. *Journal of the American Society of Nephrology* 6, 1023 (Abstract).

19. Gwathmey, J.K., Copelas, L., MacKinnon, R., Schoen, F.J., Feldman, M.D., Grossmann, W., *et al.* (1987) Abnormal intracellular calcium handling in myocardium from patients with end-stage heart failure. *Circulation Research* 61, 70–76.

20. London, G.M., Guerin, A.P. and Marchais, S.J. (1994) Pathophysiology of left ventricular hypertrophy in dialysis patients. *Blood Purification* 12, 277–283.

21. Parfrey, P.S., Foley, R.N., Harnett, J.D., Kent, G.M., Murray, D.C. and Barre, P.E. (1996) Outcome and risk factors for left ventricular disorders in chronic uremia. *Nephrology Dialysis and Transplantation* 11, 1277–1285.

22. Foley, R. and Parfrey, P. (1997) Cardiac disease in chronic uremia: clinical outcome and risk factors. *Advances in Renal Replacement Therapy* 4, 234–248.

23. London, G.M., Guerin, A.P., Marchais, S.J., Pannier, B., Safar, M.E., Day, M., *et al.* (1996) Cardiac and arterial interactions in end-stage renal disease. *Kidney International* 50, 600–608.

24. Lopez-Gomez, J.M., Verde, E. and Perez-Garcia, R. (1998) Blood pressure, left ventricular hypertrophy and long-term prognosis in hemodialysis patients. *Kidney International* 68 (Suppl.), S92–S98.

25. London, G.M. and Parfrey, P.S. (1997) Cardiac disease in chronic uremia: pathogenesis. *Advances in Renal Replacement Therapy* 4, 194–211.

26. Shichiri, M., Hiarata, Y., Ando, K., Emeri, T., Ghta, K., Kimoto, S., *et al.* (1990) Plasma endothelin levels in hypertension and chronic renal failure. *Hypertension* 15, 493–496.

27. Gross, M.L., Amann, K., Münter, K., Schwarz, U., Orth, S.R. and Ritz, E. (1997) Role of the endothelin system in uremic cardiomyopathy. *Journal of the American Society of Nephrology* 8, 616A–617A (Abstract).

28. Gross, M.L., Amann, K., Nabokov, A., Schwarz, U., Orth, S.R. and Ritz, E. (1997) Endothelin receptor antagonists prevent cardiovascular abnormalities in renal failure independent of blood pressure reduction. *Nieren- und Hochdruckkrankheiten* 9, 404 (Abstract).

29. Morishita, R., Gibbons, G., Ellison, K., Lee, W., Zharg, L., Yu, H., *et al.* (1994) Evidence for direct local effect of angiotensin in vascular hypertrophy. *In vivo* gene transfer of angiotensin converting enzyme. *Journal of Clinical Investigation* 94, 978–984.

30. Amann, K., Ritz E., Wiest, G., Klaus G. and Mall, G. (1994) The role of parathyroid hormone in the genesis of interstitial cell activation of cardiac fibroblasts in uremia. *Journal of the American Society of Nephrology* 4, 1814–1819.

31. Amann, K., Törnig, J., Flechtenmacher, C., Nabokov, A., Mall, G. and Ritz, E. (1995) Blood pressure independent wall thickening of intramyocardial arterioles in experimental uremia— evidence for a permissive action of PTH. *Nephrology Dialysis and Transplantation* 10, 2043–2048.

32. Lindner, A., Charra, B., Sherrard, D.J. and Scribner, B.H. (1974) Accelerated atherosclerosis in prolonged maintenance hemodialysis. *New England Journal of Medicine* 290, 697–701.

33. Mall, G., Rambausek, M., Neumeister, A., Kollmar, S., Vetterlein, F. and Ritz, E. (1988) Myocardial interstitial fibrosis in experimental uremia—implications for cardiac compliance. *Kidney International* 33, 804–811.

34. Rambausek, M., Ritz, E., Mall, G., Mehls, O. and Katus, H.A. (1985) Myocardial hypertrophy in rats with renal insufficiency. *Kidney International* 28, 775–782.

35. Stefanski, A., Schmidt, K.G., Waldherr, R. and Ritz, E. (1996) Early increase in blood pressure and diastolic left ventricular malfunction in patients with glomerulonephritis. *Kidney International* 50, 1321–1326.

36. Silberberg, J.S., Barre, P., Prichard, S.S. and Sniderman, A.D. (1989) Impact of left ventricular hypertrophy on survival in end-stage renal disease. *Kidney International* 36, 286–290.

37. Cannella G., Paoletti E., Delfino R., Peloso G., Rolla D. and Molinari S. (1997) Prolonged therapy with ACE inhibitors induces a regression of left ventricular hypertrophy of dialyzed uremic patients independently from hypotensive effects. *American Journal of Kidney Disease* 30; 659–664.

38. London, G.M., Pannier, B., Guerin, A.P., Marchias, S.J., Safar, M.E. and Cuche J.L. (1994) Cardiac hypertrophy, aortic compliance, peripheral resistance, and wave reflection in end-stage renal disease. Comparative effects of ACE inhibition and calcium channel blockade. *Circulation* 90, 2786–2796.

39. Silberberg, J.S., Racine, N., Barre, P. and Sniderman, A.D. (1990) Regression of left ventricular hypertrophy in dialysis patients following corrections of anemia with recombinant human erythropoietin. *Canadian Journal of Cardiology* 6, 1–4.

40. Cannella, G., La Canna, G., Sandrini, M., Gaggiotti, M., Nordio, G., Movilli, E. *et al.* (1991) Reversal of left ventricular hypertrophy following recombinant human erythropoietin treatment of anaemic dialysed uraemic patients. *Nephrology Dialysis and Transplantation* 6, 31–37.

41. Schwarz, U., Amann, K., Orth, S.R., Mall, G. and Ritz, E. (1997) Effect of ramipril on interstitial cardiac changes, myocyte hypertrophy and loss of myocytes in renal failure. *Hypertension* 30, 984a (Abstract).

42. Anversa, P. and Kajstura, J. (1998) Ventricular myocytes are not terminally differentiated in the adult mammalian heart. *Circulation Research* 83, 1–14.

43. Kajstura, J., Leri, A., Finato, N., DiLoreto, C., Beltrami, C.A. and Anversa, P. (1998) Myocyte proliferation in end-stage cardiac failure in humans. *Proceedings of the National Academy of Sciences of the United States of America* 95, 8801–8805.
44. Anversa, P., Leri, Beltrami, C.A., Guerra, S. and Kajstura, J. (1998) Myocyte death and growth in the failing heart. *Laboratory Investigation* 78, 767–786.
45. Amann, K., Kronenberg, G., Gehlen, F., Wessels, S., Orth, S.R., Münter, K., *et al.* (1998) Cardiac remodelling in experimental renal failure—an immunohistochemical study. *Nephrology Dialysis and Transplantation* 13, 1958–1966.
46. Amann, K., Wiest, G., Zimmer, G., Gretz, N., Ritz, E. and Mall, G. (1992) Reduced capillary density in the myocardium of uremic rats—a stereological study. *Kidney International* 42, 1079–1085.
47. Rambausek, M., Kollmar, S., Klug, D., Mehls, O. and Ritz, E. (1991) Regulation of myocardial isomyosin V1 in uraemic rats. *European Journal of Clinical Investigation* 21, 64–71.
48. Amann, K., Münter, K., Wagner, J., Balajew, V., Hergenröder, S., Mall, G. and Ritz, E. (1998) Beneficial effect of a selective endothelin receptor antagonist (ETA-RA) on reduced capillarisation in uremic left ventricular hypertrophy. *Journal of the American Society of Nephrology* 9, 602A (Abstract).
49. Amann, K., Rychlik, I., Miltenberger-Miltenyi, G. and Ritz, E. (1998) Left ventricular hypertrophy in renal failure. *Kidney International* 54 (Suppl. 68), S78–S85.
50. Demuth, K., Blacher, J., Guerin, A., Benoit, M.O., Moatti, N., Safar, M.E., *et al.* (1998) Endothelin and cardiovascular remodeling in end-stage renal disease. *Nephrology Dialysis and Transplantation* 13, 375–383.
51. Gross, M.L., Schneider, R., Schwarz, U., Törnig, J., Ritz, E. and Amann, K. (1998) Effect of chronic rhEPO treatment on cardiovascular changes in experimental renal failure. *Nephrology Dialysis and Transplantation* 13, 116 (Abstract).
52. Clyne, N., Lins, L.E. and Pehrsson, K.S. (1986) Occurrence and significance of heart disease in uremia. *Scandinavian Journal of Urology and Nephrology* 20, 307–311.
53. Hässler, R., Höfling, B., Castro, L., Gurland, H.J., Hillebrand, G., Land, W., *et al.* (1987) Koronare Herzkrankheit und Herzklappenerkrankungen bei Patienten mit terminaler Niereninsuffizienz. *Deutsche Medizinische Wochenschrift* 18, 714–718.
54. Ikram, H., Lynn, K.L., Bailey, R.R. and Little, P.J. (1983) Cardiovascular changes in chronic hemodialysis patients. *Kidney International* 24, 371–376.
55. Kramer, W., Wizemann, V., Lammlein, G., Thormann, J., Kindler, M., Mueller, K., *et al.* (1986) Cardiac dysfunction in patients on maintenance hemodialysis. II. Systolic and diastolic properties of the left ventricle assessed by invasive methods. *Contributions to Nephrology* 52, 110–124.
56. Kramer, W., Wizemann, V., Thormann, J., Kindler, M., Mueller, K. and Schlepper, M. (1986) Cardiac dysfunction in patients on maintenance hemodialysis. I. The importance of associated heart diseases in determining alterations of cardiac performance. *Contributions to Nephrology* 52, 97–109.
57. Manske, C.L., Thomas, W., Wang, Y. and Wilson, R.F. (1993) Screening diabetic transplant candidates for coronary artery disease: identification of a low risk subgroup. *Kidney International* 44, 617–621.
58. Bennett, M., Evan, G. and Schwartz, G. (1995) Apoptosis of human vascular smooth muscle cells derived from normal vessels and coronary atherosclerotic plaques. *Journal of Clinical Investigation* 95, 2266–2274.
59. Fuster, V., Badimon, L., Bachmon, J.J. and Chesebro, J.H. (1992) The pathogenesis of coronary artery disease and the acute coronary syndromes. *New England Journal of Medicine* 326, 310–318.
60. Fuster, V. and Badimon, J.J. (1995) Regression or stabilization of atherosclerosis means regression or stabilization of what we don't see in the arteriogram. *European Heart Journal* 16 (Suppl. E), 6–12.
61. Fuster, V. (1994) Lewis A. Conner Memorial Lecture. Mechanism leading to myocardial infarction. Insights from studies of vascular biology. *Circulation* 90, 2126–2146.

62. Flechtenmacher, C., Amann, K., Schwarz, U., Wiest, G., Stein, G., Raabe, G., *et al.* (1998) Morphology of coronary artery sclerosis in chronic renal failure. *Pathology Research and Practice* 194, 66 (Abstract).

63. Roig, E., Betriu, A., Castaner, A., Margrina, J., Sanz, G. and Navarro-Lopez, F. (1981) Disabling angina pectoris with normal coronary arteries in patients undergoing long-term hemodialysis. *American Journal of Medicine* 71, 437–444.

64. Rutsky, E. and Rostand, S.G. (1992) The management of coronary artery disease in patients with end-stage renal disease. In: Parfrey, P.S. and Harnett, J.D. (eds). *Cardiac dysfunction in chronic uremia*, pp. 231–246. Kluwer Academic.

65. Rostand, S.G. and Rutsky, E.A. (1989) Ischemic heart disease in chronic renal failure: management considerations. *Seminars in Dialysis* 2, 98–101.

66. Rostand, S.G., Kirk, K.A. and Rutsky, E.A. (1986) The epidemiology of coronary artery disease in patients on maintenance hemodialysis: implications for management. *Contributions to Nephrology* 52, 34–41.

67. Rostand, S.G., Gretes, J.C., Kirk, K.A., Rutsky, E.A. and Andreoli, T. (1979) Ischemic heart disease in patients with uremia undergoing maintenance hemodialysis. *Kidney International* 16, 600–611.

68. Rostand, S.G., Brunzell, J.D., Cannon, R.O. and Victor, R.G. (1991) Cardiovascular complications in renal failure [editorial]. *Journal of the American Society of Nephrology* 2, 1053–1062.

69. Rostand, S.G., Kirk, K.A. and Rutsky, E.A. (1984) Dialysis-associated ischemic heart disease: insights from coronary angiography. *Kidney International* 25, 653–659.

70. Opherk, D., Zebe, H., Weihe, E., Mall, G., Dürr, C., Gravert, B., *et al.* (1981) Reduced coronary dilatory capacity and ultrastructural changes of the myocardium in patients with angina pectoris but normal coronary arteriograms. *Circulation* 63, 817–825.

71. Schwartzkopff, B., Motz, W., Frenzel, H., Vogt, M., Knauer, S. and Strauer, B.E. (1993) Structural and functional alterations of the intramyocardial coronary arterioles in patients with arterial hypertension. *Circulation* 88, 993–1003.

72. Schwartzkopff, B., Motz, W., Vogt, M. and Strauer, B. (1993) Heart failure on the basis of hypertension. *Circulation* 87 (Suppl. 5), 66–72.

73. Amann, K., Neusüss, R., Ritz, E., Irzyniec, T., Wiest, G. and Mall, G. (1995) Changes of vascular architecture independent of blood pressure in experimental uremia. *American Journal of Hypertension* 8, 409–417.

74. Amann, K., Törnig, J., Nichols, C., Kronenberg, G., Zeier, M., Mall, G. and Ritz, E. (1996) Hypertrophy or hyperplasia? Wall thickening of intramyocardial arteries in experimental renal failure. *Nephrology Dialysis and Transplantation* 11, A128 (Abstract).

75. Block, G., Hulbert-Shearon, T., Levin, N.W. and Port, F.K. (1998) Association of serum phosphorus and calcium × phosphate product with mortality risk in chronic hemodialysis patients: a national study. *American Journal of Kidney Diseases* 31, 607–617.

76. Nabokov, A., Amann, K., Wessels, S., Münter, K., Wagner, J. and Ritz, E. (1999) Endothelin receptor antagonists influence cardiovascular morphology in uremic rats. *Kidney International* 55, 512–519.

77. Amann, K., Breitbach, M., Ritz, E. and Mall, G. (1998) Myocyte/capillary mismatch in the heart of uremic patients. *Journal of the American Society of Nephrology* 9, 1018–1022.

78. Amann, K., Neimeier, K.A., Schwarz, U., Törnig, J., Matthias, S., Orth, S.R. *et al.* (1997) Rats with moderate renal failure show capillary deficit in the heart but not in skeletal muscle. *American Journal of Kidney Disease* 30, 382–388.

79. Langendorf, R. and Pirani, C.L. (1947) The heart in uremia. *American Heart Journal* 33, 282–307.

80. Rössle, H. (1943) Über die serösen Entzündungen der Organe. *Virchows Archiv* 311, 252–284.

81. Wu, T.J., Ong, J.J., Hwang, C., Lee, J.J., Fishbein, M.C., Czer, L., *et al.* (1998) Characteristics of wave fronts during ventricular fibrillation in human hearts with dilated cardiomyopathy: role of increased fibrosis in the generation of reentry. *Journal of the American College of Cardiology* 32, 187–196.

82. Amann, K. and Ritz, E. (1998) Cardiovascular abnormalities in ageing and in uraemia—only analogy or shared pathomechanisms? *Nephrology Dialysis and Transplantation* 13 (Suppl. 7), 6–11.

83. Amann, K., Wolf, B., Nichols, C., Törnig, J., Schwarz, U., Zeier, M. *et al.* (1997) Aortic changes in experimental renal failure—hyperplasia or hypertrophy of smooth muscle cells? *Hypertension* 29, 770–775.

84. Barenbrock, M., Spieker, C., Laske, V., Heidenreich, S., Hohage, H., Bachmann, H.H., *et al.* (1994) Studies of the vessel wall properties in hemodialysis patients. *Kidney International* 45, 1397–1400.

85. Safar, M. and London, G. (1997) Arterial stiffness in hypertensive subjects with or without end-stage renal disease. *Kidney Blood Pressure Research* 20, 82–89.

86. London, G.M., Guerin, A.P., Pannier, B., Marchais, S., Benetos, A. and Safar, M.E. (1992) Increased systolic pressure in chronic uremia. Role of arterial wave reflection. *Hypertension* 20, 10–19.

87. London, G.M. (1994) Increased arterial stiffness in end-stage renal failure: why is it of interest to the clinical nephrologist? *Nephrology Dialysis and Transplantation* 9, 1709–1712.

88. London, G.M., Marchais, S.J., Safar, M.E., Genest, A.F., Guerin, A.P., Metivier, F., *et al.* (1990) Aortic and large artery compliance in end-stage renal failure. *Kidney International* 37, 137–142.

89. London, G.M., Zins, B., Pannier, B., Naret, C., Berthelot, J.M., Jacquot, C., *et al.* (1989) Vascular changes in hemodialysis patients in response to recombinant human erythropoietin. *Kidney International* 36, 878–882.

5

Arterial structure and function in end-stage renal failure

Gérard M. London, Sylvain J. Marchais, Alain P. Guérin, and Fabien Métivier

Introduction

Cardiovascular disease is a major cause of morbidity and mortality in patients with end-stage renal failure (ESRF).[1,2] Epidemiological and clinical studies have shown that damage of large conduit arteries is a major contributing factor. Macrovascular disease develops rapidly in ESRF patients and is responsible for the high incidence of congestive heart failure, left ventricular hypertrophy (LVH), ischemic heart disease, sudden death, cerebrovascular accidents, and peripheral artery diseases. Although the most frequent underlying cause of these complications is occlusive lesions due to atheromatous plaques, many vascular complications arise in ESRF patients in the absence of clinically significant atherosclerotic disease.[3,4] Atherosclerosis, a disease characterized by the presence of plaques, represents only one form of structural response to metabolic and hemodynamic alterations which interfere with the 'natural' process of aging.[5–8] The spectrum of arterial alterations in ESRF is broader, including large artery remodeling accompanying the growing hemodynamic burden.[9,10] The consequences of these alterations are different from those attributed to the presence of atherosclerotic plaques. In this chapter, the basic concepts of arterial remodeling and function, and their alterations in patients with ESRF, are reviewed.

Arterial remodeling and arterial function: basic concepts

Arterial remodeling

An arterial wall is a complex tissue composed of different cell populations capable of structural and functional changes in response to direct injury and atherogenic factors or to changes in long-term hemodynamic conditions.[11] The principal geometric modifications induced by hemodynamic alterations are changes in arterial lumen width and/or arterial wall thickness due to activation, proliferation, and migration of smooth muscle cells, and rearrangements of cellular elements and extracellular matrix of the vessel wall.[11–14]

The mechanical signals for arterial remodeling associated with hemodynamic overload are the cyclic tensile stress and/or shear stress.[15–18] Blood pressure is the principal determinant of arterial wall stretch and tensile stress, creating radial and tangential forces that counteract the effect of intraluminal pressure. Blood-flow alterations result in changes in shear stress— the dragging frictional force created by blood flow.[19,20] While acute changes in tensile or shear stress induce transient adjustments in vasomotor tone and in arterial diameter,[21–23] chronic alterations of mechanical forces lead to changes in the geometry and composition of the vessel walls that may be considered adaptive responses to long-lasting changes in blood flow and/or pressure.[13,14,24,25]

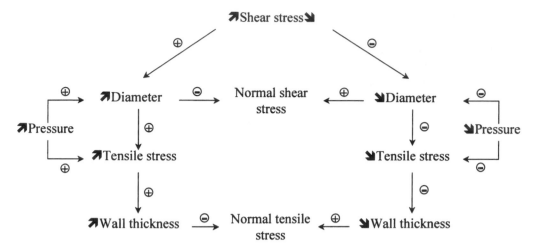

Fig. 5.1 Schematic representation of interactions between shear and tensile stresses.

According to Laplace's law, tensile stress (σ) is directly proportional to arterial transmural pressure (P) and radius (r), and inversely proportional to arterial wall thickness (h) according to the formula $\sigma = Pr/h$. In response to increased blood pressure or arterial radius, tensile stress is maintained within the physiological range by thickening of the vessel wall.

Shear stress is a function of the blood-flow pattern. In 'linear' segments of the vasculature, blood is displaced in layers moving at different velocities. The middle of the stream moves more rapidly than the side layers, generating a parabolic velocity profile. The slope of the velocity profile, i.e. the change in blood velocity per unit distance across the vessel radius, defines the shear rate. Shear stress is the product of shear rate times blood viscosity. Thus, shear stress (τ) is directly proportional to blood flow (Q) and blood viscosity (η) and inversely proportional to the radius (r) of the vessel, according to the formula $\tau = Q\eta/\pi r^3$. Increased shear stress could be the consequence of increased blood viscosity, decreased arterial diameter, or increased blood flow and blood-flow gradient applied to the vessel–blood interface. Changes of shear and tensile stresses are interrelated because any modification of arterial radius caused by alterations in blood flow and shear stress induces changes in tensile stress (unless the pressure varies in the opposite direction) (Fig. 5.1).

The processes of transmission of mechanical forces from flowing blood to the vascular wall cells and force transduction within the cells are incompletely understood. Detailed descriptions of the mechanisms of mechanotransduction and the biology of the remodeling are beyond the scope of this chapter and are available elsewhere.[17,18,26] The process of transforming mechanical forces into remodeling of the vascular system implies that there are 'sensors' that detect and transmit physical forces to effector cells. Endothelial cells are strategically situated at the blood–vessel wall interface and are the principal candidates for the role of 'sensors'.[22,26] While endothelial cells are principally involved in sensing and transducing shear stress, the experimental data have shown that endothelial mitogenesis might also be modulated by specific levels of cyclic mechanical tensile load.[27] The candidate mechanosensors are integrin–matrix–cytoskeleton interaction,[28] mechanosensitive K^+-ion channels,[29,30] G proteins,[31,32] and caveolae.[33] This mechanosensor activation results in the transduction of physical stimuli into a biochemical signal affecting arterial function through the generation of nitric oxide,[34] prostacyclin,[35] endothelium-derived hyperpolarizing factor,[30,36] endothelins,[37] adhesion molecule expression,[38,39] and activation of thrombotic and antithrombotic factors.[40–42] Endothelial cells also participate in remodeling by releasing and/or activating growth factors, such as platelet-derived growth factor,[43] fibroblast growth factor,[44] transforming growth factor-β,[45,46] and extracellular matrix regulators,[47] influencing the growth, migration,[48] phenotype, and apoptosis of vascular smooth muscle cells.[49] While shear stress acts mainly on endothelial cells, changes in tensile stress are sensed by the entire vessel wall and vascular smooth muscle cells respond directly to changes in cyclic stretch which induces vascular smooth muscle cell proliferative response, and seems essential for the maintenance of the contractile phenotype.[50] Detailed description of the mechanical influences on vascular smooth muscle function can be found elsewhere.[51]

The characteristics of arterial remodeling depend largely on the nature of hemodynamic stimuli applied to the vessel and on the presence of an intact endothelium (Fig. 5.2).[52,53] To maintain tensile stress within physiological limits, arteries respond by thickening their walls (Laplace's law). The increased tensile stress is due to the direct effect of high pressure and the pressure-dependent passive distension of the arterial lumen.[54] Studies in animals and humans have shown that this pressure-related distension of the arterial diameter is limited to central (elastic-type) arteries, being absent from peripheral (muscular-type) arteries, and

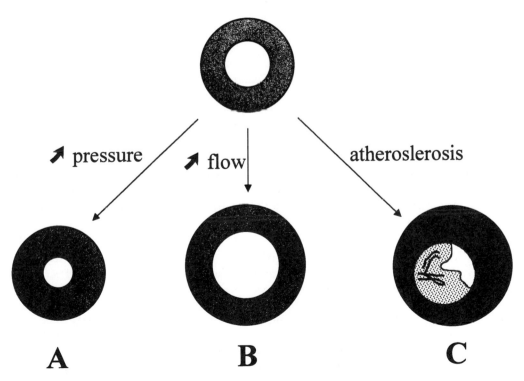

↗ pressure ↗ flow atheroslerosis

A **B** **C**

Fig. 5.2 Schematic representation of different types of arterial remodeling. (A) Arterial remodeling caused by increased tensile stress, with arterial wall hypertrophy and/or reduced diameter. (B) Increased vessel dimensions associated with chronic increase of blood flow. (C) Remodeling due to atherosclerosis or direct injury.

causes an increase of the wall-to-lumen ratio which is proportional to the pressure.[13,14,55] The limitation or absence of a pressure-dependent diameter increase efficiently maintains tensile stress within normal limits. The nature of the mechanism(s) preventing the passive 'dilatory' effect of pressure is unknown but requires the presence of an intact endothelium.[56,57]

Experimental and clinical data indicate that acute and chronic augmentations of arterial blood flow induce proportional increases in the vessel lumen, whereas decreasing flow reduces arterial inner diameter.[12,58,59] An example of flow-mediated remodeling associates arterial dilation and sustained high blood flow after the creation of an arteriovenous fistula.[25] In this situation, the lumen diameter increases to maintain shear stress within physiological limits. Increased arterial inner diameter is usually accompanied by arterial wall hypertrophy and increased intima–media cross-sectional area (following increases in the radius and wall tension). The presence of the endothelium is a prerequisite for normal vascular adaptation to chronic changes in blood flow, and experimental data indicate that flow-mediated arterial remodeling can be decreased by inhibiting nitric oxide synthase.[53,60] Although the alterations of tensile and shear stresses are interrelated, changes of tensile stress primarily induce alterations and hypertrophy of the arterial media, whereas changes of shear stress principally modify the dimensions and structure of the intima.[16,47,61]

Arterial structure is also altered in response to direct injury and atherogenic factors.[62,63] Atherosclerosis characterized by the presence of plaques is primarily an intimal disease, focal and patchy in its distribution, occurring preferentially in medium-sized conduit arteries, such as epicardial coronary arteries, femoral and iliac arteries, infrarenal aorta, carotid bulb and cerebral arteries, and usually sparing muscular type arteries in the arms, internal mammary and other arteries.[64] Mechanisms of atherogenesis are complex and include smoking, lipid disturbances, thrombogenesis, production of vasoactive substances, growth factors, and mediators of inflammation (see Chapters 8–11). Tensile stress and shear stress also influence the natural history of atherosclerotic lesions.[61,65] Evidence that enhanced tensile stress is relevant to the pathogenesis of atherosclerosis comes from the following observations: atherosclerotic plaques are virtually confined to systemic arteries where tensile stress is high, and are absent from the venous system;[66] atherosclerosis develops in autogenous venous bypass grafts, but can be prevented by applying a rigid external support to counteract the increased transmural pressure in the graft;[67] in aortic coarctation, atherosclerosis is accelerated in arteries cephalad to the coarctation,[68] while it is decreased in arteries caudal to the coarctation;[66] the frequency of atheromatous plaques is higher in patients with arterial hypertension.[54] The role of shear stress is demonstrated by the predilection of atherosclerosis for certain sites, such as ostia, branching points, bifurcations, bending, or pronounced arterial tapering.[65,69–71] These sites are characterized by flow-pattern and shear-stress disturbances; for example, low average shear stress or secondary and turbulent flows with variable shear stress over the cardiac cycle.[69,70] Although it was initially thought that atherogenesis was the consequence of injury evoked by high shear stress,[72] it was later demonstrated that atherosclerosis is uncommon in sites with high shear stress, such as at flow dividers on the inner aspects of arteries downstream from flow dividers or on the outer aspect of an arterial bend.[71,73] In these locations, the endothelial cells are aligned in the direction of flow, thereby decreasing the effective resistance to friction and 'autoregulating' shear stress.[74] The increase of shear stress promotes the secretion and synthesis of nitric oxide (NO),[23] prostacyclin,[35] and antithrombotic and antigrowth factors that mediate atheroprotection,[26] and survival of endothelial cells, which then become more adherent to the intima and less permeable to the entry of lipoproteins and monocytes.[75] At sites of low shear stress or turbulent flows (characterized by flow reversal and time-averaged shear stress approaching zero), endothelial cells secrete prothrombotic and progrowth factors, and trigger endothelial apoptosis.[49] Moreover, blood is in contact with the endothelium for longer times, thereby prolonging particle-residence time at the blood and vessel wall interface, thus favoring enhanced interaction between blood and atherogenic factors, and facilitating the diffusion of lipids or macromolecules and migration of inflammatory cells across the endothelium.[76,77]

Arterial functions

Arterial remodeling is associated with changes of arterial tree functions which are more complex than those generated by the presence of atherosclerotic plaques. The arterial system has two distinct, interrelated hemodynamic functions: (1) to deliver an adequate supply of blood from the heart to peripheral tissues, as dictated by metabolic activity (**conduit function**); and (2) to dampen blood pressure oscillations caused by intermittent ventricular ejection (**dampening function**). These two aspects of arterial function are intimately interrelated but can be dealt with independently because they have different origins and consequences. Disorders of conduit function result from the narrowing of the arterial lumen with ischemia affecting the tissues and organs downstream, while disorders of the dampening function reflect alterations of arterial wall viscoelastic properties and have deleterious effects upstream on the heart and the arteries themselves. It is beyond the scope of the present chapter to provide a detailed description of arterial hemodynamics and functions, which can be found elsewhere.[19,20]

Conduit function of arteries

The principal function of arteries is to deliver, at all times, an adequate supply of blood to peripheral tissues and organs in accordance with their metabolic needs. Conduit-function efficiency is the consequence of the width of the arteries and the very low resistance of large arteries to flow. Under normal conditions, the mean blood pressure is almost constant along the arterial tree (the mean blood pressure drops between the ascending aorta and arteries in the forearm or leg by not more than 2–3 mmHg in the supine position),[78] and conduit function is primarily dependent on the diameter of the arterial lumen. The conduit function is highly efficient and can accommodate increases in cardiac output by 5–6-fold and to increasing the flow to some tissues, such as muscle, by perhaps 10-fold. This physiological adaptability is mediated through acute changes of arterial flow velocity and/or diameter. Diameter changes are dependent on the endothelium, which responds to alterations in shear stress.[22,23] The acute endothelium-dependent vasodilation is limited in several clinical conditions; for example, atherosclerosis,[79] hypertension,[80] cardiac failure,[81] hypercholesterolemia,[82] diabetes,[83] menopause, and aging.[84,85]

Arterial remodeling associated with long-term pressure overload is characterized by a normal or slightly increased diameter of the conduit arteries under baseline conditions and, therefore, with normal baseline conductive properties.[55,86] Under conditions of long-term flow overload, the arterial diameters are enlarged and baseline arterial conductance is increased.[10,25] However, these chronic remodeling changes are frequently accompanied by inadequate responses to the demand for an acute increase in blood flow.[80,87] The principal long-term alterations of conduit function occur through narrowing or occlusion of arteries with restriction of blood flow and resulting ischemia or infarction of downstream tissues. Atherosclerosis, characterized by the presence of plaques and arterial narrowing, is the most common occlusive vascular disease that disturbs conduit function. Atherosclerosis usually narrows an artery in an irregular fashion, with focal compensatory enlargement occurring at discrete sites of narrowing immediately adjacent to more-or-less normal areas.[24] Owing to the large luminal area of conduit arteries, basal blood flow remains unchanged until the lumen diameter is narrowed by 50%. In this situation, the capacity to increase flow acutely during activity is progressively impaired, but partially compensated by arteriolar vasodilation. Beyond 70–80% reduction of the lumen diameter (critical stenosis), basal blood flow is reduced, as is the ability to increase flow during activity.[20]

Dampening function of arteries

The role of arteries is to dampen the pressure oscillations resulting from intermittent ventricular ejection (the 'Windkessel' effect) and to transform the pulsatile flow of arteries into the steady flow required in peripheral tissues and organs.[20] The large arteries can instantaneously accommodate the volume of blood ejected from the heart. Under normal conditions during systole, roughly 40% of stroke volume is forwarded directly to peripheral tissues, while the remainder is stored in capacitive arteries (mainly aorta and central arteries), distending the walls and storing the remaining 60% of stroke volume (Fig. 5.3). Approximately 10% of the energy produced by the heart is diverted for the distension of arteries and 'stored' in the walls to be available during diastole. During diastole, most of the stored energy recoils the aorta, squeezing the stored blood forward into the peripheral tissues, thereby ensuring continuous perfusion of organs and tissues. For the dampening function to

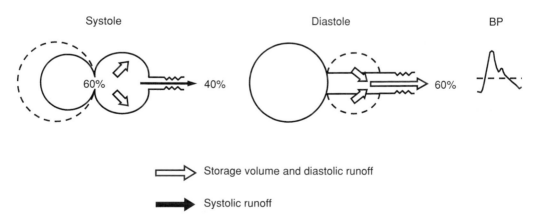

Fig. 5.3 Schematic representation of the cushioning function of the arterial system under normal conditions. During systole, approximately 40% of the stroke volume is forwarded directly into the peripheral circulation, while the other 60% is stored in the capacitive arteries, distending vessel walls and storing part of the cardiac energy. During diastole, the artery passively recoils and stored energy is used to forward the storage volume into the peripheral circulation. The final result is that the rhythmic pressure and flow pulsations induced by rhythmic contractions of the heart are converted into an almost continuous peripheral flow and pressure.

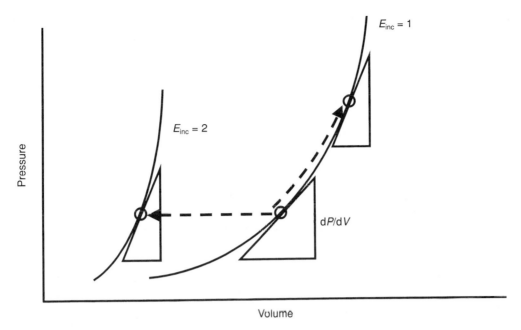

Fig. 5.4 Schematic representation of the pressure–volume relationship in cardiovascular structures with different incremental elastic moduli (E_{inc}—intrinsic stiffness of biomaterials). Increasing E_{inc} shifts the pressure–volume curve to the left, increasing the pressure effect of volume changes.

be efficient, it is essential that the energy necessary for arterial distension and recoil be as low as possible, i.e. for a given stroke volume, the pulse pressure should be as low as possible. The efficiency of the Windkessel function depends on the viscoelastic properties of arterial walls and the geometry of the arteries, including their diameter and length.[20]

The ability of arteries to accommodate the volume ejected instantaneously by the left ventricle can be described in terms of compliance, distensibility, or stiffness of the aorta or an individual artery. These terms express the contained volume of the vasculature (total or segmental) as a function of a given transmural pressure over the physiological range of pressure. Compliance is a term that describes the absolute amount of change in strain following a change in stress. In physiology, compliance (C) is defined as the change in volume (ΔV) due to a change in pressure (ΔP), that is $C = \Delta V / \Delta P$. Compliance represents the instantaneous slope of the pressure–volume relationship. The reciprocal value of compliance is the elastance ($E = \Delta P / \Delta V$) (Fig. 5.4).

The arterial media is responsible for the vessel's physical properties. Because it is composed of a 'mixture' of smooth muscle cells and connective tissue, containing elastin and collagen fibers, the pressure–volume relationship is non-linear. At a low distending pressure, the tension is borne by elastin fibers, whereas at a high distending pressure, the tension is predominantly borne by less extensible collagen fibers and the arterial wall becomes stiffer (less compliant).[20] This arrangement is advantageous because it prevents arterial blood from pooling at high pressure and protects arteries from high pressure-induced rupture.

To facilitate comparisons of viscoelastic properties of structures with different initial dimensions, compliance can be expressed relative to the initial volume as a coefficient of distensibility Di, defined as $Di = \Delta V / \Delta PV$, where $\Delta V / \Delta P$ is compliance and V is the initial volume. In contrast to distensibility or compliance which provides information about the 'elasticity' of the artery as a hollow structure, the elastic incremental modulus (E_{inc}; Young's modulus) provides direct information on the intrinsic elastic properties of the materials that compose the arterial wall independent of vessel geometry. An increased E_{inc} is characteristic of stiffer biomaterials and is responsible for the leftward shift of the pressure–volume curve (Fig. 5.4).[20] Arterial volume per unit length is equal to the arterial cross-sectional area. Arterial compliance is determined from the pressure diameter relationship as $C = \Delta D/\Delta P$, and the arterial distensibility (Di) is expressed as $Di = \Delta D/D\Delta P$ (where ΔD is the change in diameter and D is the baseline diastolic diameter induced by an increase in pressure (ΔP).[54] These different indices are usually measured by ultrasound techniques, which enable small changes of arterial diameters and arterial intima–media thickness to be determined.[88]

The stress applied to arterial segments (ΔP) is the pulse pressure. Owing to the inhomogeneity of the viscoelastic properties of successive arterial segments and the effect of arterial wave reflections (see below), pulse and systolic pressures are amplified from the aorta to the peripheral arteries and, in young and middle-aged people, peripheral pulse pressures overestimate the corresponding pressures in the aorta and central arteries (Fig. 5.5).[89] To determine the elastic properties of arterial segments accurately, the 'local' pulse pressure must be measured and taken into consideration. Pulse pressure can be assessed in central arteries, such as the aorta or carotid artery, by using applanation tonometry and a generalized transfer function.[7,90,91] As an alternative technique to ultrasound, arterial distensibility can be evaluated by measuring the pulse wave velocity (PWV) over a given arterial segment.[20,92] PWV increases

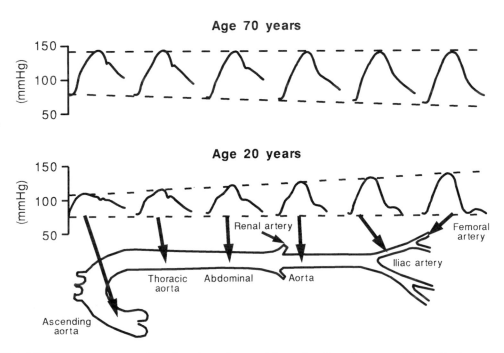

Fig. 5.5 Pressure-wave amplification along the arterial tree in old and young subjects. In the young subject, the amplitude of the pressure wave increases during wave transmission from the aorta to the arterial periphery.

Arteries as cushions

Increased TPR

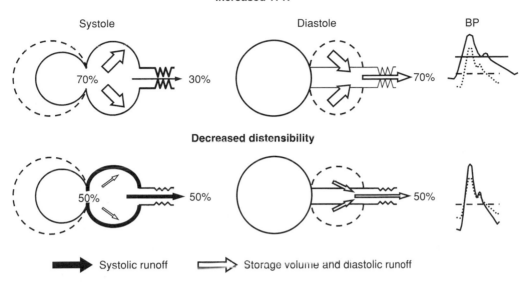

Decreased distensibility

Systolic runoff   Storage volume and diastolic runoff

Fig. 5.6 Effect of alterations of total peripheral resistance (TPR) and arterial distensibility on the cushioning function of arteries. Increased peripheral resistance results in an increase of mean blood pressure (product of TPR and cardiac output) and a pressure-dependent decrease of distensibility. The direct consequence is increased storage volume during systole and decreased diastolic runoff. The impact on the pressure wave is proportional to increases of mean and pulse pressures. Decreased arterial distensibility leads to increased pressure and decreased storage capacity during systole, with a higher part of the stroke volume directly forwarded to the peripheral circulation, and decreased diastolic recoil resulting in lower diastolic pressure. The resulting effects on the pressure wave are high systolic, low diastolic, and increased pulse pressures.

with arterial stiffness.[93] The viscoelastic properties of arterial walls determine the amplitude of pressure waves as well as their propagation and reflections along the arterial tree.[94–97]

The dampening function is altered by decreased distensibility and stiffening of arterial walls. The principal consequences of arterial stiffening are an increase in systolic and a decrease in diastolic pressures with resulting high pulse pressure.[19,20] Pulse pressure is an independent predictor of cardiovascular risk, particularly for the prediction of myocardial infarction.[98–101] Pulse pressure depends on the interaction between left ventricular (LV) ejection (stroke volume and duration of systole) and the physical properties of the arterial system that influence pulse pressure by two mechanisms. The first, direct mechanism involves the generation of a higher pressure wave by the LV ejecting into a stiff arterial system, and decreased diastolic recoil resulting in lowered diastolic pressure (Fig. 5.6).

The second, indirect mechanism acts via the influence of increased arterial stiffness on PWV and the timing of incident and reflected pressure waves.[20,66,94–96,102] Indeed, ejection of blood into the aorta generates a pressure wave that is propagated to other arteries throughout the body. This forward-traveling (incident) pressure wave is reflected at any point of structural and functional discontinuity in the arterial tree, thereby generating a reflected ('echo') wave traveling backwards towards the ascending aorta (Fig. 5.7).

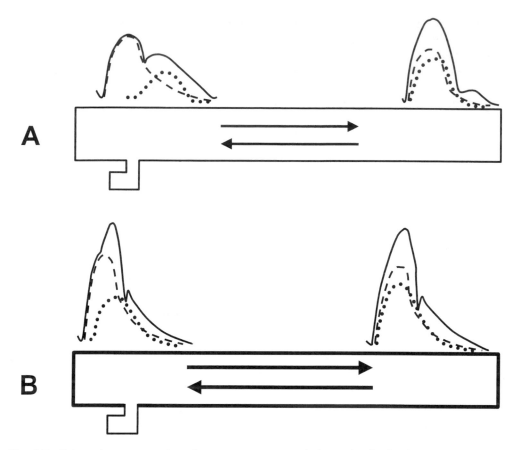

Fig. 5.7 Schematic representation of pressure-wave transmission and reflection in a tubular model of circulation. Recorded pressure wave ——; incident/forward pressure wave – – –; reflected pressure wave ……; → pulse-wave velocity. On the right, pressures waves in the peripheral circulation. On the left, the pressures waves in the aorta and central arteries are represented. (A) A distensible arterial system with low pulse-wave velocity. In the peripheral circulation, the reflected wave occurs as an almost immediate response to the impact of incident pressure wave—the two waves are 'in phase' and their sum is the measured pressure wave. The reflected wave returns at low pulse-wave velocity back to the central arteries and reaches the aorta after closure of aortic valves or during the telesystole. The reflected wave is not 'in phase' with the incident wave and has no effect on systolic pressure, but produces an additive 'boosting' effect on diastolic pressure. (B) A stiff arterial system with increased pulse-wave velocity causing the reflected wave to return towards central arteries and the aorta during ventricular ejection rather than during ventricular systole. In this situation the peripheral pressure amplification disappears (Fig. 5.5).

    Incident and reflected pressure waves interact constantly and their sum gives the measured pulse pressure wave. The final amplitude and shape of the measured pulse pressure wave are determined by the phase relationship (the timing) among the component waves.[102] The timing of incident and reflected pressure waves depends on the PWV, the traveling distance of pressure waves (i.e. body height), and the duration of LV ejection.[66,95,97,103] The shape and amplitude of measured pulse pressure waves depend on the site of pressure recording in the arterial tree (Figs 5 and 7).[7,95] Peripheral arteries are close to reflection sites, and the incident and reflected waves in these arteries are in phase and, thus, produce an additive effect. The ascending aorta and central arteries are distant from reflecting sites and, depending on the PWV and arterial length, the return of the reflected wave is variably delayed and thus the incident and reflected waves are not in phase.[102]

In young human subjects with distensible arteries and low PWV, the reflected waves affect central arteries during diastole after LV ejection has ceased (Fig. 5.7A). This timing is desirable, as the reflected wave causes an increase in ascending aortic pressure during early diastole and not during systole, resulting in aortic systolic and pulse pressures which are lower than in peripheral arteries (only mean blood pressure is almost constant throughout the arterial system).[89] This situation is physiologically advantageous because the increase in early diastolic pressure has a boosting effect on coronary perfusion without increasing LV afterload. The desirable timing is disrupted by increased PWV due to arterial stiffening. With increased PWV, the reflecting sites appear 'closer' to the ascending aorta and the reflected waves occur earlier, being more closely in phase with incident waves in this region. The earlier return means that the reflected waves affect the central arteries during systole rather than diastole, thus amplifying aortic and LV pressures during systole and reducing aortic pressure during diastole. In this situation, the pulse and systolic pressure gradients along the arterial tree tend to disappear, resulting in temporal equalization of peripheral and aortic pressures (Figs 5 and 7B).

Increased arterial stiffness is deleterious to LV function. By favoring early wave reflections, arterial stiffening increases peak- and end-systolic pressures in the ascending aorta, increasing the systolic tension-time index (STTI) and myocardial oxygen consumption, decreasing the diastolic blood pressure and diastolic tension-time index (DTTI) (Fig. 5.8), and decreasing the DTTI/STTI ratio, a determinant of subendocardial blood-flow distribution (subendocardial 'viability' index; Buckberg *et al*.[104]). Canine studies have shown that aortic stiffening directly decreases subendocardial blood flow despite an increased mean coronary flow, and that chronic aortic stiffening reduces cardiac transmural perfusion and aggravates subendocardial ischemia.[105] Furthermore, increased systolic blood pressure induces myocardial hypertrophy, and impairs diastolic myocardial function and LV ejection.[106] In addition, increased systolic blood pressure and pulse pressure accelerate arterial damage, increasing the fatigue of biomaterials, degenerative changes, and arterial stiffening, potentiating the process.[54,66]

Experimental studies have demonstrated that the endothelium plays an important role in the control of the viscoelastic properties in arterial wall. Destruction of the endothelium in arteries experimentally subjected to physiological pressure induced an increase in the arterial diameter in parallel with increases in compliance and arterial wall viscosity.[56,57] This suggests that an intact endothelium is necessary to maintain arterial compliance and distensibility within a physiologically acceptable range. While it has been shown that decreased compliance has a negative impact on LV function, the abnormal enhancement of arterial distensibility could theoretically also be detrimental to cardiac function. An abnormal increase of arterial distensibility would be responsible for increased blood pooling during systole, and alterations in pressure-wave transmission with decreased PWV and prolongation of the pressure-load transmission to peripheral circulation. In these circumstances, the displacement of the blood column in the arterial tree would be more dependent on the 'pushing' effect of the stroke volume, abnormally increasing the inertial component of the cardiac workload. Furthermore, it has been shown that endothelial injury increases arterial viscosity,

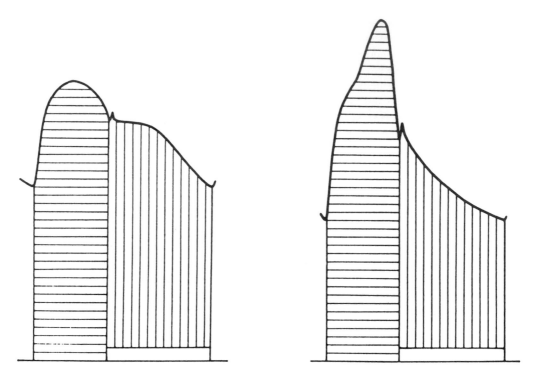

Fig. 5.8 Diagrammatic representation of the effect of arterial stiffness on systolic tension-time index (STTI, horizontally hatched area) and diastolic tension-time index (DTTI, vertically hatched area) in young (left) and old subjects (right) with similar mean blood pressure (overall pressure curve area). DTTI/STTI is an index of subendocardial perfusion (subendocardial viability index, Buckberg *et al.*[104]).

thereby increasing the hysteresis of the arterial pressure–volume relationship with two possible consequences: increased blood pooling during diastole altering diastolic recoil, or increased and inefficient dissipation of energy transmitted by the heart.[107]

The dampening function of the arterial tree is altered primarily during the aging process and in conditions associated with 'sclerotic' remodeling of arterial walls, i.e. associated with increased collagen content and modifications of extracellular matrix (arteriosclerosis).[7,8,66,92,108] Arteriosclerosis is primarily manifest as medial degeneration that is generalized throughout the thoracic aorta and central arteries, causing dilatation, diffuse hypertrophy, and stiffening of the arteries.[20,64] Arteriosclerosis is sometimes considered to be a 'physiological' aging phenomenon resulting in diffuse fibroelastic intima thickening, increased medial ground substance and collagen, and fragmentation of elastic lamellae with secondary fibrosis and calcification of the media.[5,6,8,109,110] Age-related arterial alterations leading to stiffening are heterogeneous, being more pronounced in the aorta and central, elastic-type, capacitative arteries than in the peripheral muscular-type limb arteries.[92] Changes similar to the aging process in some aspects are observed in essential hypertension. However, some differences characterize these two conditions. In hypertension, the arterial dilation is limited or absent, and the collagen content is enhanced, while aging is principally characterized by alterations in and decreased elastin content of the arterial wall.[5,111]

Taken together, atherosclerosis is a disorder that typically disturbs conduit function, while arteriosclerosis does not alter it under basal metabolic conditions.[64] However, in Western populations, these two conditions frequently coexist as both progress with aging and share several common pathogenic mechanisms, which sometimes make the distinction difficult. Moreover, increased intima–media thickness is, by itself, a condition favoring the development of atheromatous plaques and intima–media thickness has become widely regarded as a surrogate for preclinical atherosclerosis.

Arterial remodeling and function in ESRF patients

Atherosclerosis and alteration in conduit function

Atherosclerosis and arterial occlusive lesions are the most frequent causes of cardiovascular morbidity in patients with ESRF. Occlusive lesions principally involve the medium-sized conduit arteries, and coronary insufficiency, peripheral artery disease, and cerebrovascular events occupy an important place in the mortality of these patients.[112–115] The prevalence of plaques is also increased in the aorta and central, elastic-type arteries, such as the common carotid artery. However, these arteries are enlarged in ESRF patients (see below) and functionally significant occlusive lesions are rarer. The high incidence of atherosclerosis-related complications led Lindner and colleagues[116] to hypothesize that atherogenesis is accelerated in chronic hemodialysis patients. However, it remains a matter of debate whether or not the atherogenesis of dialysis patients is, indeed, accelerated and whether or not the nature of atherosclerotic plaques is similar in hemodialysis patients and the general population. Indeed, ultrasonographic studies have shown a much higher prevalence of calcified plaques in ESRF patients than in age-matched controls in whom soft plaques are more frequent.[115] The high mortality attributed to cardiovascular disease is not proof of acceleration of atherosclerosis since many factors not associated with arterial occlusive lesions contribute to cardiovascular mortality. While ESRF produces atherogenic factors essentially unique to uremia, including dyslipidemia, calcium-phosphate alterations, malnutrition, and activation of cytokines, these factors are additive to the number of risk factors observed in subjects with preserved renal function, such as age, hypertension, smoking, diabetes, male gender, and insulin resistance. Moreover, many hemodialysis patients already have significant vascular lesions before initiating dialysis and, in many patients, especially older patients, the generalized atherosclerosis can be the primary cause of renal failure (ischemic renal disease, cholesterol embolization, etc.). Indeed, risk factors present before ESRF might be of primary importance.[117]

Hemodynamic alterations could also favor the development of atherosclerotic occlusive lesions. Hypertension is a frequent complication in chronic renal diseases, and an association between high blood pressure and occlusive lesions was found in chronic hemodialysis patients. Rigorous control of hypertension at the time of incipient renal failure led to a significant decrease in the incidence of myocardial ischemia after initiation of dialysis therapy.[118,119] The role of shear-stress alterations in the development of atherosclerosis in ESRF patients has not been specifically investigated, mainly because of the difficulty of measuring the level of shear stress *in vivo* in humans. The pathophysiological mechanisms and clinical aspects of atherosclerotic disease in ESRF patients are beyond the scope of the present chapter but are addressed in other chapters of this book (see Chapters 1, 8–11, 14, 17, 18).

Table 5.1 Mean ± SD common carotid artery (CCA) geometry and arterial functional parameters in controls and end-stage renal failure (ESRF)

Parameter	Control (n = 70)	ESRF (n = 125)
Age (years)	52.2 ± 9.6	53 ± 12
Gender ({male}/{female};{male},1;{female},2)	1.43 ± 0.50	1.39 ± 0.50
BSA (m^2)	1.86 ± 0.23	1.70 ± 0.21***
Systolic blood pressure (mmHg)	147 ± 21	150 ± 31
Diastolic blood pressure (mmHg)	88 ± 12	83 ± 13**
Mean blood pressure (mmHg)	108 ± 14	105 ± 19
Heart rate (beats min^{-1})	64 ± 10	71 ± 13***
Aortic valves opening (cm)	1.85 ± 0.20	1.75 ± 0.30**
LV outflow velocity integral (cm beat^{-1})	21.9 ± 4.5	27.3 ± 7.3***
Stroke volume index (ml m^{-2})	32.3 ± 7.9	38.9 ± 12.5**
Total peripheral resistances (dyn s cm^{-5} m^2)	4260 ± 1105	3524 ± 1296**
CCA diameter (mm)	7.2 ± 0.9	7.9 ± 1.0***
CCA intima–media thickness (μm)	718 ± 97	790 ± 110***
CCA wall/lumen ratio	0.25 ± 0.03	0.25 ± 0.03
CCA distensibility (kPa^{-1} 10^{-3})	18.8 ± 6.3	16.5 ± 8.7*
CCA E_{inc} (kPa 10^3)	0.51 ± 0.22	0.71 ± 0.47***
Aortic PWV (cm s^{-1})	1029 ± 175	1104 ± 327*

*$P < 0.05$; **$P < 0.01$; ***$P < 0.001$ (London and Drüeke: Kidney International, 1997, 51:1678–95). Abbreviations: BSA, body surface area; LV, left ventricular; E_{inc}, incremental elastic modulus; PWV, pulse wave velocity.

Arteriosclerosis and alterations in dampening function

The arterial system of ESRF patients undergoes remodeling that is characterized by dilatation and, to a lesser degree, arterial intima–media hypertrophy of central, elastic-type, capac-

Table 5.2 Multivariate determinants analysis of common carotid artery (CCA) diameter and intima–media thickness

Independent variable	β coefficient	t value	P value
Dependent variable: diameter			
Age (years)	2.8	7.62	<0.0001
Gender ({male}:1; {female}:2)	−0.7	−6.00	<0.0001
Mean blood pressure (mmHg)	2.0	6.45	<0.0001
LV outflow velocity integral (cm beat^{-1})	0.04	4.47	<0.0001
	$r^2 = 0.57$ $F = 40$ ($P < 0.0001$)		
Dependent variable: intima–media thickness			
CCA diameter (mm)	43	5.45	<0.0001
Age (years)	2.47	5.90	<0.0001
Pulse pressure (mmHg)	1.00	3.42	0.0007
Body height (cm)	0.98	2.8	0.0066
	$r^2 = 0.60$ $F = 47$ ($P < 0.0001$)		

Abbreviation: LV, left ventricular.

itative arteries such as the aorta or the common carotid artery.[9,10,115,120,121] Arterial remodeling is less pronounced in peripheral, muscular-type, conduit arteries, such as the radial artery.[122,123] In ESRF patients, this remodeling is associated with arterial stiffening due to alterations of the intrinsic properties of arterial wall materials (E_{inc}) including those arteries free of atherosclerosis, such as upper arm arteries.[9,10,120,123–126] The effect of increased E_{inc} on the arterial distensibility and compliance is, in part, attenuated by the arterial dilatation, and the distensibility of capacitive arteries is less altered than E_{inc} (Table 5.1). Although some of these modifications are the consequence of mechanical load, non-hemodynamic factors could play an important role.[10,87,121,127]

Hemodynamic factors of arterial remodeling in chronic uremia

Large capacitative arteries, like the aorta or common carotid artery, are enlarged in ESRF patients in comparison with age-, sex-, and pressure-matched control subjects. Arterial enlargement is already observed at the onset of dialysis, suggesting that arterial remodeling takes place early in the course of renal failure. The internal dimensions of large arteries are influenced by many factors (Table 5.2).

Several factors, for example age, sex or mean blood pressure, are non-specific for ESRF patients, while others, such as blood-flow velocity and systemic blood flow, are more

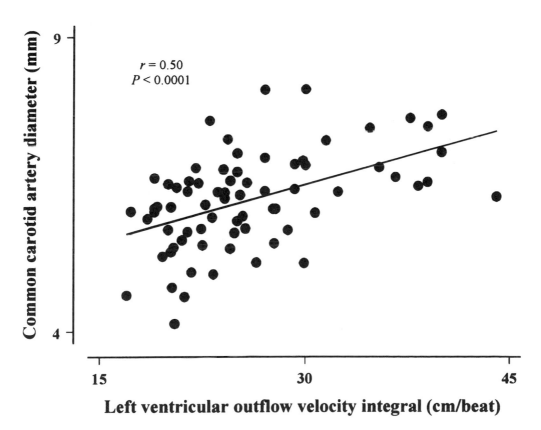

Fig. 5.9 Correlation, in hemodialyzed ESRF patients, between common carotid artery diameter and left ventricular outflow velocity integral. (Reproduced from reference 10 with permission from Blackwell Science, Inc.)

relevant for this patient population.[10,114,128] In ESRF patients, chronic volume/flow overload associated with anemia, arteriovenous shunts, and overhydration due to sodium and water retention creates conditions for arterial remodeling. This finding has been supported by cross-sectional studies showing a relationship between the diameters of the aorta and common carotid artery and LV outflow velocity integral and/or stroke volume (Fig. 5.9).[10]

The role of anemia is suggested by a negative correlation between hematocrit and LV outflow velocity (Fig. 5.10).

The role of overhydration was shown by studies indicating that arterial enlargement could be limited by adequate fluid removal during dialysis.[9] Overhydration does not only influence the internal dimensions of arterial system, but also arterial wall thickness and stiffness. In ESRF patients, sodium and water overload is a factor associated with increased blood pressure, which passively dilates the arterial system by increasing the distending pressure applied to the vessel wall.[66] This combined effect of high pressure and enlarged arterial diameter increases the circumferential tensile stress applied to the vessel wall and induces its hypertrophy. Moreover, experimental studies have shown that sodium alone can induce hypertrophy of cultured vascular smooth muscle cells and act as a direct trophic factor.[129] The effect of overhydration on the physical properties of large arteries was also demonstrated in hemodialyzed ESRF patients by the relationship between interdialysis body-weight changes and aortic PWV, which increased in proportion to salt and water balance.[130]

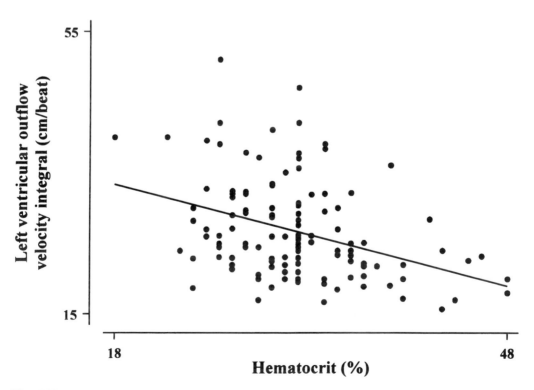

Fig. 5.10   Correlation, in hemodialyzed ESRF patients, between left ventricular outflow velocity integral and hematocrit. (Personal data.)

Unlike in blood pressure- and age-matched non-uremic patients, the arterial intima–media thickness is increased in ESRF patients.[10,121] Arterial wall thickness is influenced by non-specific factors, like age and body height, but also by factor(s) associated with the presence of uremia *per se* (Table 5.2). By contrast, the intima–media thickness is proportional to changes in diameter, with a wall-to-lumen ratio similar to that of non-uremic controls. According to Laplace's law, arterial wall hypertrophy could be considered to be a response to increased circumferential tensile stress, whereby wall tension is directly proportional to arterial radius. However, according to the same law, when the blood pressure increases, and regardless of the internal radius, the wall-to-lumen ratio should increase in order to normalize the tensile stress.[20] This increase was observed in non-uremic populations but not in ESRF patients whose wall-to-lumen ratio in large conduit arteries was not related to pressure changes.[131] The difference between the observed relationships suggests that conduit arteries could have limited capacity to hypertrophy in response to a combined flow and pressure load. This possibility was also documented by Savage and colleagues[115] who showed that, in their ESRF patients, the arterial dilation was not accompanied by arterial wall thickening. The reasons for this altered response are not clear. Dobrin and colleagues[16] demonstrated that intimal thickening occurs in response to low flow velocity, whereas medial thickening occurs in response to increased arterial wall tension and vice versa. Therefore, in ESRF patients, increased tensile stress could induce medial hypertrophy, while increased flow could decrease the intimal thickness. However, as the presently available ultrasonographic devices are unable to differentiate between intima and media, this postulate remains unproven.

Another reason for the altered hypertrophic response could be qualitative alterations of biomaterials present in 'uremic vasculopathy'. Arterial distensibility is 'pressure-dependent'[20] (Fig. 5.4) and, in essential hypertensive patients, the decreased arterial distensibility is due to higher distending blood pressure rather than to arterial wall thickening and modifications in intrinsic biomaterial stiffness.[86,132] When adjusted for differences in blood pressure (i.e. under isobaric conditions), the arterial distensibility and/or elastic modulus of essential hypertensive subjects are more distensible (in muscular conduit arteries) or similar (in elastic capacitive arteries) to those observed in normotensive control subjects.[86] These observations suggest that, in essential hypertension, the biomaterials are similar to those of normotensive subjects, with hypertrophy of the walls being due only to an increased amount of wall biomaterials.

This concept is different from the observation made in ESRF patients, in whom common carotid artery distensibility is decreased in comparison to age- and blood pressure-matched non-uremic subjects.[10] In ESRF patients, arterial hypertrophy is accompanied by alterations in the intrinsic elastic properties of arterial walls (increased E_{inc}) that contribute to creating and amplifying the pressure load. This modification affects elastic and muscular-type arteries, including arteries free of atherosclerosis, like the radial artery (Fig. 5.11).[123] The observation that the incremental modulus of elasticity is increased in ESRF patients more strongly favors altered intrinsic elastic properties or major architectural abnormalities such as those seen in experimental uremia and the arteries of uremic patients, namely fibroelastic intimal thickening, calcification of elastic lamellae, increased calcium, increased extracellular matrix, and more collagen with relatively less of the elastic fiber content[133–137] (for detailed description see Chapter 4).

Finally, abnormal endothelial function could also be responsible for the altered arterial hypertrophic process in ESRF patients. As shown experimentally by Lévy and colleagues[56,57]

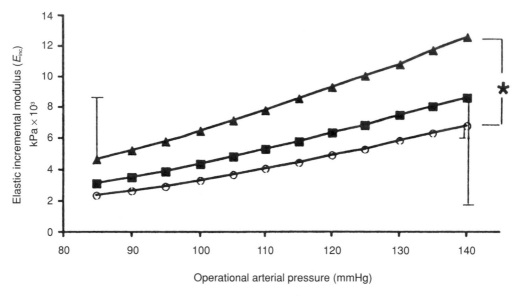

Fig. 5.11 Radial artery E_{inc}–pressure curves in ESRF (▲), control subjects (■), and patients with essential hypertension (○). The curves were evaluated within the corresponding systolic–diastolic ranges of operational pressure. At any given pressure, the E_{inc} is higher in ESRF patients. *$P < 0.01$ (Reproduced from reference 123 with permission from Lippincot and Williams-Wilkins.)

the endothelium influences the mechanical and geometric properties of large arteries, and removing the endothelium causes an increase in arterial diameter. Endothelial function is altered in ESRF patients as shown by decreased vasodilator responses of the macro- and microcirculations to various stimuli including ischemia,[87,122,138–141] hyperthermia,[142] or intravascular injections of acetylcholine.[143] In ESRF patients, the large artery alterations are associated with decreased postischemic arterial vasodilatation and flow-debt repayment, suggesting a relationship between arterial modifications and endothelial dysfunction (Fig. 5.12).[131] Joannides and colleagues[122] have demonstrated that postischemic dilation of the radial artery is almost abolished in ESRF, with blood flow increasing only secondary to increased flow velocity. Since direct vasodilatation with nitroprusside also induced a lower response in their ESRF patients than in controls, the authors concluded that endothelial (NO-mediated) function is defective or vascular sensitivity to the vasodilating action of NO is lower in uremic patients.

   The presence of generalized endothelial dysfunction in uremic patients is also suggested by higher plasma levels of von Willebrand factor, fibrinogen, endothelin, and other factors.[144–147] The endothelial dysfunction could be due to chronic 'activation' of the endothelium resulting from the chronically increased flow and shear stresses[148] or chronic proinflammatory conditions and oxidative stress.[149] By contrast, uremic medium caused endothelial cell dysfunction characterized by an alteration of the properties of the subendothelial matrix,[150] and high oxalic acid levels, like those observed in uremic patients, suppressed replication and migration of human endothelial cells *in vitro*.[151] In ESRF patients, an endogenous inhibitor(s) of the L-arginine/NO pathway accumulates.[152,153] Inhibition of NO production could also participate to enhance endothelin production, since NO inhibits

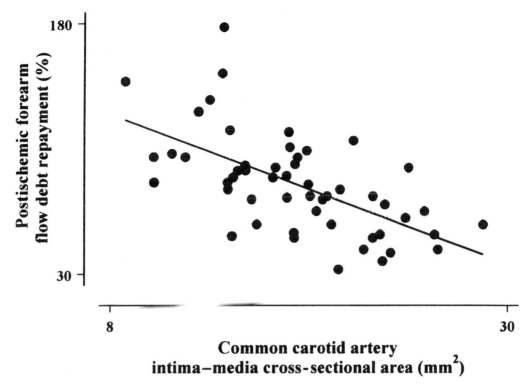

Fig. 5.12   Correlation, in ESRF patients, between common carotid artery intima–media cross-sectional area and postischemic forearm blood flow debt repayment.

endothelin production.[154] In ESRF patients, Demuth and colleagues[87] have shown a significant association between plasma endothelin levels with arterial hypertrophy and decreased postischemic vasodilation.

Hyperhomocysteinemia (tHcy) can exert a toxic effect on vascular endothelium via the promotion of oxidative damage and generation of reactive oxygen species.[155,156] Plasma homocysteine concentrations are elevated in ESRF patients.[157,158] However, tHcy principally causes atherothrombosis and its role in non-atheromatous arterial remodeling is not clear. Moreover, in ESRF patients, cross-sectional studies have not shown convincingly the type of arterial structural or functional alterations associated with tHcy.[159] In patients on peritoneal dialysis, van Guldener and co-workers[140] observed no association between the tHcy level and decreased reactive hyperemia of the brachial artery. Furthermore, the same authors did not find any attenuation of the impaired endothelial function in hemodialysis patients after long-term folic acid therapy.[141] In the study by Blacher and colleagues,[159] elevated plasma tHcy levels were associated with leg artery stiffness, but not with stiffening of the major capacitive arteries, like the aorta or carotid artery. Microcirculatory alterations are also associated with structural alterations of microvessels as shown by the analysis of cutaneous capillaries and resistance vessels.[160–162] (For detailed description of the alterations of endothelial function in ESRF patients, see Chapter 5).

Other factors

Many vasoactive substances can modulate the growth of vascular smooth muscle cells and mediate remodeling. The roles of growth promoters, such as angiotensin II, norepinephrine, vasopressin, cytokines, or reactive oxygen species, has been documented in experimental studies.[11,42,163] However, the possible participation of these factors in the arterial remodeling seen in chronic renal failure has not yet been demonstrated, and the subject is beyond the scope of the present chapter.

While the published data agree that smoking is a factor associated with arterial wall hypertrophy and stiffening in ESRF patients,[10,121] no consistent and constant associations could be established between arterial remodeling and common vascular risk factors. An association between arterial remodeling and functional alterations with lipid abnormalities is not obvious and was found only irregularly. London and colleagues[124] and Saito and co-workers[125] reported an inverse relationship between aortic PWV and HDL cholesterol. Burdick and colleagues[164] and Nishizawa and co-workers[165] described a positive relationship between carotid intima–media thickness and IDL or LDL cholesterol.

The most frequently observed factors associated with arterial stiffening in ESRF seem to be alterations in calcium and phosphate metabolism and parathyroid activity. Experimental studies suggest that some of the effects of renal failure on arterial remodeling and increased fibrogenesis depend on the permissive action of parathyroid hormone (PTH).[166,167] In hemodialyzed patients, aortic PWV was found to be associated with mediacalcinosis of conduit arteries and increased calcium-phosphate product.[124,125] Kawagishi and colleagues[121] reported that a high phosphorus level was associated with carotid artery intima media thickening, while increased serum PTH was a risk factor for increased wall thickness of femoral arteries. Studying renal transplant recipients, Barenbrock and co-workers[127] observed an association between high PTH levels and decreased common carotid artery distensibility. However, these results were not always observed by all authors and the role of calcium-phosphate and PTH alterations remain to be proven by prospective interventional studies.

Consequences of arterial alterations in ESRF patients

The principal pathophysiological consequence of vascular alterations in ESRF is decreased arterial distensibility and increased PWV with early wave reflections. The principal clinical consequences of these effects are increased systolic and pulse pressures, LV hypertrophy, and altered coronary circulation.[10,103,124,168]

For ESRF patients, significant correlations exist between vascular and cardiac parameters that reflect the influence of cardiac alterations on the arterial system and vice versa (Fig. 5.13).[10,115,128,169]

Volume/flow overload is associated with increased LV diameter and increased cardiac output whose persistence participates in arterial remodeling.[128] In turn, these alterations in arterial structure and function have a negative effect on the heart, increasing LV afterload.[10,169,170] Afterload describes the factors that oppose LV ejection.[20] Since blood pressure is the easiest measurable index of opposition to LV ejection, afterload is usually taken to be a function of the pressure generated by the LV for ejection to occur. However, blood pressure is an integrated, non-specific external load on the LV that is affected by complex interactions between arterial system properties and LV ejection characteristics. The appropriate term to define the arterial factor is aortic input impedance, a measurement of the opposition of the circulation to an oscillatory input (i.e. stroke volume). Aortic impedance is determined

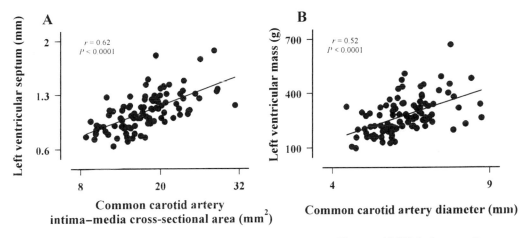

Fig. 5.13   Correlation, in ESRF patients, between common carotid artery (CCA) intima–media cross-sectional area and left ventricular septal thickness (A), and between CCA diameter and LV mass (B). (B reproduced from reference 128 with permission from W.B. Saunders Company.)

by peripheral resistance, the viscoelastic properties of the aorta and large central arteries, and the inertial forces (inertance) represented by the mass of the blood in the aorta and LV.[20] Peripheral resistance is usually not increased in ESRF patients, largely as a consequence of anemia, low blood viscosity, and the presence of arteriovenous shunts.[170] Under these conditions, increased arterial stiffness, acceleration of PWV and early wave reflections, and arterial dilation represent the major contributors to LV afterload. The principal consequences of these alterations are LV hypertrophy (Fig. 5.14). Previous studies have shown that LV hypertrophy in ESRF is correlated with increased arterial stiffness and the intensity of wave reflections.[10,163] The second important consequence of arterial stiffness in ESRF patients is compromised coronary perfusion. Cardiac ischemia and altered subendocardial perfusion are frequently observed in uremic patients despite patent coronary arteries.[3,4]

The latter was recently suggested in ESRF patients in whom the large artery structure and function changes were associated with decreased subendocardial viability index (DTTI/STTI) (Fig. 5.15),[10] an index of the propensity for subendocardial ischemia in the absence of occlusive arterial lesions.[104] In other respects, for ESRF patients, significant correlations were observed between LV septal thickness and common carotid artery intima–media thickness, and LV mass and common carotid artery diameter, suggesting a direct link between arterial dilation and LV hypertrophy (Fig. 5.13).[128] Indeed, the inertial effects are greater in enlarged arteries since larger blood-filled arteries require the heart to work harder in order to accelerate blood against larger inertial forces during ejection.[20]

In the past, the clinical consequences of arterial stiffness on cardiovascular structure and function have been poorly evaluated. Blacher and colleagues[171] applied logistic regression and Cox analyses to the characteristics of a cohort of 241 subjects with ESRF and were able to identify three significant predictors of cardiovascular mortality: aortic PWV, age, and duration of hemodialysis. After adjustment for all risk factors (age, pre-existing cardiovascular disease, blood pressure, anemia, LV hypertrophy, etc.), the odds ratio for PWV (>1227 cm/s) was 4.4 (confidence interval CI = 2.3–8.5) for all-cause mortality and 5 (CI = 2.3–10.9) for cardiovascular mortality. PWV is a complex parameter integrating arterial

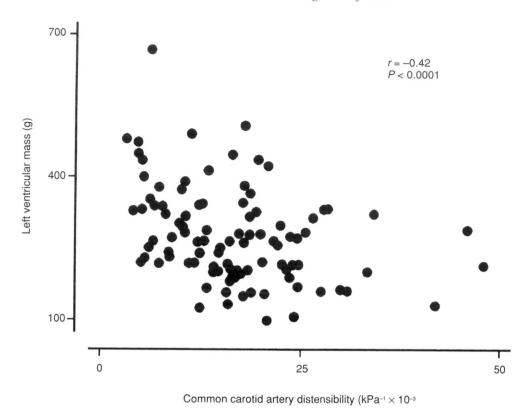

Fig. 5.14 Correlation, in ESRF patients, between left ventricular mass and common carotid artery distensibility. (Reproduced from reference 128 with permission from W.B. Saunders Company.)

geometry and intrinsic elastic properties described by the Moens–Korteweg equation, (PWV) $\leq = Eh/2r\rho$, where E is the elastic modulus (E_{inc}), r is the radius, h is the wall thickness, and ρ is the fluid density.[20] Based on Cox analyses, Blacher and colleagues[172] have shown that the principal factors associated with the PWV as a predictor of cardiovascular and all-cause mortality in ESRF were the elastic modulus and dilatation of arteries, i.e. generalized arterial disease.

In the absence of controlled studies, it is difficult to propose therapeutic interventions to prevent or treat arterial abnormalities in ESRF patients. Dialysis by itself does not increase arterial distensibility,[173] and some studies indicate that arterial function worsens with the time on dialysis.[121,164] We know from studies on essential hypertensive, non-uremic subjects that long-term antihypertensive therapy induces reverse remodeling with regression of arterial wall hypertrophy and improvement of the arterial system viscoelastic properties.[174] Until now, such controlled studies in ESRF patients have not been available. During recent years, a few controlled studies aimed at examining the effect of antihypertensive drugs on the function of large arteries have been conducted on ESRF patients on hemodialysis. It has been shown that long-term treatment with the calcium-channel blocker nitrendipine for a period of 24 weeks effectively lowered blood pressure, and significantly decreased aortic and femoral PWV.[175] The decreased aortic PWV was not due to a modification of aortic diameter, which remained unchanged. During the first 8–16 weeks of treatment, the aortic PWV

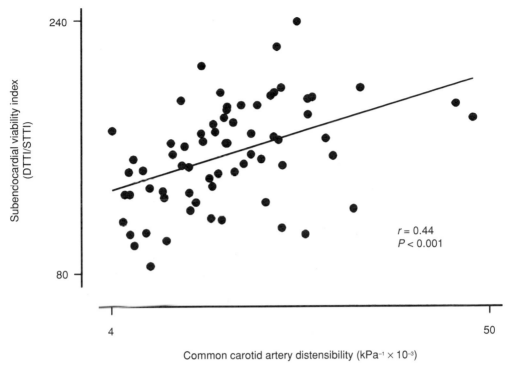

Fig. 5.15 Correlation, in ESRF patients, between common carotid artery distensibility and subendo-cardial viability index (DTTI/STTI). (Reproduced from reference 10 with permission from Blackwell Science, Inc.)

decrease paralleled the blood pressure decrease. The aortic PWV decrease continued until the end of the therapeutic trial at week 24, but these late changes in aortic distensibility that occurred between weeks 16 and 24 were no longer attributable to changes in blood pressure, which remained constant. The effect of calcium-channel blockers was more pronounced in patients with arterial mediacalcinosis.[176] These findings suggested that the long-term improvement of aortic distensibility could be a reflection of changes of elastic modulus, wall thickness, or both.[175] The same positive effect on large artery distensibility was observed in controlled studies with the angiotensin-converting enzyme (ACE) inhibitors perindopril and quinapril.[177,178] These two ACE inhibitors enhanced arterial system distensibility and had pronounced effects on wave reflections, which were decreased significantly. However, these studies did not allow us to conclude whether the improvement of elastic properties was the consequence of the lowered blood pressure or was due to reverse remodeling and to alterations in intrinsic properties of arterial walls.

In conclusion, the vascular complications in ESRF are ascribed to two different but associated mechanisms, namely atherosclerosis and arteriosclerosis. Arteriosclerosis characterized by diffuse dilation and hypertrophy of large conduit arteries and stiffening of arterial walls represents a clinical form of an accelerated aging process. These alterations are associated with several hemodynamic changes characteristic of ESRF, such as flow/volume overload and increased circumferential tensile stress due to increased arterial diameters and/or intraarterial pressure. Resulting from these arterial changes, the systolic pressure is abnormally increased in ESRF patients while diastolic pressure is usually within the normal range or even low. The main adverse affects of arterial stiffness are: (1) an increased LV afterload with development of LV hypertrophy and increased myocardial oxygen demand; and (2) altered coronary perfusion and blood flow distribution with relative subendocardial ischemia.. Epidemiological studies have demonstrated the impact of arterial abnormalities on cardiovascular disease evolution and identified arterial remodeling and stiffening as independent predictors of overall and cardiac mortality in ESRF patients.

Arterial hemodynamic indices

Tensile stress (σ)	Force exerted across an area. According to the law of Laplace, in the arteries, $\sigma = Pr/h$, where P = transmural pressure applied on arterial wall, r = the arterial radius, and h = arterial wall thickness. The product $P \times r$ is wall tension. The units of stress are dyn/cm^2.
Shear stress (τ)	Frictional force exerted by flowing blood on the arterial wall surface. $\tau = Q\eta/\pi r^3$, where Q = blood flow, η = blood viscosity, and r = arterial radius. The units of stress are dyn/cm^2.
Compliance (C)	Measure of the volume/pressure relationship, generally an absolute volume change (ΔV) for a given pressure step (ΔP): $C = \Delta V/\Delta P$ (cm^3/mmHg). The inverse of compliance is elastance. In the arteries, compliance is expressed as arterial diameter (or cross-sectional area) change (ΔD) for a given pressure step (ΔP) as $C = \Delta D/\Delta P$ (cm/mmHg; cm^2/mmHg).
Distensibility (Di)	Measure of relative volume (or diameter) change for a given pressure step. $Di = \Delta V/V\Delta P$ (mmHg^{-1}), where ΔV is absolute volume change, V is the initial volume, and ΔP is pressure change. Distensibility reflects the capacitive properties of the arteries as a hollow structure.
Elastic modulus	Elastic incremental modulus (E_{inc}). The stretching force per unit area required for 100% stretch from resting values. $E_{inc} = \Delta P \cdot V/\Delta V \cdot h$ (mmHg/cm), where ΔP is pressure step, V is initial volume (or diameter), ΔV is absolute volume (or diameter) change, and h is wall thickness. E_{inc} reflects the intrinsic elastic properties of wall material.
Pulse wave velocity	Speed of pressure wave travel along an arterial segment (cm/s). According to the Moens–Korteweg equation $(PWV)^2 = E_{inc}h/\rho D$, where E_{inc} is elastic modulus, h is wall thickness, ρ is density, and D is arterial diameter.
Units	P Pressure (1 mmHg = 1333 dyn/cm^2 = 0.13 kPa)
	Q Volumetric rate of flow (cm^3/s)

η Viscosity (poise, dyn s/cm^2)
r Radius or diameter (cm)
V Volume (cm^3)
t Time (s)

Acknowledgments

This work was supported by G.E.P.I.R. (Groupe d'Etude de Physiopathologie de l'Insuffisance Rénale) and U.M.I.F. (Union des Mutuelles de l' Ile-de-France).

References

1. Raine, A.E.G., Margreiter, R., Brunner, F.P., Ehrich, J.H.H., Geelings, W., Landais, P., *et al.* (1992). Report on management of renal failure in Europe, XXII, 1991. *Nephrology Dialysis and Transplantation*, 7(Suppl. 2), 7–35.
2. USRD: US Renal Data System. (1998). Annual Report. Bethesda, MD, The National Institute of Diabetes and Digestive and Kidney Diseases, *American Journal of Kidney Diseases*, 32(Suppl. 1), S81–8.
3. Roig, E., Betriu, A., Castaner, A., Magrina, J., Sanz, G., and Navarra-Lopez, F. (1981). Disabling angina pectoris with normal coronary arteries in patients undergoing hemodialysis. *American Journal of Medicine*, 71, 437–44.
4. Rostand, R.G., Kirk, K.A., and Rutsky, E.A. (1984). Dialysis ischemic heart disease: insight from coronary angiography. *Kidney International*, 25, 653–9.
5. Wolinsky, H. (1972). Long term effects of hypertension on rat aortic wall and their relation to concurrent aging changes: morphological and chemical studies. *Circulation Research*, 30, 301–9.
6. Fischer, G.M. (1976). Effects of spontaneous hypertension and age on arterial connective tissue in the rat. *Experimental Gerontology*, 11, 209–15.
7. Kelly, R., Hayward, C., Avolio, A., and O'Rourke, M. (1989). Noninvasive determination of age-related changes in the human arterial pulse. *Circulation*, 80, 1652–9.
8. Virmani, R., Avolio, A.P., Mergner, W.J., Robinowitz, R., Herderick, E.E., Cornhill, J.F., *et al.* (1991). Effects of aging on aortic morphology in populations with high and low prevalence of hypertension and atherosclerosis. *American Journal of Pathology*, 139, 1119–29.
9. Barenbrock, M., Spieker, C., Laske, V., Heidenreich, S, Hohage, H., Bachmann, J., *et al.* (1994). Studies of the vessel wall properties in hemodialysis patients. *Kidney International*, 45, 1397–400.
10. London, G.M., Guérin, A.P., Marchais, S.J., Pannier, B., Safar, M.E., Day, M., *et al.* (1996). Cardiac and arterial interactions in end-stage renal disease. *Kidney International*, 50, 600–8.
11. Gibbons, G.H. and Dzau, V.J. (1994). The emerging concept of vascular remodeling. *New England Journal of Medicine*, 330, 1431–8.
12. Kamiya, A. and Togawa, T. (1980). Adaptive regulation of wall shear stress to flow change in the canine carotid artery. *American Journal of Physiology*, 239, H14–21.
13. Mulvany, M.J. (1987). The structure of the resistance vasculature in essential hypertension. *Journal of Hypertension*, 5, 129–36.
14. Baunbach, G.L. and Heistadt, D.D. (1989). Remodeling of cerebral arterioles in chronic hypertension. *Hypertension*, 13, 968–72.
15. Zarins, C.K., Zatine, M.A., Giddens, D.P., Ku, D.N., and Glagov, S. (1987). Shear stress regulation of artery lumen diameter in experimental atherogenesis. *Journal of Vascular Surgery*, 5, 413–20.
16. Dobrin, P.B., Littooy, F.N., and Endean, E.D. (1989). Mechanical factors predisposing to intimal hyperplasia and medial thickening in autogenous vein grafts. *Surgery*, 105, 393–400.
17. Davies, P.F. and Tripathi, S.C. (1993). Mechanical stress mechanisms and the stress to flow change in the canine carotid artery. *Circulation Research*, 72, 235–9.

18. Davies, P.F. (1995). Flow-mediated endothelial mechanotransduction. *Physiological Review*, **75**, 519–60.

19. Milnor, W.R. (1989). *Hemodynamics*, 2nd edn. Williams and Wilkins, Baltimore.

20. Nichols, W.W. and O'Rourke, M.F. (1998). Vascular impedance. In *McDonald's blood flow in arteries: theoretical, experimental and clinical principles*, 4th edn. Edward Arnold, London.

21. Hull, S.S.J., Kaiser, L., Jaffe, M.D., and Sparks, H.V.J. (1986). Endothelium-dependent flow-induced dilatation of canine femoral and saphenous arteries. *Blood Vessels*, **23**, 183–98.

22. Pohl, U., Holtz, J., Busse, R., and Bassenge, E. (1986). Crucial role of endothelium in the vasodilatator response to increased flow *in vivo*. *Hypertension*, **8**, 37–44.

23. Moncada, S., Palmer, R.M.J., and Higgs, A. (1991). Nitric oxide: physiology, pathophysiology and pharmacology. *Pharmacological Review*, **43**, 109–42.

24. Glagov, S., Weisenberg, E., Zarins, C.K., Stankunavicius, R., and Kolettis, G.J. (1987). Compensatory enlargement of human atherosclerotic coronary arteries. *New England Journal of Medicine*, **316**, 1371–5.

25. Girerd, X., London, G., Boutouyrie, P., Mourad, J.J., Laurent, S., and Safar, M. (1996). Remodelling of radial artery and chronic increase in shear stress. *Hypertension*, **27**(Part 2), 799–803.

26. Traub, O. and Berk, B.C. (1998). Laminar shear stress: mechanisms by which endothelial cells transduce an atheroprotective force. *Arteriosclerosis Thrombosis and Vascular Biology*, **18**, 677–85.

27. Upchurch, G.R. Jr., Loscalzo, J., and Banes. A.J. (1997). Changes in the amplitude of cyclic load biphasically modulate endothelial cell DNA synthesis and division. *Vascular Medicine*, **2**, 19–24.

28. Schwartz, M.A., Schaller, M.D., and Ginsberg, M.H. (1995). Integrins: emerging paradigms of signal transduction. *Annual Review of Cellular and Developmental Biology*, **11**, 549–99.

29. Olesen, S.P., Clapham, D.E., and Davies, P.F. (1988). Haemodynamic shear stress activates a K^+ current in vascular endothelial cells. *Nature*, **331**, 168–70.

30. Cooke, J.P., Rossitch, E., Andon, N., Loscalzo, J., and Dzau, V.J. (1991). Flow activates an endothelial potassium channel to release an endogenous nitrovasodilator. *Journal of Clinical Investigation*, **88**, 1663–71.

31. Kuchan, M.J., Jo, H., and Frangos, J.A. (1994). Role of G protein in shear stress-mediated nitric oxide production by endothelial cells. *American Journal of Physiology*, **267**, C753–8.

32. Redmond, E.M., Cahill, P.A., and Sitzmann, J.V. (1998). Flow-mediated regulation of G-protein expression in cocultured vascular smooth muscle and endothelial cells. *Arteriosclerosis Thrombosis and Vascular Biology*, **18**, 75–83.

33. Schnitzer, J.E., Liu, J., and Oh, P. (1995). Endothelial caveolae have the molecular transport machinery for vesicle budding, docking, and fusion including VAMP, NSF, SNAP, annexins, and GTPases. *Journal of Biological Chemistry*, **270**, 14399–404.

34. Cooke, J.P., Stamler, J.S., Andon, N., Davies, P.F., McKinley, J., and Loscalzo, J. (1990). Flow stimulates endothelial cells to release a nitrovasodilator that is potentiated by reduced thiols. *American Journal of Physiology*, **259**, H804–12.

35. Koller, A., Sun, D., Huang, A., and Kaley, G. (1994). Corelease of nitric oxide and prostaglandins mediates flow-dependent dilatation of rat gracilis muscle arterioles. *American Journal of Physiology*, **267**, H326–32.

36. Nakache, M. and Gaub, H.E. (1988). Hydrodynamic hyperpolarization of endothelial cells. *Proceedings of National Academy of Science USA*, **85**, 1841–3.

37. Kuchan, M.J. and Frangos, J.A. (1993). Shear stress regulates endothelin-1 release via protein kinase C and cGMP in cultured endothelial cells. *American Journal of Physiology*, **264**, H150–6.

38. Walpola, P.L., Gotlieb, A.I., Cybulsky, M.I., and Langille, B.L. (1995). Expression of ICAM-1 and VCAM-1 and monocyte adherence in arteries exposed to altered shear stress. *Arteriosclerosis Thrombosis and Vascular Biology*, **15**, 2–10.

39. Chiu, J.J., Wung, B.S., Shyy, J.Y.J., Hsieh, H.J., and Wang, D.L. (1997). Reactive oxygen species are involved in shear stress-induced intercellular adhesion molecule-1 expression in endothelial cells. *Arteriosclerosis Thrombosis and Vascular Biology*, **17**, 3570–7.

40. Diamond, S.L., Sharefrin, J.B., Dieffenbach, C., Frasier, S.K., McIntire, L.V., and Eskin, S.G. (1990). Tissue plasminogen activator messenger RNA level increase in cultured human endothelial cells exposed to laminar shear stress. *Journal of Cellular Physiology*, 143, 364–71.

41. Malek, A.M., Jackman,R., Rosenberg, R.D., and Izumo, S. (1994). Endothelial expression of thrombomodulin is reversibly regulated by fluid shear stress. *Circulation Research*, 74, 852–60.

42. Okada, H., Woodcock-Mitchell, J., Mitchell, J., Sakamoto, T., Marutsuka, K., Sobel, B.E., *et al.* (1998). Induction of plasminogen activator inhibitor type 1 and collagen type 1 expression in rat cardiac microvascular endothelial cells by interleukin-1 and its dependence on oxygen-centered free radicals. *Circulation*, 97, 2175–82.

43. Hsieh, H.J., Li, N.Q., and Frangos, J.A. (1992). Shear-induced platelet-derived growth factor gene expression in human endothelial cells is mediated by protein kinase C. *Journal of Cellular Physiology*, 150, 552–8.

44. Hassid, A., Arabshahi, H., Bourcier, T., Dhaunsi, G.S., and Matthews, C. (1994). Nitric oxide selectively amplifies FGF-2 induced mitogenesis in primary rat aortic smooth muscle cells. *American Journal of Physiology*, 267, H1040–8.

45. Battegay, E.J., Raines, E.W., Seifert, R.A., Bowen-Pope, D.F., and Ross, R. (1990). TGF-β induces bimodal proliferation of connective tissue cells via complex control of autocrine PDGF loop. *Cell*, 63, 515–24.

46. Gibbons, G.H., Pratt, R.E., and Dzau, V.J. (1992). Vascular smooth muscle cell hypertrophy vs. hyperplasia: autocrine transforming growth factor-β1 expression determine growth response to angiotensin II. *Journal of Clinical Investigation*, 90, 456–61.

47. Bassiouny, H.S., Song, R.H., Hong, X.F., Singh, A., Kocharyan, H., and Glagov, S. (1998). Flow regulation of 72-kD collagenase IV (MMP-2) after experimental arterial injury. *Circulation*, 98, 157–63.

48. Dzau, V.J. (1993). The role of mechanical and humoral factors in growth regulation of vascular smooth muscle and cardiac myocytes. *Current Opinion in Nephrology and Hypertension*, 2, 27–32.

49. Kaiser, D., Freyberg, M.A., and Friedl, P. (1997). Lack of hemodynamic forces triggers apoptosis in vascular endothelial cells. *Biochemical and Biophysical Research Communications*, 231, 586–91.

50. Birukov, K.G., Bardy, N., Lehoux, S., Merval, R., Shirinsky, V.P., and Tedgui, A. (1998). Intraluminal pressure is essential for the maintenance of smooth muscle calmodesmon and filamin content in aortic organ culture. *Arteriosclerosis Thrombosis and Vascular Biology*, 18, 922–7.

51. Williams, B. (1998). Mechanical influences on vascular smooth muscle cell function. *Journal of Hypertension*, 16, 1921–9.

52. Tozzi, C.A., Poiani, G.J., Harangozo, A.M., Boyd, C.D., and Riley, D.J. (1989). Pressure-induced connective tissue synthesis in pulmonary artery segments is dependent on intact endothelium. *Journal of Clinical Investigation*, 84, 1005–12.

53. Tronc, F., Wassef, M., Esposito, B., Henrion, D., Glagov, S., and Tedgui, A. (1996). Role of NO in flow-induced remodeling of the rabbit common carotid artery. *Arteriosclerosis Thrombosis and Vascular Biology*, 16, 1256–62.

54. Safar, M.E. and London, G.M. (1994). The arterial system in human hypertension. In *Textbook of hypertension* (ed. J.D. Swales), pp. 85–102. Blackwell Scientific, London.

55. Boutouyrie, P., Laurent, S., Girerd, X., Benetos, A., Lacolley, P., Abergel, E., *et al.* (1995). Common carotid artery stiffness and patterns of left ventricular hypertrophy in hypertensive patients. *Hypertension*, 25(Part 1), 651–9.

56. Lévy, B.I., Benessiano, J., Poitevin, P., and Safar, M.E. (1990). Endothelium-dependent mechanical properties of carotid artery in WKY and SHR: role of angiotensin converting enzyme inhibition. *Circulation Research*, 66, 321–8.

57. Lévy, B.I., El Fertak, L., Pieddeloup, Ch., Barouki, F., and Safar, M.E. (1993). Role of the endothelium in the mechanical response of the carotid arterial wall to calcium blockade in spontaneously hypertensive and Wistar–Kyoto rats. *Journal of Hypertension*, 11, 57–63.

58. Guyton, J.R. and Hartley, C.J. (1985). Flow restriction of one carotid artery in juvenile rats inhibits growth of arterial diameter. *American Journal of Physiology*, **248**, H540–6.

59. Langille, B.L. and O'Donnell, F. (1986). Reductions in arterial diameters produced by chronic decrease in blood flow are endothelium-dependent. *Science*, **231**, 405–7.

60. Tohda, K., Masuda, H., Kawamura, K., and Shozawa, T. (1992). Difference in dilatation between endothelium-preserved and -desquamated segments in the flow-loaded rat common carotid artery. *Arteriosclerosis and Thrombosis*, **12**, 519–28.

61. Bassiouny, H.S., Zarins, C.K., Kadowaki, M.H., and Glagov, S. (1994). Hemodynamic stress and experimental aortoiliac atherosclerosis. *Journal of Vascular Surgery*, **19**, 426–34.

62. Ross, R. (1999). Atherosclerosis—an inflammatory disease. *New England Journal of Medicine*, **340**, 115–26.

63. Selhub, J., Jacques, P.F., Bostom, A.G., D'Agostino, R.B., Wilson, P.W.F., Belanger, A.F., *et al.* (1995). Association between plasma homocysteine concentration and extracranial carotid-artery stenosis. *New England Journal of Medicine*, **332**, 286–91.

64. O'Rourke, M.F. (1995). Mechanical principles in arterial disease. *Hypertension*, **26**, 2–9.

65. Glagov, S., Zarins, C., Giddens, D.P., and Ku, D.N. (1988). Hemodynamics and atherosclerosis: insights and perspectives gained from the studies of human arteries. *Archives of Pathology and Laboratory Medicine*, **112**, 1018–31.

66. O'Rourke, M.F. (1982). *Arterial function in health and disease*. Churchill Livingstone, Edinburgh.

67. Batellier, J., Wassef, M., Merval, R., Duriez, M., and Tedgui, A. (1993). Protection from atherosclerosis in vein grafts by rigid external support. *Arteriosclerosis and Thrombosis*, **13**, 374–9.

68. Owens, G.K. and Reidy, M.A. (1985). Hyperplastic growth response of vascular smooth muscle cells following induction of acute hypertension in rats by aortic coarctation. *Circulation Research*, **57**, 695–705.

69. Ku, D.N., Giddens, D.P., Zarins, C.K., and Glagov, S. (1985). Pulsatile flow and atherosclerosis in the human carotid bifurcation: positive correlation between plaque location and low oscillating shear stress. *Arteriosclerosis*, **5**, 293–302.

70. Asakura, T. and Karino, T. (1990). Flow patterns and spatial distribution of atherosclerotic lesions in human coronary arteries. *Circulation Research*, **66**, 1045–66.

71. Moore, J.E. Jr., Xu, C., Glagov, S., Zarins, C.K., and Ku, D.N. (1994). Fluid wall shear stress measurements in a model of the human abdominal aorta: oscillatory behavior and relationship to atherosclerosis. *Atherosclerosis*, **110**, 225–40.

72. Fry, D.L. (1968). Acute vascular endothelial changes associated with increased blood flow velocity gradients. *Circulation Research*, **22**, 165–97.

73. Glagov, S. and Zarins, C.K. (1989). Is intimal hyperplasia an adaptive response or a pathologic process? Observations on the nature of nonatherosclerotic intimal thickening. *Journal of Vascular Surgery*, **10**, 571–3.

74. Barbee, K.A., Davies, P.F., and Lal, R. (1994). Shear stress-induced reorganization of the surface topography of living endothelial cells imaged by atomic force microscopy. *Circulation Research*, **74**, 163–71.

75. Sprague, E.A., Steinbach, B.L., Nerem, R.M., and Schwartz, C.J. (1987). Influence of a laminar steady-state fluid-imposed wall shear stress on the binding, internalization, and degradation of low-density lipoproteins by cultured arterial endothelium. *Circulation*, **76**, 648–56.

76. Caro, C.C. and Nerem, R.M. (1973). Transport of 14 C-4-cholesterol between serum and wall in the perfused dog common carotid artery. *Circulation Research*, **32**, 187–205.

77. Berceli, S.A, Warty, W.S., How, T., Merhi, Y., King, M., Guidoin, R., *et al.* (1990). Hemodynamics and low density lipoprotein metabolism: rates of low density lipoprotein incorporation and degradation along medial and lateral walls of the rabbit aortoiliac bifurcation. *Arteriosclerosis*, **10**, 686–94.

78. Krooker, E.J. and Wood, E.H. (1955). Comparison of simultaneously recorded central and peripheral arterial pressure pulses during rest, exercise and tilted position in man. *Circulation Research*, 3, 623–32.

79. Föstermann, U., Mügge, A., Albheid, U., Haverich, A., and Frölich, J.C. (1988). Selective attenuation of endothelium-mediated vasodilatation in atherosclerotic human coronary arteries. *Circulation Research*, 62, 185–90.

80. Panza, J.A., Quyyumi, A.A., Brush, J.E. Jr., and Epstein, S.E. (1990). Abnormal endothelium-dependent vascular relaxation in patients with essential hypertension. *New England Journal of Medicine*, 323, 22–7.

81. Kubo, S.H., Rector, T.S., Bank, A.J., Williams, R.E., and Heifetz, F.M. (1991). Endothelium-dependent vasodilation is attenuated in patients with heart failure. *Circulation*, 84, 1589–96.

82. Egashira, K., Horooka, Y., Kai, H., Sugimachi, M., Suzuki, S., Inou, T., *et al.* (1994). Reduction in serum cholesterol with pravastatin improves endothelium-dependent coronary vasomotion in patients with hypercholesterolemia. *Circulation*, 89, 2519–24.

83. Williams, S.B., Cusco, J.A., Roddy, M.A., Johnstone, M.T., and Creager, M.A. (1996). Impaired nitric oxide-mediated vasodilation in patients with non-insulin dependent diabetes mellitus. *Journal of the American College of Cardiology*, 27, 567–74.

84. Bush, D.E., Jones, C.E., Bass, K.M., Walters, G.K., Bruza, J.M., and Ouyang, P. (1998). Estrogen replacement reverses endothelial dysfunction in postmenopausal women. *American Journal of Medicine*, 104, 552–8.

85. Taddei, S, Virdin, A., Mattei, P., Ghiadoni, L., Gennari, A., Fasolo, C.B., *et al.* (1995). Aging and endothelial function in normotensive subjects and patients with essential hypertension. *Circulation*, 91, 1981–7.

86. Laurent, S., Girerd, X., Mourad, J.J., Lacolley, P., Beck, L., Boutouyrie, P., *et al.* (1994). Elastic modulus of the radial artery wall material is not increased in patients with essential hypertension. *Arteriosclerosis and Thrombosis*, 14, 1223–31.

87. Demuth, K., Blacher, J., Guérin, A.P., Benoit, M.-O., Moatti, N., Safar, M.F., *et al.* (1998). Endothelin and cardiovascular remodelling in end-stage renal disease. *Nephrology Dialysis Transplantation*, 13, 375–83.

88. Hoeks, A P.G., Brands, P.J., Smeets, F.A.M., and Reneman, R.S. (1990). Assessment of distensibility of superficial arteries. *Ultrasound in Medicine and Biology*, 16, 121–8.

89. Nichols, W.W., Avolio, A.P., Kelly, R.P., and O'Rourke, M.F. (1993). Effects of age and of hypertension on wave travel and reflections. In: *Arterial vasodilatation: mechanisms and therapy* (ed. M. O'Rourke, M. Safar, and V. Dzau), pp. 23–40. Edward Arnold, London.

90. Karamanoglu, M., O'Rourke, M.F., Avolio, A.P., and Kelly, R.P. (1993). An analysis of the relationship between central aortic and peripheral upper limb pressure waves in man. *European Heart Journal*, 14, 160–7.

91. Chen, C.H., Nevo, E., Fetics, B., Pak, P.H., Yin, F.C.P., Maughan, L., *et al.* (1997). Estimation of central aortic pressure waveform by mathematical transformation of radial tonometry pressure. Validation of generalized transfer function. *Circulation*, 95, 1827–36.

92. Avolio, A.O., Chen, S.G., Wang, R.P., Zhang, C.I., Li, M.F., and O'Rourke, M.F. (1983). Effects of aging on changing arterial compliance and left ventricular load in a northern Chinese urban community. *Circulation*, 68, 50–8.

93. Bramwell, J.V. and Hill, A.V. (1922). Velocity of transmission of the pulse wave and elasticity of arteries. *Lancet*, 1, 891–2.

94. Murgo, J.P., Westerhof, N., Giolma, J.P., and Altobelli, S.A. (1980). Aortic input impedance in normal man: relationship to pressure wave forms. *Circulation*, 62, 105–16.

95. Latham, R.D., Westerhof, N., Sipkema, P., Rubal, B.J., Reuderink, P., and Murgo, J.P. (1985). Regional wave travel and reflections along the human aorta: a study with six simultaneous micromanometric pressures. *Circulation*, 72, 1257–69.

96. O'Rourke, M.F. and Kelly, R.P. (1993). Wave reflections in systemic circulation and its implications in ventricular function. *Journal of Hypertension*, **11**, 327–37.

97. London, G.M. and Yaginuma, T. (1993). Wave reflections: clinical and therapeutic aspects. In *The arterial system in hypertension* (ed. M.E. Safar and M.F. O'Rourke), pp. 221–37. Kluwer Academic, Dordrecht.

98. Darne, B., Girerd, X., Safar, M., Cambien, F., and Guise, L. (1989). Pulsatile versus steady component of blood pressure: a cross-sectional analysis and prospective analysis on cardiovascular mortality. *Hypertension*, **13**, 392–400.

99. Madhavan, S., Ooi, W.L., Cohen, H., and Aldermen, M.H. (1994). Relation of pulse pressure and blood pressure reduction to the incidence of myocardial infarction. *Hypertension*, **23**, 395–401.

100. Benetos, A., Safar, M., Rudnichi, A., Smulyan, H., Richard, J.L., Ducimetiere, P., *et al.* (1997). Pulse pressure: a predictor of long-term cardiovascular mortality in a French male population. *Hypertension*, **30**, 1410–15.

101. Mitchell, G.F., Moye, L.M., Braunwald, E., Rouleau, J.-L., Bernstein, V., Geltman, E.M., *et al.* (1997). Sphygmomanometrically determined pulse pressure is a powerful independent predictor of recurrent events after myocardial infarction in patients with impaired left ventricular function. *Circulation*, **96**, 4254–60.

102. Burattini, R., Knowlen, G.G., and Campbell, K.B. (1991). Two arterial effective reflecting sites may appear as one to the heart. *Circulation Research*, **68**, 85–99.

103. London, G.M., Guerin, A.P., Pannier, B., Marchais, S.J., Benetos, A., and Safar, M.E. (1992). Increased systolic pressure in chronic uremia: role of arterial wave reflections. *Hypertension*, **20**, 10–19.

104. Buckberg, G.D., Towers, B., Paglia, D.E., Mulder, D.G., and Maloney, J.V. (1972). Subendocardial ischemia after cardiopulmonary bypass. *Journal of Thoracic and Cardiovascular Surgery*, **64**, 669–87.

105. Watanabe, H., Ohtsuka, S., Kakihana, M., and Sugishita, Y. (1993). Coronary circulation in dogs with an experimental decrease in aortic compliance. *Journal of the American College of Cardiology*, **21**, 1497–506.

106. Chang, K.C., Tseng, Y.Z., Kuo, T.S., and Chen, H.I. (1994). Impaired left ventricular relaxation and arterial stiffness in patients with essential hypertension. *Clinical science*, **87**, 641–7.

107. Boutouyrie, P., Bezie, Y., Lacolley, P., Challande, P., Chamiot-Clerc, P., Benetos, A., *et al.* (1997). *In vivo/in vitro* comparison of rat abdominal aorta wall viscosity: influence of endothelial function. *Arteriosclerosis Thrombosis and Vascular Biology*, **17**, 1346–55.

108. Vaitkevicius, P.V., Fleg, J.L., Engel, J.H., O'Connor, F.C., Wright, J.G., Lakatta, L.E., *et al.* (1993). Effects of age and aerobic capacity on arterial stiffness in healthy adults. *Circulation*, **88**(Part 1), 1456–62.

109. Feldman, S.A. and Glagov, S. (1971). Transmedial collagen and elastin gradient in human aortas: reversal with age. *Atherosclerosis*, **13**, 385–94.

110. Guyton, J.R., Lindsay, K.L., and Dao, D.T. (1983). Comparison of aortic intima and inner media in young adults versus aging rats. *American Journal of Pathology*, **111**, 234–6.

111. Tedgui, A. and Lévy, B. (1994). Influence des facteurs mécaniques sur la biologie du vaisseau. In *Biologie de la paroi artérielle: aspects normaux et pathologiques*, pp. 35–43. Masson, Paris.

112. Rossi, A., Bonfante, L., Giacomini, A, Calabro, A., Rossi, G., Saller, A., *et al.* (1996). Carotid artery lesions in patients with nondiabetic chronic renal failure. *American Journal of Kidney Diseases*, **27**, 58–66.

113. Pascazio, L., Bianco, F., Giorgini, A., Galli, G., Curri, G., and Panzetta, G. (1996). Echo color doppler imaging of carotid vessels in hemodialysis patients: evidence of high levels of atherosclerotic lesions. *American Journal of Kidney Diseases*, **28**, 713–20.

114. London, G.M. and Drüeke, T.B. (1997). Atherosclerosis and arteriosclerosis in chronic renal failure. *Kidney International*, **51**, 1678–95.

115. Savage, T., Clarke, A.L., Giles, M., Tomson, C.R.V., and Raine, A.E.G. (1998). Calcified plaque is common in the carotid and femoral arteries of dialysis patients without clinical vascular disease. *Nephrology Dialysis Transplantation*, **13**, 2004–12.

116. Lindner, A., Charra, B., Sherrard, D., and Scribner, B.M. (1974). Accelerated atherosclerosis in prolonged maintenance hemodialysis. *New England Journal of Medicine*, **290**, 697–702.

117. Joki, N., Nakamura, R., and Yamaguchi, T. (1997). Onset of coronary artery disease prior to initiation of haemodialysis in patients with end-stage renal disease. *Nephrology Dialysis Transplantation*, **12**, 718–23.

118. Vincenti, F., Amend, W.J., Abele, J., Feduska, N.J., and Salvatierra, O. Jr. (1980). The role of hypertension in hemodialysis-associated atherosclerosis. *American Journal of Medicine*, **68**, 363–9.

119. Parfrey, P.S., Foley, R.N., Harnett, J.D., Kent, M.G., Murray, D.C., and Barre, P.E. (1996). Outcome and risk factors of ischemic heart disease in chronic uremia. *Kidney International*, **49**, 1428–34.

120. Barenbrock, M., Spieker, C., Laske, V., Baumgart, P., Hoeks, A.P.G., Zidek, W., et al. (1993). Effect of long-term hemodialysis on arterial compliance in end-stage renal failure. *Nephron*, **65**, 249–53.

121. Kawagishi, T., Nishizawa, Y., Konishi, T., Kawasaki, K., Emoto, M., Shoji, T., et al. (1995). High-resolution B-mode ultrasonography in evaluation of atherosclerosis in uremia. *Kidney International*, **48**, 820–6.

122. Joannides, R., Bakkali, E.H., Le Roy, F., Rivault, O., Godin, M., Moore, N., et al. (1997). Altered flow-dependent vasodilatation of conduit arteries in maintenance haemodialysis. *Nephrology Dialysis Transplantation*, **12**, 2623–8.

123. Mourad, J.J., Girerd, X., Boutouyrie, P., Laurent, S., Safar, M.E., and London, G.M. (1997). Increased stiffness of radial artery wall material in end-stage renal disease. *Hypertension*, **30**, 1425–30.

124. London, G.M., Marchais, S.J., Safar, M.E., Genest, A.F., Guerin, A.P., Métivier, F., et al. (1990). Aortic and large artery compliance in end-stage renal failure. *Kidney International*, **37**, 137–42.

125. Saito, Y., Shirai, K., Uchino, J., Okazawa, M., Hattori, Y., Yoshida, T., et al. (1990). Effect of nifedipine administration on pulse wave velocity (PWV) of chronic hemodialysis patients 2-year trial. *Cardiovascular Drug Therapy*, **4**, 987–90.

126. Luik, A.J., Spek, J.J., Charra, B., van Bortel, L.M.A.B., Laurent, G., and Leunissen, K.M.L. (1997). Arterial compliance in patients on long-time dialysis. *Nephrology Dialysis Transplantation*, **12**, 2629–32.

127. Barenbrock, M., Hausberg, M., Kosch, M., Kisters, K., Hoeks, A.P.G., and Rahn, K.-H. (1998). Effect of hyperparathyroidism on arterial distensibility in renal transplant recipients. *Kidney International*, **54**, 210–15.

128. London, G.M. and Parfrey, P.S. (1997). Cardiac disease in chronic uremia: pathogenesis. *Advances in Renal Replacement Therapy*, **4**, 194–211.

129. Gu, J.W., Anand, V., Shek, E.W., Moore, M.C., Brady, A.L., Kelly, W.C., et al. (1998). Sodium induces hypertrophy of cultured myocardial myoblasts and vascular smooth muscle cells. *Hypertension*, **31**, 1083–7.

130. Safar, M.E., Asmar, R.G., Benetos, A., London, G.M., and Lévy, B.I. (1992). Sodium, large arteries and diuretic compounds in hypertension. *Journal of Hypertension*, **10**(Suppl. 6), S133–6.

131. Guérin, A.P., Pannier, B., Marchais, S.J., Métivier, F., and London, G.M. (1998). Arterial remodeling and cardiovascular function in end-stage renal disease. In *Advances in Nephrology*, Vol. 27 (ed. J.P. Grünfeld, J.F. Bach, H. Kreis, and M.H. Maxwell), pp. 105–9. Mosby-Year Book, Inc., St Louis.

132. Hayoz, D., Rutschmann, B., Perret, F., Niederberger, M., Tardy, Y., Mooser, V. et al. (1992). Conduit artery compliance and distensibility are not necessarily reduced in hypertension. *Hypertension*, **20**, 1–6.

133. Ibels, L.S., Alfrey, A.L., Huffer, W.E., Craswell, P.W., Anderson, J.T., and Weil, R. (1979). Arterial calcification and pathology in uremic patients undergoing dialysis. *American Journal of Medicine*, **66**, 790–6.

134. Meema, H.E. and Oreopoulos, D.G. (1986). Morphology, progression, and regression of arterial and periarterial calcifications in patients with end-stage renal disease. *Radiology*, **158**, 671–7.

135. Amann, K., Neusüß, R., Ritz, E., Irzyniec, T., Wiest, G., and Mall, G. (1995). Changes of vascular architecture independent of blood pressure in experimental uremia. *American Journal of Hypertension*, **8**, 409–17.

136. Amann, K., Törnig, J., Flechtenmacher, C., Nabokov, A., Mall, G., and Ritz, E. (1995). Blood-pressure-independent wall thickening of intramyocardial arterioles in experimental uremia: evidence for a permissive action of PTH. *Nephrology Dialysis Transplantation*, **10**, 2043–8.

137. Amann, K., Wolf, B., Nichols, C., Törnig, J., Schwartz, U., Zeier, M., *et al.* (1997). Aortic changes in experimental renal failure: hyperplasia or hypertrophy of smooth muscle cells? *Hypertension*, **29**, 770–5.

138. Bradley, J.R., Evans, D.B., and Cowley, A.J. (1988). Abnormalities in the peripheral circulation in patients with chronic renal failure. *Nephrology Dialysis Transplantation*, **3**, 412–16.

139. van Guldener, C., Lambert, J., Janssen, M.J., Donker, A.J., and Stehouwer, C.D. (1997). Endothelium-dependent vasodilatation and distensibility of large arteries in chronic hemodialysis patients. *Nephrology Dialysis Transplantation*, **12**(Suppl. 2), S14–18.

140. van Guldener, C., Janssen, M.J.F., Lambert, J., Steyn, M., Donker, A.J.N., and Stehouwer, C.D.A. (1998). Endothelium-dependent vasodilatation is impaired in peritoneal dialysis patients. *Nephrology Dialysis Transplantation*, **13**, 1782–6.

141. van Guldener, C., Janssen, M.J., Lambert, J., ter Wee, P.M., Jakobs, C., Donker, A.J., *et al.* (1998). No change in impaired endothelial function after long-term folic acid therapy of hyperhomocysteinemia in hemodialysis patients. *Nephrology Dialysis Transplantation*, **13**, 106–12.

142. Wilkinson, S.P., Spence, V.A., and Stewart, W.K. (1989). Arterial stiffening and reduced cutaneous hyperaemic response in patients with end-stage renal failure. *Nephron*, **52**, 149–53.

143. Hand, M.F., Haynes, W.G., and Webb, D.J. (1998). Hemodialysis and L-arginine, but not D-arginine, correct renal failure-associated endothelial dysfunction. *Kidney International*, **53**, 1068–77.

144. Nakayama, M., Yamada, K., Yamamoto, Y., Yokoyama, K., Nakano, H., Kubo, H., *et al.* (1994). Vascular endothelial dysfunction in patients on regular dialysis treatment. *Clinical Nephrology*, **42**, 117–20.

145. Gris, J.C., Branger, B., Vécina, F., Sabadani, B.A., Fourcade, J., and Schved, J.F. (1994). Increased cardiovascular risk factors and features of endothelial activation and dysfunction in dialyzed uremic patients. *Kidney International*, **46**, 807–13.

146. Haaber, A.B., Eidemak, I., Jensen, T., Feldt-Rasmussen, B., and Strandgaard, S. (1995). Vascular endothelial cell function and cardiovascular risk factors in patients with chronic renal failure. *Journal of American Society of Nephrology*, **5**, 1581–4.

147. Tomura, S., Nakamura, Y., Doi, M., Ando, R., Ida, T., Chida, Y., *et al.* (1996). Fibrinogen, coagulation factor VII, tissue plasminogen activator, plasminogen activator inhibitor-1, and lipid as cardiovascular risk factors in chronic hemodialysis and continuous ambulatory peritoneal dialysis patients. *American Journal of Kidney Diseases*, **27**, 848–54.

148. Yoshizumi, M., Kurihara, H., Sugiyama, T., Takaku, F., Yanagisawa, M., Masaki, T., *et al.* (1989). Hemodynamic shear stress stimulates endothelin production by cultured endothelial cells. *Biochemical and Biophysical Research Communications*, **161**, 859–64.

149. Witko-Sarsat, V., Friedlander, M., Capeillère-Blandin, Ch., Nguyen-Khoa, T., Nguyen, A.T., Zingraff, J., *et al.* (1996). Advanced oxidation protein products as a novel marker of oxidative stress in uremia. *Kidney International*, **49**, 1304–13.

150. Aznar-Salatti, J., Escolar, G., Cases, A., Gomez-Ortiz, G., Anton, P., Castillo, R., *et al.* (1995). Uraemic medium causes endothelial cell dysfunction characterized by an alteration of the properties of its subendothelial matrix. *Nephrology Dialysis Transplantation*, **10**, 2199–204.

151. Levin, R.I., Kantoff, P.W., and Jaffe, E.A. (1990). Uremic levels of oxalic acid suppress replication and migration of human endothelial cells. *Arteriosclerosis*, **10**, 198–207.

152. Vallance, P., Leone, A., Calver, A., Collier, J., and Moncada, S. (1992). Accumulation of an endogenous inhibitor of nitric oxide synthesis in chronic renal failure. *Lancet*, **339**, 572–5.

153. Arese, M., Strasly, M., Ruva, C., Costamagna, C., Ghigo, D., MacAllister, R., et al. (1995). Regulation of nitric oxide synthesis in uraemia. *Nephrology Dialysis Transplantation*, **10**, 1386–97.

154. Boulanger, C., and Lüscher, T.F. (1990). Release of endothelin from the porcine aorta. Inhibition of endothelium-derived nitric oxide. *Journal of Clinical Investigation*, **85**, 587–90.

155. Woo, K.S., Chook, P., Lolin, Y.I., Cheung, A.S.P., Chan, L.T., Sun, Y.Y., et al. (1997). Hyperhomocyst(e)inemia is a risk factor for arterial endothelial dysfunction in humans. *Circulation*, **96**, 2542–4.

156. Welch, G.N. and Loscalzo, J. (1998). Homocysteine and atherothrombosis. *New England Journal of Medicine*, **338**, 1042–50.

157. Chauveau, P., Chadefaux, B., Coudé, M., Aupetit, J., Hannedouche, T., Kamoun, P., et al. (1992). Increased plasma homocystcine concentration in patients with chronic renal failure. *Mineral and Electrolyte Metabolism*, **18**, 196–8.

158. Bostom, A.G. and Lathrop, L. (1997). Hyperhomocysteinemia in end-stage renal disease: prevalence, etiology, and potential relationship to arteriosclerotic outcomes. *Kidney International*, **52**, 10–20.

159. Blacher, J., Demuth, K., Guerin, A.P., Safar, M.E., Moatti, N., and London GM. (1998). Influence of biochemical alterations on arterial stiffness in patients with end-stage renal disease. *Arteriosclerosis Thrombosis and Vascular Biology*, **18**, 535–41.

160. Gilchrest, B.A., Rowe, J.W., and Mihm, M.C. (1980). Clinical and histological skin changes in chronic renal failure: evidence for a dialysis-resistant, transplant-responsive microangiopathy. *Lancet*, **2**, 1271–5.

161. Aalkjaer, C., Pedersen, E.B., Danielsen, H., Fjeldborg, O., Jespersen, B., Kjaer, T., et al. (1986). Morphological and functional characteristics of isolated resistance vessels in advanced uraemia. *Clinical Science*, **71**, 657–63.

162. Ichimaru, K. and Horie, A. (1987). Microangiopathic changes of subepidermal capillaries in end-stage renal failure. *Nephron*, **46**, 144–9.

163. Li, P.F., Dietz, R., and von Harsdorf, R. (1997). Differential effect of hydrogen peroxide and superoxide anion on apoptosis and proliferation of vascular smooth muscle cells. *Circulation*, **96**, 3602–9.

164. Burdick, L., Periti, M., Salvaggio, A., Bertoli, S., Mangiarotti, R., Castagnone, D., et al. (1994). Relation between carotid artery atherosclerosis and time on dialysis. A non-invasive study *in vivo*. *Clinical Nephrology*, **42**, 121–6.

165. Nishizawa, Y., Shoji, T., Kawagishi, T., and Morii, H. (1997). Atherosclerosis in uremia: possible roles of hyperparathyroidism and intermediate density lipoprotein accumulation. *Kidney International*, **52**(Suppl. 2), S90–2.

166. Amann, K., Wiest, G., Klaus, G., Ritz, E., and Mall, G. (1994). The role of parathyroid hormone in the genesis of interstitial cell activation in uremia. *Journal of the American Society of Nephrology*, **4**, 1814–19.

167. Schluter, K.D. and Piper, H.M. (1998). Cardiovascular action of parathyroid hormone and parathyroid hormone-related peptide. *Cardiovascular Research*, **37**, 34–41.

168. Marchais, S.J., Guérin, A.P., Pannier, B.M., Lévy, B.I., Safar, M.E., and London, G.M. (1993). Wave reflections and cardiac hypertrophy in chronic uremia: influence of body size. *Hypertension*, **22**, 876–83.

169. London, G.M. (1998). The concept of ventricular/vascular coupling: functional and structural alterations of the heart and arterial vessels go in parallel. *Nephrology Dialysis Transplantation*, **13**, 250–3.

170. London, G.M., Guérin, A.P., and Marchais, S.J. (1999). Hemodynamic overload in end-stage renal disease. *Seminars in Dialysis*, **12**, 77–83.

171. Blacher, J., Guérin, A.P., Pannier, B., Marchais, S.J., Safar, M.E., and London, G.M. (1999). Impact of aortic stiffness on survival in end-stage renal disease. *Circulation*, **99**, 2434–39.

172. Blacher, J., Pannier, B., Guerin, A.P., Marchais, S.J., Safar, M.E., and London, G.M. (1998). Carotid arterial stiffness as a predictor of cardiovascular and all-cause mortality in end-stage renal disease. *Hypertension*, **32**, 570–7.

173. Marchais, S., Guérin, A., Safar, M., and London, G. (1989). Arterial compliance in uremia. *Journal of Hypertension*, **7**(Suppl. 6), S84–5.

174. Girerd, X., Giannattassio, C., Moulin, C., Safar, M., Mancia, G., and Laurent, S. (1998). Regression of radial artery wall hypertrophy and improvement of carotid artery compliance after long-term antihypertensive treatment in elderly patients. *Journal of the American College of Cardiology*, **31**, 1063–73.

175. London, G.M., Marchais, S.J., Guerin, A.P., Métivier, F., Safar, M.E., Fabiani, F., *et al.* (1990). Salt and water retention and calcium blockade in uremia. *Circulation*, **82**, 105–13.

176. Marchais, S.J., Boussac, I., Guerin, A.P., Delavaux, G., Métivier, F., and London, G.M. (1991). Arteriosclerosis and antihypertensive response to calcium antagonists in end-stage renal failure. *Journal of Cardiovascular Pharmacology*, **18**(Suppl. 5), S14–18.

177. London, G.M., Pannier, B., Guerin, A.P., Marchais, S.J., Safar, M.E., and Cuche, J.L. (1994). Cardiac hypertrophy, aortic compliance, peripheral resistance, and wave reflection in end-stage renal disease: comparative effects of ACE inhibition and calcium channel blockade. *Circulation*, **90**, 2786–96.

178. London, G.M., Pannier, B., Vicaut, E., Guérin, A.P., Marchais, S.J., Safar, M.E., *et al.* (1996). Antihypertensive effects and arterial haemodynamic alterations during angiotensin converting enzyme inhibition. *Journal of Hypertension*, **14**, 1139–46.

6

Endothelial function in end-stage renal failure

Helene L. Glassberg and Joseph Loscalzo

The vascular endothelium regulates vascular function through synthesis and local release of several substances, including endothelium-derived relaxing factor (EDRF)/nitric oxide (NO), prostacyclin, and endothelium-derived hyperpolarizing factor (EDHF), that modulate vascular tone and vascular remodeling. Through elaboration of these factors, the normal endothelium supports vasodilation, inhibition of platelet activation, and inhibition of leukocyte adhesion and intimal proliferation, and helps to maintain blood fluidity and tissue perfusion.

Alteration in the production or activity of these regulatory effectors or frank injury to the endothelium, however, can substantially contribute to the pathophysiology of many vascular diseases. In patients with renal failure, coronary artery disease and other atherosclerotic and thrombotic vascular complications are a major cause of morbidity and mortality. In the presence of end-stage renal failure (ESRF), significant perturbations in normal endothelial mechanisms can occur. Independent of the traditional cardiovascular risk factors that are frequently present in patients with renal failure, endothelial dysfunction or injury directly related to the specific pathobiology of ESRF may provide an explanation for the excess burden of atherothrombotic disease that occurs in these patients. In this chapter, we will review both the normal and pathophysiological states of the endothelium and how each relates to the development of the vascular complications of ESRF.

Normal endothelial function (Table 6.1)

EDRF/NO

EDRF, as first described by Furchgott and Zawadzki[1] in 1980, was shown to account for the vascular smooth muscle relaxation response to muscarinic agonists in isolated rabbit aorta.

Table 6.1

Normal endothelial function
Maintain vascular tone
Modulate intimal growth and vascular remodeling
Regulate hemostasis and thrombosis
Mediate inflammation and immune mechanisms
Inhibit leukocyte and platelet adherence
Modulate lipid oxidation and oxygen-derived free radical production

Furthermore, these investigators noted that removing the endothelium from isolated blood vessels prevented acetylcholine-induced relaxation. They subsequently showed that acetylcholine released a soluble factor from the endothelium, termed endothelium-derived relaxing factor (EDRF). EDRF was later identified as nitric oxide (NO)[2,3] or a closely related redox form of NO.[4] Nitric oxide, which is derived from the oxidative metabolism of L-arginine, relaxes vascular smooth muscle by activating soluble guanylyl cyclase and increasing intracellular cyclic 3',5'-guanosine monophosphate (cGMP) concentration. Physiological stimuli (e.g. shear stress) and endogenous mediators (e.g. serotonin, thrombin, acetylcholine, bradykinin, substance P, and α-adrenergic agonists) that act through specific endothelial cell membrane receptors lead to increased release of NO, resulting in vasodilation and maintenance of vascular patency.[5] There are many actions of NO beyond its role as a vasodilator that are important for normal vascular homeostasis, including inhibition of platelet activation and thrombosis[6,7,8] and impairment of leukocyte adhesion.[9-12]

NO is a reactive free radical species that is synthesized during the oxidation of L-arginine to L-citrulline in endothelial cells.[13] The reaction is catalyzed by the enzyme family, the NO synthases (NOS). There are two main isoform classes of NOS. One is a constitutive enzyme (cNOS) class, which is made up of the endothelial form (eNOS) and the neuronal form (nNOS). In the endothelium, agonists such as acetylcholine and bradykinin activate the phosphoinositide second messenger system, stimulating inositol (1,4,5)-trisphosphate (IP$_3$) production and binding to receptors on the endoplasmic reticulum.[14] Calcium is then released from intracellular stores, binds to calmodulin, and activates cNOS, which produces NO until calcium levels decrease.[15-17] Owing to the continuous production of NO in the basal state, cNOS helps to maintain resting vascular tone.[18]

The other main isoform of NOS is an inducible enzyme (iNOS) found in macrophages,[19] neutrophils,[20] and many other cell types. The expression of iNOS is induced by inflammatory stimuli, such as bacterial endotoxin and cytokines.[21] iNOS is not affected by intracellular calcium levels owing to the effectively irreversible complexation of calcium–calmodulin to the enzyme, and is capable of generating significantly greater amounts of NO than cNOS.[22]

A key mechanism by which vascular diseases may influence endothelial NO production is by promoting protein kinase C (PKC) activation, which phosphorylates NOS and thereby reduces NOS catalytic activity.[23] PKC also inhibits the increase in calcium after endothelial cell stimulation.[24-26]

In addition, there exists an endogenous NO inhibitor, asymmetric dimethylarginine (ADMA), which may modulate endothelial NO production and action. In rats, central administration of N-l-ω-nitro-L-arginine methylester (L-NAME), an exogenous NOS inhibitor, and ADMA inhibited the baroreflex, indicating a central role for NO in regulating baroreflex function. By contrast, peripheral intravenous administration of ADMA increases mean arterial blood pressure similar to L-NAME, indicating that ADMA inhibits endothelial NO production by eNOS. This finding suggests that ADMA both inhibits NO production and contributes to regulating cardiovascular function by central mechanisms.[27]

Shear stress and stretch forces exerted on endothelial cells by blood flow and pressure, respectively, also modulate NO release. An increase in blood flow appears to activate shear-sensitive calcium-dependent potassium channels to induce NO release.[28-32] Under normal physiological conditions, shear stress and stretch are probably responsible for tonic, basal release of NO. Direct evidence for the continuous release of NO is provided by the observation that inhibitors of NO synthesis, such as N^G-monomethyl-L-arginine (L-NMMA), cause vasoconstriction and hypertension.[33-36] This finding suggests that continuous endothelial production of NO is involved in regulating vascular tone and blood pressure. Nishida and co-workers[37] showed that shear stress upregulates steady-state eNOS mRNA levels in cultured bovine aortic endothelial cells. Furthermore, Awolesi and colleagues[38] showed that subjecting cultured bovine aortic endothelial cells to cyclic strain increases eNOS gene expression, protein, and activity. The clinical implication of these findings is that not only do shear stress and stretch contribute to the tonic release of NO, but also strain-induced increases in eNOS may contribute to the beneficial effect of exercise on cardiovascular disease. Chronic exercise in dogs increases coronary vascular NO production, and the enhanced NO production is associated with an increase in eNOS expression in aortic endothelial cells, suggesting that exercise-related elevations of vascular flow rates can upregulate eNOS production.[39] By increasing the release of NO, shear stress augments endothelium-dependent vasodilation and potentially inhibits processes involved in atherogenesis.

There is also evidence for the tonic release of NO by arterial endothelium even in the absence of humoral or physical stimuli:[40,41] inhibition of NO or removal of the endothelium leads to greater smooth muscle contraction in response to submaximal stimuli while maximal response is maintained.[40-43] NO plays a major role in regulating the vascular tone of coronary resistance vessels,[44] as well as the mesenteric, carotid, and renal arterial beds.[45] It also appears to be involved in the autoregulation of blood flow in the heart, brain, and kidney.[46]

In addition to the basal release of NO, endothelial cells produce NO in response to several physiological stimuli, including thrombin, substances released from activated platelets, changes in oxygen tension, and, as already mentioned, shear stress. Shear stress stimulates NO release via calcium-sensitive potassium channels on the endothelium that act as mechanochemical receptors, and NO activity appears to be highest in large-diameter arteries subject to the greatest changes in flow and shear stress.[29,31,47]

NO may also participate in the regulation of vascular tone by the autonomic nervous system. NO has been identified in the parasympathetic nerves of the cerebral and retinal arteries, where it probably contributes to the neural regulation of vascular tone.[48] Balligand and co-workers[49] showed that NO modulates rat myocytes' responsiveness to adrenergic and cholinergic stimuli, and that NOS inhibition enhances the inotropic effect of the β-agonist isoproterenol.

In addition to its direct effect as a vasodilator, NO also regulates vascular tone by mediating the expression of growth factors with acute effects on vascular tone.[50] Hypoxia induces the production and secretion of endothelin (ET-1)[51] and platelet-derived growth factor (PDGF-B),[52] both mitogens with vasoconstrictive properties. NO both regulates the expression of these substances and suppresses their production.[50]

NO also helps to maintain blood flow and tissue perfusion by inhibiting platelet aggregation. The production and release of NO is stimulated by products released from activated platelets (e.g. serotonin, ADP) or by coagulation determinants, such as thrombin.[53] NO diffuses into the vessel lumen and interacts with platelets, inhibiting their function by activating guanylyl cyclase and increasing cGMP.[54]

There is increasing evidence that NO also plays a role in inhibiting neutrophil aggregation[55] and leukocyte adhesion to the endothelium.[10] The effects of NO on neutrophils are related to inactivation of the superoxide anion.[56] The superoxide anion activates mast cells, causing degranulation and leukocyte adhesion to the vascular endothelium.[57,58] NO inhibits this process by reacting with and inactivating the superoxide anion, producing peroxynitrite in the process. When production of the superoxide anion is excessive, however, the availability and action of NO are attenuated. Recent studies suggest that an important mechanism of impaired NO action in atherosclerosis is increased oxidative stress.[59] Increased production of reactive oxygen species, including the superoxide anion and lipid peroxyl radicals, and oxidation of low-density lipoprotein (LDL) by these species may lead to impaired NO action through several mechanisms. The superoxide anion reacts with NO, limiting its biological activity.[60-62] Furthermore, in several disease states it has been shown that superoxide anion scavengers improve the abnormal endothelium-dependent responses.[63-69]

The vascular endothelium also regulates cell growth in the vascular wall, and several endothelial factors promote or inhibit smooth muscle cell proliferation. Mechanical removal of the endothelium is followed by proliferation of the intima.[70,71] Furthermore, the extent of intimal proliferation following femoral balloon injury in hypercholesterolemic rabbits is inversely correlated with the degree of relaxation in response to acetylcholine.[72] This finding suggested that the release of EDRF or other endothelium-dependent vasodilators may contribute to suppression of intimal growth. NO may inhibit smooth muscle cell proliferation by a variety of mechanisms, including inhibition of ribonucleotide reductase, which is rate-limiting for nucleic acid synthesis,[73] impairment of electron transport, and impairment of aerobic glycolysis by promoting ADP-ribosylation of glyceraldehyde-3-phosphate dehydrogenase (GAPDH).[74]

The ability of NO to inhibit intimal growth is both a primary action and a consequence of the inhibition of platelet aggregation and leukocyte adhesion. L-Arginine, the substrate for NOS in the production of NO, has been demonstrated to inhibit intimal proliferation after balloon injury in rats.[75] Schwarzacher and co-workers[76] showed that a single intramural administration of L-arginine enhanced NO production and reduced intimal thickening due to suppression of macrophage accumulation at the site of balloon injury in rabbits. In hypercholesterolemic rabbits, dietary arginine reduced intimal thickening in balloon-injured vessels and substantially inhibited macrophage accumulation in the lesion.[77] Finally, the endothelium may inhibit intimal growth through the synthesis of heparan sulfate proteoglycans.[78]

Other vasorelaxant factors (Table 6.2)

In addition to EDRF/NO, the vascular endothelium also produces other vasorelaxing factors, such as prostacyclin and EDHF. Prostaglandins are produced when arachidonic acid is liberated from calcium-activated phospholipase A_2. Arachidonic acid is then converted to prostaglandin G_2 and prostaglandin H_2 by cyclooxygenase and, subsequently, to other prostaglandins. The most abundant prostanoid product of this pathway, prostacyclin, relaxes vascular smooth muscle and inhibits platelet aggregation by activating adenylyl cyclase and increasing cyclic $3',5'$-adenosine monophosphate (cAMP). The prostanoids all have vasoconstricting capability; however, the most potent vasoconstrictors are thromboxane A_2 and the endoperoxide intermediate prostaglandins (PGs) PGG_2 and PGH_2. EDRF/NO and prosta-

Table 6.2

Vasodilators	Vasoconstrictors
NO	TXA_2
Prostacyclin	PGG_2 and PGH_2
EDHF	endothelin
	Angiotensin II

cyclin indirectly limit the vasoconstrictor effect of thromboxane A_2 by inhibiting platelet activation and adhesion.

Another vasoactive mediator released from the endothelium by a calcium-dependent process similar to that for NO is EDHF,[79–82] which hyperpolarizes vascular smooth muscle cells by stimulating potassium efflux through potassium channels causing vasodilation. Hyperpolarization of the cell membrane inhibits calcium entry into the cells, thereby causing vasorelaxation.[83,84]

In addition to these mediators, endothelial cells also produce vasoconstrictor substances, including endothelin, endothelium-derived constricting factor (EDCF), and angiotensin II. All of these factors act in combination with EDRF to modulate vasomotor tone and vascular structure.

Other factors regulating hemostasis and thrombosis

The endothelium also participates in the regulation of hemostasis and fibrinolysis. Circulating platelets, coagulation factors, and the endothelial wall are the three major determinants of hemostasis. The intact endothelial lining possesses effective antithrombotic properties physiologically critical for maintaining blood fluidity. However, injury to endothelial cells can promote hemostasis by releasing von Willebrand factor (vWF) and plasminogen activator inhibitor type-1 (PAI-1), expressing procoagulant molecules including tissue factor, and binding some of the coagulation factors. Tissue-type plasminogen activator (tPA), which converts plasminogen to plasmin, thereby promoting degradation of fibrin, is a 72-kDa serine protease that is synthesized and secreted basally by endothelial cells.[85] t-PA receptors on endothelial cells localize plasminogen activation to the endothelial surface and enhance local antithrombotic effects.[86] PAI-1, a 52 kDa glycoprotein synthesized by endothelial cells[87] and platelets,[88] acts to inhibit t-PA in plasma.[89] The endothelium also regulates thrombosis through the synthesis of vWF, which carries factor VIII in plasma. vWF mediates platelet adhesion to injured vessel surfaces, incorporating platelets into evolving thrombi.[90] Other anticoagulation functions of the endothelium include the production of heparan sulfate proteoglycans[91] and enhanced activation of protein-C by thrombin when the latter is bound to thrombomodulin on the endothelial cell surface.[92]

The endothelium regulates platelet activity through the release of NO and prostacyclin. Disruption of the endothelium attracts platelets, which adhere to the vessel wall, primarily mediated by vWF.[93] Exposure of subendothelial collagen and loss of NO activity promote this process of platelet adhesion. Activated platelets then release products that promote further platelet activation, recruitment, and formation of a platelet plug. Factors that impair NO vasodilator activity may lead to increased platelet aggregation, promoting thrombus formation and potentially furthering the development of atherothrombotic disease.

Endothelial regulation of hemostasis and fibrinolysis is altered in hypercholesterolemia and atherosclerosis. Increased circulating levels of t-PA were associated with an increased risk for myocardial infarction in healthy males in the Physicians' Health Study.[94] In a group of patients with documented coronary artery disease and angina, t-PA levels predicted cardiovascular events.[95] PAI-1 level and activity are also increased in patients with coronary artery disease, suggesting a predisposition for thrombosis.

Vaughan and colleagues[97] demonstrated that the vascular renin–angiotensin system also influences fibrinolysis. Angiotensin II induces the release of PAI-1 from cultured endothelial cells[96] and increases circulating levels of PAI-1 in hypertensive subjects. Two clinical trials examining outcomes of patients with left ventricular dysfunction following myocardial infarction treated with an angiotensin-converting enzyme inhibitor showed a reduction in recurrent myocardial infarction, possibly by reducing coronary thrombosis through diminished angiotensin II formation, thereby reducing PAI-1 release.[98,99]

Finally, vascular endothelial cells modulate hemostasis by releasing tissue factor, a membrane protein that activates coagulation through association with factor VII. Typically, levels of tissue factor are undetectable in normal endothelial cells, but can be induced in cultured cells by a variety of agonists, cytokines, and oxidized LDL.[100]

Endothelial function, NO, and the kidney

The endothelium plays a major role in the regulation of renal hemodynamics, sodium handling, natriuresis, and excretory function. The normal endothelium's ability to maintain the appropriate balance of vasorelaxing and vasodilating mediators and to influence hemostasis

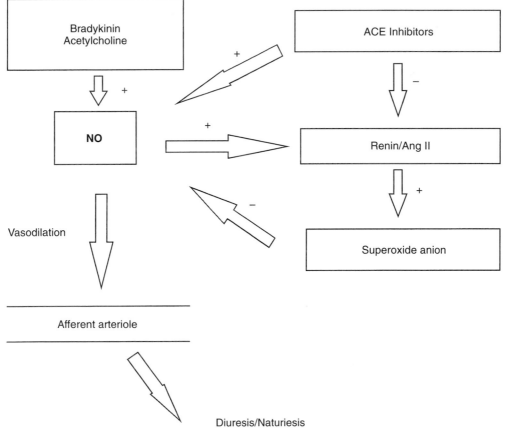

Fig. 6.1 Effects of nitric oxide (NO) on renal function. ACE, angiotensin-converting enzyme; Ang II, angiotensin II.

and cellular proliferative responses significantly contributes to regulating renal function. Importantly, EDRF/NO participates in local modulation of afferent arteriolar tone and relaxation of the mesangium, and thereby contributes to regulation of glomerular perfusion. Its antiplatelet and antithrombotic actions also help to prevent thrombosis within the glomerular capillaries. When NO synthesis/release is decreased in the glomerulus, an increase in glomerular thrombosis and cellular proliferation occurs.

NO also participates in regulating renal sodium excretion and renin release. The sodium concentration at the macula densa regulates both glomerular arteriolar resistance and the secretion of renin. Tubuloglomerular feedback regulates distal sodium delivery and, thus, salt excretion in response to changes in total body sodium. Sodium reabsorption at the macula densa increases afferent arteriolar tone and results in a decrease in glomerular filtration rate.[101] With chronic alterations in sodium concentration at the macula densa, control of renin release by the macula densa dominates. NO released from the macula densa may modulate tubuloglomerular feedback by affecting afferent arteriolar tone and modulating renin secretion. Bradykinin and acetylcholine increase NO synthesis and induce renal vasodilation, leading to enhanced diuresis and natriuresis. Blockade of NO synthesis has been shown to decrease renal blood flow and sodium excretion. Inhibition of intrarenal NO synthesis reduces the sodium excretion response to changes in renal arterial pressure without affecting autoregulation. Nakamura and colleagues[102] showed that intravenous infusion of L-NAME in rats resulted in a reduction in renal plasma flow and glomerular filtration rate; however, autoregulatory responses to renal perfusion pressure were maintained. Furthermore, NO synthesis may play a significant role in renal adaptation to increased sodium intake. Bech and co-workers[103] demonstrated a decrease in renal plasma flow and fractional excretion of sodium (FENa), as well as an increase in mean arterial pressure, with L-NMMA treatment in 12 healthy subjects during high sodium intake. However, during low sodium intake, L-NMMA induced a reduction in plasma renin not noted with high sodium intake, and the effect of L-NMMA on FENa was abolished.[103] Welch and Wilcox[104,105] showed that L-NMMA perfusion into the loop of Henle and macula densa potentiated tubuloglomerular feedback responses in rats receiving high salt, but was ineffective in rats on low salt. They also showed that delivery and/or cellular uptake of L-arginine limits macula densa NO generation and its blunting action on tubuloglomerular feedback in salt-restricted rats.[106]

The glomerular basement membrane (GBM) is lined by endothelial cells which regulate permselectivity. At the point where the mesangium is closest to the glomerular arterioles, the GBM is absent, and a single layer of endothelium separates the mesangial and endothelial cells. The mesangial cells contain receptors for vasoactive substances, including angiotensin II, endothelin-1, and thromboxane A_2. Modulation of glomerular blood flow and filtration occurs through contraction/relaxation of mesangial cells and consequent changes in arteriolar tone.[107–109]

Rat mesangial cells co-incubated with endothelial cells and agonists of NO synthesis have increased cGMP levels, but do not when incubated without endothelial cells or when exposed to L-NMMA.[110] Tolins and colleagues[111] showed that administration of acetylcholine produced hypotensive and renal vasodilatory effects accompanied by an increase in urinary excretion of cGMP. L-NMMA inhibited this effect, but did not inhibit the effects of endothelium-independent vasodilators such as nitroprusside or PGI_2. In addition, L-NMMA administration resulted in an increase in blood pressure, confirming the role of NO in maintaining basal vascular tone.[33,111]

Interactions between angiotensin II and NO

There is a clear association between the local renin–angiotensin system and the pathogenesis of vascular disease.[112] Thus, the balance between NO and angiotensin II is crucial for vascular homeostasis. Indirect effects of NO on renal vascular tone probably occur by inhibiting the release of renin from juxtaglomerular cells and, thereby, decreasing the production of angiotensin II.[113] The inhibition of NO synthesis may actually be a result of the effects of unopposed angiotensin II.[114]

Chronic inhibition of NO synthesis induces glomerular injury[115] as well as structural myocardial and coronary vascular changes associated with an increase in angiotensin-converting enzyme expression.[116] Angiotensin II has been shown to activate NADPH/NADP oxidase in vascular smooth muscle[117] and mesangial cells,[118] leading to generation of superoxide anion, thereby inactivating NO.[119] Coadministration of L-NMMA and an angiotensin II blocker attenuates the hemodynamic effects of inhibiting NO synthesis alone.[114] In isolated rabbit glomeruli, NO modulates the effect of angiotensin II on the afferent arteriole.[120] In addition to its vasomotor actions, NO has also been shown to inhibit mesangial cell proliferation.[121,122] The renin–angiotensin system, and angiotensin II specifically, may be viewed as the functional antagonist to NO, promoting vasoconstriction and cell growth. ET-1 stimulates mesangial cell proliferation.[109] In addition to acting as potent vasoconstrictors in the renal vascular bed,[122,123] both angiotensin II and ET-1 have been shown to reduce glomerular filtration rate (GFR) and glomerular plasma flow.

It remains unclear how NO provides protection for the renal vasculature against angiotensin II-induced vasoconstriction. One possibility is that angiotensin II enhances the production of NO, which then counteracts the vasoconstrictor effect of angiotensin II. Deng and colleagues[124] showed that an acute infusion of angiotensin II increases the urinary excretion of NO metabolites (nitrite and nitrate), suggesting an upregulation in NO production; however, chronic angiotensin II had no such effect. Hennington and co-workers[125] demonstrated that the acute perturbation in intrarenal hemodynamics produced by angiotensin II administration is associated with increased renal eNOS mRNA production; and longer-term increases in angiotensin II result in increased eNOS protein synthesis, suggesting that angiotensin II can chronically increase NO production in the kidney.

In addition to the direct effect on the generation of angiotensin II, angiotensin-converting enzyme (ACE) also cleaves bradykinin,[126–129] and ACE inhibition may, therefore, increase bradykinin-mediated vasodilation. Bradykinin is a potent vasodilator that exerts this effect mainly through endothelial release of NO,[130,131] and this bradykinin-mediated vasodilation is potentiated in the presence of ACE inhibitors.[132,133] ACE is identical to kininase II, an enzyme that degrades bradykinin. This suggests that the beneficial cardiovascular effects of ACE inhibitors may not only be related to a reduction in angiotensin II, but also to an increase in bradykinin. Furthermore, probably through a similar mechanism of decreasing angiotensin II and an amplification of NO release induced by increased bradykinin, this dual benefit of ACE inhibitors helps to restore vascular and intrarenal homeostasis. Frohlich[134] showed that alterations in renal dynamics, proteinuria, and renal pathological lesions can be prevented or reversed with ACE inhibitor treatment in spontaneously hypertensive rats, an effect not seen with hydrochlorothiazide treatment despite similar anti-hypertensive effects.

In combination, NO, PGI_2, angiotensin II, and ET-1 modulate renal hemodynamics. This complex interplay among potent vasodilators and vasoconstrictors may be important in renal disease, particularly in renal ischemia, where NO-dependent effects are impaired[135] and ET-1 synthesis is increased.[136]

As discussed above, evidence suggests that NO plays a role in sodium excretion. Antagonists of NO synthesis and release lead to increases in renin release.[113] Infusion of NOS inhibitors into the renal artery results in inhibition of sodium excretion.[137] Natriuresis induced by NO probably occurs secondary to antagonism of the effects of angiotensin II on sodium reabsorption in the proximal tubule[138] and by inhibiting sodium reabsorption in the cortical collecting duct.[139] Inhibition of sodium excretion with NOS inhibitors is enhanced by cyclooxygenase inhibitors, suggesting an interaction between NO and intrarenal prostaglandins.[140] Salt loading in rats has been shown to increase urinary excretion of NO metabolites,[141] which suggests that altered NO production may play a role in salt-sensitive hypertension.[142]

Chen and Sanders[142,143] showed that salt-sensitive hypertension in Dahl/Rapp rats was prevented by administration of L-arginine. They also suggested that an increase in dietary salt increased the production of NO in salt-resistant (R), but not salt-sensitive (S), rats. Hu and Manning[144] showed that Dahl S rats had impaired production of NO over a wide range of salt intakes. Administration of L-arginine increased the NO production of Dahl S rats to that of Dahl R rats, and a high dose of L-arginine prevented the hypertensive shift in the long-term pressure–natriuresis relationship in these animals, again suggesting that a deficiency in NO production may contribute to the development of salt-sensitive hypertension in this animal model.

Ikeda and colleagues[145] found that nNOS activity was decreased in Dahl S rats given a high-salt diet, but eNOS and iNOS were unchanged. Furthermore, salt loading regulates the gene expression of nNOS in Sprague-Dawley rats.[146] Raij and Hayakawa found that NOS activity is linked with end-organ disease and that impaired NOS may be more common in salt-sensitive hypertension.[115,147,148] Human studies suggest that salt-sensitive hypertensives seem to be more prone to end-organ damage, such as left ventricular hypertrophy and fibrosis, and renal disease.[149,150]

Most forms of glomerular injury involve platelet activation and fibrin deposition within the glomerular capillaries.[151,152] Thus, the antithrombotic actions of NO may play an important role in preventing glomerular injury. Within the glomerulus, platelet-activating factor and cytokines, such as IL-1 and tumor necrosis factor-α, may be released locally by activated mesangial cells and/or circulating macrophages.[109,153] These mediators induce the release of tissue factor and plasminogen activator inhibitors, thereby enhancing platelet activation and coagulation.[109,154] In this setting, NO and PGI_2 may play an important role in preventing glomerular thrombosis.

NO also inhibits cellular proliferative responses to vascular injury. In the presence of hypertension, NO may act in the kidney to inhibit mesangial cell hypertrophy and hyperplasia, which are effects antagonistic to those of angiotensin II.[112,155]

It is apparent that stimulation of NO activity results in renal vasodilation and increased sodium and water excretion. Conversely, inhibition of NO production/release results in a decrease in glomerular filtration, renal vasoconstriction, and decreased sodium and water excretion.

Endothelial dysfunction

In animal studies and patients with vascular disease states, including hypercholesterolemia and atherosclerosis, endothelial control of vascular tone and blood flow is impaired.[156] In arteries isolated from patients with coronary artery disease, impaired endothelium-dependent relaxation has been demonstrated:[157,158] furthermore the extent of atherosclerosis in both

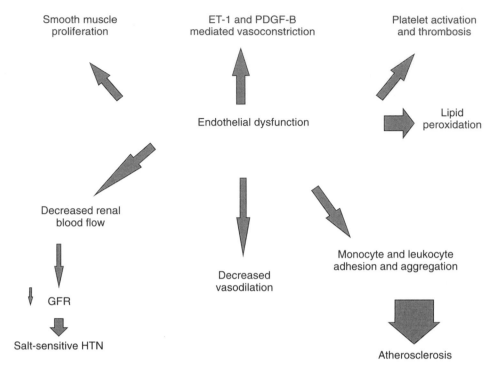

Fig. 6.2 Effects of endothelial dysfunction that promote hypertension and atherosclerosis. ET-1, endothelin-1; PDGF-B, platelet derived growth factor-B; GFR, glomerular filtration rate; HTN, hypertension.

human and animal arteries correlates with the impairment of endothelium–dependent relaxation.[157,159,160]

Most studies suggest that vascular relaxation to exogenous nitrovasodilators remains unimpaired in these disease states, suggesting that the defect is a consequence of a reduction in NO production or bioavailability rather than an intrinsic defect in the vascular smooth muscle's ability to relax. At least three mechanisms in the NO pathway may lead to the endothelial dysfunction of atherosclerosis: NOS dysfunction secondary to substrate or cofactor deficiency;[161,162] increased destruction of NO;[163,164] or decreased expression of NOS.[165]

Endothelial regulation of vascular tone is impaired in other disease states, including hypertension and diabetes mellitus. Panza and co-workers[166] recently showed that hypertensive patients have a defect in NO release under basal conditions and during endothelial activation, which appears to be a consequence of impaired NO synthesis and/or release. Conversely, animal studies have shown that treatment of hypertension corrects the impairment of endothelium-dependent vasodilation, suggesting that hypertension itself may actually induce endothelial dysfunction.[167] There is also evidence that in addition to impaired EDRF production, the release of EDCFs may contribute to altered vascular tone in hypertension.[168,169]

Barton and colleagues[170] demonstrated that in Dahl S rats hypertension is associated with increased aortic tissue ET-1, aortic hypertrophy, and endothelial dysfunction. Endothelial dysfunction was inversely correlated with vascular ET-1 content. Furthermore, ET-1 receptor blockade only partially reduced blood pressure, but normalized ET-1 levels and prevented vascular hypertrophy and dysfunction induced by a high sodium diet.

Endothelial dysfunction is also present in patients with diabetes mellitus. Impaired endothelium–dependent relaxation was observed in animals made diabetic with streptozotocin[171] and alloxan.[172] Several studies suggest a role for increased production and action of vasoconstrictor prostaglandins in diabetic animals and in isolated arteries exposed to high glucose concentrations.[173]

Mechanisms of impaired endothelial function

Several potential causes of impaired NO bioactivity in endothelial dysfunction include a reduction in production/release of NO, enhanced degradation of NO, overproduction of vasoconstrictors, and altered end-organ sensitivity. The factors that influence these alterations in NO action and endothelial function in patients with ESRF will be discussed next.

An increasingly recognized mechanism of EDRF impairment and contributor to atherogenesis is oxidative stress.[174] The production of oxygen-derived free radicals and oxidative modification of LDL may lead to impaired EDRF action and initiate the atherosclerotic process.[175] A major source of oxidative stress is the superoxide anion, which arises from activated macrophages and other components of the vascular wall. There is increased production of the superoxide anion in hypercholesterolemia,[119,174,176] and this free radical and derivative radicals may contribute to endothelial dysfunction by reacting with and inactivating NO. In a study of cholesterol-fed rabbits, a reduction in plasma cholesterol was associated with a decrease in superoxide anion production and an improvement in endothelial function.[177] In patients with coronary atherosclerosis, the administration of ascorbic acid, a potent scavenger of the superoxide anion, improved flow-mediated brachial artery dilation.[178] Evidence suggests that hyperlipoproteinemia, even in the absence of histologic evidence of atherosclerosis, impairs endothelial function.[179] Vita and co-workers[180] demonstrated that infusion of acetylcholine in patients with coronary risk factors but angiographically normal coronary arteries produced a 'paradoxical' vasoconstrictor response, probably a consequence of the unopposed direct effects of muscarinic agonists on smooth muscle cell tone.

The superoxide anion and NO react to form peroxynitrite, which can initiate lipid peroxidation.[119] In the setting of limited L-arginine substrate or tetrahydrobiopterin cofactor, NOS itself is capable of generating the superoxide anion.[181] The superoxide anion can undergo dismutation to hydrogen peroxide (H_2O_2), which might impair EDRF production[182] and mediate endothelial injury.[183]

Oxidized lipids contained within LDL stimulate monocyte adhesion[184] and migration into the subendothelial space where they participate in the early stages of atherogenesis. The activated endothelium expresses cell-surface adhesion molecules that further facilitate the attachment of circulating leukocytes to the endothelial surface, and a deficiency of NO enhances the expression of these adhesion molecules.[185] The recruitment of leukocytes in the vascular wall by oxidized LDL leads to the release of oxygen-derived free radicals that can not only degrade NO,[186-190] but also directly produce endothelial cytotoxicity and impairment of NO release.[191] Thus, elevated levels of oxidized LDL probably not only initiate the development of the atherosclerotic lesions, but also promote accelerated atherogenesis by inhibiting the production and release of NO.

Endothelium-derived vasoconstrictors may also be increased in hypercholesterolemia. In patients with atherosclerosis, plasma levels of ET-1 are higher than in normals,[192] and oxidized lipoproteins increase the expression of ET-1 in cultured endothelial cells.[193]

Antioxidants, such as probucol and α-tocopherol, which prevent lipoprotein oxidation, reduce atherosclerosis,[194] supporting the hypothesis that oxidized lipoproteins are an important component of the atherosclerotic process. Furthermore, probucol[160] and α-tocopherol[195] appear to normalize endothelium-dependent relaxation prior to slowing atherogenesis.

Oxidative stress also contributes to impairment of EDRF in other vascular diseases, including that associated with diabetes mellitus and hypertension. In severely diabetic rats, response to nitrovasodilators may be decreased.[196] Free radical scavengers, such as superoxide dismutase (SOD), can restore endothelium-dependent relaxation in isolated diabetic vessels.[63,66] Catalase, a scavenger of H_2O_2, and desferrioxamine, a chelator of iron and a hydroxyl-radical scavenger, also restore diabetic endothelial function.[63] The superoxide anion has also been implicated in the development of endothelial dysfunction in animal models of hypertension.[69] Acutely induced hypertension in cats has been shown to induce superoxide generation, which can then be reversed with SOD administration.[197] Furthermore, treatment with SOD[198] or oxypurinol, the inhibitor of xanthine oxidase, lowers blood pressure in spontaneously hypertensive rats, but not in controls.[69] Taddei and colleagues[199] showed that in essential hypertensive human subjects, treatment with the antioxidant vitamin C improved endothelium-dependent vasodilation, at least in part, by preserving the L-arginine–NO pathway, supporting the concept that the superoxide anion participates in endothelial dysfunction in essential hypertension.

An interesting hypothesis suggests that differences in growth factors account for the more frequent and severe hypertension and nephrosclerotic ESRF that exist in the Black population,[200–202] and that growth factors might play a significant role in the pathogenesis of atherosclerosis, hypertension, and renal disease.[203] This hypothesis derives from evidence that the fibroblasts of keloids, which exist almost exclusively in Blacks, have different growth patterns from normal skin,[204] and that those patients with keloids also appear to have altered cytokine production by peripheral blood mononuclear cells.[205] Furthermore, the sensitivity of the renal vasculature of Blacks to hypertensive damage might represent a racial difference in the response of kidney cells to growth factors similar to that of keloid fibroblasts. Evidence suggests that the racial differences in the severity of hypertension and its associated vascular disease is at least partially explained by differences in cytokines affecting vascular smooth muscle cell growth.

Determinants of endothelial dysfunction in ESRF

Homocysteine

Homocysteine and oxidative stress

An increasingly recognized source of oxidative stress that is particularly relevant to patients with ESRF is homocysteine, an intermediate amino acid formed during the metabolism of methionine. Homocysteine is believed to injure endothelial cells through a number of mechanisms, including the generation of H_2O_2 during its oxidation to homocysteine. An elevated plasma homocysteine concentration is an independent risk factor for atherosclerosis and thrombosis, and more recently identified as an independent risk factor for endothelial dysfunction in healthy subjects.[206] First described in patients with an inborn error of metabolism, McCully[207] reported postmortem findings of extensive atherosclerosis in several patients with elevated plasma homocysteine concentrations who were deficient in cystathionine-β-synthase. He concluded that hyperhomocysteinemia can cause atherosclerotic vascular disease. Since McCully's observation, abundant data have emerged linking elevated homocysteine levels to coronary artery, peripheral, and cerebrovascular atherothrombotic disease.

The Horland Homocysteine Study found that elevated homocysteine levels were associated with unfavorable cardiovascular risk factors, including male gender, increased age, tobacco use, hypertension, hypercholesterolemia, and physical inactivity.[208] According to the Physicians' Health Study,[209] patients with myocardial infarction had only a 6% higher mean plasma homocysteine level than controls, but the relative risk was 3.3 in subjects with levels greater that 15.8 μM. An increased homocysteine level confers an independent risk of vascular disease similar to that of hypercholesterolemia and smoking, and significantly further increases the risk associated with smoking and hypertension.[210]

Plasma homocysteine levels are a strong predictor of overall morbidity and mortality due to cardiovascular causes among patients with angiographically confirmed coronary artery disease.[211] Further support of this finding resulted from a prospective study of serum homocysteine levels and ischemic heart disease in which homocysteine levels were significantly higher in men who died of ischemic heart disease than in men who did not. The risk of ischemic heart disease among men in the highest quartile was 3.7 times the risk of the men in the lowest. Furthermore, there was a dose–response relationship, with risk increasing by 33% for each 5 μM increase in serum homocysteine concentration after adjusting for apolipoprotein B and blood pressure.[212]

Homocysteine metabolism

Homocysteine is a sulfur-containing amino acid formed during the metabolism of methionine, an essential amino acid derived from dietary protein. Once synthesized, homocysteine can undergo remethylation or enter the trans-sulfuration pathway. In remethylation, homocysteine is recycled to methionine, a reaction catalyzed by methionine synthase using 5,10-methyltetrahydrofolate as a methyl donor; cobalamin (vitamin B_{12}) is an essential cofactor for this reaction. In the presence of excess methionine or when cysteine synthesis is required, homocysteine can enter the trans-sulfuration pathway. Homocysteine and serine form cystathionine, a rate-limiting reaction requiring pyridoxal 5'-phosphate (vitamin B_6). Cystathionine is subsequently hydrolyzed to form cysteine, which can be incorporated in glutathione or metabolized to sulfate.

Factors that affect homocysteine levels

Plasma homocysteine levels are primarily determined by enzymes in the metabolic pathways for sulfur-containing amino acids and vitamin cofactors, several disease states, nutritional status, age, gender, and medication. Patients with hereditary homocystinuria typically have enzyme defects in either the remethylation or trans-sulfuration pathways. The most common cause of homocystinuria is cystathionine β-synthase deficiency, an autosomal recessive disorder; the homozygous trait often results in death from atherothrombotic vascular disease during childhood and adolescence.

Homocysteine concentrations also increase with age and are greater in men than in women. Medication with theophylline and phenytoin alters vitamin B_6 and folate metabolism, respectively, and can alter homocysteine concentrations. Concentration differences in age, gender, and nutritional status are apparently related to levels of the vitamin cofactors B_{12}, B_6, and folate. Selhub and co-workers[213] have suggested that most individuals with hyperhomocysteinemia have deficiencies of one or more of these vitamins, and that up to 40% of the general population does not consume enough folate to maintain normal homocysteine levels. Vitamin supplementation has been shown to normalize homocysteine levels;[214,215] however, effects of supplementation on clinical endpoints have not yet been evaluated. Several disease states, including hypothyroidism and a variety of carcinomas, have been linked to hyperhomocysteinemia.[216,217] The two major acquired causes of hyperhomocysteinemia, however, are chronic renal failure and deficiencies of B_{12}, B_6, and folate.

Prevalence of hyperhomocysteinemia in renal failure

An important association between hyperhomocysteinemia and ESRF exists such that hyperhomocysteinemia may be an important determinant of the high prevalence of accelerated atherosclerosis that has long been reported in renal failure patients. Hyperhomocysteinemia is quite common in ESRF,[218–221] and it has been suggested that elevated homocysteine levels may partly explain the accelerated atherothrombotic disease of chronic uremia.

A variety of studies have shown that the prevalence of increased homocysteine concentration is high in patients with chronic renal failure,[219–233] particularly those with vascular complications[220] In patients with ESRF, homocysteine levels reach up to 3–4 times the normal range of 5–15 μM. Hyperhomocysteinemia is found in patients with varying degrees of renal failure, as well as those on chronic hemodialysis or peritoneal dialysis.[220,226,228–231,234] Homocysteine levels decrease approximately 40% during hemodialysis, but may remain above the normal range in patients who are adequately dialyzed.[219–221,224] The high prevalence of hyperhomocysteinemia in ESRF compares with the prevalence rates of 18–30% in coronary artery disease,[235–237] 42% in angina among men,[238] 40–42% in cerebrovascular disease,[236,239,240] and 19–28% in peripheral vascular disease.[236,241]

Data from the Framingham Offspring Study suggest that an elevated homocysteine level had a greater prevalence than any other traditional atherothrombotic risk factors in ESRF patients. Furthermore, ESRF patients were 33-fold more likely to be hyperhomocysteinemic than matched controls.[232] Chauveau and colleagues[220] studied 79 patients with non-dialysis-dependent renal failure and reported significantly higher homocysteine values in patients with prior histories of occlusive arterial disease than in patients without such histories. Furthermore, hyperhomocysteinemia increases in parallel with progression of renal failure, with only partial correction following chronic hemodialysis. Dennis and Robinson[242] studied 176 patients with ESRF and showed that higher homocysteine levels were associated with an increase in atherosclerotic and thrombotic complications independent of other traditional risk factors and length of time to dialysis. Moustapha and colleagues[243] prospectively observed 167 patients with ESRF and confirmed hyperhomocysteinemia as an independent risk factor for cardiovascular morbidity and mortality with an increased relative risk of 1% per 1 μM increase in total homocysteine concentration. Although homocysteine levels positively correlate with serum creatinine concentration, it is unclear whether this is secondary to impaired metabolism or reduced renal excretion. Reduced excretion of homocysteine may not necessarily be the major cause of elevated homocysteine levels since the daily renal excretion of homocysteine is 3.5–10 micromoles, which is approximately 0.1% of total homocysteine production.[244]

Levels of other sulfur-containing amino acids also increase in chronic renal failure, which reflect alterations in amino acid metabolism seen in patients with renal disease. Wilcken and colleagues[218,223] showed increased homocysteine–cysteine mixed disulfide concentrations, as well as increased cystine and taurine, but not methionine.

Homocysteine-induced endothelial dysfunction

Evidence suggests that the atherosclerotic effects of homocysteine are a result of endothelial injury or dysfunction. Lentz and colleagues[245] showed that diet-induced hyperhomocysteine-

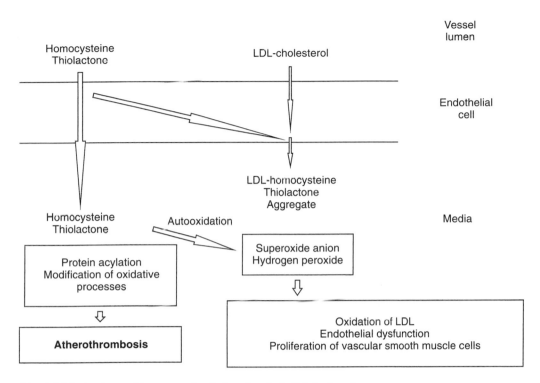

Fig. 6.3 Mechanisms of homocysteine-induced endothelial dysfunction.

mia in primates led to impaired responses of resistance vessels to endothelium-dependent vasodilators, providing evidence for the deleterious effects of homocysteine in the absence of underlying vascular disease. In addition to blunted vasodilation, they also demonstrated depressed thrombomodulin activity and moderately reduced vascular smooth muscle responses to nitrovasodilators *ex vivo*.

The primary toxic effect of homocysteine appears to involve oxidative damage to the endothelium. Homocysteine readily autooxidizes in plasma, forming the reactive oxygen derivatives superoxide and H_2O_2. The oxidative stress created by the generation of these derivatives accounts for the endothelial damage from homocysteine. As just discussed, these free radicals impair the actions of EDRF and oxidize LDL, promoting atherogenesis. A major by-product of dysregulated homocysteine metabolism, homocysteine thiolactone, can react with LDL to form LDL–homocysteine thiolactone aggregates, which are taken up by macrophages and incorporated into foam cells,[246] promoting the development of atherosclerotic plaques.

Endothelial dysfunction secondary to homocysteine exposure occurs by several other mechanisms. Homocysteine increases Factor XI and Factor V activity and depresses protein C activation, creating a more prothrombotic endothelial environment. Homocysteine also inhibits heparan sulfate and thrombomodulin expression, induces tissue factor expression, and reduces the binding of tissue-type plasminogen activator to its endothelial receptor.

Homocysteine alters the vasodilator properties of the endothelium by affecting NO production. Normal endothelial cells detoxify homocysteine by releasing NO or a related

S-nitrosothiol, which forms a non-toxic adduct with homocysteine.[247] S-nitrosation of homocysteine prevents homocysteine's oxidative generation of H_2O_2; in addition, it acts as a vasodilator and platelet inhibitor. With chronic exposure, persistently elevated homocysteine levels eventually damage the endothelium such that NO production is impaired and the oxidative damage from homocysteine is unopposed.

Autooxidation of homocysteine generates several oxygen-derived free radicals. It is likely that H_2O_2 is primarily involved in endothelial injury. After formation, H_2O_2 crosses cell membranes and is reduced to H_2O by catalase or glutathione peroxidase. Glutathione peroxidase, an antioxidant enzyme, reduces H_2O_2 and lipid peroxides to alcohols in a reaction involving the oxidation of glutathione. Four isoforms of the enzyme exist, including intracellular, extracellular, phospholipid hydroperoxide, and gastrointestinal isoforms. The cellular isoform acts as a major enzymatic intracellular buffering system against oxidative stress, and the extracellular isoform is the principal antioxidant enzyme in the extracellular space. The reduction of H_2O_2 and lipid peroxides to alcohols prevents inactivation of NO by hydroxyl and peroxyl derivatives.[248] In addition, high concentrations of homocysteine inhibit glutathione peroxidase activity *in vitro* and decrease mRNA levels of the intracellular isoform.[249]

Glutathione peroxidase contains a selenium atom at the active site in the form of selenocysteine.[250] Plasma glutathione peroxidase (GPx) activity is low in partially nephrectomized uremic rats[251–253] and in hemodialysis patients. The kidney is the main source of extracellular GPx, specifically the renal tubular cell.[254–256] Yoshimura and colleagues[257] showed that creatinine levels in non-dialyzed chronic renal failure patients correlate highly negatively with plasma GPx activity, indicating that plasma GPx activity depends largely on normal renal mass. Furthermore, significantly lower GPx activity was noted in chronic ambulatory peritoneal dialysis patients compared with hemodialysis patients. Erythrocytic GPx activity in hemodialysis patients has been reported as low,[253,258,259] normal,[260] or high.[254] Selenium deficiency has been implicated in reports showing low levels of activity of all isoenzymes, although selenium deficiency has not been convincingly proven in uremia. However, the importance of selenium (Se) as an essential trace element has been increasingly recognized, and, frequently, Se blood levels are low in ESRF patients. Geographic factors have frequently complicated the determination of the Se status in uremic patients owing to a wide range of methods of Se measurements. Bonomini and co-workers[261] documented a significant difference in blood Se levels between two groups of healthy controls from two different countries in Europe. Furthermore, Se concentrations were significantly lower in chronic renal failure (CRF) and hemodialysis (HD) patients than in their corresponding controls, but no difference was found between CRF and HD. That same group had previously suggested that dialysis-mediated Se depletion was an unlikely mechanism for Se deficiency in uremia, as they showed a significant increase in Se plasma levels after hemodialysis.[262] Furthermore, Girelli and colleagues[263] reported a low Se concentration in chronic renal failure patients independent of dialysis, and that chronic renal failure patients with cardiovascular complications showed a further significant reduction in both serum Se concentration and platelet glutathione peroxidase activity compared with the patients without cardiovascular complications. Koenig and colleagues[264] also documented profoundly decreased concentrations of Se in plasma and of glutathione and glutathione peroxidase activity in hemodialysis patients, and that selenium supplementation improved the status of all these factors; however, the clinical outcomes of Se supplementation and a possibly improved oxygen radical scavenger system have not yet been evaluated. A small number of reports suggest that there is no difference in Se concentration between chronic renal failure patients and controls, and that no change in Se concentration occurs during dialysis.[265]

Basal release of NO from the endothelium inhibits smooth muscle proliferation. Homocysteine has been shown to increase vascular smooth muscle DNA synthesis and proliferation *in vitro* independently by activating cyclin A and D1 expression.[266]

Pathophysiology in renal disease

Eighty per cent of homocysteine is protein-bound, and the remaining free homocysteine is filtered by the glomerulus. In rat studies, measurements of arteriovenous differences in homocysteine concentrations demonstrate adequate renal uptake and metabolism with low urinary clearance, suggesting that a reduction in excretion is not the primary cause of hyperhomocysteinemia.[267] In fact, as renal function worsens, the fractional clearance of homocysteine actually increases.[221]

The cause of increased serum homocysteine levels in chronic renal failure has not yet been clearly defined, although it is likely to be multifactorial. One hypothesis suggests a decrease in plasma serine, given that both remethylation and trans-sulfuration consume serine.[268] Alteration in enzyme activities within the kidney may also contribute, as remethylation enzymes are present in the renal tubule, and cystathionone β-synthase activity has been shown to be reduced.[269–271]

In patients with chronic renal failure, methionine challenge (a standard oral dose of methionine is administered and homocysteine level is measured 4 hours later) increases homocysteine levels, consistent with impaired trans-sulfuration.[221] Impaired hepatic metabolism related to uremia has also been implicated, as the liver has the capacity to carry out remethylation and trans-sulfuration but does not eliminate the excess homocysteine of uremia. This inability may be due to diminished hepatic uptake of homocysteine, decreased availability of cofactors and substrate,[216] or endogenous enzyme inhibitors.[223]

As discussed earlier, vitamin deficiencies play a prominent role in hyperhomocysteinemia. Patients with renal failure are also at risk for B_6 and folate deficiencies, although they typically receive supplementation. In addition, deficiencies have not been consistently demonstrated in patients with ESRF and hyperhomocysteinemia.[230,231] Robinson and colleagues[230] showed that B_{12} and folate levels were higher in patients with ESRF than in a control population, and mean B_6 levels were similar. Only folate deficiency was present in 2% of ESRF patients; however, B_6 deficiency was present in 18% of ESRF patients versus 2% of controls.

Hyperhomocysteinemia may persist in ESRF patients on chronic hemodialysis or peritoneal dialysis, although concentrations tend to decrease during hemodialysis. Bostom and colleagues[272] studied 73 maintenance peritoneal dialysis or hemodialysis patients and found that hyperhomocysteinemia continued to be an independent risk factor for cardiovascular morbidity and mortality.

L-Arginine

Another mechanism of endothelial dysfunction involves availability of L-arginine, the substrate for NO synthesis. In cholesterol-fed rabbits, acute and chronic L-arginine administration improves endothelium-dependent dilation.[273,274] In patients with hypercholesterolemia, intra-arterial L-arginine corrected endothelial dysfunction in coronary resistance vessels, but not the epicardial vasodilator responses to acetylcholine.[275] Recently, Lerman and colleagues[276] have shown that long-term L-arginine supplementation for 6 months in subjects free of significant coronary artery disease by angiography improves coronary small-vessel endothelial function, and is associated with improved symptoms and a decrease in plasma ET-1 concentrations. Thorne and co-workers[277] demonstrated varying responses to intravenous L-arginine on brachial artery flow-mediated dilation in three groups with isolated risk factors—hypercholesterolemia, smoking, and insulin-dependent diabetes mellitus. Flow-mediated dilation improved in hypercholesterolemic subjects and smokers, but was unchanged in diabetics, suggesting a different underlying pathophysiology of endothelial dysfunction.

Schwarzacher and colleagues[76] showed that local intramural administration of L-arginine enhances vascular NO generation and inhibits lesion formation after balloon injury. Furthermore, Wolf and co-workers[278] demonstrated that L-arginine supplementation in hypercholesterolemic subjects can attenuate platelet reactivity. Candipan and colleagues[279] found that supplemental L-arginine in rabbits with pre-existing intimal lesions restored NO activity, reduced the generation of superoxide, and induced regression of lesions.

In the setting of acute renal ischemia/reperfusion in uninephrectomized rabbits, L-arginine and superoxide dismutase synergistically improve renal function and block ischemia/reperfusion-dependent neutrophil accumulation. However, these immediate protective effects were short-lived and no longer present at 24 and 48 hours.[280]

L-Arginine appears to play a beneficial role in progressive renal failure after subtotal nephrectomy in rats. Reyes and co-workers[281] showed that in rats with 85–90% of their renal mass surgically ablated, oral administration of L-arginine increased renal perfusion pressure and glomerular filtration rate without altering mean arterial pressure or urine protein excretion rate. Furthermore, there was a lesser degree of glomerulosclerosis in these animals. Other studies suggest that L-arginine has beneficial effects on renal hemodynamics and end-organ damage in diabetes mellitus. In streptozotocin-induced diabetes, oral administration of L-arginine to rats reduced proteinuria, and glomerular filtration rate approached normal.[282] Furthermore, Weninger and colleagues[283] demonstrated a decrease in the accumulation of advanced glycosylation end-products in the glomerular basement membrane of diabetic mice fed oral L-arginine.

Other mechanisms of disruption of NO metabolism potentially exist in hypertension and renal failure, including inhibitors of NO synthases, some of which are produced endogenously. As mentioned earlier, ADMA is an L-arginine analog with asymmetric dimethyl substitution of a guanidinium nitrogen atom. Vallance and co-workers[284] have suggested that its accumulation promotes hypertension in dialysis patients. That group showed that intravenous infusion of this compound into guinea pigs increased blood pressure in a dose-dependent fashion. However, the clinical significance of this intermediate remains uncertain. Other guanidino compounds besides creatinine also accumulate in renal failure that may inhibit the synthesis of NO. Chen and Sanders[143] and Hecker and colleagues[285] found that L-homoarginine can also serve as a substrate for NO synthesis. MacAllister and colleagues[286] showed that of the guanidino compounds which accumulate in renal failure, only ADMA is a potent inhibitor of NO synthesis; guanidinosuccinic acid, guanidinopropionic acid, and methylguanidine did not demonstrate any antagonist or agonist effect. Thus, the endogenous accumulation of ADMA in renal failure is the only guanidino compound to have been shown to inhibit the L-arginine–NO pathway.

Another inhibitor of NO synthesis discussed previously, L-NMMA, has been shown to normalize bleeding time when given to uremic rats, suggesting that NO is a probable mediator of the bleeding tendency of uremia.[287] This effect of L-NMMA on bleeding time was completely reversed by the administration of L-arginine. Possible mechanisms of the pathobiological role of NO include its potent vascular relaxing effects, which may counter the vasoconstrictor response to vascular injury, and its inhibition of platelet adhesion to the vascular endothelium. This observation ultimately may have clinical therapeutic implications in the management of bleeding disorders associated with chronic renal failure. Yet, its precise molecular mechanism and the relationship of this mechanism to ADMA-induced vasoconstriction remain poorly defined.

Factors influenced by dialysis

It is worth mentioning that some differences in endothelial function and dysfunction do exist between non-dialysis-dependent patients and those on maintenance dialysis. Several vascular endothelial cell markers are altered by dialysis. Takagi and colleagues[288] reported increased levels of thrombomodulin, PAI-1, and vWF before dialysis, although not of t-PA. Compared with levels before dialysis, t-PA and vWF were significantly increased after hemodialysis, both 1 hour into dialysis and at the end of dialysis. Thrombomodulin was elevated at 1 hour, and PAI-1 was decreased at the end of dialysis. Thrombomodulin and vWF were negatively correlated with the number of years on hemodialysis. They concluded that hemodialysis may actually cause endothelial damage and that increases in thrombomodulin, PAI-1, and vWF before hemodialysis, and a decrease in thrombomodulin and vWF thereafter, might be caused by endothelial activation or damage from long-term uremia or hemodialysis itself.[288]

In addition, Ceballos-Picot and colleagues[289] showed that alterations in the glutathione antioxidant system occurred gradually, increasing with the degree of renal failure and then further with peritoneal dialysis, and eventually was almost completely abolished in hemodialysis patients. These observations suggest that dialysis exacerbates oxidative stress in renal failure patients. Alterations in antioxidant enzymes and trace elements exist in hemodialysis patients, some of which dialysis seemed to improve, while at the same time also inducing some deleterious oxidant effects. Chen and colleagues[290] showed that reduced levels of SOD, catalase, and glutathione peroxidase exist in chronic renal failure patients if measured prior to hemodialysis; catalase and glutathione peroxidase were lower after hemodialysis than controls, but plasma glutathione peroxidase was significantly higher after a single hemodialysis than prior to dialysis.

Therapeutic implications

NO donors

Evidence suggests that exogenous NO donors might provide clinical therapeutic benefits. Organic nitrates/nitrovasodilators serve as exogenous sources of NO and exert similar effects, including vasorelaxation and reduced platelet aggregation. Nitrovasodilators have been effective in ischemic coronary syndromes, probably because of these actions.[291] In addition, nitrovasodilators inhibit vascular smooth muscle growth, suggesting a potential role in vascular interventions, such as coronary angioplasty.

Lipid lowering

Cholesterol-lowering therapy has clearly been shown to reduce total and cardiovascular mortality in patients with coronary artery disease.[292,293] A meta-analysis of 22 primary and secondary prevention trials shows that every 10% reduction in total cholesterol resulted in a 20% reduction in cardiovascular mortality.[292] The lack of significant lesion regression as an explanation for these mortality benefits suggests that other mechanism are involved. Possibilities include reduced susceptibility to plaque rupture and improved endothelial function.[156,294] Evidence from animal and human studies shows that endothelial vasodilation improves with lipid-lowering therapy.[295–298] Furthermore, Wilson and colleagues[299] demonstrated that fenofibrate prevents hypertension in Dahl S rats, and even though minimal antihypertensive effects occurred, pravastatin exhibited renoprotective effects on glomeruli and renal arterioles. Thus, improvements in endothelial vasodilator and antithrombotic activities may partly explain the benefits observed with lipid-lowering therapy.

Antioxidants

Evidence suggests that reducing oxidative stress with dietary antioxidants has beneficial effects in coronary disease. In the Health Professional Follow-Up Study of 39 910 men, increasing intake of α-tocopherol was associated with a reduced risk of coronary artery disease.[300] In the Nurses' Health Study, α-tocopherol supplementation was associated with a 34% reduction in the risk of coronary artery events,[301] and plasma levels of retinol and α-tocopherol have been shown to correlate inversely with mortality from coronary artery disease.[302] In cholesterol-fed rabbits with impaired endothelial vasomotor function, supplementation with β-carotene or α-tocopherol led to preservation of endothelium-dependent dilation in response to acetylcholine.[303] In essential hypertensive patients, the antioxidant ascorbate improves endothelium-dependent vasodilation, probably by scavenging oxygen-derived free radicals and thereby restoring the efficacy of the L-arginine–NO pathway.[199]

Antioxidants can also be useful in reducing homocysteine-induced oxidative stress. α-Tocopherol and ascorbate may be useful in improving the antioxidant capacity of the endothelium in patients with hyperhomocysteinemia. Furthermore, elevated homocysteine levels can be normalized with folate alone or in combination with B_{12} and B_6 vitamin supplementation.[216,217,224,234,239,304–307]

Folate administration reduces homocysteine levels in patients with chronic renal disease, even in the presence of normal folate levels. Wilcken and colleagues[224] showed that folate, but not B_6 or B_{12}, decreased homocysteine levels by approximately 40% in patients who had undergone renal transplantation. The same group showed a reduction in homocysteine levels by 40–50% with administration of 5 mg folate daily for 15 days in non-dialysis-dependent patients with chronic renal failure. Bostom and colleagues[307] used a higher dose of folate (15 mg) combined with 100 mg of vitamin B_6 and 1 mg of B_{12}, which reduced homocysteine by 30%, but few patients actually achieved normal values. It remains unclear to what extent hyperhomocysteinemia in ESRF is correctable, and whether or not it will have an effect on the prevalence of atherothrombotic vascular complications.

Finally, in patients on chronic hemodialysis, Se deficiency has been implicated in the reduced antioxidative capacity in these patients. Koenig and co-workers[264] showed that Se supplementation increased Se concentration in plasma and erythrocytes as well as erythrocyte glutathione peroxidase activity in these patients.

Exercise

Although the cardiovascular benefits of exercise are multifactorial, one potential outcome may be improved endothelium-dependent vasodilation. Wang and co-workers[309] showed an improvement in endothelium-dependent epicardial vasodilation after 7 days of treadmill exercise in dogs. Exercise training enhanced acetylcholine-stimulated nitrite production in dogs, reflecting an increase in NO synthesis and in mRNA levels for eNOS.[309] Furthermore, exercise-induced increases in blood flow and shear stress have been observed to enhance vasodilator function.

The effects of a sedentary lifestyle on renal function have not been adequately studied. However, sedentary individuals have a 20–50% increased risk of developing hypertension,[310] suggesting a potential beneficial effect of exercise in hypertension and the associated endothelial dysfunction in this disorder.

L-Arginine

Supplemental L-arginine provides a substrate for the synthesis of NO and appears to improve vasodilation by enhancing NO activity, reducing the generation of oxygen-derived free radicals, and potentially inducing the regression of intimal lesions. These beneficial effects of L-arginine suggest a potential therapeutic benefit of dietary supplementation, although further clinical investigation is necessary in patients with and without renal disease.

Antihypertensive therapy/ACE inhibition

Epidemiological studies have shown that in hypertensive patients, increased creatinine levels,[311] proteinuria,[312] and microalbuminuria[313] are independent predictors of increased cardiovascular morbidity and mortality. Furthermore, myocardial ischemia and infarction in ESRF patients on chronic hemodialysis are nearly 20 times that of the general population.[314] The association between increased activity of the renin–angiotensin system and vascular pathophysiology was discussed earlier. In Dahl S rats, ACE inhibitor therapy prevented hypertension, a decrease in NOS, abnormal vasodilation, left ventricular hypertrophy, and renal injury.[148]

Clinical trials examining ACE inhibitor therapy in post-myocardial infarction patients with left ventricular dysfunction have demonstrated a reduction in recurrent myocardial infarction.[98,99] It has been hypothesized that ACE inhibitors reduced coronary thrombosis by decreasing the formation of angiotensin II and reducing the release of PAI-1.[315] It has also been shown that patients with hypertension and elevated circulating renin concentrations, and, therefore, increased angiotensin II concentrations, have an increased risk of sustaining a myocardial infarction compared with those with normal or low renin concentrations.[316] ACE inhibitors also interfere with the breakdown of bradykinin[317] and, thereby, potentially increase the release of EDRF/NO by this peptide.

ACE inhibitors, originally developed as antihypertensive agents, are now thought to exert a major influence on the endothelium. ACE inhibitors can prevent the progression of atherosclerosis.[318] In hypertensive rats, ACE inhibitors reduce medial thickness and smooth muscle mass and reduce macrophage accumulation.[319,320] Inhibition of the actions of angiotensin II with ACE inhibitors limits vasoconstriction, smooth muscle hyperplasia, generation of toxic oxygen metabolites, and monocyte accumulation.[321] Inhibition of angiotensin II may also prevent the breakdown of bradykinin.[322] In patients with several risk factors, administration of the ACE inhibitor quinapril significantly reversed coronary artery endothelial dysfunction.[323] Brenner and co-workers[324] demonstrated a positive effect of the use of ACE inhibitors in preventing the progression of renal failure in the rat, and subsequent studies have shown a positive effect in preventing potentially deleterious effects of angiotensin II by ACE inhibitors.[325,326] This improvement in renal hemodynamics and attenuation of the rate of progression of azotemia in pre-dialysis patients with the use of ACE inhibitors is likely to be secondary to improving endothelial function.

Conclusion

In summary, abundant evidence indicates that endothelial dysfunction is an important mechanism in the development of vascular diseases. Alteration in any of the activities of the endothelium may accelerate the pathophysiology of many disease states, including atherosclerosis, hypertension, diabetes mellitus, coronary artery disease, and renal failure. A reduction in EDRF/NO activity may result in unopposed vasoconstriction, platelet aggregation, intravascular thrombosis, and smooth muscle proliferation. In addition, an increased production of oxygen-derived free radicals further enhances vascular pathogenicity.

Several treatment modalities may potentially ameliorate the deleterious effects of endothelial dysfunction, including lipid-lowering therapy, antioxidant/vitamin supplementation, and ACE inhibitor therapy. Further investigations designed to elucidate the mechanisms of endothelial dysfunction in ESRF will help to identify new therapeutic strategies directed at attenuation of endothelial pathophysiology.

References

1. Furchgott RF, Zawadzki JV (1980). The obligatory role of endothelial cells in the relaxation of arterial smooth muscle by acetylcholine. *Nature* 288, 373–6.
2. Ignarro LJ, Buga GM, Wood, Byrns, RE, Chauhuri G (1987). Endothelium-derived relaxing factor produced and released from artery and vein is nitric oxide. *Proceedings of the National Academy of Science* USA 84, 9265–9.
3. Palmer RM, Ferrige AG, Moncada S (1987). Nitric oxide release accounts for the biological activity of endothelial-derived relaxing factor. *Nature* 327, 524–6.
4. Stamler JS, Singel DJ, Loscalzo J (1992). Biochemistry of nitric oxide and its redox-activated forms. *Science* 258, 1898–902.
5. Cooke JP, Theilmeier G (1996). Endothelium-derived nitric oxide: an atherogenic molecule. *Resident Staff Physician* 42, 13–25.
6. Stamler JS, Loscalzo J (1991). The antiplatelet effects of organic nitrates and related nitroso compounds *in vitro* and *in vivo* and their relevance to cardiovascular disorders. Journal of *American College of Cardiology* 18, 1529–36.
7. Radomski MW, Palmer RM, Moncada S (1991). Modulation of platelet aggregation by an L-arginine–nitric oxide pathway. *Trends in Pharmacologic Science* 12, 87–8.
8. Radomski MW, Palmer RM, Moncada S (1990). An L-arginine/nitric oxide pathway present in human platelets regulates aggregation. *Proceedings of the National Academy of Science USA* 87, 5193–7.
9. Bath PM, Hassall DG, Gladin AM, Palmer RM, Martin JF (1991). Nitric oxide and prostacyclin. Divergence of inhibitory effects on monocyte chemotaxis and adhesion to endothelium *in vitro*. *Arteriosclerosis and Thrombosis* 88, 254–60.

10. Kubes P, Suzuki M, Granger DN (1991). Nitric oxide: an endogenous modulator of leukocyte adhesion. *Proceedings of the National Academy of Science USA* 88, 4651–5.

11. Vidal MJ, Zocchi MR, Poggi A, Pellegatta F, Churchia SL (1992). Involvement of nitric oxide in tumor cell adhesion to cytokine-activated endothelial cells. *Journal of Cardiovascular Pharmacology* 20, S155–9.

12. Ma XL, Weyrich AS, Lefer DJ, Lefer AM (1993). Diminished basal nitric oxide release after myocardial ischemia and reperfusion promotes neutrophil adherence to coronary endothelium. *Circulation Research* 72, 403–12.

13. Nathan C (1992). NO as a secretory product of mammalian cells. FASEB Journal 6, 3051–64.

14. Dinerman JL, Lowenstein CJ, Snyder SH (1993). Molecular mechanisms and nitric oxide regulation. *Circulation Research* 73, 217–22.

15. Bredt DS, Snyder SH (1990). Isolation of nitric oxide synthase, a calmodulin-requiring enzyme. *Proceedings of the National Academy of Science USA* 87, 682–5.

16. Busse R, Mulsch A (1990). Calcium-dependent nitric oxide synthesis in endothelial cytosol is mediated by calmodulin. *FEBS Lett* 265, 133–6.

17. Mayer B, Schmidt K, Jumbert P, Bohme E (1989). Biosynthesis of endothelium-derived relaxing factor: a cytosolic enzyme in porcine endothelial cells. Ca^{2+} dependently converts L-arginine into an activator of soluble guanylyl cyclase. *Biochemical and Biophysical Research Communications* 164, 678–85.

18. Ignarro LJ (1989). Biological actions and properties of endothelium-derived nitric oxide formed and released from artery and vein. *Circulation Research* 65, 1–21.

19. Marletta MA, Yoon PS, Iyengar R, Leaf CD, Wishnok JS (1988). Macrophage oxidation of L-arginine to nitrite and nitrate:nitric oxide is an intermediate. *Biochemistry* 27, 8706–11.

20. Yui Y, Hattori R, Kosuga K, Eizawa H, Hiki K, Ohkawa S, *et al.* (1991). Calmodulin-independent nitric oxide synthase from rat polymorphonuclear neutrophils. *Journal of Biological Chemistry* 266, 3369–71.

21. Drapier JC, Hibbs JB Jr (1988). Differentiation of murine macrophages express nonspecific cytotoxicity for tumor cell results in L-arginine-dependent inhibition of mitochondrial iron-sulfur enzymes in the macrophage effector cells. *Journal of Immunology* 140, 2829–38.

22. Welch G, Loscalzo J (1994). Nitric oxide and the cardiovascular system. *Journal of Cardiac Surgery* 9, 361–71.

23. Bredt DS, Ferris CD, Snyder SH (1992). NOS regulatory sites. Phosphorylation by cyclic AMP dependent protein kinase, protein C kinase, and calcium/calmodulin protein kinase, identification of flavin and calmodulin binding sites. *Journal of Biological Chemistry* 267, 10976–81.

24. Lewis MJ, Henderson, AH (1987). A phorbol ester inhibits the release of endothelium-derived relaxing factor. *European Journal of Pharmacology* 137, 167–71.

25. Freay A, Johns A, Adams DJ, Ryan US, Van Breeman C (1989). Bradykinin and inositol 1,4,5-trisphosphate-stimulated calcium release from intracellular stores in cultured bovine endothelial cells. *Pflugers Archives European Journal of Physiology* 414, 377–84.

26. Flavahan NA, Shimokawa H, Vanhoutte PM (1991). Inhibition of endothelium-dependent relaxation by phorbol myristate acetate in canine coronary arteries: role of a pertussis toxin-sensitive G-protein. *Journal of Pharmacology and Experimental Therapeutics* 256, 50–5.

27. Jin JS, D'Alecy LG (1996). Central and peripheral effects of asymmetric dimethylarginine, an endogenous nitric oxide synthetase inhibitor. *Cardiovascular Pharmacology* 28, 439–46.

28. Rubanyi GM, Romero JC, Vanhoutte PM (1986). Flow-induced release of endothelium-derived relaxing factor. *American Journal of Physiology* 250, 1145–9.

29. Olesen SP, Clapham DE, Davies PF (1988). Haemodynamic shear stress activates a K^+ current in vascular endothelial cells. *Nature* 331, 168–70.

30. Pohl U, Lamontagne D (1988). Impaired tissue perfusion after inhibition of endothelium-derived nitric oxide. *Basic Research in Cardiology* 86, 97–105.

31. Cooke JP, Stamler J, Andon N, Davies PF, McKinley G, Loscalzo J (1990). Flow stimulates endothelial cells to release nitrovasodilator that is potentiated by reduced thiol. *American Journal of Physiology* 259, H804–12.

32. Cooke JP, Rossitch E Jr, Andon N, Loscalzo J, Dzau VJ (1991). Flow activates an endothelial potassium channel to release endogenous nitrovasodilator. *Journal of Clinical of Investigation* 88, 1663–71.

33. Rees D, Palmer RM, Moncada S (1989). Role of endothelium-derived nitric oxide in the regulation of blood pressure. *Proceedings of the National Academy of Science USA* 86, 3375–8.

34. Fozard JR, Part M (1991). Haemodynamic responses to NG-monomethyl-L-arginine in spontaneously hypertensive and normotensive Wistar-Kyoto rats. *British Journal of Pharmacology* 102, 823–6.

35. Aisaka K, Gross SS, Griffith OW, Levi R (1989). NG-monomethyl arginine, an inhibitor of endothelium-derived nitric oxide synthesis, is a potent pressor agent in the guinea pig: does nitric oxide regulate blood pressure *in vivo*. *Biochemical and Biophysical Research Communications* 160, 881–6.

36. Vallance P, Collier JG, Moncada S (1989). Effect of endothelium-derived nitric oxide on peripheral arteriolar tone in man. *Lancet* 28, 997–1000.

37. Nishida K, Harrison DG, Navas JP, Fisher AA, Dockery SP, Uematsu M, *et al.* (1992). Molecular cloning and characterization of the constitutive bovine endothelial cell nitric oxide synthase. *Journal of Clinical Investigation* 90, 2092–3.

38. Awolesi MA, Widmann MD, Sessa WC, Sumpio BE (1994). Cyclic strain increases endothelial nitric oxide synthase activity. *Surgery* 116, 439–44.

39. Sessa W, Pritchard K, Seyedi N, Wang J, Hintze T (1994). Chronic exercise in dogs increases coronary vascular nitric oxide production and endothelial cell nitric oxide synthase gene expression. *Circulation Research* 74, 349–53.

40. Martin W, Villani GM, Jothianandan D, Furchgott RF (1985). Selective blockade of endothelium-dependent and glyceryl trinitrate—induced relaxation by hemoglobin and by methylene blue in rabbit aorta. *Journal of Pharmacology and Experimental Therapeutics* 232, 708–16.

41. Martin W, Furchgott RF, Villani GM, Jothianadan D (1986). Depression of contractile responses in rat aorta by spontaneously released endothelium-derived relaxing factor. *Journal of Pharmacology and Experimental Therapeutics* 237, 529–38.

42. Cohen RA, Zitnay KM, Weisbrod RM, Tesfamariam B (1988). Influence of the endothelium on tone and the response of isolated pig coronary artery to norepinephrine. *Journal of Pharmacology and Experimental Therapeutics* 244, 550–5.

43. Tesfamariam B, Weisbrod RM, Cohen RA (1987). Endothelium inhibits responses of rabbit carotid artery to adrenergic nerve stimulation. *American Journal of Physiology* 22, H792–8.

44. Kelm M, Feelisch M, Spahr R, Piper HM, Noack E, Schrader J (1988). Quantitative and kinetic characterization of nitric oxide and ERF release from cultured endothelial cells. *Biochemical and Biophysical Research Communications* 154, 237–44.

45. Gardiner SM, Compton AM, Bennett T, Palmer RM, Moncada S (1990). Control of regional blood flow by endothelium-derived nitric oxide. *Hypertension* 15, 486–92.

46. Lowenstein CJ, Dinerman JL, Snyder SH (1994). Nitric oxide: a physiologic messenger. *Annals of Internal Medicine* 120, 227–37.

47. Griffith TM, Edwards DH, Davies RL, Harrison TJ, Evans KT (1987). EDRF coordinates the behavior of vascular resistance vessels. *Nature* 329, 442–5.

48. Nozaki K, Moskowitz MA, Maynard KI, Koketsu N, Dawson TM, Bredt DS, *et al.* (1993). Possible origins and distribution of immunoreactive nitric oxide synthase-containing nerve fibers in cerebral arteries. *Journal of Cerebral Blood Flow and Metabolism* 13, 70–9.

49. Balligand JL, Kelly RA, Marsden PA, Smith TW, Michel T (1993). Control of cardiac muscle cell function by an endogenous nitric oxide signalling system. *Proceedings of the National Academy of Science USA* 90, 347–51.

50. Kourembanas S, McQuillan LP, Leung GK, Faller DV (1993). Nitric oxide regulates the expression of vasoconstrictors and growth factors by vascular endothelium under both normoxia and hypoxia. *Journal of Clinical Investigation* 92, 99–104.

51. Kourembanas S, Morsden PA, McQuillan LP, Faller DV (1991). Hypoxia induces endothelium gene expression and secretion in cultured human endothelium. *Journal of Clinical Investigation* 88, 1054–7.

52. Kourembanas S, Hannan RL, Faller DV (1990). Oxygen tension regulates the expression of the platelet-derived growth factor-B chain gene in human endothelial cells. *Journal of Clinical Investigation* 86, 670–4.

53. Luscher TF, Diederich D, Siebenmann R, Lehman K, Stutz P, vonSegesser L, *et al.* (1988). Difference between endothelium-dependent relaxation in arterial and in venous coronary bypass graft. *New England Journal of Medicine* 319, 462–7.

54. Ignarro LJ (1984). Association between cyclic GMP accumulation and acetylcholine-elicited relaxation of bovine intrapulmonary artery. *Journal of Pharmacology and Experimental Therapeutics* 228, 682–90.

55. Salvemini D, de Nucci G, Gryglewski RJ, Vane JR (1989). Human neutrophils and mononuclear cells inhibit platelet aggregation by releasing a nitric oxide-like factor. *Proceedings of the National Academy of Science USA* 86, 6328–32.

56. Gaboury J, Woodman RC, Granger DN, Reinhardt P, Kubes P (1993). Nitric oxide prevents leukocyte adherence: role of superoxide. *American Journal of Physiology* 265, H862–5.

57. Del Maestro RF, Planker M, Arfors KE (1982). Evidence for the participation of superoxide anion radical in altering the adhesive interaction between granulocytes and endothelium, *in vivo*. *International Journal of Microcirculation Clinical and Experimental* 1, 105–20.

58. Kubes P, Kanwar S, Niu X, Gaboury JP (1993). Nitric oxide inhibition induces leukocyte adhesion via superoxide and mast cells. *FASEB Journal* 7, 1293–9.

59. Keaney JF Jr, Vita JA (1995). Atherosclerosis, oxidative stress and antioxidant protection in EDRF action. *Progress in Cardiovascular Disease* 38, 129–54.

60. Gryglewski RJ, Palmer RM, Moncada S (1986). Superoxide anion is involved in the breakdown of endothelium derived vascular relaxing factor. *Nature* 320, 454–6.

61. Rubanyi GM, Vanhoutte PM (1986). Superoxide anions and hypoxia inactivate endothelium-derived relaxing factor. *American Journal of Physiology* 250, H822–7.

62. Omar HA, Cherry PD, Martelliti MP, Burke-Wolin T, Wolin MS (1991). Inhibition of coronary artery superoxide dismutase attenuates endothelium-dependent and -independent nitrovasodilator relaxation. *Circulation Research* 69, 601–8.

63. Tesfamariam B, Cohen RA (1992). Free radicals mediate endothelial cell dysfunction caused by elevated glucose. *American Journal of Physiology* 263, H321–6.

64. Mugge A, Elwell JH, Peterson TE, Hofmeyer TG, Heistad DD, Harrison DG (1991). Chronic treatment with polyethylene-glycolated superoxide dismutase partially restores endothelium-dependent vascular relaxation in cholesterol-fed rabbits. *Circulation Research* 69, 1293–300.

65. Abrahamsson T, Brat U, Marklund SL, Sjoqvist PO (1992). Vascular bound recombinant extracellular superoxide dismutase type C protects against the detrimental effects of superoxide radical on endothelium-dependent arterial relaxation. *Circulation Research* 70, 264–71.

66. Hattori Y, Kawasaki H, Abe K, Kanno M (1991). Superoxide dismutase recovers altered endothelium-dependent relaxation in diabetic rat aorta. *American Journal of Physiology* 261, H1086–94.

67. Cameron NE, Cotter MA, Maxfield EK (1993). Anti-oxidant treatment prevents the development of peripheral nerve dysfunction in streptozotocin-diabetic rats. *Diabetologia* 36, 299–304.

68. Martin DB, Granger DN, McCord JM, Parker JC, Taylor AR (1982). The protective effects of superoxide dismutase on pulmonary endothelial damage associated with antu. *Microvascular Research* 23, 265.

69. Nakazono K, Watanabe N, Matsuno K, Sasaki J, Sato T, Inoue M (1991). Does superoxide underlie the pathogenesis of hypertension? *Proceedings of the National Academy of Science USA* 88, 10045–8.

70. Clowes AW, Reidy MA, Clowes MM (1983). Kinetics of cellular proliferation after arterial injury. Smooth muscle growth in the absence of endothelium. *Laboratory Investigation* 49, 327–33.

71. Reidy MA (1985). Biology of disease A reassessment of endothelial injury and arterial lesion formation. *Laboratory Investigation* 53, 513–20.

72. Weidinger FF, McLenaehan JM, Cybulsky MI, Gordon JB, Rennke HG, Hollenberg NK, *et al.* (1990). Persistent dysfunction of regenerated endothelium after balloon angioplasty of rabbit iliac artery. *Circulation* 81, 1667–79.

73. Lepoivre M, Flaman JM, Henry Y (1992). Early loss of the tyrosyl radical of ribonucleotide reductase of adenocarcinoma cells producing nitric oxide. *Journal of Biology and Chemistry* 267, 22994–3000.

74. Molina y Vedia L (1993). Nitric oxide S-nitrosylation of glyceraldehyde-3-phosphate dehydrogenase inhibits enzymatic activity and increases endogenous ADP-ribosylation. *Journal of Biology and Chemistry* 267, 24929–32.

75. Taguchi J, Abe J, Okazaki H, Takuwa Y, Yurokawa K (1993). L-Arginine inhibits neointimal formation following balloon injury. *Life Sciences* 53, PL387–92.

76. Schwarzacher SP, Lim TT, Wang B, Kernoff RS, Niebauer J, Cooke JP, *et al.* (1997). Local intramural delivery of L-arginine enhances nitric oxide generation and inhibits lesion formation after balloon angioplasty. *Circulation* 95, 1863–9.

77. Wang BY, Candipan RC, Arjomandi M, Hsiun PT, Tsao PS, Cooke JP (1996). Arginine restores nitric oxide activity and inhibits monocyte accumulation after vascular injury in hypercholesterolemic rabbits. *Journal of the American College of Cardiology* 28, 1573–9.

78. Castellot JJ Jr, Addonizio ML, Rosenberg R, Karnovsky MJ (1981). Cultured endothelial cells produce a heparin-like inhibitor of smooth muscle cell growth. *Journal of Cell Biology* 90, 372–9.

79. Chen G, Suzuki H (1990). Calcium dependency of the endothelium-dependent hyperpolarization in smooth muscle cells of the rabbit carotid artery. *Journal of Physiology* 421, 521–34.

80. Suzuki H, Chen G, Yamamoto Y (1992). Endothelium-derived hyperpolarizing factor (EDHF). *Japanese Circulation Journal* 56, 170–4.

81. Chen G, Suzuki H, Weston AH (1988). Acetylcholine releases endothelium-derived hyperpolarizing factor and EDRF from rat blood vessels. *British Journal of Pharmacology* 95, 1165–74.

82. Nagao T, Vanhoutte PM (1993). Endothelium-derived hyperpolarizing factor and endothelium-dependent relaxation. *American Journal of Respiratory Cell Molecular Biology* 8, 1–6.

83. Taylor SG, Weston AH (1988). Endothelium-derived hyperpolarizing factor: a new endogenous inhibitor from the vascular endothelium. *Trends in Pharmacologic Science* 9, 272–4.

84. Weston AH, Edwards G (1992). Recent progress in potassium channel opener pharmacology. *Biochemistry and Pharmacology* 43, 47–54.

85. Hekman CM, Loskutoff DJ (1987). Fibrinolytic pathways and the endothelium. *Seminars in Thrombosis and Hemostasis* 13, 514–27.

86. Hajjar KA, Hamel NM (1990). Identification and characterization of human endothelial cell membrane binding sites for tissue plasminogen activator and urokinase. *Journal of Biology and Chemistry* 265, 2908–16.

87. Loskutoff D, Edgington TE (1977). Synthesis of a fibrinolytic activator and inhibitor by endothelial cells. *Proceedings of the National Academy of Science USA* 74, 3903–7.

88. Erickson LA, Heckman CM, Loskutoff DJ (1985). The primary plasminogen-activator inhibitors in endothelial cells, platelets, serum, and plasma are immunologically related. *Proceedings of the National Academy of Science USA 82*, 8710–14.

89. Sprengers ED, Kluft C (1987). Plasminogen activator inhibitors. *Blood* 69, 381–7.

90. Turitto VT, Weiss HJ, Baumgartner HR (1984). Platelet interaction with rabbit subendothelium in von Willebrand disease: altered thrombus formation distinct from defective platelet adhesion. *Journal of Clinical Investigation* 74, 1730–41.

91. Marcum JA, Rosenberg RD (1985). Heparin-like molecules with anticoagulant activity are synthesized by cultured endothelial cells. *Biochemical and Biophysical Research Communications* 126, 365–72.

92. Esmon NL, Owen WG, Esmon CT (1982). Isolation of membrane-bound cofactor for thrombin-catalyzed activation of protein C. *Journal of Biology and Chemistry* 257, 859–64.

93. Meyer D, Baumgartner HR (1983). Role of von Willebrand factor in platelet adhesion to the subendothelium. *British Journal of Haematology* 54, 1–9.

94. Ridker PM, Vaughan DE, Stampfer MJ, Manson JE, Hennekens CH (1993). Endogenous tissue-type plasminogen activator and risk of myocardial infarction. *Lancet* 341,1165–8.

95. Jansson JH, Nilsson TK, Olofsson BO (1991). Tissue plasminogen activator and other risk factors as predictors of cardiovascular events in patients with severe angina pectoris. *European Heart Journal* 12, 157–61.

96. Vaughan DE, Lazos SC (1992). Angiotensin II induces plasminogen activator inhibitor (PAI-1) *in vitro*. *Circulation* 86 (Suppl 1), I-557.

97. Ridker PM, Gaboury CL, Conlin PR, Seely EW, Williams GH, Vaughan DE (1993). Stimulation of plasminogen activator inhibitor *in vivo* by infusion of angiotensin II. Evidence of a potential interaction between the renin–angiotensin system and fibrinolytic function. *Circulation* 87, 1969–73.

98. Pfeffer MA, Braunwald E, Moye LA, Bastal, Brown EJ Jr, Cuddy TE, et al. (1992). Effect of captopril on mortality and morbidity in patients with left ventricular dysfunction after myocardial infarction. Results of the survival and ventricular enlargement trial The SAVE Investigators. *New England Journal of Medicine* 327, 676–7.

99. The SOLVD Investigators (1991). Effects of enalapril on survival in patients with reduced left ventricular ejection fractions and congestive heart failure. *New England Journal of Medicine* 325, 293–302.

100. Fei H, Berliner JA, Parhami F, Drake TA (1993). Regulation of endothelial cell tissue factor expression by minimally oxidized LDL and lipopolysaccharide. *Arteriosclerosis and Thrombosis* 23, 1711.

101. Briggs JP, Schnermann J (1995). Control of renin release and glomerular vascular tone by the juxtaglomerular apparatus. *Hypertension: Pathophysiology, Diagnosis, and Management* (ed. Laragh JH, Brenner BM), pp. 1359–84. Raven Press, New York.

102. Nakamura T, Alberola AM, Salazar FJ, Saito Y, Kurashina T, Granger JP, et al. (1998). Effects of renal perfusion pressure on renal interstitial hydrostatic pressure and Na+ excretion: role of endothelium-derived nitric oxide. *Nephron* 78, 104–11.

103. Bech JN, Nielsen CB, Ivarsen P, Jensen KT, Pedersen EB (1998). Dietary sodium affects systemic and renal hemodynamic response to NO inhibition in healthy humans. *American Journal of Physiology* 274, F914–23.

104. Wilcox CS, Welch WJ (1996). TGF and nitric oxide: effects of salt intake and salt-sensitive hypertension. *Kidney International* 49, S9–13.

105. Welch WJ, Wilcox CS (1993). Independent effects of salt intake and angiotensin II on the macula densa-nitric oxide signalling pathway. *Journal of American Society of Nephrology* 4, 572.

106. Welch WJ, Wilcox CS (1997). Macula densa arginine delivery and uptake in the rat regulates glomerular capillary pressure: effects of salt intake. *Journal of Clinical Investigation* 100, 2235–42.

107. Raij L, Keane WF (1985). Glomerular mesangium: its function and relationship to angiotensin II. *American Journal of Medicine* 79 (Suppl 36), 24–30.

108. Schlondorff D (1987). The glomerular mesangial cell: an expanding role for specialized pericyte. *FASEB Journal* 1, 272–81.

109. Mene P, Simonson MS, Dunn MJ (1989). Physiology of mesangial cell. *Physiology Review* 69, 1347–424.

110. Schultz PJ, Shorer AE, Raij L (1990). Effects of endothelium derived relaxing factor and nitric oxide in rat mesangial cells. *American Journal of Physiology* 258, F162–7.

111. Tolins JP, Palmer RM, Moncada S, Raij L (1990). Role of endothelium-derived relaxing factor in regulation of renal hemodynamic responses. *American Journal of Physiology* 258, H655–62.

112. Gibbons GH, Dzau VJ (1994). The emerging concept of vascular remodeling. *New England Journal of Medicine* 330, 1431–8 (Review).

113. Vidal MJ, Romero JC, Vanhoutte PM (1988). Endothelium-derived relaxing factor inhibits renin release. *European Journal of Pharmacology* 149, 401–2.

114. Tolins JP, Raij L (1991). Effects of amino acid infusion on renal hemodynamics: Role of endothelium-derived relaxing factor. *Hypertension* 17, 1045–51.

115. Hayakawa H, Raij L (1998). Nitric oxide synthase activity and renal injury in genetic hypertension. *Hypertension* 31, 266–70.

116. Takemoto M, Egashira K, Usui M, Numaguchi K, Tomita H, Tsutsui H, *et al.* (1997). Important role of tissue angiotensin-converting enzyme activity in the pathogenesis of coronary vascular and myocardial structural changes induced by long-term blockade of nitric oxide synthesis in rats. *Journal of Clinical Investigation* 99, 278–87.

117. Griendling KK, Minieri CA, Ollerenshaw JD, Alexander RW (1994). Angiotensin II stimulates NADH and NADPH oxidase activity in cultured vascular smooth muscle cells. *Circulation Research* 74, 1141–8.

118. Galceran JM, Jaimes EA, Raij L (1996). Pathogenetic role of angiotensin II in glomerular injury: is superoxide the missing link? *Journal of American Society of Nephrology* 7, 1631.

119. White CR, Brock TA, Chang L-Y, Crapo J, Briscoe P, Ku D (1994). Superoxide and peroxynitrite in atherosclerosis. *Proceedings of the National Academy of Science* USA 91, 1044–48.

120. Ito S, Johnson CS, Carretero OA (1991). Modulation of angiotensin II-induced vasoconstriction by endothelium-derived relaxing factor in the isolated microperfused rabbit afferent arteriole. *Journal of Clinical Investigation* 87, 1656–63.

121. Garg UC, Hassid A (1989). Inhibition of rat mesangial cell mitogenesis by nitric oxide-generating vasodilation. *American Journal of Physiology* 237, F60–6.

122. Schultz P, Ruble D, Raij L (1990). S-Nitroso-n-acetylpenicillamine (SNAP) inhibits mitogen-induced mesangial cell proliferation. *Kidney International* 37, 203.

123. Vanhoutte PM, Rubany GM, Millre VM, Houston DS (1986). Modulation of vascular smooth muscle contraction by endothelium. *Annual Review of Physiology* 48, 307–20.

124. Deng X, Welch WJ, Wilcox CS (1996). Role of nitric oxide in short-term and prolonged effects of angiotensin II on renal hemodynamics. *Hypertension* 27, 1173–9.

125. Hennington BS, Zhang H, Miller MT, Granger JP, Reckelhoff JF (1998). Angiotensin II stimulates synthesis of endothelial nitric oxide synthase. *Hypertension* 31, 283–8.

126. Zanzinger J, Zheng X, Bassenge E (1994). Endothelium dependent vasomotor responses to endogenous agonists are potentiated following angiotensin converting enzyme inhibition by a bradykinin dependent mechanism. *Cardiovascular Research* 28, 209–14.

127. Wiemer G, Scholkens BA, Becker RH, Busse R (1991). Ramiprilat enhances endothelial autocoid formations by inhibiting breakdown of endothelium-derived bradykinin. *Hypertension* 18, 558–63.

128. Skidgel RA, Erdos EG (1987). The broad substrate specificity of human angiotensin I converting enzyme. *Clinical and Experimental Hypertension Part A. Theory and Practice* 9, 243–59.

129. Dorer FE, Kahn JR, Lentz KE, Levine M, Skeggs LT (1974). Hydrolysis of bradykinin by angiotensin-converting enzyme. *Circulation Research* 34, 824–7.

130. Cockcroft JR, Chowienczyk PJ, Brett SE, Ritter JM (1994). Effect of NG-monomethyl-L-arginine on kinin-induced vasodilation in the human forearm. *British Journal of Clinical Pharmacology* 38, 307–10.

131. O'Kane KP Webb DJ, Collier JG, Vallance RJ (1994). Local L-NG-monomethylarginine attenuates the vasodilator action of bradykinin in the human forearm. *British Journal of Clinical Pharmacology* 38, 311–15.

132. Mombouli JV, Vanhoutte PM (1992). Heterogeneity of endothelium-dependent vasodilator effects of angiotensin-converting inhibitors: role of bradykinin generation during ACE inhibition. *Journal of Cardiovascular Pharmacology* 20, S74–82.

133. Kiowski W, Linder L, Kleinbloesem C, van Brummelen P, Buhler FR (1992). Blood pressure control by the renin–angiotensin system in normotensive subjects. Assessment by angiotensin converting enzyme and renin inhibition. *Circulation* 85, 1–8.

134. Frohlich ED (1997). Arthus C. Corcoran Memorial Lecture. Influence of nitric oxide and angiotensin II on renal involvement in hypertension. *Hypertension* 29, 188–93.

135. Conger JD, Robinette, JB, Schrier RW (1988). Smooth muscle calcium and endothelium-derived relaxing factor in the abnormal vascular responses of acute renal failure. *Journal of Clinical Investigation* 82, 532–7.

136. Firth JD, Ratcliffe PJ (1992). Organ distribution of the three rat endothelin messenger RNAs and the effects of ischemia on renal gene expression. *Journal of Clinical Investigation* 90, 1023–31.

137. Romero JC, Lahera V, Salom MG, Biondi ML (1992). Role of endothelium-dependent relaxing factor nitric oxide on renal function. *Journal of the American Society of Nephrology* 2, 1371–87.

138. De Nicola L, Blantz RC, Gabbai FB (1992). Nitric oxide and angiotensin II. Glomerular and tubular interaction in the rat. *Journal of Clinical Investigation* 89, 1248–56.

139. Stoos BA, Carretero OA, Farhy RD, Scicli G, Garvin JL (1992). Endothelium-derived relaxing factor inhibits transport and increased cGMP content in cultured mouse cortical collecting duct cells. *Journal of Clinical Investigation* 89, 761–5.

140. Henrich WL, McAllister FA, Smith PB, Campbell WB (1988). Guanosine 3'5'-cyclic monophosphate as a mediator of inhibition of renin release. *American Journal of Physiology* 255, F474–8.

141. Schultz PJ, Tolins JP (1993). Adaptation to increased dietary salt intake in the rat. Role of endogenous nitric oxide. *Journal of Clinical Investigation* 91, 642–50.

142. Chen PY, Sanders PW (1991). L-Arginine abrogates salt-sensitive hypertension in Dahl/Rapp rats. *Journal of Clinical Investigation* 88, 1559–67.

143. Chen PY, Sanders PW (1993). Role of nitric oxide synthesis in salt-sensitive hypertension in Dahl/Rapp rats. *Hypertension Dallas* 22, 812–18.

144. Hu L, Manning RD Jr (1995). Role of nitric oxide in regulation of long-term pressure-natriuresis relationship in Dahl rats. *American Journal of Physiology* 268, H2375–83.

145. Ikeda Y, Saito K, Kim JI, Yokoyama M (1995). Nitric oxide synthase isoform activities in kidney for Dahl salt-sensitive rats. *Hypertension* 26, 1030–4.

146. Mattson DL, Higgins DJ (1996). Influence of dietary sodium intake on renal medullary nitric oxide synthase. *Hypertension* 27, 688–92.

147. Hayakawa H, Raij L (1997). The link among nitric oxide synthase activity, endothelial function, and aortic and ventricular hypertrophy in hypertension. *Hypertension* 29, 235–41.

148. Hayakawa H, Coffee K, Raij L (1997). Endothelial dysfunction and cardiorenal injury in experimental salt-sensitive hypertension: effects of antihypertensive therapy. *Circulation* 96, 2407–13.

149. Campese VN, Tawadrous M, Bigazzi R, Bianchi S, Mann AS, Oparil, S, *et al.* (1996). Salt intake and plasma atrial natriuretic peptide and nitric oxide in hypertension. *Hypertension* 28, 335–40.

150. Campese VM (1994). Salt sensitivity in hypertension. Renal and cardiovascular implications. *Hypertension* 23, 531–5.

151. Wilson CB (1991). The renal response to immunologic injury. In: *The kidney*, 4th edn (ed. Brenner and Rector), pp. 1062–181. WB Saunders, Philadelphia.

152. Raij L (1994). Glomerular thrombosis in pregnancy: role of L-arginine–nitric oxide pathway. *Kidney International* 45, 775–81.

153. Giroir BP, Johnson JH, Brown T, Allen GL, Beutler B (1992). The tissue distribution of tumor necrosis factor biosynthesis during endotoxemia. *Journal of Clinical Investigation* 90, 693–8.

154. van der Poll T, Buller HR, ten Cate H, Wortel CH, Bauer KA, *et al.* (1990). Activation of coagulation after administration of tumor necrosis factor to normal subjects. *New England Journal of Medicine* 322, 1622–7.

155. Raij L, Baylis C (1995). Glomerular actions of nitric oxide. *Kidney International* 48, 20–32.
156. Levine GN, Keaney JF Jr, Vita JA (1995). Cholesterol reduction in cardiovascular disease. Clinical benefits and possible mechanisms. *New England Journal of Medicine* 332, 512–21.
157. Bossallar C, Habib GB, Yamamoto H, Williams C, Wells S, Nemy PD (1987). Impaired muscarinic endothelium-dependent relaxation and cyclic guanosine 5′-monophosphate formation in atherosclerotic human coronary artery and rabbit aorta. *Journal of Clinical Investigation* 62, 185–90.
158. Forstermann U, Mugge A, Alheid U, Haverich A, Frolich JC (1988). Selective attenuation of endothelium-mediated vasodilation in atherosclerotic human coronary arteries. *Circulation Research* 62, 185–90.
159. Verbeuren TJ, Jordaens FJ, Zonnekeyn LL, VanHovi CE, Coene MC, Herman AG (1986). Effect of hypercholesterolemia on vascular reactivity in the rabbit. Endothelium-dependent and endothelium-independent contraction and relaxations in isolated arteries of control and hypercholesterolemic rabbits. *Circulation Research* 58, 552–64.
160. Simon BC, Haudenschild CC, Cohen RA (1993). Preservation of endothelium-dependent relaxation in atherosclerotic rabbit aorta by probucol. *Journal of Cardiovascular Pharmacology* 21, 893–901.
161. Cooke JP, Dzau VJ (1997). Nitric oxide synthase: role in the genesis of vascular disease. *Annual Review in Medicine* 48, 489–509.
162. Stroes E, Kastelein J, Cosentino F, Erkelens W, Wever R, Koomans H, *et al.* (1997). Tetrahydrobiopterin restores endothelial function in hypercholesterolemia. *Journal of Clinical Investigation* 99, 41–6.
163. Harrison DG, Freiman PC, Armstrong ML, Marcus ML, Heistad DD (1987). Alterations of vascular reactivity in atherosclerosis. *Circulation Research* 61, 1174–80.
164. Minor RL Jr, Myers PR, Guerra R Jr, Bates JN, Harrison DG (1990). Diet-induced atherosclerosis increases the release of nitrogen oxides from rabbit aorta. *Journal of Clinical Investigation* 86, 2109–16.
165. Oemar BS, Tschudi MR, Godoy N, Brovkovich V, Malinski T, Luscher TF (1998). Reduced endothelial nitric oxide synthase expression and production in human atherosclerosis. *Circulation* 97, 2494–8.
166. Panza JA, Quyumi AA, Brush JE Jr, Epstein SE (1990). Abnormal endothelium-dependent vascular relaxation in patients with essential hypertension. *New England Journal of Medicine* 323, 22–7.
167. Tschudi MR, Criscione L, Novosel D, Pfeiffer K, Lusher TF (1994). Antihypertensive therapy augments endothelium-dependent relaxation in coronary arteries of spontaneously hypertensive rats. *Circulation* 89, 2212–18.
168. Luscher TF, Vanhoutte PM. (1986). Endothelium-dependent contractions to acetylcholine in the aorta of the spontaneously hypertensive rat. *Hypertension* 8, 344–8.
169. Diederich D, Yang ZH, Buhler FR, Luscher TF (1990). Impaired endothelium-dependent relaxations in hypertensive resistance arteries involve cyclooxygenase pathway. *American Journal of Physiology* 258, H445–51.
170. Barton M, d'Uscio LV, Shaw S, Meyer P, Moreau P, Luscher TF (1998). ET-1 receptor blockade prevents increased tissue ET-1, vascular hypertrophy and endothelial dysfunction in salt-sensitive hypertension. *Hypertension* 31, 499–504.
171. Tesfamariam B, Jakabowski JA, Cohen RA (1989). Contraction of diabetic rabbit aorta due to endothelium-derived PGH2/TXA2. *American Journal of Physiology* 257, H1327–33.
172. Oyama Y, Kawasaki H, Hattori Y, Kanno M (1986). Attenuation of endothelium-dependent relaxation in aorta from diabetic rats. *European Journal of Pharmacology* 132, 75–8.
173. Tesfamariam B, Brown ML, Deykin D, Cohen RA (1990). Elevated glucose promotes generation of endothelium-derived vasoconstrictor prostanoids in rabbit aorta. *Journal of Clinical Investigation* 85, 929–32.

174. Keaney JF Jr, Xu A, Cunningham D, Jackson T, Frei B, Vita JA (1995). Dietary probucol preserves endothelial function in cholesterol fed rabbits by limiting vascular oxidative stress and superoxide production. *Journal of Clinical Investigation* 95, 2520–9.

175. Steinberg D, Parthasarathy S, Carew TE, Khoo JC, Witzum JL (1989). Beyond cholesterol. Modifications of low density lipoprotein that increase its atherogenecity. *New England Journal of Medicine* 320, 915–24.

176. Ohara Y, Peterson TE, Harrison DG (1993). Hypercholesterolemia increases endothelial superoxide anion production. *Journal of Clinical Investigation* 91, 2546–51.

177. Ohara Y (1993). Dietary treatment of hypercholesterolemia normalizes endothelial superoxide production. *Circulation* 88, I-467.

178. Levine GN, Frei B, Koulouris SN, Gerhar MD, Keaney JF Jr, Vita JA (1996). Ascorbic acid reverses endothelial function in patients with coronary artery disease. *Circulation* 93, 1107–13.

179. Cohen RA, Zitnay KM, Haudenschild CC, Cunningham LD (1988). Loss of selective endothelial cell vasoactive functions caused by hypercholesterolemia in pig coronary arteries. *Circulation Research* 63, 903–10.

180. Vita JA, Treasure CB, Nabel EG, McLenachan JM, Fish RD, Yeung AC, *et al.* (1990). Coronary vasomotor response to acetylcholine relates to risk factors for coronary artery disease. *Circulation* 81, 491–7.

181. Pou S, Pou WS, Bredt DS, Snyder SH, Rosen GM (1992). Generation of superoxide by purified brain nitric oxide synthase. *Journal of Biological Chemistry* 267, 24173–6.

182. Wei EP, Kontos HF (1990). H_2O_2 and endothelium-dependent cerebral arteriolar dilation. Implications for the identity of endothelium-derived relaxing factor generated by acetylcholine. *Hypertension* 16, 162–9.

183. Weiss SJ, Young J, LoBuglio AF, Slivka A, Nimeh NF (1981). Role of hydrogen peroxide in neutrophil-mediated destruction of cultured endothelial cells. *Journal of Clinical Investigation* 68, 714–21.

184. Kume N, Cybulsky MI, Gimbrone MA Jr (1992). Lysophosphatidylcholine, a component of atherogenic lipoproteins, induces mononuclear leukocyte adhesion molecules in cultured human and rabbit arterial endothelial cells. *Journal of Clinical Investigation* 90, 1138–44.

185. Libby P, Geng YJ, Aikawa M, Schoenbeck U, Mach F, Clinton SK, *et al.* (1996). Macrophages and atherosclerotic plaque stability. *Current Opinions in Lipidology* 7, 330–5.

186. Cushing SD, Berliner JA, Valente AJ, Territo MC, Navab, M, Parhami F, *et al.* (1990). Minimally modified low density lipoprotein induces monocyte chemotactic protein 1 in human endothelial cells and smooth muscle cells. *Proceedings in National Academy of Science USA* 87, 5134–8.

187. Cybulsky MI, Gimbrone MA Jr (1991). Endothelial expression of mononuclear leukocyte adhesion molecule during atherogenesis. *Science* 251, 788–91.

188. McNally AK, Chisolm GM, Morel DW, Cathcart MK (1990). Activated human monocytes oxidize low-density lipoprotein by a lipooxygenase-dependent pathway. *Journal of Immunology* 145, 254–9.

189. Hiramatsu K, Rosen H, Heinicke JW, Wolfbauer G, Chait A (1986). Superoxide initiates oxidation of low density lipoproteins by human monocytes. *Arteriosclerosis* 7, 55–60.

190. Negre-Salvayre A, Pieraggi MT, Mabile L, Salvayre R (1992). Protective effect of 17-beta estradiol against the cytotoxicity of minimally oxidized LDL to cultured bovine aortic endothelial cells. *Atherosclerosis* 99, 207–17.

191. Kugiyama K, Kerns SA, Morrisette JD, Roberts R, Henry PD (1990). Impairment of endothelium-dependent arterial relaxation by lysolecithin in modified low-density lipoproteins. *Nature* 344, 160–2.

192. Lerman A, Edwards BS, Hallett JW, Heublein DM, Sandberg SM, Burnett JC Jr (1991). Circulating and tissue endothelin immunoreactivity in advanced atherosclerosis. *New England Journal of Medicine* 325, 997–1001.

193. Boulanger CM, Tanner FC, Bea ML, Hahn AW, Werner A, Luscher TF (1992). Oxidized low-density lipoproteins induce mRNA expression and release from human and porcine endothelium. *Circulation Research* 70, 1191–7.

194. Steinberg D (1991). Antioxidants and atherosclerosis. A current assessment. *Circulation* 84, 1420–5.

195. Keaney JF Jr, Gaziano JM, Xu A, Frei B, Curran-Celentano J, Shwaery G, *et al.* (1994). Low-dose alpha-tocopherol improves and high-dose alpha-tocopherol worsens endothelial vasodilator function in cholesterol-fed rabbits. *Journal of Clinical Investigation* 93, 844–51.

196. Bucala R, Tracey, KJ, Cerami A (1991). Advanced glycosylation products quench nitric oxide and mediate defective endothelium-dependent vasodilation in experimental diabetes. *Journal of Clinical Investigation* 87, 432–8.

197. Wei EP, Kontos HA, Christman CW, DeWitt DS, Povlishock JT (1985). Superoxide generation and reversal of acetylcholine-induced cerebral arteriolar dilatation after acute hypertension. *Circulation Research* 57, 781–7.

198. Omar BA, Flores SC, McCord JM (1992). Superoxide dismutase: pharmacological developments and applications. *Advances in Pharmacology* 23, 109–61.

199. Taddei S, Virdis A, Ghiadoni L, Magagna A, Salvetti A (1998). Vitamin C improves endothelium-dependent vasodilation by restoring nitric oxide activity in essential hypertension. *Circulation* 97, 2222–9.

200. Final Report of the Subcommittee on Definition and Prevalence of the 1984 National Joint Committee (1985). Hypertension prevalence and the states of awareness, treatment, and control in the United States. *Hypertension* 7, 457–68.

201. Burt VL, Whelton P, Roccella EJ, Brown C, Cutler JA, Higgins M, *et al.* (1995). Prevalence of hypertension in the US adult population. Results from the Third National Health and Nutrition Examination Survey, 1988–1991. *Hypertension* 25, 305–13.

202. Rostand SG, Kirk KA, Rutsky EA, Pate BA (1982). Racial differences in the incidence of treatment for end-stage renal disease. *New England Journal of Medicine* 306, 1276–9.

203. Dustan HP (1995). Does keloid pathogenesis hold the key to understanding black/white differences in hypertension severity? *Hypertension* 26, 858–62.

204. Russell SB, Trupin KM, Rodriguez-Eaton S, Russell JD, Trupin JS (1988). Reduced growth-factor requirement of keloid-derived fibroblasts may account for tumor growth. *Proceedings of the National Academy of Science USA* 85, 587–91.

205. McCauley RL, Chopra V, Li Y-Y, Herndon D, Robson MC (1992). Altered cytokine production in black patients with keloids. *Journal of Clinical Immunology* 12, 300–8.

206. Woo KS, Chook P, Lolin YI, Cheung AS, Chan LT, Sun YY, *et al.* (1997). Hyperhomocysteinemia is a risk factor for arterial endothelial dysfunction in humans. *Circulation* 96, 2542–4.

207. McCully KS (1969). Vascular pathology of homocysteinemia: implications for the pathogenesis of arteriosclerosis. *American Journal of Pathology* 56, 111–28.

208. Nygard O, Vollset SE, Refsum H, Stensvold I, Tverdal A, Nordrehaug JE, *et al.* (1995). Total plasma homocysteine and cardiovascular risk profile. The Horland Homocysteine Study. *Journal of American Medical Association* 274, 1526–33.

209. Stampfer MJ, Malinow MR, Willett WC, Newcomer LM, Upson B, Ullman D, *et al.* (1992). A prospective study of plasma homocyst(e)ine and risk of myocardial infarction in US physicians. *Journal of American Medical Association* 268, 877–81.

210. Graham IM, Daly LE, Refsum HM, Robinson K, Brattstrom LE, Ueland PM, *et al.* (1997). Plasma homocysteine as a risk factor for vascular disease. The European Concerted Action Project. *Journal of American Medical Association* 277, 1775–81.

211. Nygard O, Nordrehaug JE, Refsum HM, Ueland PM, Farstad M, Vollset SE (1997). Plasma homocysteine levels and mortality in patients with coronary artery disease. *New England Journal of Medicine* 337, 230–6.

212. Wald NJ, Watt HC, Law MR, Weir DG, McPartlin J, Scott JM (1998). Homocysteine and ischemic heart disease: results of a prospective study with implications regarding prevention. *Archives of Internal Medicine* 158, 862–7.

213. Selhub J, Jacques PF, Wilson PW, Rush D, Rosenberg IH (1993). Vitamin status and intake as primary determinants of homocysteinemia in an elderly population. *Journal of American Medical Association* 270, 2693–8.

214. Ubbink, JB Vermaak WJ, van der Merwe A, Becker PJ (1993). Vitamin B12, vitamin B6, and folate nutritional status in men with hyperhomocysteinemia. *American Journal of Clinical Nutrition* 57, 47–53.

215. Wilcken DE, Wilcken B, Dudman NP, Tyrell PA (1983). Homocysteinuria—the effects of betaine in the treatment of patients not responsive to pyridoxine. *New England Journal of Medicine* 309, 448–53.

216. Ueland PM, Refsum H, Brattstrom L (1982). Plasma homocysteine and cardiovascular disease. In: *Atherosclerotic cardiovascular disease, hemostasis, and endothelial function* (ed. Francis RB Jr), pp. 183. Marcel Dekker, New York.

217. Mayer EM, Jacobsen DW, Robinson K (1996). Homocysteine and coronary atherosclerosis. *Journal of American College of Cardiology* 27, 517–27.

218. Wilcken DE, Gupta VJ, Reddy SG (1980) Accumulation of sulphur-containing amino acids including cysteine–homocysteine disulfide in patients on maintenance haemodialysis, *Clinical Science* 58, 427.

219. Kang SS, Wong PW, Didani A, Milanez S (1983). Plasma protein-bound homocyst(e)ine in patients requiring chronic haemodialysis. *Clinical Science* 65, 335–6.

220. Chauveau P, Chadefaux B, Coude M, Aupetit J, Hannendouche T, Kamoun P, *et al.* (1993). Hyperhomocysteinemia a risk factor for atherosclerosis in chronic uremic patients. *Kidney International* 41, S72–7.

221. Hultberg B, Andersson A, Sterner G (1993). Plasma homocysteine in renal failure. *Clinical Nephrology* 40, 230–5.

222. Cohen BD, Patel H, Kornhauser RS (1977). Alternate reasons for atherogenesis in uremia. *Proceedings of Dialysis Transplant Forum* 7, 178–80.

223. Wilcken DE, Gupta VJ (1979). Sulfur containing amino acids in chronic renal failure with particular reference to homocysteine and cysteine–homocysteine mixed disulfide. *European Journal of Clinical Investigation* 9, 301–7.

224. Wilcken DE, Gupta VJ, Betss AK (1981). Homocysteine in the plasma of renal transplant recipients: effects of cofactors for methionine metabolism. *Clinical Science* 61, 743–9.

225. Soria C, Chadefaux B, Coude M, Gaillard O, Kamoun P (1990). Concentrations of total homocysteine in plasma in chronic renal failure. *Clinical Chemistry* 36, 2137–8.

226. Kim SS, Hirose S, Tamura H, Nagasawa R, Tokushima H, Mitarai T, *et al.* (1994). Hyperhomocysteinemia as a possible role for atherosclerosis in CAPD patients. *Advances in Peritoneal Dialysis* 10, 282–5.

227. Massy ZA, Chadefaux-Vekemans B, Chevalier A, Bader CA, Drueke TB, Legendre C, *et al.* (1994). Hyperhomocysteinaemia: a significant risk factor for cardiovascular disease in renal transplant patients. *Nephrology Dialysis Transplant* 9, 1103–8.

228. Bachmann J, Tepel M, Raidt H, Riezler R, Graefe U, Langer K, *et al.* (1995). Hyperhomocysteinemia and the risk for vascular disease in hemodialysis patients. *Journal of American Society of Nephrology* 6, 121–5.

229. Hultberg B, Andersson A, Arnadottir M (1995). Reduced, free and total fractions of homocysteine and other thiol compounds in plasma from patients with renal failure. *Nephron* 70, 62–7.

230. Robinson K, Gupta A, Dennis V, Arheart K, Chaudhary D, Green R, *et al.* (1996). Hyperhomocysteinemia confers an independent increased risk of atherosclerosis in end-stage renal disease and is closely linked to plasma folate and pyridoxine concentrations. *Circulation* 94, 2743–8.

231. Bostom AG, Shemin D, Nadeau MR, Shih V, Stabler SP, Allen RH, *et al.* (1995). Short term betaine therapy fails to lower elevated fasting total plasma homocysteine concentrations in hemodialysis patients maintained on chronic folic acid supplementation. *Atherosclerosis* 113, 129–32.

232. Bostom AG, Shemin D, Lapane KL, Miller JW, Sutherland P, Nadeau M, *et al.* (1995). Hyperhomocysteinemia and traditional cardiovascular disease risk factors in end-stage renal disease patients on dialysis: a case-control study. *Atherosclerosis* 114, 93–103.

233. Arnadottir M, Hultberg B, Vladov V, Nilsson-Ehle P, Thysell H (1996). Hyperhomocysteinemia in cyclosporin-treated renal transplant recipients. *Transplantation* 61, 509–12.

234. Wilcken DE, Dudman NP, Tyrrell PA, Robertson MR (1988). Folic acid lowers elevated plasma homocysteine in chronic renal insufficiency: possible implications for prevention of vascular disease. *Metabolism* 37, 697–701.

235. Genest JJ Jr, McNamara JR, Upson B, Salem DN, Ordovas JM, Schaefer EJ, *et al.* (1991). Prevalence of familial hyperhomocysteinemia in men with premature coronary artery disease. *Arteriosclerosis and Thrombosis* 11, 1129–36.

236. Clarke R, Daly L, Robinson K, Naughten E, Cahalane S, Fowler B, *et al.* (1991). Hyperhomocysteinemia: an independent risk factor for vascular disease. *New England Journal of Medicine* 324, 1149–55.

237. Wu LL, Wu J, Hunt SC, James BC, Vincent GM, Williams RR, *et al.* (1994). Plasma homocys(e)ine as a risk factor for early familial coronary artery disease. *Clinical Chemistry* 40, 552–61.

238. Ubbink JB, Vermaak WJH Bennett JM, Becker PJ, van Staden DA, Bissbort S (1991). The prevalence of homocysteinemia and hypercholesterolemia in angiographically defined coronary heart disease. *Klinische Wochenschrift* 69, 527–34.

239. Brattstrom L, Israelsson B, Norrving B, Bergqvist D, Thorne J, Hultberg B, *et al.* (1990). Impaired homocysteine metabolism in early-onset cerebral and peripheral occlusive arterial disease, effects of pyridoxine and folic acid treatment. *Atherosclerosis* 81, 51–60.

240. Brattstrom L, Lindgren A, Isrealsson B, Malinow MR, Norrving B, Upson B, *et al.* (1992). Hyperhomocysteinemia in stroke: prevalence, cause, and relationship to type of stroke and stroke risk factors. *European Journal of Clinical Investigation* 22, 214–21.

241. Fermo I, Vigano D'Angelo S, Paroni R, Mazzola G, Calori G, *et al.* (1995). Prevalence of moderate hyperhomocysteinemia in patients with early-onset venous and arterial occlusive disease. *Annals of Internal Medicine* 123, 747–53.

242. Denies VOW, Robinson K (1996). Homocysteinemia and vascular disease in end-stage real disease. *Kidney International* 57, S11–17.

243. Moustapha A, Naso A, Nahlawi M, Gupta A, Arheart K, Jacobsen DW, *et al.* (1998). Prospective study of hyperhomocysteinemia as an adverse cardiovascular risk factor in end-stage renal disease. *Circulation* 97, 138–41.

244. Ueland PM, Refsum H (1989). Plasma homocysteine, a risk factor for vascular disease: plasma levels in health, disease and drug therapy. *Journal of Laboratory and Clinical Medicine* 114, 473–501.

245. Lentz SR, Sobey CG, Piegors DJ, Bhopatkar MY, Faraci FM, Malinow MR, *et al.* (1996). Vascular dysfunction in monkeys with diet-induced hyperhomocyst(e)inemia. *Journal of Clinical Investigation* 98, 24–9.

246. Jakubowski H (1997). Metabolism of homocysteine thiolactone in human cell cultures Possible mechanism for pathological consequences of elevated homocysteine levels. *Journal of Biology and Chemistry* 272, 1935–42.

247. Stamler JS, Osborne JA, Jaraki O, Rabbani LE, Mullins M, Singel D, *et al.* (1993). Adverse vascular effects of homocysteine are modulated by endothelium-derived relaxing factor and related oxides of nitrogen. *Journal of Clinical Investigation* 91, 308–18.

248. Freedman JE, Loscalzo J, Benoit SE, Valeri CR, Barnard MR, Michelson AD (1996). Decreased platelet inhibition by nitric oxide in two brothers with a history of arterial thrombosis. *Journal of Clinical Investigation* 97, 979–87.

249. Upchurch GR Jr, Welch GN, Freedman JE, Loscalzo J (1995). Homocysteine attenuates endothelial glutathione peroxidase and thereby potentiates peroxide-mediated cell injury. *Circulation* 92, I-228.

250. Sunde RA (1990). Molecular biology of selenoproteins. *Annual Review Nutrition* 10, 451–74.

251. Mizuiri S, Hirata K, Izumi S, Komatsu N, Yoshimura S, Watanabe K (1989). Immunocytochemical localization of glutathione peroxidase in uremic rat kidney. In: *Nephrotoxicity* (ed. Bach PH, Lock EA), pp. 699–704. Plenum Publishing, New York.

252. Imura T, Kuroda M. (1984). Clinical significance of glutathione peroxidase analysis in biochemical laboratory analysis. *Nippon Rinsho—Japanese Journal of Clinical Medicine* 48, 274–6.

253. Saint-Georges MD, Bonnefont DJ, Bourely BA, Jaudon MLT, Cereze P, Chaumeil P, *et al.* (1989). Correction of selenium deficiency in hemodialyzed patients. *Kidney International* 27, S274–7.

254. Avissar N, Ornt DB, Yagil Y, Horowitz S, Watkins RH, Kerl EA, *et al.* (1994). Human kidney proximal tubules are the main source of plasma glutathione peroxidase. *American Journal of Physiology* 266, C367–75.

255. Yoshimura S, Watanabe K, Suemizu H, Onozawa T, Mizoguchi J, Tsuda K, *et al.* (1991). Tissue specific expression of the plasma glutathione peroxidase gene in rat kidney. *Journal of Biochemistry* (Tokyo) 109, 918–23.

256. Yoshimura S, Suemizu H, Taniguchi Y, Wantanabe K, Nomoto Y, Katsuoka Y, *et al.* (1992). Tissue specific expression of human plasma glutathione peroxidase gene in kidney and decreased production of the enzyme in patients with chronic renal failure. In: *Oxygen radicals* (ed. Yagi K, Kondo M, Niki E, Yoshikawa T), pp. 545–48. Elsevier, Tokyo.

257. Yoshimura S, Suemizu H, Nomoto Y, Sakai H, Katsuoka Y, Kawamura N, *et al.* (1996). Plasma glutathione peroxidase deficiency caused by renal dysfunction. *Nephron* 73, 207–11.

258. Paul LJ, Sall ND, Soni T, Poignet JL, Lindenbaum A, Man MK, *et al.* (1993). Lipid peroxidation abnormalities in hemodialyzed patients. *Nephron* 64, 106–9.

259. Richard MJ, Arnaud J, Jurkovitz C, Hachache T, Meftahi H, Laporte F, *et al.* (1991). Trace elements and lipid peroxidation abnormalities in patients with chronic renal failure. *Nephron* 57, 10–15.

260. Muller E, Blumberg A, Marti HR (1975). The activity of erythrocyte glutathione peroxidase in chronic renal failure. *Klinische Wochenschrift* 53, 879–80.

261. Bonomini M, Forster S, Manfrini V, De Risio F, Steiner M, Vidovich MI, *et al.* (1996). Geographic factors and plasma selenium in uremia and dialysis. *Nephron* 72, 197–204.

262. Bonomini M, Manfrini V, Marini A, De Risio F, Niri L, Klinkmann H, *et al.* (1995). Hemodialysis with regenerated cellulosic membranes does not reduce plasma selenium levels in chronic uremic patients. *Artificial Organs* 19, 81–5.

263. Girelli D, Olivieri O, Stanzial AM, Azzini M, Lupo A, Bernich P, *et al.* (1993). Low platelet glutathione peroxidase activity and serum selenium concentration in patients with chronic renal failure: relations to dialysis treatments, diet and cardiovascular complications. *Clinical Science* 84, 611–17.

264. Koenig JS, Fischer M, Bulant E, Tiran B, Elmadfa I, Druml W (1997). Antioxidant status in patients on chronic hemodialysis therapy: impact of parenteral selenium supplementation. *Wien Klin Wochenschr* 109, 13–19.

265. Milly K, Wit L, Diskin C, Tulley R (1992). Selenium in renal failure patients. *Nephron* 61, 139–44.

266. Tsai JC, Perrella MA, Yoshizumi M, Hsieh CM, Haber E, Schlegel R, *et al.* (1994). Promotion of vascular smooth muscle cell growth by homocysteine: a link to atherosclerosis. *Proceedings of the National Academy of Science USA* 91, 6369–73.

267. Bostom A, Brosnan JT, Hall B, Nadeau MR, Selhub J (1995). Net uptake of plasma homocysteine by the rat kidney *in vivo*. *Atherosclerosis* 116, 59–62.

268. Dudman NP, Tyrrell PA, Wilcken DE (1987). Homocysteinemia: depressed plasma serine levels. *Metabolism* 36, 198–201.

269. Sturman JA, Gaull GE, Niemann WH (1976). Activities of some enzymes involved in homocysteine methylation in brain, liver and kidney of the developing rhesus monkey. *Journal of Neurochemistry* 27, 425–31.

270. Gaull GE, Von Berg W, Raiha NC, Sturman JA (1973). Development of methyltransferase activities of human fetal tissues. *Pediatric Research* 7, 527–33.

271. Sturman JA, Rassin DK, Gaull GE (1970). Distribution of transsulphuration enzymes in various organs and species. *International Journal of Biochemistry* 1, 251–3.

272. Bostom AG, Shemin D, Verhoef P, Nadeau MR, Jaques PF, Selhub J, *et al.* (1997). Elevated fasting total plasma homocysteine levels and cardiovascular disease outcomes in maintenance dialysis patients. A prospective study. *Arteriosclerosis Thrombosis Vascular Biology* 17, 2554–8.

273. Cooke JP, Singer AH, Tsao P, Zera P, Rowan RA, Billingham ME (1992). Antiatherogenic effects of L-arginine in the hypercholesterolemic rabbit. *Journal of Clinical Investigation* 90, 1168–72.

274. Girerd XJ, Hirsch AT, Cooke JP, Dzau VJ, Creager MI (1990). L-Arginine augments endothelium-dependent vasodilation in cholesterol-fed rabbits. *Circulation Research* 67, 1301–8.

275. Drexler H, Zeiher AM, Memzer K, Just H (1991). Correction of endothelial dysfunction in coronary microcirculation of hypercholesterolaemic patients by L-arginine. *Lancet* 338, 1546–50.

276. Lerman A, Burnett JC Jr, Higano ST, McKinley LJ, Holmes DR Jr (1998). Long-term L-arginine supplementation improves small-vessel coronary endothelial function in humans. *Circulation* 97, 2123–8.

277. Thorne S, Mullen M, Clarkson P, Donald A, Deanfield JE (1998). Early endothelial dysfunction in adults at risk from atherosclerosis: different responses to L-arginine. *Journal of the American College of Cardiology* 32, 110–16.

278. Wolf A, Zalpour C, Theilmeier, G, Wang BY, Ma A, Anderson B, *et al.* (1997). Dietary L-arginine supplementation normalizes platelet aggregation in hypercholesterolemic humans. *Journal of the American College of Cardiology* 29, 479–85.

279. Candipan RC, Wang BY, Buitrago R, Tsao PS, Cooke JP (1996). Regression or progression. Dependency on vascular nitric oxide. *Arteriosclerosis Thrombosis Vascular Biology* 16, 44–50.

280. Caramelo C, Espinosa G, Namzarbeitia F, Cernadas MR, Perez Tejerizo G, Tan G, *et al.* (1996). Role of endothelium-related mechanisms in the pathophysiology for renal ischemia/reperfusion in normal rabbits. *Circulation Research* 79, 1031–8.

281. Reyes AA, Purkerson ML, Karl I, Klahr S (1992). Dietary supplementation with L-arginine ameliorates the progression of renal disease in rats with subtotal nephrectomy. *American Journal of Kidney Disease* 20, 168–76.

282. Reyes AA, Kark IE, Kissane J, Klahr S (1993). L-Arginine administration prevents glomerular hyperfiltration and decreases proteinuria in diabetic rats. *Journal of American Society of Nephrology* 4, 1039–45.

283. Weninger M, Xi Z, Lubee B, Szalay S, Hoger H, Lubec G (1992). L-Arginine reduces glomerular basement membrane collagen N epsilon-carboxymethyllysine in the diabetic db/db mouse. *Nephron* 62, 80–3.

284. Vallance P, Leone A, Calver A, Collier J, Moncada S (1992). Accumulation of an endogenous inhibitor of nitric oxide synthesis in chronic renal failure. *Lancet* 339, 572–5.

285. Hecker M, Walsh DT, Vane JR (1991). On the substrate specificity of nitric oxide synthase. *FASEB Journal.* 294, 221–4.

286. MacAllister RJ, Whitley GS, Vallance P (1994) Effects of guanidino and uremic compounds on nitric oxide pathways. *Kidney International* 45, 737–42.

287. Remuzzi G, Perico N, Zoja C, Corna D, Macconi D, Vigano G (1990). Role of endothelium-derived nitric oxide in the bleeding tendency uremia. *Journal of Clinical Investigation* 86, 1768–71.

288. Takagi M, Wada H, Mukai K, Kihira H, Yano S, Minamikawa Y, Wakita Y, *et al.* (1994). Increased vascular endothelial cell markers in patients with chronic renal failure on maintenance haemodialysis. *Blood Coagulation Fibrinolysis* 5, 713–17.

289. Ceballos-Picot I, Witko-Sarsat V, Merad-Boudia M, Ngyen AT, Thevenin M, Jaudon MC, *et al.* (1996). Glutathione antioxidant system as a marker of oxidative stress in chronic renal failure. *Free Radical Biology and Medicine* 21, 845–53.

290. Chen CK, Liaw JM, Juang JG, Lin TH (1997). Antioxidant enzymes and trace elements in hemodialyzed patients. *Biological Trace Element Research* 58, 149–57.

291. Loscalzo J (1992). Antiplatelet and antithrombotic effects of organic nitrates. *American Journal of Cardiology* 70, 18B–22B.

292. Yusuf S, Wittes J, Friedman L (1988). Overview of results of randomized clinical trials in heart disease. II. Unstable angina, heart failure, primary prevention with aspirin, and risk factor modification. *Journal of the American Medical Association* 260, 2259–63.

293. Scandinavian Simvastatin Survival Study Group. (1994). Randomised trial of cholesterol lowering in 4444 patients with coronary heart disease: the Scandinavian Simvastatin Survival Study (4S). *Lancet* 344, 1383–9.

294. Loscalzo J (1990). Regression of coronary atherosclerosis. *New England Journal of Medicine* 323, 1337 9.

295. Harrison DG, Armstrong ML, Freiman PC, Heistad DD (1987). Restoration of endothelium-dependent relaxation by dietary treatment of atherosclerosis. *Journal of Clinical Investigation* 80, 1808–11.

296. Leung WH, Lau CP, Wong CK (1993). Beneficial effect of cholesterol-lowering therapy on coronary endothelium-dependent relaxation in hypercholesterolemic patients. *Lancet* 341, 1496–500.

297. Treasure CB, Klein JL, Weintraub WS, Tally JD, Stillabown ME, Kosinski AS, *et al.* (1995) Beneficial effects of cholesterol-lowering therapy on the coronary endothelium in patients with coronary artery disease. *New England Journal of Medicine* 332, 481–7.

298. Anderson TJ, Meredith IT, Yeung AC, Frei B, Selwyn AP, Ganz P (1995). The effect of cholesterol lowering and antioxidant therapy on endothelium-dependent coronary vasomotion. *New England Journal of Medicine* 332, 488–93.

299. Wilson TW, Alonso-Galicia M, Roman RJ (1998). Effects of lipid-lowering agents in the Dahl salt-sensitive rat. *Hypertension* 31, 225–31.

300. Rimm EB, Stampfer MJ, Ascherio A, Giovannucci E, Colditz GA, Willet WC (1993). Vitamin E consumption and the risk of coronary heart disease in men. *New England Journal of Medicine* 328, 1450–6.

301. Stampfer MJ, Hennekens CH, Manson JE, Colditz GA, Rosner B, Willett WC (1993). Vitamin E consumption and the risk of coronary heart disease in women. *New England Journal of Medicine* 328, 1444–9.

302. Gey KF, Puska P (1989). Plasma vitamins E and A are inversely correlated to mortality from ischemic heart disease in cross-cultural epidemiology. *Annals of the New York Academy of Science* 570, 268–82.

303. Keaney JF Jr, Gaziano JM, Xu A, Frei B, Curran-Celentano J, Shwaery GT, *et al.* (1993). Dietary antioxidants preserve endothelium-dependent vessel relaxation in cholesterol-fed rabbits. *Proceedings of the National Academy of Science USA* 90, 11880–4.

304. Arnadottir M, Brattstrom L, Simonsen O, Thysell H, Hultberg B, Andersson A, *et al.* (1993). The effect of high-dose pyridoxine and folic acid supplementation on serum lipid and plasma homocysteine concentrations in dialysis patients. *Clinical Nephrology* 40, 236–40.

305. vanGuldener CV, Janssen MJ, deJong GM, vandenBerg M, Stehouwer CD (1996). Folic acid treatment of hyperhomocysteinemia in peritoneal dialysis patients. *Mineral and Electrolyte Metabolism* 22, 110–4.

306. vanGuldener C, Janssen MJ, Lambert J, terWee PM, Donker AJ, Stehouwer CD (1998). Folic acid lowers elevated homocysteine concentrations in chronic dialysis patients. No change in endothelial function after long-term therapy. *Peritoneal Dialysis International* 18, 282–9 (Abstract).

307. Bostom AG, Shemin D, Lapane KL, Hume AL, Yoburn D, Nadeau MR, et al. (1996). High dose B-vitamin treatment of hyperhomocysteinemia in dialysis patients. *Kidney International* 49, 147–52.

308. Wang J, Wolin MS, Hintze TH (1993). Chronic exercise enhances endothelium-mediated dilation of epicardial coronary artery in conscious dogs. *Circulation Research* 73, 829–38.

309. Sessa WC, Pritchard K, Seyedi N, Wang J, Hintze TH (1994). Chronic exercise in dogs increases coronary vascular nitric oxide production and endothelial cell nitric oxide synthase gene expression. *Circulation Research* 74, 349–53.

310. Blair SN, Goodyear NN, Gibbons LW, Cooper KH (1989). Physical fitness and incidence of hypertension in healthy normotensive men and women. *Journal of the American Medical Association* 252, 487–90.

311. Shulman NB, Ford CE, Hall WD, Blaufox MD, Simon D, Langford HG, et al. (1989). Prognostic value of serum creatinine and effect of treatment of hypertension on renal function. Results from the hypertension detection and follow-up program. The Hypertension Detection and Follow-up Program Cooperative Group. *Hypertension* 13, 180–93.

312. Kannel WB, Stampfer MJ, Castelli WP, Verter J (1984). The prognostic significance of proteinuria: the Framingham Study. *American Heart Journal* 108, 1347–52.

313. Parving HH (1996). Microalbuminuria in essential hypertension and diabetes. *Journal of Hypertension* 14, S89–93.

314. Raine AE, Margreiter R, Brunner FG, Ehrich JH, Geelings W, Landais P, et al. (1992). Report on management of renal failure in Europe XXII 1991. *Nephrology Dialysis Transplant* 7, 7–35.

315. Vaughan DE, Lazos SC (1992). Angiotensin II induces plasminogen activator inhibitor (PAI-1) *in vitro*. *Circulation* 86(Suppl 1), I-557.

316. Alderman MH, Madhavan S, Ooi WL, Cohen H, Sealey JE, Laragh JH (1991). Association of the renin-sodium profile with the risk of myocardial infarction in patients with hypertension. *New England Journal of Medicine* 324, 1098–104.

317. Williams GH, Hollengerg NK (1977). Accentuated vascular and endocrine response to SQ 20881 in hypertension. *New England Journal of Medicine* 297, 184–8.

318. Chobanian AV, Haudenschild CC, Nickerson C, Drago R (1990). Antiatherogenic effect of captopril in the Watanabe heritable hyperlipidemic rabbit. *Hypertension* 15, 327–31.

319. Schiffrin EL (1996). Correction of remodeling and function of small arteries in human hypertension by clazapril, an angiotensin I-converting enzyme inhibitor. *Journal of Cardiovascular Pharmacology* 27, S13–18.

320. Clozel M, Kuhn H, Baumgartner HR (1993). ACE inhibition and the vascular intima in hypertension. *Journal of Cardiovascular Pharmacology* 22, S15–18.

321. Zhang X, Xie Y-W, Nasjletti A, Xu X, Wolin MS, Hintze TH (1997). ACE inhibitors promote nitric oxide accumulation to modulate myocardial oxygen consumption. *Circulation* 95, 176–82.

322. Vanhoutte PM, Boulanger CM, Illiano SC, Nagao T, Vidal M, Mombouli JV (1993). Endothelium-dependent effects of converting enzyme inhibitors. *Journal of Cardiovascular Pharmacology* 22, S10–16.

323. Mancini GB, Henry GC, Macaya C, O'Neill BJ, Pucillo AL, Carere RG, et al. (1996). Angiotensin-converting enzyme inhibition with quinipril improves endothelial vasomotor dysfunction in patients with coronary artery disease. The TREND (Trial of Reversing Endothelial Dysfunction) Study. *Circulation* 94, 258–65.

324. Brenner BM, Meyer TW, Hosetter TH (1982). Dietary protein intake and the progressive nature of kidney disease: the role of hemodynamically mediated glomerular injury in the pathogenesis of progressive glomerular sclerosis in aging, renal ablation, and intrinsic renal disease. *New England Journal of Medicine* 307, 652–9.

325. Parving HH, Andersen AR, Smidt UM, Svendsen PA (1983). Early aggressive antihypertensive treatment reduces rate of decline in kidney function in diabetic nephropathy. *Lancet* 1, 1175–9.

326 Mimran A, Insua A, Ribstein J, Monnier L, Bringer J, Mirouze J (1988). Contrasting effects of captopril and nifedipine in normotensive patients with incipient diabetic nephropathy. *Journal of Hypertension* 6, 919–23.

7

Cardiac hypertrophy in end-stage renal failure

Claudio Rigatto, Patrick S. Parfrey, and Gérard M. London

Introduction

Cardiac hypertrophy is highly prevalent among patients with end-stage renal failure (ESRF). It may present as concentric left ventricular hypertrophy (LVH) or LV dilatation with or without compensatory parietal hypertrophy. These abnormalities result in varying degrees of diastolic and systolic dysfunction which in turn predispose to congestive heart failure, a strong independent predictor of early death among dialysis patients. These structural alterations are now known to begin in the pre-dialysis phase, progress in parallel with the deterioration of renal function, and partially regress subsequent to renal transplantation. They are influenced by a variety of risk factors which may themselves change as the renal failure evolves. This chapter will summarize the nature, pathophysiology, and clinical consequences of LVH in the pre-dialysis, dialysis, and transplant phases of ESRF. Particular emphasis will be placed on modifiable risk factors for LVH and their appropriate clinical management.

Echocardiographic definitions

Echocardiography is the most widely available method to estimate LV volume, mass index and function. Systolic dysfunction is defined as an ejection fraction of <40%, indicating impaired myocardial contractility. It is often associated with LV dilatation, sometimes defined echocardiographically as LV cavity volume index >90 ml/m^2.[1] Concentric LVH is characterized by a thickened LV wall with normal cavity volume. LV mass index (LVMI) is a calculated parameter that reflects the degree of muscular hypertrophy in the LV. Epidemiological studies in non-renal patients have established that the upper limits of LVMI as 130 g/m^2 for adult men and 102 g/m^2 for adult women.[2] Values above these limits indicate hypertrophy.

Diastolic dysfunction results from impaired diastolic compliance and is associated with concentric LVH. Diastolic LV function can be assessed non-invasively using pulsed Doppler analysis of flow across the mitral valve during diastole. Normally, as the mitral valve opens, ventricular relaxation occurs, with a rapid increase in flow leading to an E (or 'early') peak, followed by a later increase, the A (or 'atrial') peak, which reflects atrial contraction. Assuming normal atrial function, the increased stiffness of the hypertrophic LV leads to a smaller E peak and a larger A peak, expressed conveniently as a decreased E/A ratio.

Table 7.1 Important causes of volume and pressure overload

Volume overload	Pressure overload
Salt and water retention	Hypertension
AV fistulae	Arteriosclerosis
Anemia	Calcific aortic stenosis

Pathogenesis

Pressure and volume overload

LVH is an adaptive process occurring in response to long-term increase in myocardial work caused by pressure or volume overload, and results from the interaction between mechanical stimuli and locally generated growth factors and vasoactive substances.[3] LVH usually develops in a pattern specific to the inciting mechanical stress.[3,4] Pressure overload results in parallel addition of new sarcomeres and is characterized by an unchanged or smaller internal diameter of the LV and an increased wall thickness (concentric hypertrophy). Volume overload results in addition of new sarcomeres in series, leading to LV dilatation. Wall thickening accompanies dilatation and is a second-order adaptive mechanism which reduces wall stress.[3] The term eccentric hypertrophy is often used to describe this phenomenon. Table 7.1 summarizes some important causes of pressure and volume overload.

Both dilatation and hypertrophy are initially beneficial. Dilatation permits an increase in stroke volume without an increase in the inotropic state of the myocardium and as such is an efficient adaptation to volume overload.[4] It also permits the maintenance of a normal stroke volume and cardiac output in the presence of decreased contractility. The trade-off in either case is an increase in parietal wall tension. This is a consequence of Laplace's law, which states that wall tension is proportional to ventricular diameter. Assuming a spherical ventricle, Laplace's equation takes the form $T = PD/4$, where T = parietal tension, P = ventricular pressure, and D = LV internal diameter. It should be noted that T is also directly proportional to P, the intraventricular pressure. Factors that increase P, such as systemic hypertension and aortic stenosis, also increase T. The ventricular response to increased wall tension is to increase wall thickness (hypertrophy) by the parallel addition of new sarcomeres. This remodeling distributes the increased wall tension over a larger cross-sectional area, resulting in lower wall stress (defined as T/cross-sectional area) and hence lower energy consumption per unit muscle.

As was mentioned above, the normal adaptation to increased wall stress, whether the result of volume or pressure overload, is an increase in wall thickness, or hypertrophy. When the increase in LV mass is appropriate to the LV volume for a given ventricular pressure, the ratio of LV mass to volume is linearly correlated with systolic pressure. Regression equations have been derived for the normal population, as well as for physiological situations of volume and pressure overload.[5] 'Inadequate hypertrophy' is the term used to describe an LV mass to volume ratio that is less than predicted for a given systolic pressure. This occurs in hemodialysis patients and may be associated with an adverse outcome. In dialysis patients with LV dilatation, adverse survival is associated with a low LV mass to volume ratio, whereas in patients with concentric LV hypertrophy, the opposite occurs and adverse survival is associated with a high LV mass to volume ratio.[6]

Myocyte death

The detrimental effects of LVH are consequences of the structural adaptations described above. Hypertrophy is accompanied by decreased capillary density, decreased coronary reserve, impaired subendocardial perfusion and, ultimately, myocyte death and myocardial fibrosis.[3,7-10] The earliest consequences of these alterations are electrophysiological abnormalities and abnormal ventricular relaxation. Impaired relaxation due to slow re-uptake of calcium by sarcoplasmic reticulum and decreased passive compliance of the hypertrophied wall cause diastolic dysfunction.[11] In the later phases of chronic and sustained overload, progressive myocyte death occurs, leading to development of fibrosis and LV failure. Overstretching of papillary muscles is coupled with oxidant stress, programmed cell death, architectural rearrangement of myocytes, and impaired force generation in the myocardium.[12] The death of myocytes in chronic uremia may be exacerbated by diminished perfusion, malnutrition, hyperparathyroidism, and inadequate dialysis.[3,13] Such cell death in the presence of LVH and continuing pressure and volume overload may be catastrophic, leading to further LV dilatation and eventually systolic dysfunction.

Myocardial fibrosis

Concomitant with myocardial hypertrophy, an expansion of the cardiac interstitium also occurs.[14] It is more marked in pressure overload than in volume overload. The causes of myocardial fibrosis are multifactorial and include senescence, ischemia, and effects of hormones such as catecholamines, angiotensin II, and aldosterone.[14,15] Recent studies have demonstrated that parathyroid hormone is a permissive factor in the genesis of cardiac interstitial fibrosis.[16] The extensive intramyocardial fibrosis in ESRF patients with elevated parathyroid hormone could be responsible for attenuation of the hypertrophic response to pressure overload and the development of high-stress cardiomyopathy and cardiac failure.[3] Interstitial myocardial fibrosis is a prominent finding in uremia. Clinical studies have shown that the extent of myocardial fibrosis in ESRF patients is more marked than in patients with diabetes mellitus or essential hypertension with similar LV mass.[17]

Arteriosclerosis

Structural changes in the ventricle are intimately related to changes occurring in the blood vessels.[18,19-21] In ESRF, conduit arteries undergo several structural and functional changes. Key among these is a process of diffuse intimal–medial hypertrophy, which radically decreases arterial compliance.[18,22] These arterial changes resemble those that occur in age-related arteriosclerosis and must be distinguished from atherosclerosis, which is focal, non-uniformly distributed, primarily intimal, and induces occlusive lesions and compensatory focal enlargement of arterial diameters.[23,24]

The causes of this remodeling are incompletely understood. Experimental and clinical studies have shown that chronically increased arterial flow leads to increased internal arterial dimensions and arterial wall remodeling, with a compensatory increase in arterial wall thickness.[25,26] The hemodynamic consequence of this arterial remodeling is an early, amplified, reflected arterial pressure wave, which leads to increased pulse pressure and increased pressure load on the LV. Studies in humans have shown that decreased arterial compliance and an early return of arterial wave reflections are independent predictors of the extent of LVH.[18]

Relationship with coronary vascular disease

Coronary vascular disease, ischemia, and cardiac hypertrophy are distinct but closely linked phenomena. It is well known that coronary vascular disease can cause changes in cardiac geometry. Myocardial infarction and angina result from myocardial ischemia. Infarction leads to loss of myocardium, scar formation, and remodeling of the ventricle. Contractile function may be diminished, and the compensatory dilatation may or may not be accompanied by adequate muscular hypertrophy. Epidemiological studies have shown that symptomatic ischemic heart disease is an independent predictor of LV dilatation.[13]

Although manifestations of ischemic heart disease are most often due to the presence of coronary artery disease,[27] they can also result from non-atherosclerotic disease.[18,27,28] The decreased capillary density and impaired ventricular relaxation associated with LVH compromise myocardial perfusion during diastole, especially in the subendocardium. Diastolic perfusion is critical since the LV is not perfused during systole as a consequence of the high systolic intramyocardial pressure. An increased ventricular mass increases total myocardial oxygen demand. To accommodate the increased demand for oxygen, the coronary vasculature dilates above baseline, compromising its ability to dilate further in response to further increases in myocardial oxygen consumption. This limitation may be exacerbated by pre-existing pathological changes (e.g. atherosclerosis) in the large or small coronary vessels. The small vessel smooth muscle hypertrophy and endothelial abnormalities described in experimental LVH would further exacerbate ischemia.[14] Peripheral arterial remodeling has been associated with an increased risk for subendocardial ischemia even in the absence of coronary lesions.[18]

Epidemiology

Chronic renal failure

It has become increasingly evident that disorders of LV geometry begin well before the initiation of renal replacement therapy. In a cross-sectional study conducted by Greaves and co-workers, patients with chronic renal failure (serum creatinine >3.4 mg/dl) had a mean LVMI of 120 g/m^2, which was intermediate between that of gender- and age-matched controls (79 g/m^2) and dialysis patients (136 g/m^2).[29] An abnormal echocardiogram was observed in 63% of chronic renal failure patients versus 72% of dialysis patients, suggesting a relationship between LV morphology and worsening renal function. The major abnormality found was LVH. Levin and colleagues have reported a prevalence of LVH of 26.7% in patients with creatinine clearances >50 ml/min, 30.8% in those with clearances of 25–49 ml/min, and 45.2% in those with clearances <25 ml/min. In the prospective arm of this study, a similar association between rising LVMI and falling glomerular filtration rate was observed.[30] Another cross-sectional study has yielded comparable results.[31]

Little has been reported in the literature regarding LV dilatation, systolic and diastolic dysfunction, and congestive heart failure in the chronic renal failure period. Little is known as well about determinants of LVH, although anemia and hypertension may be risk factors for myocardial hypertrophy in this population.[32] The results of ongoing prospective cohort studies are needed to help define risk factors and establish targets for intervention in this group.

Dialysis

The overall prevalence of increased LV mass is 75% in patients beginning dialysis.[6,33-36] In a large prospective cohort study, only 16% had normal echocardiograms at inception. Fifteen percent had systolic dysfunction, 28% had dilatation with preserved contractility, and 41% had concentric LVH.[13] The presence of concentric LVH, LV dilatation with normal contractility, and systolic dysfunction at baseline were associated with progressively worse survival (Fig. 6.1). This survival gradient, arising in association with increasing severity of LV structural abnormality, is consistent with the known evolution of LVH (see Pathophysiology). All three abnormalities were associated with increased risk for the development of heart failure (Fig. 6.2). Moreover, the presence of congestive heart failure at baseline was a powerful independent predictor of poor survival (Fig. 6.3), whereas the presence of clinical ischemic heart disease, adjusted for age, gender diabetes, and heart failure, was not. The implication of these observations is that pump failure is a major mediator of death in dialysis patients.

LV structure does not remain static but continues to evolve with time on dialysis. In a subset of dialysis patients who underwent four consecutive echocardiograms at yearly inter-

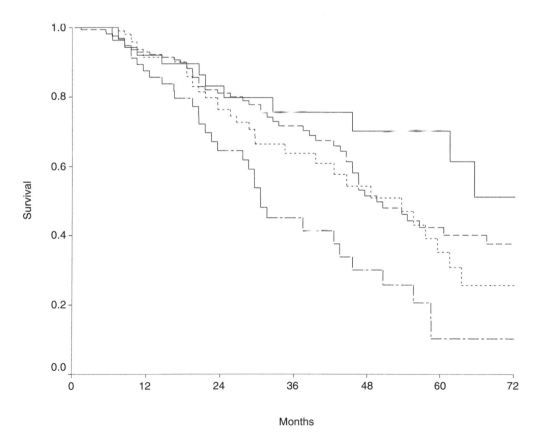

Fig. 6.1 Survival in patients with normal LV (———), concentric LV hypertrophy (– – –), LV dilatation (-----), and systolic dysfunction (———) at baseline. Adapted from Parfrey *et al.*[13]

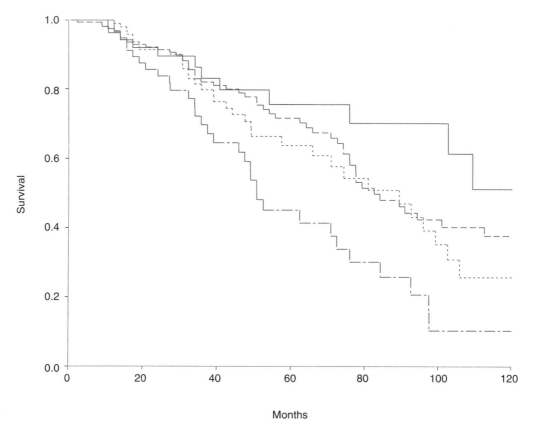

Fig. 6.2 Time to first onset of congestive heart failure in patients with normal LV (———), concentric LV hypertrophy (– – –), LV dilatation (······), and systolic dysfunction (—·—) at baseline. Adapted from Parfrey *et al.*[13]

vals from the initiation of dialysis onward, LVMI and LV cavity volume progressively increased. LV mass to volume ratios did not change. The biggest increase in mass and volume indices occurred between baseline and year 1, with smaller but progressive increases after the first year. Hemodialysis (as opposed to peritoneal dialysis) and anemia predicted progressive LV enlargement. Partial correction of anemia with erythropoietin induced regression of LV cavity volume.[38]

Although there is much overlap, risk factors differ slightly among patients with different LV structural abnormalities. When dialysis patients with LV dilatation were compared with those with normal echocardiograms, independent predictors of higher LV volumes included ischemic heart disease, anemia, hypertension, and hypoalbuminemia.[13] Furthermore, low serum albumin levels were significantly associated with progressive LV dilatation between baseline and follow-up echocardiograms 1 year later.[36] This is consistent with the hypothesis that diminished perfusion, as defined by the presence of ischemic symptoms, and malnutrition, as suggested by low serum albumin levels, may predispose to myocyte death and consequent LV dilatation. It is also possible that hypoalbuminemia reflects systemic inflammation, which may predispose to arterial disease via alterations in endothelial function.

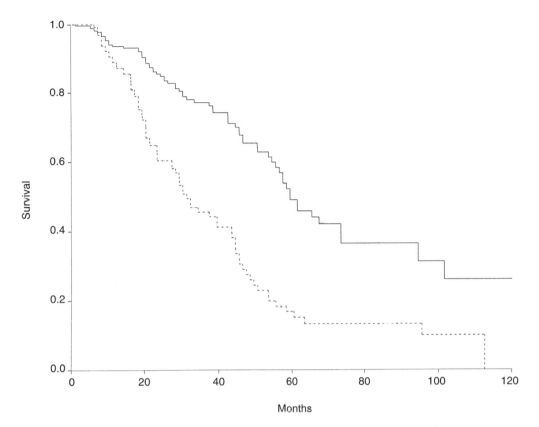

Fig. 6.3 Survival in patients with (---) and without (—) congestive heart failure at baseline. Adapted from Harnett *et al.*[37]

Transplantation

Of the choices available for ESRF therapy, renal transplantation provides the most physiological and complete reversal of the uremic state. Parfrey and co-workers examined the impact of transplantation on echocardiographic manifestations of uremic cardiomyopathy in a large cohort of dialysis patients.[39] Over the period of observation, 102 of 433 patients were transplanted. The transplanted patients were younger and had less cardiovascular morbidity than the entire cohort, but the distribution of echocardiographic abnormalities was similar: normal 17% (vs. 16%), concentric LVH 41% (vs. 41%), dilatation 32% (vs. 28%), and systolic dysfunction 12% (vs. 15%). At 1 year, the proportion of patients with normal studies doubled to 36% and systolic function normalized in all patients with fractional shortening <25%. LV mass and volume indices regressed by 17% and 19%, respectively. A subsequent analysis of yearly echocardiograms in the transplanted cohort showed that regression of concentric hypertrophy and dilatation continued beyond the first year after transplantation, reached a nadir at 2 years, and persisted into the third and fourth post-transplant years.[40] Further studies must be done to clarify the etiology and prognosis of LV morphology on morbidity and survival in the renal transplant population.

Risk factors and prevention

Non-modifiable risk factors

Although age and gender are not amenable to intervention, they are important clinical markers of risk. In the general population, increasing age is associated with increasing prevalence of cardiovascular disease. In the ESRF population, numerous studies have shown a positive association between age and prevalence of coronary artery disease,[27,41,42] LVH, and congestive heart failure (CHF).[37]

In the general population, male gender confers higher risk for all cardiac outcomes and mortality. In the ESRF population, male gender is associated with increased prevalence of coronary artery disease and decreased survival. The role of gender as a risk factor for LVH and CHF is less clear. In a registry-based study, women were found to be more likely to have radiographic cardiomegaly or a history of CHF and less likely to exhibit electrocardiographic or echocardiographic evidence of LVH than men.[43] In contrast to this result, a large prospective cohort study of patients beginning dialysis found no relationship between gender and development of heart failure. Moreover, female gender was associated with concentric LVH, whereas male gender was predictive of LV dilatation and CHF.[37] These contradictory findings may relate to differences in sample size (5000 in Ref. 43 vs. 432 in Ref. 37), design (prospective cohort in Ref. 37 vs. retrospective cohort in Ref. 43), and criteria for LV geometry.

Hypertension

Chronic renal insufficiency

The prevalence of hypertension in patients with chronic renal insufficiency is about 80%, and it varies with the cause of renal disease. In the Modification of Diet in Renal Disease study,[44] although 91% of patients were treated with antihypertensive agents only 54% had blood pressure ≤140/90 mmHg. Hypertension was associated with increased risk of progression of renal disease and onset of dialysis. A lower than usual target blood pressure (<125/75 mmHg) was more effective in delaying renal decline than the usual goal (<140/90 mmHg) in patients with proteinuria (>1 gm/day), but not in patients without proteinuria.[45]

The impact of hypertension on the heart in chronic renal failure is less clearly established. Levin and colleagues showed that hypertension was associated with LVH in a cross-sectional analysis of chronic renal failure patients.[32] It seems reasonable to assume that slowing progression of renal failure and controlling hypertension will mitigate cardiac hypertrophy in pre-dialysis patients. Cohort studies underway may clarify the issue but ultimately clinical trials must be performed to establish efficacy.

Dialysis patients

The prevalence of hypertension is about 80% in hemodialysis patients and 50% in peritoneal dialysis patients.[46] The 1996 Core Indicators project reported that 53% of adult hemodialysis patients had pre-dialysis systolic blood pressures ≥150 mmHg, and 17% had pre-dialysis diastolic blood pressures ≥90 mmHg. The comparable rates in peritoneal dialysis patients were 29% and 18%. In dialysis patients, each 10 mmHg increment in blood pressure is associated with a 48% higher chance of having LVH, a 39% higher risk of *de novo* ischemic heart disease, and a 44% higher risk of *de novo* cardiac failure.[46] It is paradoxical, therefore, that low blood pressure has been so frequently linked with increased mortality in cross-sectional studies.[47,48] The resolution of this paradox may lie in the observation that low blood pressure is more likely to be the result, not the cause, of pump failure, which is known to predispose to death.

Transplantation

Data are sparse in this patient group. The prevalence of hypertension among transplant recipients is 79% to 80%.[49] Elevated blood pressure has been associated with shortened graft and patient survival, as well as higher rates of coronary artery disease.[50,51] However, a recent retrospective study of a large transplant cohort did not find an association between hypertension and mortality after adjustment for age, diabetes, tobacco use, and time on dialysis prior to transplantation.[52] Only one study has examined the natural history of cardiomyopathy after transplantation.[40] In this analysis low blood pressure was associated with regression of LVH in patients with echocardiographically defined concentric hypertrophy.

Treatment

Consensus guidelines for the treatment of hypertension in uremia have been developed.[49] These recommendations are aimed at limiting all adverse renal and cardiovascular outcomes, but are probably relevant to the prevention of LVH as well. In chronic renal insufficiency and renal transplant recipients, target blood pressure should be less than 125/75 mmHg in proteinuric and less than 130/85 mmHg in non-proteinuric individuals. Regimens containing angiotensin-converting enzyme (ACE) inhibitors are recommended, since ACE inhibitor-based regimens appear to be more effective in improving renal outcomes than antihypertensive regimens not including ACE inhibitors.[53,54]

In dialysis patients, a target blood pressure <140/90 mmHg is recommended. Although no specific class of agent is preferred by the guidelines, one small trial in dialysis patients has shown that ACE inhibitors, but not calcium blockers, induce regression of LVH.[55] Moreover, ACE inhibitors have been clearly shown to improve symptoms, morbidity, and survival in non-uremic individuals with heart failure, systolic dysfunction, or diastolic dysfunction. It seems reasonable, therefore, to recommend their use in dialysis patients also, particularly if there is clinical evidence of heart failure or echocardiographic evidence of either systolic or diastolic dysfunction. Ultimately, the validity of each of the recommendations above must be established by clinical trials.

Diabetes mellitus

In non-renal patients, diabetes mellitus is an independent risk factor for the development of heart failure and coronary artery disease. Diabetic patients have more widespread coronary artery disease than age- and gender-matched controls.[56] Some diabetic patients with ESRF have impairment of LV function despite normal coronary arteries ('diabetic cardiomyopathy'). In addition to coronary artery disease and systolic dysfunction, echocardiographic LVH is probably a more frequent finding in hypertensive diabetic patients than in hypertensive non-diabetic patients. In diabetic patients, this increased LV mass seems to be closely related to the level of blood pressure. A comparison of the pathological spectrum of hypertensive, diabetic, and hypertensive–diabetic heart disease shows that the latter group had a significantly higher heart weight and a higher total fibrosis score than either of the other two groups.[56]

In a cohort of dialysis patients who survived at least 6 months following the initiation of dialysis, 15% had insulin-dependent diabetes and 12% non-insulin-dependent diabetes.[57]

Compared with non–diabetic patients, diabetic patients had a higher baseline prevalence of concentric LVH (50% vs. 38%), clinically diagnosed ischemic heart disease (32 vs. 18%), and cardiac failure (48 vs. 24%). After adjustment for age and gender, diabetic patients had similar rates of progression of echocardiographic disorders and *de novo* cardiac failure. However, a threefold higher risk of *de novo* ischemic heart disease (RR 3.2) and a two- to threefold higher risk for overall mortality (RR 2.3) and cardiovascular mortality (RR 2.6) were observed. Older age, left ventricular hypertrophy, smoking, clinically diagnosed ischemic heart disease, cardiac failure, and hypoalbuminemia were independently associated with mortality in diabetic dialysis patients.[57]

Treatment

The role of intensive glycemic control in diabetic renal failure has been reviewed extensively.[58] In patients with chronic renal insufficiency due to diabetic renal disease, strict glycemic control may slow the progression of renal disease, and in transplant recipients it may slow the recurrence of diabetic renal disease. Therefore, intensive glucose control may be beneficial in these two groups. However, in these two patient groups, strict glycemic control is more difficult, the risk of hypoglycemia is greater, and the consequences of hypoglycemia are more severe. Aggressive glycemic control may not be appropriate in patients with established coronary artery disease or limited awareness of hypoglycemia. It must be emphasized that these recommendations are aimed at preserving renal function. The impact of strict glycemic control on LVH and other cardiac disorders in these patients is unknown. In dialysis patients, the risk to benefit ratio of strict control is likely to be less favorable. In these patients, strict control cannot be generally recommended.

Anemia

Anemia is associated with LV dilatation and LVH in chronic renal insufficiency and in dialysis patients. It is a risk factor for the development of *de novo* cardiac failure and death in dialysis patients.[59] Partial correction of anemia is associated with regression of hypertrophy in cohort studies.

Recently, two trials have compared the normalization of hemoglobin with partial correction. A large randomized controlled clinical trial was undertaken in the USA in hemodialysis patients with pre-existing ischemic heart disease or cardiac failure, in which normalization of hemoglobin with erythropoietin was compared with partial correction. The primary outcome was death or myocardial infarction. The trial was stopped early because the results of an interim analysis precluded the possibility of demonstrating survival benefit in the normalization group by the end of the trial.[60] Increased mortality and increased access loss were observed among patients randomized to normalization. In a Canadian trial, hemodialysis patients without symptomatic cardiac disease were allocated to normalization of hemoglobin with erythropoietin or to partial correction of anemia.[61] Normalization of hemoglobin failed to induce regression of LV dilatation in patients with dilated hearts at baseline, but appeared to prevent progressive LV dilatation in those with normal cardiac volumes at baseline. These two studies suggest that full correction of anemia is not beneficial in patients with established cardiac disease. It remains to be established whether hemoglobin normalization at an earlier stage in the evolution of uremic cardiomyopathy may be beneficial. This last hypothesis needs to be tested in a randomized controlled trial. For the moment, partial correction (target hemoglobin 11.0–12.0 g/L) must remain the accepted norm.[62]

Coronary artery disease

The risk factors for and management of coronary artery disease are discussed elsewhere (see Chapters 3 and 10). Nevertheless, it is worthwhile emphasizing that coronary artery disease is an important cause of systolic and diastolic dysfunction, and, therefore, constitutes a logical target for intervention.

Mode and quantity of ESRF therapy

Renal transplantation provides the most physiological and complete reversal of uremia. Renal transplantation appears to induce normalization of systolic dysfunction and regression of concentric LVH and LV dilatation. This effect seems to persist for at least 3 years post-transplantation.[39,40] It is not known which adverse risk factors characteristic of the uremic state have been corrected to produce the improvement in LV contractility. In contrast, hemodialysis and peritoneal dialysis provide only partial reversal of the uremic state. Analyses of data from multiple large prospective studies have shown that there exists a threshold dialysis dose below which mortality increases sharply. These inflection points have been used to formulate targets for Kt/V_{urea} for both peritoneal dialysis (weekly $Kt/V > 2.0$) and hemodialysis (per treatment $Kt/V > 1.2$).[63,64] Whether higher dosing targets will result in improved cardiac outcomes is not known. The HEMO study in the USA will compare high ($Kt/V = 1.5$) vs. standard ($Kt/V = 1.2$) dialysis dose in hemodialysis patients and may shed light on this question. There is no evidence to suggest that continuous ambulatory peritoneal dialysis (CAPD) is better than hemodialysis in prolonging life in those with cardiac disease, or in predisposing to the development of cardiac diseases. The preponderance of evidence suggests equivalence between the two techniques. For the moment, the NKF–DOQI guidelines for dialysis dosing remain the accepted standard.

Hypoalbuminemia

Several studies have shown that hypoalbuminemia is a powerful predictor of poor outcome in ESRF patients. Hypoalbuminemia has been associated with LV dilatation and predisposes to *de novo* cardiac failure and ischemic heart disease.[65] The mechanisms underlying this association are unknown. Hypoalbuminemia is associated with a hypercoagulable state and may therefore predispose to myocardial infarction and ischemic cardiomyopathy. Alternatively, it may be a marker for malnutrition, inadequate dialysis, vitamin deficiency, or a chronic inflammatory state, all of which could hypothetically accelerate myocyte death and the development of cardiomyopathy. Further research is needed to clarify the mechanisms and identify targets for intervention.

Hypoalbuminemia is more frequently encountered in peritoneal dialysis than in hemodialysis, but carries a higher risk for development of CHF in hemodialysis.[65] Given this difference in outcomes it is plausible that the causes of hypoalbuminemia and the mechanisms of its effects differ in the two types of dialysis.

Abnormal divalent ion metabolism

Foley and colleagues found that hypocalcemia was strongly associated with ischemic heart disease and mortality, even after adjustment for age, diabetes, blood pressure, hemoglobin, and other predictors.[65] The effect was similar in peritoneal dialysis and hemodialysis patients, and was only partly explained by the relationship between mean serum calcium and time spent on dialysis therapy. Secondary hyperparathyroidism is frequently associated with hypocalcemia. High parathyroid hormone levels may promote myocyte death and myocardial fibrosis.[16] Extensive fibrosis may be responsible for attenuation of the hypertrophic response to pressure overload, and may contribute to the development of dilated cardiomyopathy and heart failure in subjects with secondary hyperparathyroidism.[66,67] The cardiovascular impact of hyperparathyroidism in the chronic renal failure and renal transplant populations is unclear.

Although the circumstantial evidence supports a role for abnormalities of divalent ion metabolism in the development of cardiac disease in dialysis patients, the implications for patient care are less obvious. The absence of large cohort studies precludes the precise identification of risk factors, which would permit studies of relevant interventions. Current practice is to aggressively treat abnormalities in divalent ion metabolism in order to prevent or treat uremic bone disease in its multiple manifestations. This practice may attenuate the frequency of full-blown hyperparathyroidism, rendering the issue of parathyroid hormone cardiotoxicity a moot point. For the present, there are no defined 'cardiac' indications for the treatment of divalent ion abnormalities.

Even though aluminum may be cardiotoxic, the use of aluminum-based phosphate binders has been sharply curtailed because of its known central nervous system and bone toxicities, and it is unlikely to be an important cause of cardiomyopathy in future.

Aortic stenosis

Acquired aortic stenosis may occur in a minority of patients[68] and may induce concentric LVH. Calcification of the aortic valve has been observed in 28–55% of dialysis patients in various series, whereas hemodynamically important stenosis has been reported in 3–13%. Progression at times may be extremely rapid. The major factors predisposing to aortic valve calcification appear to be hyperparathyroidism, duration of dialysis, and degree of elevation of calcium × phosphate product.

Salt and water overload

Salt and water overload is a persistent problem in dialysis patients and is problematic to a lesser extent in chronic renal failure and transplant patients. Blood volume correlates directly with LV diameter in hemodialysis patients,[69] as does the magnitude of interdialytic weight changes.[70] LV diameter decreases with volume contraction during hemodialysis.[71] Keeping the patient's dry weight optimal[72] can minimize the degree of enlargement of the LV. Despite these associations, it is difficult to clearly discern cause and effect. Salt and water overload is by definition blood volume overload and hence probably plays a causal role in the development of LVH. However, it is possible that salt and water retention is induced by pre-existing systolic or diastolic dysfunction in some patients.

Arteriovenous (AV) fistulae

AV fistulae and grafts used for hemodialysis access cause significant peripheral AV shunting of blood. The cardiac consequences of this shunting are primarily due to volume overload secondary to increased venous return, although decreases in peripheral resistance and increased inotropic state also play a role.[23] Increases in cardiac output result in increased flow in the conduit arteries which promotes arterial remodeling, decreasing arterial compliance and increasing the amplitude and velocity of the reflected pressure wave. As discussed in the section on Arteriosclerosis, these changes promote myocardial hypertrophy and compromise subendocardial perfusion. High output failure with cardiomegaly is well known to occur with high flow fistulae and grafts, and often responds to ligation of the shunt.[73]

At the time of renal transplantation, the AV access is usually not ligated. Many fistulas undoubtedly thrombose over time but a proportion may remain patent. It is not known how many remain patent or what effect persistent AV shunting has on the heart of transplant patients, although it is unlikely to be beneficial.

Summary

The prevalence of LVH in uremia is high and its clinical impact grave. Although studies have traditionally focused on the dialysis population, it has become increasingly evident that risk factors for LVH and their initial consequences to the heart are already evident during the pre-dialysis phase and persist despite significant amelioration in the transplant phase. Even so, our knowledge of these risks and consequences remains sketchy. We hope that some of these gaps will be filled, as the results of research currently underway become available.

The dearth of experimental evidence is particularly acute with regard to therapy. Although many data exist on the impact of risk factor modification and therapy of congestive heart failure for the non-renal population, as a general rule corresponding trials in the renal population have not been done. In the interim, it is useful to remember that many of the risks for cardiac dysfunction are common to both renal and non-renal patients, that many of these risks are higher in the renal failure population, and that the absolute benefit of any intervention tends to increase with increasing risk. It is likely, therefore, that the validity of extrapolations from the general population will be vindicated in future trials. The most logical approach at present seems to be to treat according to recommendations for the non-renal population unless there is a compelling contraindication, or there are convincing data from studies in the renal failure population. Ultimately, this approach will have to be validated by clinical trials of adequate statistical power. This goal will remain an invigorating challenge in the years to come.

References

1. Pombo JF, Troy BL, Russell RO Jr. (1971) Left ventricular volumes and ejection fractions by echocardiography. *Circulation* 43:480–490.
2. Levy D, Savage DD, Garrison RJ, Anderson KM, Kannel WB, Castelli WP. (1987) Echocardiographic criteria for left ventricular hypertrophy: the Framingham Heart Study. *American Journal of Cardiology* 59:956–960.
3. London GM, Parfrey PS. (1997) Cardiac disease in chronic uremia: pathogenesis. *Advances in Renal Replacement Therapy* 4:194–211.
4. Grossman W. (1980) Cardiac hypertrophy: useful adaptation or pathological process? *American Journal of Medicine* 69:576–584.
5. Koren MJ, Devereux RB, Casale PN, Savage DD, Laragh JH. (1991) Relation of left ventricular mass and geometry to morbidity and mortality in uncomplicated essential hypertension. *Annals of Internal Medicine* 114:345–352.

6. Foley RN, Parfrey PS, Harnett JD, Kent GM, Murray DC, Barre PE. (1995) The prognostic importance of left ventricular geometry in uremic cardiomyopathy. *Journal of the American Society of Nephrology* 5:2024–2031.

7. Anversa P, Olivetti G, Melissari M, Loud AV. (1980). Stereological measurement of cellular and subcellular hypertrophy and hyperplasia in the papillary muscle of the adult rat. *Journal of Molecular and Cellular Cardiology* 12:781–795.

8. Hoffman JI. (1987) Transmural myocardial perfusion. *Progress in Cardiovascular Disease* 29:429–464.

9. Brilla CG, Janicki JS, Weber KT. (1991) Impaired diastolic function and coronary reserve in genetic hypertension. Role of interstitial fibrosis and medial thickening of intramyocardial coronary arteries. *Circulation Research* 69:107–115.

10. Weber KT. (1989) Cardiac interstitium in health and disease: the fibrillar collagen network. *Journal of the American College of Cardiology* 13:1637–1652.

11. Rozich JD, Smith B, Thomas JD, Zile MR, Kaisen J, Mann DL. (1991) Dialysis induced alterations in left ventricular filling: mechanisms and clinical significance. *American Journal of Kidney Diseases* 3:277–285.

12. Cheng W, Li B, Kajstura J, Li P, Wolin MS, Sonnenblick EH, *et al.* (1995). Stretch induced programmed myocyte death. *Journal of Clinical Investigation* 96:2247–2259.

13. Parfrey PS, Foley RN, Harnett JD, Kent GM, Murray DC, Barre PE. (1996). The outcome and risk factors for left ventricular disorders in chronic uremia. *Nephrology, Dialysis and Transplantation* 11:1277–1285.

14. Amann K, Ritz E. (1997) Cardiac disease in chronic uremia: pathophysiology. *Advances in Renal Replacement Therapy* 4:212–224.

15. Suzuki H, Schaefer L, Ling H, Schafer RM, Dammrich J, Teschner M, *et al.* (1995) Prevention of cardiac hypertrophy in experimental chronic renal failure by long term ACE inhibitor administration: potential role of lysosomal proteinases. *American Journal of Nephrology* 15:129–136.

16. Amann K, Ritz E, Wiest G, Klaus G, Mall G. (1994) The role of parathyroid hormone for the activation of cardiac fibroblasts in uremia. *Journal of the American Society of Nephrology* 4:1814–1819.

17. Mall G, Huther W, Schneider J, Lundin P, Ritz E. (1990) Diffuse intermyocardiocytic fibrosis in uremic patients. *Nephrology, Dialysis and Transplantation* 5:39–44.

18. London GM, Guerin AP, Marchais SJ, Pannier B, Safar ME, Day M, *et al.* (1996) Cardiac and arterial interactions in end stage renal disease. *Kidney International* 50:600–608.

19. London GM, Marchais SJ, Safar ME, Genest AF, Guerin AP, Métivier F, *et al.* (1990) Aortic and large artery compliance in end stage renal failure. *Kidney International* 37:137–142.

20. London GM, Guerin AP, Pannier B, Marchais S, Benetos A, Safar M. (1992) Increased systolic pressure in chronic uremia: role of arterial wave reflections. *Hypertension* 20:10–19.

21. Marchais SJ, Guerin AP, Pannier B, Levy BI, Safar ME, London GM. (1993) Wave reflections and cardiac hypertrophy in chronic uremia: influence of body size. *Hypertension* 22:876–883.

22. Kawagishi T, Nishizawa Y, Konishi T, Kawasaki K, Emoto M, Shoji T, *et al.* (1994) High resolution B-mode ultrasonography in evaluation of atherosclerosis in uremia. *Kidney International* 48:820–826.

23. London GM, Drueke TB. (1997) Atherosclerosis and arteriosclerosis in chronic renal failure. *Kidney International* 51:1678–1695.

24. O'Rourke M. (1995) Mechanical principles in arterial disease. *Hypertension* 26:2–9.

25. Kamiya A, Togawa T. (1980) Adaptive regulation of wall shear stress to flow change in the canine carotid artery. *American Journal of Physiology* 239:H14–H21.

26. Langille BL, O'Donnell F. (1986) Reductions in arterial diameters produced by chronic decrease in flow are endothelium dependent. *Science* 231:405–407.

27. Rostand RG, Kirk KA, Rutsky EA. (1984) Dialysis-associated ischemic heart disease: insights from coronary angiography. *Kidney International* 25:653–659.

28. Roig E, Betriu A, Castaner A, Magrina J, Sanz G, Novarro-Lopez E. (1981) Disabling angina pectoris with normal coronary arteries in patients undergoing long-term hemodialysis. *American Journal of Medicine* 71:437–444.

29. Greaves SC, Gamble GD, Collins JF, Whalley GA, Sharpe GN. (1994) Determinants of left ventricular hypertrophy and systolic dysfunction in chronic renal failure. *American Journal of Kidney Diseases* 24:768–776.

30. Levin A, Ethier J, Carlisle E, Burgess E, Mendelssohn D, Tobe S, *et al.* (1996) for the Canadian Nephrology investigators group. Anemia in renal insufficiency promotes left ventricular growth. *Journal of the American Society of Nephrology* 7:1391(Abstract).

31 Tucker B, Fabbian F, Giles M, Thuraisingham RC, Raine AE, Baker LR. (1997) Left ventricular hypertrophy and ambulatory blood pressure monitoring in chronic renal failure. *Nephrology, Dialysis and Transplantation* 12:724–728.

32. Levin A, Singer J, Thompson CR, Ross H, Lewis M. (1996) Prevalent left ventricular hypertrophy in the predialysis population: opportunities for intervention. *American Journal of Kidney Diseases* 27:347–354.

33. Silberberg JS, Barre PE, Prichard SS, Sniderman AD. (1989) Impact of left ventricular hypertrophy on survival in end-stage renal disease. *Kidney International* 286–290.

34. Foley RN, Parfrey PS, Harnett JD, Kent GM, Martin CJ, Murray DC, *et al.* (1995) Clinical and echocardiographic disease in patients starting end stage renal disease therapy. *Kidney International* 47:186–192.

35. Covic A, Goldsmith DJ, Georgescu G, Venning MC, Ackrill P. (1996) Echocardiographic findings in long-term long hour hemodialysis patients. *Clinical Nephrology* 45:104–110.

36. Dahan M, Siohan P, Viron B, Michel C, Paillole C, Gourgon R, *et al.* (1997) Relationship between left ventricular hypertrophy, myocardial contractility, and load conditions in hemodialysis patients: an echocardiographic study. *American Journal of Kidney Diseases* 30:780–785.

37. Harnett JD, Foley RN, Kent GM, Barre PB, Murray DC, Parfrey PS. (1995) Congestive heart failure in dialysis patients: prevalence, incidence, prognosis and risk factors. *Kidney International* 47:884–890.

38. Foley RN, Parfrey PS, Kent GM, Harnett JD, Murray DC, Barre PE. (1998) The long term evolution of cardiomyopathy in dialysis patients. *Kidney International* 54:1720–1725.

39. Parfrey PS, Harnett JD, Foley RN, Kent GM, Murray DC, Barre PE, *et al.* (1995) Impact of renal transplantation on uremic cardiomyopathy. *Transplantation* 60:908–914.

40. Rigatto C, Foley RN, Parfrey PS, Kent GM, Barre PE, Murray DC. (1999) Long-term evolution of uremic cardiomyopathy. *Journal of the American Society of Nephrology* 10:A3766.

41. Disney AP, editor. (1996) *ANZDTA Report, Australia and New Zealand Dialysis and Transplant Registry*. Adelaide, South Australia.

42. *CORR Annual Report* (1996) Volume 1: Dialysis and renal transplantation. Canadian Organ Replacement Registry, Canadian Institute for Health Information, Don Mills, Ontario.

43. Bloembergen WE, Carroll C, Gillespie B. (1996) Why do males with ESRD have higher mortality than females? *Journal of the American Society of Nephrology* 7:1440.

44. Buckalew VM Jr, Berg RL, Wang SR, Porush JG, Rauch S, Schulman G. (1996) Prevalence of hypertension in 1795 subjects with chronic renal disease: the Modification of Diet in Renal Disease Study baseline cohort. *American Journal of Kidney Diseases* 28:811–821.

45. Klahr S, Levey AS, Beck GJ, Caggiula AW, Hunsicker L, Kusek JW, Striker G. (1994) The effects of dietary protein restriction and blood pressure control on the progression of chronic renal disease. Modification of Diet in Renal Disease Study Group. *New England Journal of Medicine* 330:877–884.

46. Foley RN, Parfrey PS, Harnett JD, Kent GM, Murray DC, Barre PE. (1996) Impact of hypertension on cardiomyopathy, morbidity, and mortality in end-stage renal disease. *Kidney International* 49:1379–1385.

47. Zager PG, Nikolic J, Brown RH, Campbell MA, Hunt WC, Peterson D, *et al.* (1998) 'U' curve association of blood pressure and mortality in hemodialysis patients. Medical Directors of Dialysis Clinic, Inc. *Kidney International* 54:561–569.
48. Lowrie EG, Lew NL. (1992) Commonly measured laboratory variables in hemodialysis patients: relationships among them and to death risk. *Seminars in Nephrology* 12:276–283.
49. Mailloux LU, Levey AS. (1998) Hypertension in patients with chronic renal disease. *American Journal of Kidney Diseases* 32(Suppl 3):S120–S141.
50. Opelz G, Wujciak T, Ritz E. (1998) Association of chronic kidney graft failure with recipient blood pressure. Collaborative Transplant Study. *Kidney International* 53:217–222.
51. United States Renal Data Systems: *USRDS (1998) Annual Data Report.* US Department of Health and Human Services. The National Institute of Health, National Institute of Diabetes and Digestive and Kidney Diseases, Bethesda, MD.
52. Cosio FG, Alamir A, Yim S, Pesavento TE, Falkenhain ME, Henry ML, *et al.* (1998) Patient survival after renal transplant: I. The impact of dialysis pre-transplant. *Kidney International* 53:762–772.
53. Lewis EJ, Hunsicker LG, Bain RP, Rohde RD. (1993) The effect of angiotensin converting enzyme inhibition on diabetic nephropathy. Collaborative Transplant Study. *New England Journal of Medicine* 329:1456–1462.
54. Giatras I, Lau J, Levey AS. (1997) Effect of angiotensin converting enzyme inhibitors on progression of nondiabetic renal disease: a meta-analysis of randomized trials. *Annals of Internal Medicine* 127:337–345.
55. London GM, Pannier B, Guerin AP, Marchais SJ, Safar ME, Cuche JL. (1994) Cardiac hypertrophy, aortic compliance, peripheral resistance, and wave reflection in ESRD: comparative effects of ACE inhibition and calcium channel blockade. *Circulation* 90:2786–2796.
56. Grossman E, Messerli FH. (1996) Diabetic and hypertensive heart disease. *Annals of Internal Medicine* 125:304–310.
57. Foley RN, Culleton BF, Parfrey PS, Harnett JD, Kent GM, Murray DC, *et al.* (1997) Cardiac disease in diabetic end-stage renal disease. *Diabetologia* 40:1307–1312.
58. Manske CL. (1998) Hyperglycemia and intensive glycemic control in diabetic patients with chronic renal disease. *American Journal of Kidney Diseases* 32(Suppl 3):S157–S171.
59. Foley RN, Parfrey PS, Harnett JD, Kent GM, Murray DC, Barre PE. (1996) The impact of anemia on cardiomyopathy, morbidity and mortality in end stage renal disease. *American Journal of Kidney Diseases* 28:53–61.
60. Besarab A, Bolton WK, Browne JK, Egrie JK, Nissenson AR, Okamoto DM, *et al.* (1998) The effects of normal as compared with low hematocrit values in patients with cardiac disease who are receiving hemodialysis and epoietin. *New England Journal of Medicine* 339:584–590.
61. Foley RN, Parfrey PS, Morgan J. (1998) A randomized controlled trial of complete vs. partial correction of anemia in hemodialysis patients with asymptomatic concentric LV hypertrophy or LV dilatation. *Journal of the American Society of Nephrology* 9:208A.
62. NKF–DOQI (1997) Clinical practice guidelines for the treatment of anemia of chronic renal failure. National Kidney Foundation–Dialysis Outcomes Quality Initiative. *American Journal of Kidney Diseases* 30:S192–S240.
63. CANUSA (1996) Canada–USA adequacy of dialysis and nutrition in continuous peritoneal dialysis: association with clinical outcomes. Peritoneal Dialysis Study Group. *Journal of the American Society of Nephrology* 7:198–207.
64. Gotch F, Levin N, Port F, Wolfe R, Uehlinger D. (1997) Clinical outcome relative to dose of dialysis is not what you think: the fallacy of the mean. *American Journal of Kidney Diseases* 30:1–15.
65. Foley RN, Parfrey PS, Harnett JD, Kent GM, Murray DC, Barre PE. (1996) Hypoalbuminemia, cardiac morbidity and mortality in end stage renal disease. *Journal of the American Society of Nephrology* 7:728–736.

66. London GM, Fabiani F, Marchais SJ, de Vernejoul MC, Guerin AP, Safar ME, *et al.* (1987) Uremic cardiomyopathy: an inadequate left ventricular hypertrophy. *Kidney International* 31:973–980.
67. London GM, de Vernejoul MC, Fabiani F, Marchais SJ, Guerin AP, Métivier F, *et al.* (1987) Secondary hyperparathyroidism and cardiac hypertrophy in hemodialysis patients. *Kidney International* 32:900–907.
68. Raine AE. (1994) Acquired aortic stenosis in dialysis patients. *Nephron* 68:159–168.
69. Chaignon M, Chen WT, Tarazi RC, Bravo El, Nakamoto S. (1981) Effect of hemodialysis on blood volume distribution and cardiac output. *Hypertension* 3:327–332.
70. London GM, Marchais SJ, Guerain AP. (1991) Cardiovascular function in hemodialysis patients. In: Grunfeld JP, Bach JF, Funck-Brentano JL, Maxwell MH, editors. *Advances in nephrology*, vol. 20. St Louis, MO:Mosby Year Book,
71. Harnett JD, Murphy B, Collingwood P, Purchase L, Kent G, Parfrey PS. (1993) The reliability and validity of echocardiographic measurement of left ventricular mass in hemodialysis patients. *Nephron* 65:212–214.
72. Huting J, Kramer W, Schutterle G, Wizemann V. (1988) Analysis of left ventricular changes associated with chronic hemodialysis: a non-invasive follow-up study. *Nephron* 49:284–290.
73. Ahearn DJ, Maher JF. (1972) Heart failure as a complication of hemodialysis arteriovenous fistula. *Annals of Internal Medicine* 70:201–204.
74. Foley RN, Parfrey PS. (1997) Cardiac disease in chronic uremia: clinical outcome and risk factors. *Advances in Renal Replacement Therapy* 4:234–248.

8

Lipoprotein abnormalities in end-stage renal failure

Florian Kronenberg

Physiological lipoprotein metabolism

Characterization of lipoproteins

Cholesterol and triglycerides are hydrophobic substances that can be transported in plasma only as lipoproteins. Therefore, lipoproteins are essential 'couriers' which deliver lipids where they are needed and remove them from peripheral cells when in excess. Lipoproteins are macromolecular complexes with a core of hydrophobic triglycerides and cholesteryl esters. The surface of lipoproteins is mainly composed of a monolayer of phospholipids in contact with the lipids of the lipoprotein core on the endofacial aspect and with the plasma compartment on the exofacial aspect. Apolipoproteins are interspersed in this surface and are necessary for the stability and integrity of particles, the activation or inhibition of enzymes, and the interaction of lipoproteins with their receptors. Most apolipoproteins (except apoB-48, apoB-100, and apo(a)) are able to exchange readily between lipoprotein classes. This continuous redistribution enhances many metabolic processes of lipoproteins.

The five major lipoprotein fractions are defined by physicochemical properties and are known as chylomicrons, very-low-density lipoproteins (VLDLs), intermediate-density lipoproteins (IDLs), low-density lipoproteins (LDLs), and high-density lipoproteins (HDLs) (Fig. 8.1). Chylomicrons and VLDLs transport most plasma triglycerides; LDLs and HDLs are enriched in cholesterol and protein and less in triglycerides. An additional lipoprotein called lipoprotein(a) [Lp(a)] is distinct from other lipoproteins by its unique apoprotein moiety and will be discussed later in detail.

Lipoprotein pathways

Exogenous pathway

In the exogenous pathway (Fig. 8.2), chylomicrons transport absorbed dietary fat, cholesterol, and fat-soluble nutrients from the intestine via lymph into the systemic circulation. Chylomicrons are triglyceride-rich and normally catabolized within minutes by lipoprotein lipase (LPL), thereby generating free fatty acids (FFAs) which are taken up by liver, muscle, and adipose tissue. During this catabolic process, chylomicrons diminish in size and become chylomicron remnants, which are taken up by the liver mediated by the LDL receptor and the LDL receptor-related protein (LRP).

Endogenous pathway

In the endogenous pathway (Fig. 8.2) the liver assembles and secretes triglyceride-rich VLDL particles which transport triglycerides from the liver to peripheral tissues and which

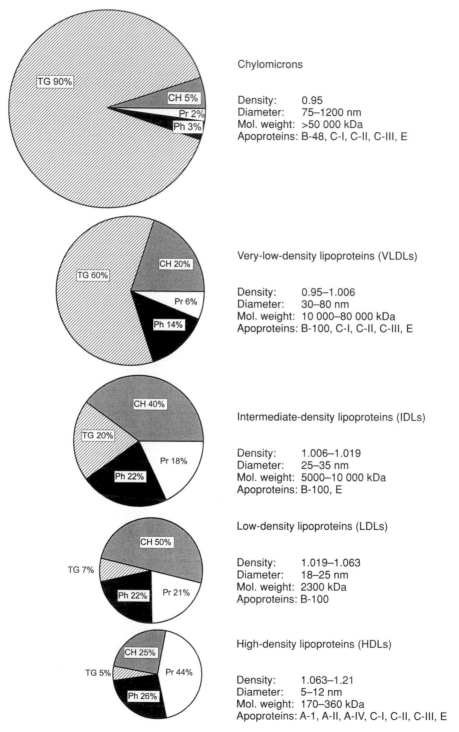

Chylomicrons

Density: 0.95
Diameter: 75–1200 nm
Mol. weight: >50 000 kDa
Apoproteins: B-48, C-I, C-II, C-III, E

Very-low-density lipoproteins (VLDLs)

Density: 0.95–1.006
Diameter: 30–80 nm
Mol. weight: 10 000–80 000 kDa
Apoproteins: B-100, C-I, C-II, C-III, E

Intermediate-density lipoproteins (IDLs)

Density: 1.006–1.019
Diameter: 25–35 nm
Mol. weight: 5000–10 000 kDa
Apoproteins: B-100, E

Low-density lipoproteins (LDLs)

Density: 1.019–1.063
Diameter: 18–25 nm
Mol. weight: 2300 kDa
Apoproteins: B-100

High-density lipoproteins (HDLs)

Density: 1.063–1.21
Diameter: 5–12 nm
Mol. weight: 170–360 kDa
Apoproteins: A-1, A-II, A-IV, C-I, C-II, C-III, E

Fig. 8.1 Characteristics of human plasma lipoproteins. TG, triglycerides; CH, cholesterol; Ph, phospholipids; Pr, proteins.

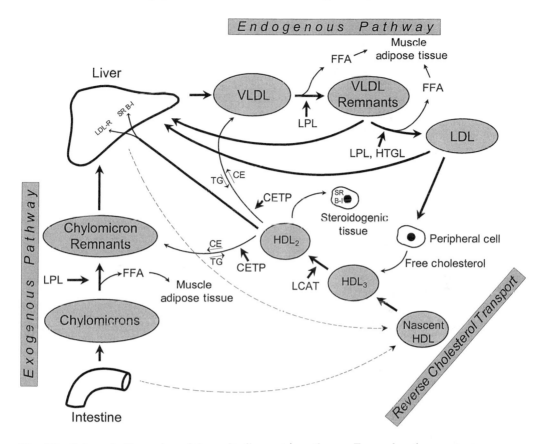

Fig. 8.2 Schematic illustration of the major lipoprotein pathways. For explanation, see text.

are hydrolyzed by LPL. Apo C-II and C-III play an important step in the regulation of LPL: apo C-II is a cofactor for LPL activation and apo C-III decreases the stimulation of LPL (Table 8.1). VLDL particles are reduced in size by triglyceride hydrolysis to VLDL remnants (also called IDL), which can be taken up by the liver or can be further hydrolysed to LDL particles. During this conversion, the particles become depleted of triglycerides and surface components but retain considerable amounts of cholesterol[1] (Fig. 8.1).

LDL transports cholesterol primarily to hepatocytes but also to peripheral tissues. ApoB-100 is responsible for the recognition and uptake of LDL by the LDL receptor, which clears approximately 60–80% of LDL in normal subjects. The remaining LDL is removed by other specific receptors, such as LRP, or by scavenger receptors.[2] Oxidized LDL, in particular, can be taken up by scavenger receptors on cells like macrophages and vascular smooth muscle cells. When these macrophages become overloaded with cholesteryl esters they develop into foam cells, which is a major step in the development of atherosclerosis.[2] When LDL becomes lipid-depleted, small, dense LDL is generated which interacts less well with the LDL receptor and is more susceptible to oxidative modification. Thus, small, dense LDLs are believed to be more atherogenic than larger LDL particles.[3]

LDL is the main external source of cholesterol for cells. After binding to the LDL receptor, the LDL-receptor complex is internalized and cholesterol will, depending on the tissue,

Table 8.1 Characteristics and function of apolipoproteins and concentrations in hemodialysis (HD) and continuous ambulatory peritoneal dialysis (CAPD) patients

Apoprotein	Molecular weight (Da)	Metabolic function	HD	CAPD
A-I	28016	Major apolipoprotein of HDL; activates LCAT	↓	↔
A-II	17414	Enhances HTGL activity	↓	↔
A-IV	46465	Participates in reverse cholesterol transport; probably involved in activation of LCAT and LPL	↑↑	↑↑
B-48	264000	Major apolipoprotein of chylomicrons; assembly and secretion of chylomicrons		
B-100	540000	Assembly and secretion of VLDL, major apolipoprotein of VLDL, IDL, and LDL; ligand for LDL receptor	↔→↑	↑
C-I	6630	Activates LCAT	↔	↑
C-II	9900	Activates LPL	↑	↑↑
C-III	8800	Inhibitor of LPL	↑↑	↑
E	34145	Ligand for several members of the LDL receptor gene family	↔→↑	↑↑
Apo(a)	300000– >800000	Unknown; independent predictor of coronary artery disease	↑	

↔ = no significant change; ↑ = increased; ↑↑ = markedly increased; ↓ = decreased.
HDL, high-density lipoprotein; IDL, intermediate-density lipoprotein; LDL, low-density lipoprotein; VLDL, very-low-density lipoprotein; LCAT, lecithin:cholesterol acyltransferase; HTGL, hepatic triglyceride lipase; LPL, lipoprotein lipase.

either be stored or used for the production of bile salts, cell membranes, or hormones. Cells are also capable of *de novo* synthesis of cholesterol. When body cholesterol is sufficient, this synthesis will be inhibited and the LDL receptor will be downregulated, reducing the binding and cellular uptake of exogenous cholesterol.

HDL plays an important role in reverse cholesterol transport, which means the transport of cholesterol from different peripheral cells to the liver[4] (Fig. 8.2). HDL precursor particles are secreted as disc-shaped structures by the liver and intestine (nascent HDL) and can absorb free cholesterol from cell membranes, a process mediated by apoA-IV[5] and eventually facilitated by the scavenger receptor B-I (SR B-I).[6] ApoA-I is the major apolipoprotein of HDL and activates the enzyme lecithin:cholesterol acyltransferase (LCAT), which esterifies the accepted free cholesterol. By acquisition of additional apolipoproteins, cholesteryl esters, and triglycerides, HDL_3 particles are transformed into spherical HDL_2 particles.[7] Reverse cholesterol transport can take three different routes. First, large HDL particles with multiple copies of apoE can be taken up by the liver via the LDL receptor.[4] Second, the accumulated cholesteryl esters from HDL can be selectively taken up by the liver mediated by SR B-I.[8] This receptor is expressed primarily in liver and non-placental steroidogenic tissues. Third, cholesteryl esters are transferred by the cholesteryl ester transfer protein (CETP) from HDL to triglyceride rich lipoproteins.[4] HDL cholesterol levels are influenced by the complexity of these reverse cholesterol transport processes and its contributing components. Disturbances in the concentrations of apoproteins, function of enzymes, transport proteins, receptors, other lipoproteins, and the clearance from plasma can have a major impact on the antiatherogenic properties in HDL.

Lipoprotein abnormalities in hemodialysis patients

Lipids and lipoproteins

Total and LDL cholesterol concentrations are usually normal or subnormal in hemodialysis patients when compared with healthy controls.[9–15] Many studies have described hypertriglyceridemia as the most common lipid abnormality in hemodialysis patients with a prevalence of 25–75%[10–13,15–18] and it is associated with increased VLDL levels[12,19,20] and a Frederickson type-IV pattern of hyperlipidemia. HDL cholesterol values are markedly reduced in hemodialysis patients.[9,10,12,14,15,21]

Figure 8.3 shows the results from a recent multicenter study including 256 controls, 534 hemodialysis patients, and 168 continuous ambulatory peritoneal dialysis (CAPD) patients.[15] The most noticeable changes in hemodialysis patients were low HDL cholesterol levels: nearly 60% of the patients showed levels in the range of the lowest quintile of the control group. Mean values were 38.3 mg/dL compared with 50.3 mg/dL in the control group ($p <$ 0.001). These dramatic changes might be of major importance in light of the growing evidence that HDL cholesterol has strong antiatherogenic properties. Triglyceride concentrations were elevated in hemodialysis patients, but only 25% of them showed values higher than 200 mg/dL. Total and LDL cholesterol values were significantly lower than in controls, with nearly 60% and approximately 40%, respectively, of the patients in the lowest quintile of the control group (Fig. 8.3). More than 30% of patients were in the highest quintile for the ratio of total/HDL cholesterol, which was higher than 5.6 in the total group.

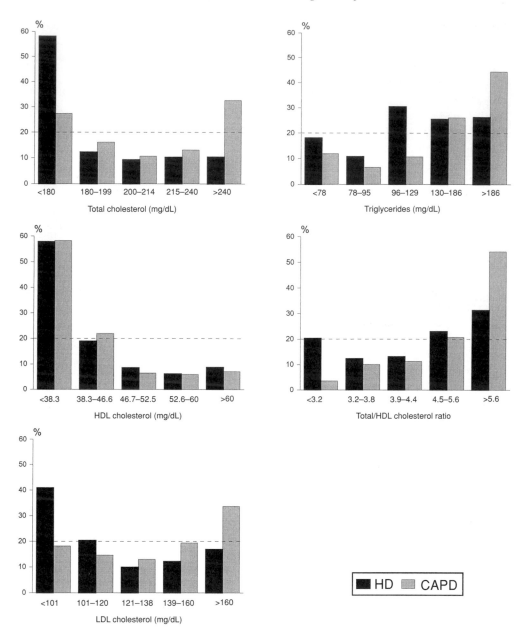

Fig. 8.3 Frequency distribution of total, high-density lipoprotein (HDL), and low-density lipoprotein (LDL) cholesterol and triglyceride values, as well as the total/HDL ratio, in 534 hemodialysis (HD) patients and 168 patients treated by continuous ambulatory peritoneal dialysis (CAPD) in relation to the corresponding quintiles of a control group of 256 individuals. Data are calculated from reference 15.

The underlying reason for renal failure has a strong influence on lipoprotein concentrations in early stages of renal disease. This influence may be determined principally by the degree of proteinuria.[22] Once dialysis treatment has started, plasma lipid and apolipoprotein concentrations become independent of the primary etiology for renal failure.[23]

Apolipoproteins

The apolipoprotein profile of hemodialysis patients shows major deviations from healthy controls (Table 8.1). Concentrations of apoA-I and apoA-II are reduced.[15,19,20,24,25] Reports on apoB concentrations are contrasting, ranging from decreased[12,15] to normal[24,25] to increased concentrations.[19,20] Elevated levels are reported for apoC-II and apoC-III, and the relative increase is more pronounced for apoC-III,[19,20,25,26] resulting in a decreased apoC-II/apoC-III ratio. These changes in apolipoprotein concentrations might be important since apoA-I activates LCAT, apoC-II activates LPL, and apoC-III inhibits LPL, which results in decreased activity of both LPL and LCAT.

ApoA-IV was demonstrated to be markedly elevated in hemodialysis and peritoneal dialysis patients.[15,27,28] The function of apoA-IV is not completely known, but *in vitro* studies support the participation in several steps of the reverse cholesterol transport. It binds to peripheral cells, promotes cholesterol efflux, and enhances the formation of small HDL particles[5] by activating LCAT,[29] and it might be involved in the binding and uptake of HDL lipoproteins by hepatocytes. Furthermore, apoA-IV modulates the activation of lipoprotein lipase and the CETP-mediated transfer of cholesteryl esters from HDL to LDL.[30] Two recent studies in mice transgenic for human apoA-IV[31] or mice overexpressing mouse apoA-IV[32] demonstrated a significant reduction of aortic atherosclerotic lesions compared with control mice, both in the setting of an atherogenic diet. This effect was apparent even when human apoA-IV was expressed in apoE-deficient mice.[31] If this observation holds true in humans, the markedly elevated levels in dialysis patients may be a counteracting response to the 'atherogenic' environment in these patients.

The changes in apolipoprotein profile in hemodialysis patients are not necessarily associated directly with hyperlipidemia. They are considered, however, as atherogenic owing to their influence on lipolytic activity and lipoprotein metabolism.

Underlying mechanisms for metabolic disturbances

Triglyceride-rich lipoproteins

The mechanisms causing hypertriglyceridemia in hemodialysis patients are not understood precisely. Increased production or decreased removal of these lipoproteins might contribute to the dyslipidemic state. Thus, the arterial wall of these patients is exposed to high levels of postprandial circulating chylomicron remnants for long periods of time.

An increased production of triglyceride-rich lipoproteins is possibly a consequence of stimulated hepatic VLDL synthesis or impaired carbohydrate tolerance.[22] By contrast, fat-loading tests showed a severe defect in the clearance of postprandial chylomicron remnants in hemodialysis patients irrespective of their fasting triglyceride levels.[33] Turnover studies revealed impaired triglyceride removal in uremia,[18,34] which is enhanced by the impaired LPL activity.[34–36] It is conceivable that this reduced activity is caused by a decreased enzyme synthesis, an inhibitor against the enzyme, or a depletion of the enzyme pool induced by frequent heparinization in hemodialysis patients[37] (see below). Decreased synthesis of LPL is possibly related to secondary hyperparathyroidism, which is a common abnormality in hemodialysis patients. Increased parathyroid hormone (PTH) levels suppress insulin release, which results in carbohydrate intolerance. Since insulin is a potent stimulator of LPL synthesis,[38] hyperparathyroidism indirectly causes decreased synthesis of LPL with accompanying increased triglyceride concentrations. A correlation of high PTH and triglyceride values was observed in several clinical[39] and experimental investigations.[40] Recent studies in rats with chronic renal failure demonstrated that parathyroidectomy completely normalized LPL mRNA, LPL protein mass, and enzymatic activity of LPL, and partially ameliorated the hypertriglyceridemia caused by chronic renal failure.[41] Interestingly, one clinical study in hemodialysis patients demonstrated that intravenous $1,25(OH)_2D_3$ therapy corrected glucose intolerance, insulin resistance, and hypoinsulinemia as well as hypertriglyceridemia, although PTH was not suppressed.[42]

Studies in chronic experimental renal failure showed that the impaired triglyceride removal might also be accentuated by the downregulation of the expression of the VLDL receptor.[43]

LDL metabolism

In vivo turnover studies demonstrated decreased clearance of *in vitro* mildly carbamylated LDL in healthy humans and a decreased fractional catabolic rate of uremic LDL when injected into rabbits.[44] Similar turnover studies in hemodialysis patients revealed a slightly decreased clearance of LDL.[45] Several mechanisms have been proposed for this observation. LDL particles isolated from uremic patients show impaired binding to the LDL receptor,[46] which could be caused by chemical modification of LDL-apoB in the uremic state.[44]

There is evidence that the lipid and apolipoprotein components of LDL in patients with end-stage renal failure (ESRF) are modified by advanced glycation end-products (AGEs).[47] Infusion of AGE-modified albumin in normal animals provided evidence that AGEs have atherogenic potential.[48] AGE-peptides are cleared by the healthy human kidney, and patients with ESRF, therefore, have markedly elevated concentrations.[49] These AGE-peptides are able to crosslink covalently with plasma proteins such as apoB,[47,49] which results in significantly impaired LDL-receptor mediated clearance of LDL.[47] In accordance, LDL concentrations significantly decreased when aminoguanidine, an inhibitor of advanced glycation, was administered.[47] Recent investigations identified epitopes close to the apoB LDL receptor-binding site that are modified by AGE and that might be responsible for the inhibited cellular uptake.[50]

The abnormal composition of LDL in uremia consisting of an increased triglyceride-to-cholesterol ratio[9] or the presence of small dense LDL particles[51,52] may alter the clearance of LDL. The triglyceride content of the LDL particle has an influence on the conformation of the LDL receptor binding domain,[53] which results in poor catabolism of triglyceride-rich LDL in human fibroblasts.[54] This observation is supported by *in vitro* experiments demonstrating enhanced degradation of cholesteryl ester-enriched LDL by cultured human dermal fibroblasts.[55]

A further possibility is that the LDL receptor itself is influenced by uremia. LDL receptors are reportedly reduced in uremic patients, caused either by downregulation of transcription, reduced LDL receptor mRNA stability, or increased LDL receptor mRNA degradation.[56] Furthermore, manifold changes in the fatty acid profiles are described in uremic patients[57,58] that possibly alter the cell membrane lipid composition or membrane fluidity, which might influence the LDL receptor function.[59,60]

Despite the decreased clearance of LDL, normal or subnormal values of LDL are observed in hemodialysis patients. This might be explained by the concomitant decrease in the rate of LDL production.[45]

HDL metabolism

Kinetic studies in patients with chronic renal failure have attributed the low HDL level to a decreased synthesis.[61] Others have described an association of decreasing HDL cholesterol levels with hypertriglyceridemia,[62] a view that is supported by an increase in HDL choles-terol and a decrease in triglycerides in hemodialysis patients under clofibrate therapy.[63]

The decrease of HDL in hemodialysis patients is more pronounced in the HDL_2 than the HDL_3 density range.[64,65] LCAT esterifies free cholesterol in HDL and, thereby, transforms HDL_3 to HDL_2.[7] Decreased cholesterol esterification and cholesterol transfer rate to VLDL and LDL have been observed in hemodialysis patients,[9] which could explain the abnormal HDL_2/HDL_3 ratio in these patients. HDL particles carry up to 50% less cholesterol, and the triglyceride content is elevated.[65] In addition, a reversed net transport of free cholesterol from hemodialysis plasma to cultured fibroblasts was observed, which was in contrast to controls that showed cholesterol efflux from cells to the plasma. This effect was a conse-quence of the significantly different lipid composition of apoB-containing lipoproteins and was interpreted as a manifestation of an abnormal reverse cholesterol transport system.[9]

Oxidation of lipoproteins

Oxidation of lipids and lipoproteins has been shown to be an important pathogenic step in the development of atherosclerosis.[66] Modified lipoproteins are taken up by macrophages leading to the formation of foam cells, the initial lesions in atherosclerosis. Studies on the oxidation of lipoproteins in hemodialysis patients are contrasting. Enhanced lipid peroxidation[67] and an increased susceptibility to oxidation were described for VLDL[68] and LDL[69] but not observed consistently in other studies.[70,71] However, methodological issues of the direct measurement of uremia-related oxidative changes to LDL make the interpretation of the results difficult. Alternative approaches used a murine monoclonal antibody recognizing oxidized products of phosphatidylcholine and determined an eightfold increase of oxidized LDL in hemodialysis patients when compared with normal controls.[72] Maggi and colleagues observed increased titers of autoantibodies against oxidized LDL, which were more pronounced in hemodialysis than in CAPD patients.[73] These approaches support the hypothesis of increased levels of oxi-dized LDL. Whether this plays indeed an important role in the accelerated atherosclerosis in renal patients has yet to be investigated in clinical and epidemiological studies.

The influence of heparins on lipid metabolism

The chronic administration of heparin during hemodialysis has been suggested as a possible reason for dyslipidemia in hemodialysis patients. Heparin is a mixture of polysaccharides of different weight-average molecular weights, ranging from 2000 to 25 000 Da. The specific antithrombotic effect is most efficient in fractions from 4000 to 6000 Da. Fractions with higher molecular weight account for lipolytic effects[74] by the activation of LPL with subse-quent depletion of LPL from its endothelial surface-binding site and, therefore, accumula-tion of chylomicrons.[75] Low-molecular-weight heparins (LMWHs) have a mean molecular weight of 4000 to 7000 Da and are, therefore, expected to have a favorable effect on lipid metabolism compared with unfractionated heparin. Clinical trials, however, revealed conflicting results, showing either a beneficial effect of LMWH on lipid metabolism,[76–81] no effect,[82,82a] or even an adverse effect.[83–85]

Several reasons might be responsible for the discrepancies and should be further eluci-dated in future studies. First, the different LMWH preparations are heterogeneous in mole-cular weight. The inclusion of fractions with higher molecular weight could result in increased activation and depletion of LPL. Second, drug administration procedures seem to influence the effect of LMWH; most of the studies which described a beneficial effect administered LMWH in a bolus injection at commencement of the dialysis session followed by a continuous infusion during the entire session of LMWH.[76–79] Studies which did not observe a beneficial effect administered LMWH only as a single bolus.[82–85] Third, some studies suggest that the beneficial effect of LMWH can only be observed after 1 year or more of use. Finally, dyslipidemic and especially hypertriglyceridemic patients seem to benefit more than normolipidemic patients from administration of LMWH.

In conclusion, LMWH might have a beneficial effect after long-term use and especially in hyperlipidemic patients. Owing to considerable differences among available preparations, a general recommendation cannot be given at this time.

Erythropoietin

Reports on the effect of erythropoietin on lipoprotein metabolism are contrasting. One large study including 81 hemodialysis patients and 31 CAPD patients observed a decrease of total cholesterol, triglycerides, and apoB,[86] but this was not confirmed in a study including 102 hemodialysis patients.[87] Allegra and colleagues suggested that the changes in lipid profile are dependent on energy intake; patients who increased their food intake under erythropoietin therapy showed an increase in total and LDL cholesterol and apoB, whereas those with stable energy intake showed a decrease of these parameters.[88] An investigation in hemodialysis patients suggested that erythropoietin supplement therapy may reduce remnant-like particles-cholesterol levels by increasing plasma LPL and HTGL levels[88a]. A study in adolescent dialysis patients observed not only a decrease of total and LDL cholesterol and triglycerides, but a significant improvement of insulin sensitivity.[89] None of these studies, however, corrected the changes of lipoproteins for the marked increase in hematocrit, which was recently shown to have a major impact on the interpretation of results.[90]

Antihypertensive agents

Most knowledge about the influence of antihypertensive drugs on lipoprotein metabolism originates from studies in non-renal patients. Diuretics and β-blockers tend to influence the lipid profile negatively, whereas the peripherally acting α-blocking agents show beneficial effects.[91,92] Thiazides and chlorthalidone increase total and LDL cholesterol as well as triglycerides without affecting HDL cholesterol. Loop diuretics increase total and LDL cholesterol, and potassium-sparing diuretics seem to have a minimal effect on lipoprotein metabolism. Selective and non-selective β-blockers increase triglycerides and decrease HDL cholesterol, whereas β-blockers with intrinsic sympathomimetic activity and combined α- and β-blockers have no significant influence on lipid levels. Alpha-blockers were reported to decrease triglycerides, total and LDL cholesterol, and to increase HDL cholesterol. Centrally acting agents, calcium channel blockers, and angiotensin-converting enzyme (ACE) inhibitors seem to be neutral. The mechanisms responsible for the observed changes in lipoprotein metabolism are probably the influence of these drugs on LPL activity and worsening of insulin resistance.

Dialysis membranes

Prospective controlled trials clearly indicate that the use of dialysis membranes has a pronounced influence on lipid parameters. Triglyceride levels in patients dialysed using high-flux membranes were about 60–70% of those in patients using conventional dialysis membranes.[93] LPL activity increased significantly during dialysis with high-flux membranes,[93,94] and serum from patients dialysed with these membranes inhibited LPL much less than serum from those dialysed with saponified cellulose ester membranes.[94] An LPL-inhibiting substance, which is not dialyzable with cellulose membranes and which is removed with high-flux membranes, is thought to be responsible.[37] This view is supported by the observation that low-flux cellulose acetate membranes with a good clearance of mid-range molecular weight molecules may also be associated with an improvement of the lipoprotein profile.[95] The LPL-inhibiting apoC-III could be one of these factors. ApoC-III decreased and apoC-II, a cofactor for LPL activation, remained stable during long-term treatment with high-flux membranes, which might be responsible for the observed increase in LPL activation.[96]

High-flux membranes have two further advantages: first, a lower dosage of heparin is necessary, which significantly decreases triglycerides and LDL cholesterol levels and the LDL/HDL ratio.[97] Second, they reduce AGEs during a dialysis session which results after long-term use in lower steady-state serum levels of AGE,[49] AGE-apoB, and total apoB.[98] This was explained by a decreased exposure of apoB to AGE and, therefore, reduced crosslinking which might otherwise result in decreased recognition and clearance of LDL by the LDL receptor-pathway.[98]

Lipoprotein abnormalities in CAPD patients

Lipids and lipoproteins

The lipid abnormalities in CAPD patients are investigated less intensively and differ in many ways from those in hemodialysis patients. These differences are obviously caused by the differences in treatment modalities. Generally, CAPD is associated with a more atherogenic lipoprotein profile when compared with hemodialysis patients. The lipoprotein subfractions show markedly increased concentrations of triglyceride-rich particles.[99] After several months of CAPD treatment, about half of the patients develop hypertriglyceridemia.[15,100–102] Furthermore, total, VLDL, and LDL cholesterol levels increase during the first months[101,102] and are higher than in hemodialysis patients.[15] Most studies found low concentrations of HDL cholesterol in these patients.[15,100–102]

A recent study investigated lipoproteins and apolipoproteins in 168 CAPD patients[15] (Fig. 8.3). About 45% of these patients had triglyceride levels in the highest quintile when compared with healthy controls. This percentage is also markedly higher than in hemodialysis patients. Significantly higher total and LDL cholesterol levels were observed in CAPD compared with hemodialysis patients (221.5 vs. 174.4 mg/dL and 145.4 vs. 113.3 mg/dL, respectively, $p < 0.001$). The frequency distribution of total cholesterol was markedly different from that of hemodialysis patients (Fig. 8.3). CAPD patients showed a mean level and distribution of HDL cholesterol similar to hemodialysis patients, and both had significantly lower levels than controls. More than 50% of the CAPD patients had total/HDL cholesterol ratios in the highest quintile of the control group. As in hemodialysis patients, plasma lipid and apolipoprotein concentrations were independent of the underlying etiology of renal failure.

Apolipoproteins

ApoA-I and apoA-II concentrations are normal in CAPD patients.[103] ApoA-IV concentrations are twice that of controls but are not different from hemodialysis patients.[15] ApoB and apoE are higher than in controls as well as in hemodialysis patients.[15,103] ApoC-II and apoC-III are elevated as in hemodialysis patients[103] (Table 8.1).

Underlying mechanisms for metabolic disturbances

In contrast to hemodialysis patients, the mechanisms for hyperlipidemia in CAPD patients seem to be determined more by increased production than by decreased removal of triglycerides. Approximately 100–200 g glucose are absorbed per day from dialysis fluid, which is taken up by the liver. Elevated blood glucose and fasting insulin levels are observed following the instillation of a hypertonic glucose-containing dialysis fluid, which probably stimulates triglyceride synthesis.[104] On the other hand, tremendous amounts of proteins, including lipoproteins and apolipoproteins, are lost in dialysis fluid by a molecular sieving effect of the peritoneum. The daily loss of proteins in CAPD patients is about 8 to 15 g per day,[15,105,106] comparable to a severe nephrotic syndrome. Kagan and colleagues[106] found VLDL, IDL, HDL, LDL, and apoB in the peritoneal fluid, and these lipoproteins showed a lipid and apolipoprotein composition similar to plasma lipoproteins. The peritoneal clearance of these lipoproteins correlated with their molecular weight, plasma concentration, and dialysis dwell time. The clearance of total protein correlated positively with plasma triglycerides and LDL and negatively with HDL levels.[106] Taken together, these results suggest that the low plasma levels of total protein and albumin in CAPD patients trigger an increased non-specific production of proteins, including lipoproteins, which is similar to the situation in nephrotic syndrome.[107] In addition to the increased production of lipoproteins, the clearance of LDL is reported to be decreased markedly compared with controls and is also lower than in hemodialysis patients.[45] The low HDL levels are probably caused by their high loss through peritoneal clearance, which was estimated to be about one-third of the normal daily synthesis rate.[106]

Lipoprotein(a)

Structure, synthesis, and metabolism of Lp(a)

Lp(a) differs in structure from LDL by the highly polymorphic glycoprotein apolipoprotein(a), which is covalently linked to the apoB of an LDL by a disulfide bridge.[108] Apo(a) shows a high degree of homology to plasminogen,[108] which contains five so-called kringle structures (K-I–K-V). Instead of K-I–K-III, apo(a) has a variable number of copies of the plasminogen-like K-IV. The exact physiological function of Lp(a) is still unclear. Owing to the high homology with plasminogen, a relation between Lp(a) and the fibrinolytic system has been suggested.[109]

Lp(a) is synthesized primarily in the liver.[110] The site and mechanism of catabolism are controversial. Although Lp(a) contains apoB-100, the catabolism of Lp(a) by the LDL-receptor is not of major importance, at least under physiological conditions. The rate of Lp(a) catabolism does not correlate with Lp(a) plasma concentrations, which suggests that plasma levels are controlled by synthesis rather than by clearance.[111,112]

Several observations argue for a role for the kidney in the metabolism of Lp(a). A recent study[113] measured Lp(a) in the aorta and in the renal vein of 100 patients without renal disease undergoing coronary angioplasty. A large arteriovenous difference of about 9% with lower values in the renal vein was observed, which demonstrated that the kidney is able to remove large amounts of Lp(a) from the systemic circulation.[113] The role of the kidney in the metabolism of Lp(a) is also supported by the observation that apo(a) fragments of various sizes are found in urine.[114–116] Furthermore, plasma apo(a) fragments larger in size than urinary fragments have been described.[117] Intravenous injection of these purified plasma fragments into mice, a species that does not produce apo(a), resulted in detection of smaller fragments in mouse urine that were similar to those found in human urine.[117] Obviously, the plasma apo(a) fragments are the source of the (smaller) urinary fragments. The precise molecular mechanism for renal catabolism of Lp(a), however, remains to be elucidated.

Genetic control of Lp(a) plasma concentrations

The mean and median concentrations of Lp(a) are about 15 mg/dL and 8 mg/dL, respectively, with an extremely broad range from <0.1 mg/dL to >300 mg/dL.[118] The distribution of Lp(a) plasma concentrations in the general Caucasian population is skewed, and most individuals express low Lp(a) concentrations.[119]

A genetic size polymorphism of apo(a) with six isoforms was described in 1987[119] and is determined by the apo(a) gene locus on chromosome 6q26-q27. In sodium dodecyl sufate (SDS)–polyacrylamide gel electrophoresis, the molecular weight of isoforms ranged from 300 to >800 kDa. They were designated F, B, S1, S2, S3, and S4 according to their relative mobility compared with apoB-100 (F stands for fast, B for the position of apoB-100, and S for slow) and are inherited in a codominant manner.[119] Technical refinements in identifying the polymorphic forms of apo(a) later allowed more than 30 isoforms to be distinguished.[120–122] Analyses of genomic DNA have shown that the protein size polymorphism is caused by a varying number of K-IV repeats in the apo(a) gene.[123,124]

A negative correlation exists between the molecular weight of apo(a) and the Lp(a) plasma concentrations.[119] Individuals with low-molecular-weight (LMW) isoforms like F, B, S1, and S2 (correspond to 11–22 K-IV repeats) on average have high Lp(a) concentrations, whereas those with high-molecular-weight (HMW) isoforms like S3 and S4 (>22 K-IV repeats) express low Lp(a) values (Fig. 8.4). About 45–70% of the broad variability of Lp(a) plasma concentrations in Caucasian populations can be explained by apo(a) size polymorphism.[125,126] Several further sequence variations at or near the apo(a) gene contribute to the variation in Lp(a) concentrations, resulting in a very high heritability of Lp(a) concentrations.[126] Besides some rare genetic disorders, several non-genetic diseases also have an effect on Lp(a) plasma concentrations, as discussed elsewhere.[127,128]

Lp(a) and atherosclerosis

Numerous retrospective and prospective case-control studies have reported significantly higher Lp(a) levels in patients with coronary artery disease (CAD), cerebrovascular disease, and peripheral atherosclerosis compared with controls (discussed in detail in reference 128). Armstrong and colleagues calculated a 2.7-fold higher risk for CAD in patients with Lp(a) plasma concentrations >30 mg/dL compared with patients with Lp(a) <5 mg/dL. The combination of high Lp(a) plasma concentrations with LDL cholesterol levels above the group median increased the risk to 6.0.[129] A recent study revealed that high plasma Lp(a) concentrations increase the risk of familial CAD only if the total/HDL cholesterol ratio was elevated.[130] Apparently the interaction of Lp(a) with other lipoproteins triggers or enhances its atherogenic properties.

A cross-sectional study determined apo(a) phenotypes and Lp(a) plasma concentrations in six different ethnic populations with CAD.[131] The LMW isoforms B, S1, and S2 with their associated high Lp(a) plasma concentrations were significantly more frequent in the patient groups from all six populations. Regression analysis demonstrated that the apo(a) phenotype is a significant predictor of CAD, independent of total and HDL cholesterol but not of Lp(a)

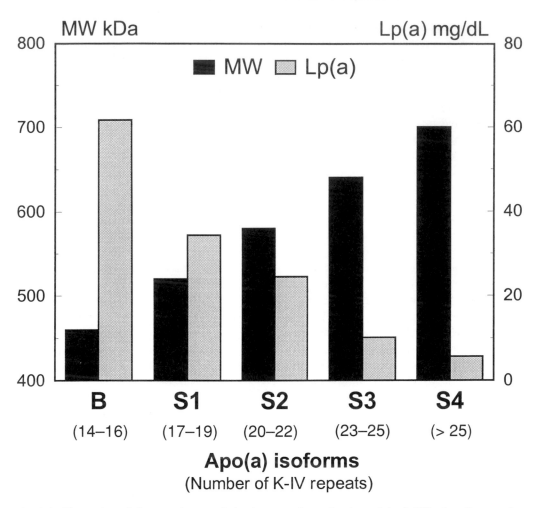

Fig. 8.4 Illustration of the negative correlation between the molecular weight (MW) of apolipoprotein [apo(a)] isoforms and lipoprotein(a) [Lp(a)] plasma concentrations. Individuals with low-molecular-weight isoforms (B, S1, and S2) show high Lp(a) levels; individuals with high-molecular-weight isoforms (S3 and S4) express low Lp(a) concentrations. The corresponding number of kringle-IV (K-IV) repeats is provided. Data from reference 191. Reprinted and adapted from reference 127 with permission of the authors.

plasma concentrations. This suggests that the apo(a) gene locus determines the risk for CAD through its control of Lp(a) plasma concentration. Therefore, the association of genetic variations at the apo(a) gene locus with CAD supports Lp(a) as a primary genetic risk factor for CAD.[131] There are only two prospective studies in the general population available, which considered and confirmed the apo(a) size polymorphism as a risk factor for CAD.[132,133]

Several mechanisms have been proposed by which Lp(a) promotes atherosclerosis. High Lp(a) concentrations impair activation of transforming growth factor-β by downregulation of plasmin generation, thereby contributing to smooth muscle cell proliferation.[134,135] Experiments in rabbit arteries indicate that oxidized Lp(a) impairs endothelium-dependent dilation more markedly than oxidized LDL.[136] Recent studies demonstrated that Lp(a) induces chemotactic activity to human monocytes in a dose-dependent fashion.[137,138] Lp(a) enhances the expression of intercellular adhesion molecule-1 (ICAM-1) critical for the adhesion and transendothelial migration of monocytes.[139] Since Lp(a) accumulates in the subendothelial space of the vessel wall,[140] it may act as a potent chemoattractant for these cells in human atherosclerosis. Others observed that the apo(a) size polymorphism influences the effect of Lp(a) on fibrinolysis in that only LMW apo(a) isoforms showed high-affinity binding to fibrin surfaces, thereby acting as a prominent competitive antagonist to plasminogen.[141,142] These *in vitro* findings suggest that high concentrations of Lp(a) of LMW should have the most pronounced influence on fibrinolysis, and are in line with results from the prospective, population-based Bruneck Study.[142a] LMW apo(a) phenotypes with a putatively high antifibrinolytic capacity emerged as one of the strongest risk preedictors of advanced stenotic carotid atherosclerosis especially when associated with high Lp(a) plasma concentrations.

Pitfalls in epidemiological studies

Epidemiological studies of Lp(a) are extremely contrasting, ranging from no change of Lp(a) up to 1000% higher Lp(a) levels in patients with renal disease compared with controls.[127] There may be several reasons. First, the more than 1000-fold range of Lp(a) levels among individuals and the highly skewed distribution make case-control studies very prone to random deviations. The strong genetic control of Lp(a) levels by the apo(a) gene locus makes it even harder to detect deviations of Lp(a) levels caused by non-genetic factors. It is known from simulation studies that case-control studies must include a minimum of 100 cases and controls in order to detect a 'real' difference of about 30–50% between two groups at $p <$ 0.05.[15,127] Often reported group sizes of 50 individuals or less do not allow reliable conclusions and even with 100 individuals 'false positive' results may occur. Therefore, it is mandatory to determine apo(a) phenotypes, especially in small groups, to identify possible random deviations in the apo(a) isoform distribution and the resulting deviations in Lp(a) levels.

Second, the measurement of Lp(a) is not yet standardized.[128,143] A concentration of 30 mg/dL (often referred as threshold for increased coronary risk) measured in one assay may be determined to be two or three times higher or lower in another assay. Many assays might be influenced by the number of K-IV repeats and, therefore, measure Lp(a) not independently of apo(a) isoforms. Uremic plasma conditions can probably further influence the measurement. For these reasons, results are divergent and are often not comparable among different studies.

Lipoprotein(a) in ESRF

Most case-control studies of Lp(a) in ESRF reported significantly elevated Lp(a) plasma concentrations in hemodialysis and CAPD patients (for review see reference 127). The observed differences between controls and patients were extremely broad, ranging from a decrease of 31% to an increase of more than 400% for hemodialysis patients and from a decrease of 49% to an increase of more than 1000% in CAPD patients. Only approximately 10% of the case-control studies investigated about 100 patients and controls and consistently showed an elevation of Lp(a) plasma concentrations which were, however, less than 100%[15,144–150] (Table 8.2).

One of the most important questions is whether the elevation of Lp(a) in patients with ESRF is secondary and, therefore, caused by renal disease or whether high Lp(a) levels in these patients are caused by an overrepresentation of LMW apo(a) isoforms coding for high Lp(a) levels. Two observations clearly demonstrated that Lp(a) levels are increased sec-

Table 8.2 Case-control studies investigating Lp(a) concentrations in patients with end-stage renal failure treated by hemodialysis (HD) or continuous ambulatory peritoneal dialysis (CAPD). Only studies including a control group and at least about 100 patients and controls are considered

Author	HD or CAPD	Number of		Mean Lp(a) mg/dL, U/dL			Median Lp(a) mg/dL, U/dL		
		Controls	Patients	Controls	Patients	% of change[a]	Controls	Patients	% of change[a]
Kronenberg et al.[15]	HD	256	534	18.4	23.4	27	8.2	14.0	71
Zimmermann et al.[144]	HD	160	280	16.3	25.5	56	9.2	13.6	48
Kronenberg et al.[15]	CAPD	256	168	18.4	34.6	88	8.2	19.9	143
Dieplinger et al.[145]	HD	236	138	12.1	20.1	66	–	–	
Hirata et al.[146]	HD	421	104	14.9	26.4	77	–	–	
Fiorini et al.[150]	HD	104	104	17.1	30.1	76	–	–	
Auguet et al.[147]	HD	101	101	12.0	17.0	42	–	–	
Webb et al.[148]	HD	146	99	–	–	–	9.4	17.4	85
Barbagallo et al.[149]	HD	90	93	18.2	35.2	93	–	–	

[a]Relative change of Lp(a) concentrations compared to the mean and median, respectively, of the respective control group. Changes between patients and controls were significantly different.

ondary to the disease; first, no difference in the apo(a) isoform distribution and, in particular, no overrepresentation of LMW apo(a) isoforms were observed in patients compared with controls.[15,145] And, second, Lp(a) decreased significantly after restoration of kidney function following renal transplantation.[151,152]

The dialysis modality strongly influences the Lp(a) concentrations; patients treated by CAPD show markedly higher levels of Lp(a) than those treated by hemodialysis.[15,148] Consequently, CAPD patients experience a significantly greater decrease of Lp(a) than hemodialysis patients after successful renal transplantation.[152]

The cause of renal failure no longer influences the amount of Lp(a) elevation once patients have stabilized on dialysis treatment. There was no significant difference between the increased Lp(a) plasma concentrations between patients who acquired ESRF because of glomerulonephritis, polycystic kidney disease, pyelonephritis, or diabetic nephropathy.[15,23,153]

It is an interesting phenomenon that Lp(a) is significantly elevated only in hemodialysis and CAPD patients with HMW apo(a) phenotypes.[15,145] Hemodialysis patients with LMW apo(a) phenotypes had nearly the same Lp(a) levels as controls with the same apo(a) types; CAPD patients with LMW apo(a) types showed a trend to higher levels which did not, however, reach significance (Fig. 8.5). The observation in hemodialysis patients is based on the investi-

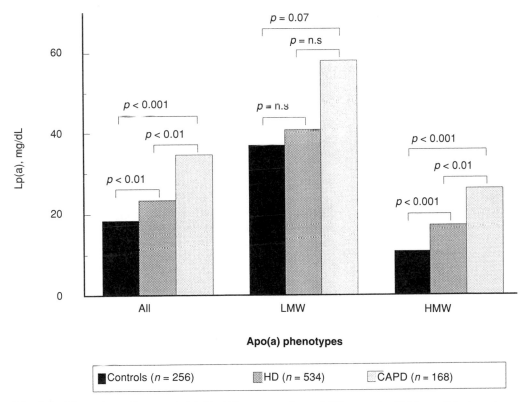

Fig. 8.5 Mean plasma lipoprotein(a) [Lp(a)] concentrations of 256 controls, 534 hemodialysis patients (HD), and 168 patients treated by continuous ambulatory peritoneal dialysis (CAPD). The Lp(a) levels are also calculated separately for low-molecular-weight (LMW) and high-molecular-weight (HMW) apolipoprotein(a) [apo(a)] phenotypes. Data from reference 15.

gation of nearly 1000 patients and about 650 controls in three studies[15,144,145] but was not confirmed by three other much smaller studies in different populations using different phenotyping methods, Lp(a) assays, and cut-points for categorization of LMW and HMW apo(a) phenotypes.[146,147,154] It is, however, supported by a decrease of Lp(a) plasma levels following transplantation only in patients with HMW apo(a) phenotypes.[151,152] This phenomenon of an apo(a) phenotype-specific elevation of Lp(a) is not restricted to dialysis patients and can be observed at all levels of renal dysfunction even in the earliest stage of non-nephrotic renal disease when glomerular filtration rate is still normal (>90 mL/min/1.73 m^2).[152a]

The reason for the selective elevation of Lp(a) levels in HMW apo(a) isoforms is unclear at present. Kario and colleagues reported high levels of C-reactive protein (CRP), sialic acid, and interleukin-6 to be closely related to the elevated Lp(a) levels in a small group of hemodialysis patients without considering the apo(a) size polymorphism.[155] This relation seemed to be an intriguing explanation for the elevated Lp(a) levels in these patients as several interleukin-6-responsive elements were described in the 5′ flanking regulatory region of the apo(a) gene[156] and some studies described Lp(a) as responding as an acute phase reactant.[157,158] Zimmermann and colleagues recently suggested that the apo(a) phenotype-specific elevation of Lp(a) in hemodialysis patients might be explained by an inflammatory condition also resulting in elevated CRP and serum amyloid A levels.[144] They also observed, however, an elevation of Lp(a) in those patients with HMW apo(a) phenotypes and normal CRP and serum amyloid A levels, which was still significant compared with controls, but less pronounced than in those with elevated CRP and serum amyloid A levels. An acute phase reaction might therefore have, at most, a modifying effect but cannot explain this phenomenon.

The underlying reason for the elevation of Lp(a) seems to differ between hemodialysis and CAPD patients. The Lp(a) concentrations in healthy controls are determined by synthesis rather than by catabolism.[112] In hemodialysis patients, a catabolic block is supported by the arteriovenous differences observed in the renovascular bed.[113] Cell-culture studies showed that the assembly of Lp(a) is not disturbed in hemodialysis patients.[159] In CAPD patients, non-specifically increased hepatic synthesis seems to be an additional possibility, which might be triggered by the high loss of proteins via dialysate and the resulting low serum albumin concentrations.[107,160] This is in line with a negative correlation between Lp(a) and plasma albumin concentrations in CAPD patients ($r = -0.17$, $p < 0.05$).[15] In accordance with this, a recent study demonstrated that rising albumin in hypoalbuminic CAPD patients by infusion of albumin results in an impressive decrease of Lp(a) plasma concentrations.[161] However, only turnover studies with a stable isotope technique will finally clarify whether the elevation of Lp(a) in hemodialysis and CAPD patients is caused by synthesis and/or catabolism.

All prospective studies investigating the influence of a successful renal transplantation clearly showed a decrease of Lp(a) following transplantation.[151,152a,162,163] Cross-sectional studies in patients who underwent transplantation many years ago, however, described contrasting results and some of them reported higher Lp(a) levels in patients treated with cyclosporin.[164] However, several other studies, especially those with a longitudinal study design, argue against this finding.[151,152,165,166] Recently, a dose-dependent influence of azathioprine on the relative decrease of Lp(a) levels was reported in a large prospective study during a follow-up of 4 years.[152]

Lipoproteins and cardiovascular risk in ESRF

Some studies noted significantly higher levels of triglycerides, VLDL cholesterol, and/or lower HDL cholesterol concentrations in hemodialysis patients with CAD or atherosclerotic complications when compared with those without.[10,11,62,167,168] On the other hand, Rostand and colleagues investigated in a retrospective analysis 320 hemodialysis patients without ischemic heart disease prior to the onset of hemodialysis. Thirty-nine of these patients developed ischemic heart disease and, in contrast to hypertension, triglyceride values were not found to be a significant risk factor.[169] Koch and colleagues followed 412 diabetic dialysis patients for 3 years. They observed that apoA-I, fibrinogen, age, and previous stroke, but not lipids, were independent predictors for cardiac and non-cardiac death.[170] Owing to these contrasting results, the predictive value of lipids was questioned.[171] Attman and Alaupovic suggested that the atherogenic potential of dyslipidemia in renal disease depends more on apolipoprotein than lipid abnormalities and may not always be recognized by measurement of lipids alone.[19] They studied a small group of 68 patients in different stages of renal impairment and observed in those 17 patients with vascular disease significantly higher apoB, apoC-II, and apoE values and lower apoC-III concentrations than in those without.[19]

The elevated Lp(a) concentrations in patients with ESRF raised the hope that it could be a predictive parameter for atherosclerotic disease in these patients. This was supported by the first prospective study by Cressman and colleagues who followed 129 hemodialysis patients for 48 months.[172] Lp(a) levels were significantly higher in 26 patients who developed an atherosclerotic event compared with those without (78.9 vs. 35.4 mg/dL, $p < 0.001$), and patients in the quartile with the highest Lp(a) levels (>73 mg/dL) suffered more than half of the events. Total, LDL, and HDL cholesterol did not significantly contribute to the occurrence of atherosclerotic events.

Subsequent studies on Lp(a) were contrasting (reviewed in reference 127) and it turned out that the apo(a) phenotype might have higher predictive value than Lp(a) concentrations. The first of these studies screened the extracranial carotid arteries of 167 hemodialysis patients for the occurrence of atherosclerotic plaques by B-mode ultrasound.[173] Patients with plaques had three times the frequency of LMW apo(a) phenotypes than those without plaques (26.9 vs. 8.5%, $p < 0.05$). Lp(a) increased significantly with the degree of atherosclerosis and in patients with LMW apo(a) phenotypes significantly more arterial sites were affected by plaques (3.62 vs. 2.08, $p < 0.001$). Moreover, patients with LMW isoforms were on average 10 years younger than patients with HMW types with the same degree of atherosclerosis of the carotid arteries. In the multivariate analysis, age, angina pectoris, and the apo(a) type were the only significant predictors for the degree of atherosclerosis.[173]

A study in CAPD patients found 67% of the patients with CAD to have an LMW apo(a) phenotype compared with only 31% in patients without CAD.[174] Webb and colleagues reported symptomatic arterial disease in 92 out of 325 patients heterogeneous in terms of renal replacement therapy. The symptomatic patient group had significantly higher Lp(a) plasma concentrations and a higher frequency of LMW apo(a) phenotypes.[175]

Two large-scale studies, one cross-sectional and one prospective, supported the apo(a) phenotype as risk factor for CAD, applying stringent diagnostic criteria in two independent patient groups. The first one[176] found a CAD prevalence of 26% in 607 hemodialysis patients. Lp(a) in patients with CAD showed only a tendency to higher levels without reaching significance compared with patients without CAD. The frequency of LMW apo(a) isoforms, however, was significantly higher in the group with CAD (Fig. 8.6). In multivariate analysis the following variables were independently associated with CAD: apoB, the LMW apo(a) phenotype, male sex, age, fibrinogen, and diabetes mellitus.[176] The second study[177] prospectively followed major coronary events in 440 unselected hemodialysis patients for a period of 5 years (Fig. 8.6). Cox proportional hazards multiple regression analysis found age and the apo(a) phenotype to be the best predictors for coronary events

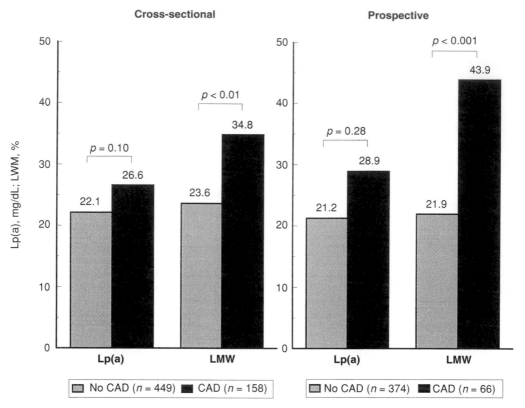

Fig. 8.6 Mean lipoprotein(a) [Lp(a)] plasma concentrations and frequency of low-molecular-weight (LMW) apolipoprotein(a) phenotypes in hemodialysis patients with, compared to those without, coronary artery disease (CAD) in a cross-sectional study including 607 patients[176] and in a prospective study which followed 440 patients for a period of 5 years.[177]

during the observation period, independently of whether patients with pre-existing CAD, or an age >65 years at study entry, or both were excluded from the analysis (Fig. 8.7). Triglycerides or other lipoproteins or apolipoproteins were not significantly associated with the incidence of CAD.[177]

The observation that the apo(a) phenotype is a better predictor for CAD in hemodialysis patients is in contrast to the general population, where the Lp(a) concentration dominates in the prediction of CAD.[131,132,178] Therefore, a model (Fig. 8.8) was proposed[173,176,177] which explains this difference based on the above-described apo(a) isoform-specific elevation of Lp(a).[15,145] In hemodialysis patients with HMW apo(a) phenotypes Lp(a) concentrations

Fig. 8.7 Coronary event-free survival in 440 hemodialysis patients with high- (HMW) and low-molecular-weight (LMW) apolipoprotein(a) [apo(a)] phenotypes. Panel A shows the results for the whole patient group, panel B includes only patients free of coronary events at the start of the study. Adjusted results are obtained from a multiple Cox proportional hazards regression analysis. Numbers near the survival curves represent the number of patients with HMW and LMW apo(a) phenotypes at risk at 0, 12, 24, 36, 48, and 60 months. Reprinted from reference 177 with permission of the authors.

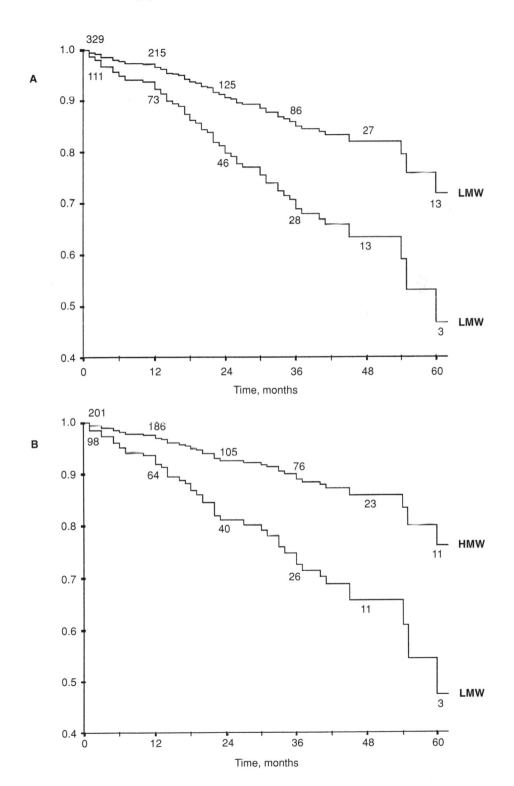

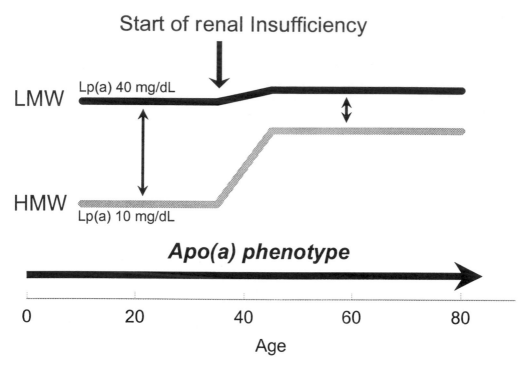

Fig. 8.8 Model to illustrate the predictive value of the apolipoprotein(a) [apo(a)] phenotype for atherosclerosis risk in hemodialysis patients; before the development of end-stage renal failure (ESRF), the risk for atherosclerosis can be estimated by the lipoprotein(a) [Lp(a)] plasma concentrations which had been present over the previous lifespan. With the start of renal insufficiency, Lp(a) plasma concentrations of high-molecular-weight (HMW) apo(a) phenotypes come closer to those of low-molecular-weight (LMW) phenotypes. Therefore, the risk for atherosclerotic complications can no longer be discriminated by means of Lp(a) concentrations. The genetically determined apo(a) phenotype is a more powerful predictor because it reflects predisease Lp(a) levels and takes into account baseline atherosclerosis risk before the development of ESRF. It is conceivable that patients with an LMW apo(a) phenotype and a more pronounced atherosclerotic risk burden develop a 'galloping' atherosclerosis after commencement of renal insufficiency or hemodialysis treatment. Reprinted from reference 192 with permission of the author.

increase and come closer to the concentrations seen in patients with LMW apo(a) phenotypes. Therefore, the risk for atherosclerotic complications can no longer be discriminated by means of Lp(a) concentrations. The apo(a) phenotype, however, gives approximate information about the contribution of Lp(a) to the risk for atherosclerosis before renal insufficiency started. This is probably more important since the predisease period with its specific atherosclerosis risk lasted longer in most of the patients than did the time of renal disease. It is, furthermore, conceivable that patients with an LMW apo(a) phenotype and a more pronounced atherosclerosis preload develop a 'galloping' atherosclerosis after commencement of renal insufficiency or hemodialysis treatment.[173,176,177]

    Compared with biochemical or clinical parameters, a genetic parameter such as the apo(a) phenotype has a major advantage for the evaluation of atherosclerosis risk as it will not change with disease or environmental influences. This is especially important in patients with renal disease because during the various stages of disease they show pronounced and manifold changes in their biochemical parameters,[22] such as Lp(a) concentrations.[127,179]

Therapy

Cholesterol and triglycerides

ESRF patients treated by CAPD might need therapeutic intervention more often than hemodialysis patients. Unfortunately, no large prospective intervention trials are available that prove the antiatherogenic effect of lipid-lowering therapy in these patients. However, the cardiovascular risk in these patients is elevated tremendously, which demands a preventive approach. The following is based on the recommendations of the National Kidney Foundation (NKF),[180] which uses the National Cholesterol Educational Program (NCEP) Adult Treatment Panel II (ATP II) general population guidelines:[181] patients with chronic renal failure should be considered at the highest risk for CAD.[182] Therefore, LDL cholesterol ≥100 mg/dL and ≥130 mg/dL should be the thresholds for starting diet and drug therapy, respectively. LDL cholesterol should be decreased to ≤100 mg/dL. Step 1 NCEP diet is recommended, which consists of 15% proteins (≈1.2 g/kg/day), 55% carbohydrates, <30% fat, 8–10% saturated fat, and less than 300 mg/day cholesterol. The protein intake in CAPD patients has to be adjusted to accommodate the protein loss into dialysate. For drug treatment, 3-hydroxy-3-methylglutaryl–coenzyme A (HMG–CoA) reductase inhibitors should be the first choice in cases of elevated LDL cholesterol levels. Fibric acid analogs are also effective for patients with increased LDL and triglyceride levels, but dosage has to be reduced due to impaired renal function. Myositis may occur as a side-effect, especially with high doses and/or combination therapy. The effects of other therapies as well as diet were not consistent in a recent meta-analysis.[183] It is not clear whether the most prevalent finding, high triglyceride or low HDL cholesterol levels, should be treated by drugs. There is no recommendation for treatment by the NCEP guidelines when no concomitant increase of LDL is observed. The NKF Task Force, however, admits that it is difficult to make recommendations and that individual judgement should be used. It should also be noted critically that hemodialysis patients usually have low total cholesterol concentrations which, according to the findings of Lowrie and colleagues,[184] are associated with an increased relative risk of mortality. Only those with very high concentrations (>350 mg/dL) are also at increased risk of death. It might be worth investigating whether the above guidelines for starting diet and drug therapy should be used only for secondary prevention in ESRF patients with known CAD and not for primary intervention. Neglecting the often-present malnutrition in these patients by focusing on lowering lipid levels could lead to adverse outcomes. Furthermore, it is highly questionable whether chronic dialysis patients are able to adopt the dietary advice under the circumstance of their chronic illness without exposing them to the risk of malnutrition.

Besides these NKF recommendations, using high-flux dialysis membranes might be a valuable trial in hemodialysis patients. A recent 1-year, open-labeled trial of sevelamer hydrochloride, a non-aluminium and non-calcium-containing phosphate binder, in haemodialysis patients demonstrated an average 30% decrease of LDL cholesterol and a 15% increase in HDL cholesterol without significant changes in PTH over the treatment period. Changes in LDL and HDL cholesterol were dependent on the starting LDL cholesterol concentrations and were most pronounced in those with the highest LDL cholesterol levels.[184a] The concentration of glucose in dialysate of CAPD patients should be reduced, if possible. Control of diabetes mellitus in both patient groups probably improves the lipid profile. Lipid apheresis is a successful option in otherwise therapy-refractory hyperlipidemia.

Lipoprotein(a)

There are no official guidelines available for Lp(a) lowering therapy and also no satisfactory and simple means of reducing Lp(a). Recent studies recommended measuring Lp(a) in all patients with renal disease. In the case of high Lp(a) plasma concentrations, apo(a) phenotyping should be performed. Patients with LMW apo(a) phenotypes and high Lp(a) values are exposed to a higher risk,[173,174,176,177] and should, therefore, be examined at regular intervals to detect and, if possible, to correct atherosclerotic changes before they have caused irreversible damage. Other atherosclerosis risk factors such as hypertension, diabetes mellitus, hyperlipidemia, and hyperhomocysteinemia should be managed even more strictly in all patients with an LMW apo(a) phenotype and high Lp(a) values.

Recently, promising investigations described the influence of adrenocorticotrophic hormone (ACTH) in steroid-treated hyperlipemic[185] as well as in hemodialysis patients.[186,187] This hormone was found to decrease Lp(a) up to 65% and also resulted in lower values for apoB, total and LDL cholesterol. In contrast to healthy individuals and steroid-treated patients, triglycerides remained elevated in hemodialysis patients;[185,186] however, this treatment is still experimental.

Small clinical trials showed the nicotinic acid derivates Niceritol and Acipimox to be effective in reducing Lp(a).[188,189] Large controlled trials are, however, still unavailable. A single-blind placebo-controlled trial observed that 6 mg/day of D-thyroxine reduced Lp(a) levels significantly in hemodialysis patients without causing clinical symptoms of hyperthyroidism.[190]

Acknowledgments

I wish to thank Dr Martin Auinger (Lainz Hospital, Vienna, Austria), Dr Hans Dieplinger (Institute of Medical Biology and Human Genetics, Innsbruck, Austria), Dr Steven C. Hunt (Cardiovascular Genetics, University of Utah, Salt Lake City, USA) and Dr Michael Koch (Nephrology Center Mettmann, Germany) for helpful comments and critical reading of the manuscript. The excellent cooperation with several dialysis units is appreciated.

F. Kronenberg is supported by the 'Austrian Programme for Advanced Research and Technology' (APART) of the Austrian Academy of Science. Studies from our group mentioned in this article were supported by grants from the Austrian 'Fonds zur Förderung der wissenschaftlichen Forschung', the Austrian Nationalbank and the D. Swarovski/Raiffeisen Foundation.

References

1. Eisenberg S, Bilheimer DW, Lindgren FT, Levy RI (1973) On the metabolic conversion of human plasma very low density lipoprotein to low density lipoprotein. *Biochimica et Biophysica Acta* 326:361–377.
2. Brown MS, Goldstein JL (1983) Lipoprotein metabolism in the macrophage: implications for cholesterol deposition in atherosclerosis. *Annual Review of Biochemistry* 52:223–261.
3. Austin MA, King M-C, Vranizan KM, Krauss RM (1990) Atherogenic lipoprotein phenotype: a proposed genetic marker for coronary heart disease risk. *Circulation* 82:495–506.
4. Bruce C, Chouinard RA Jr, Tall AR (1998) Plasma lipid transfer proteins, high-density lipoproteins, and reverse cholesterol transport. *Annual Review of Nutrition* 18:297–330.

5. Steinmetz A, Barbaras R, Ghalim N, Clavey V, Fruchart J-C, Ailhaud G (1990) Human apolipoprotein A-IV binds to apolipoprotein A-I/A-II receptor sites and promotes cholesterol efflux from adipose cells. *Journal of Biological Chemistry* 265:7859–7863.
6. Ji Y, Jian B, Wang N, Sun Y, Moya ML, Phillips MC, *et al.* (1997) Scavenger receptor BI promotes high density lipoprotein-mediated cellular cholesterol efflux. *Journal of Biological Chemistry* 272:20982–20985.
7. Dieplinger H, Zechner R, Kostner GM (1985) The *in vitro* formation of HDL2 during the action of LCAT: the role of triglyceride-rich lipoproteins. *Journal of Lipid Research* 26:273–282.
8. Acton S, Rigotti A, Landschulz KT, Xu S, Hobbs HH, Krieger M (1996) Identification of scavenger receptor SR-BI as a high density lipoprotein receptor. *Science* 271:518–520.
9. Dieplinger H, Schoenfeld PY, Fielding J (1986) Plasma cholesterol metabolism in end-stage renal disease: difference between treatment by hemodialysis or peritoneal dialysis. *Journal of Clinical Investigation* 77:1071–1083.
10. Hahn R, Oette K, Mondorf H, Finke K, Sieberth HG (1983) Analysis of cardiovascular risk factors in chronic hemodialysis patients with special attention to the hyperlipoproteinemias. *Atherosclerosis* 48:279–288.
11. Ponticelli C, Barbi G, Cantaluppi A, Donati C, Annoni G, Brancaccio D (1978) Lipid abnormalities in maintenance dialysis patients and renal transplant recipients. *Kidney International* 13(Suppl 8):S72–S78.
12. Senti M, Romero R, Pedro-Botet J, Pelegrí A, Nogués X, Rubiés-Prat J (1992) Lipoprotein abnormalities in hyperlipidemic and normolipidemic men on hemodialysis with chronic renal failure. *Kidney International* 41:1394–1399.
13. Feussner G, Wey S, Bommer J, Deppermann D, Grützmacher P, Ziegler R (1992) Apolipoprotein E phenotypes and hyperlipidemia in patients under maintenance hemodialysis. *Human Genetics* 88:307–312.
14. Shoji T, Nishizawa Y, Kawagishi T, Tanaka M, Kawasaki K, Tabata T, *et al.* (1997) Atherogenic lipoprotein changes in the absence of hyperlipidemia in patients with chronic renal failure treated by hemodialysis. *Atherosclerosis* 131:229–236.
15. Kronenberg F, König P, Neyer U, Auinger M, Pribasnig A, Lang U, *et al.* (1995) Multicenter study of lipoprotein(a) and apolipoprotein(a) phenotypes in patients with end-stage renal disease treated by hemodialysis or continuous ambulatory peritoneal dialysis. *Journal of the American Society of Nephrology* 6:110–120.
16. Chan MK, Varghese Z, Moorhead JF (1981) Lipid abnormalities in uremia, dialysis, and transplantation. *Kidney International* 19:625–637.
17. Grützmacher P, März W, Peschke P, Gross W, Schoeppe W (1988) Lipoproteins and apolipoproteins during the progression of chronic renal disease. *Nephron* 50:103–111.
18. Cattran DC, Fenton SS, Wilson DR, Steiner G (1976) Defective triglyceride removal in lipemia associated with peritoneal dialysis and hemodialysis. *Annals of Internal Medicine* 85:29–33.
19. Attman P-O, Alaupovic P (1991) Lipid and apolipoprotein profiles of uremic dyslipoproteinemia. Relation to renal function and dialysis. *Nephron* 57:401–410.
20. Zambon S, Zambon A, Stabellini N, Tarroni G, Gilli P, Crepaldi G, *et al.* (1993) Lipoprotein abnormalities in hypertriglyceridaemic patients on long-term haemodialysis. *Journal of Internal Medicine* 234:217–221.
21. Avram MM, Fein PA, Antignani A, Mittman N, Mushnick RA, Lustig AR, *et al.* (1989) Cholesterol and lipid disturbances in renal disease: the natural history of uremic dyslipidemia and the impact of hemodialysis and continuous ambulatory peritoneal dialysis. *American Journal of Medicine* 87:5-55N–5-60N.
22. Appel G (1991) Lipid abnormalities in renal disease. *Kidney International* 39:169–183.
23. Kronenberg F, Dieplinger H, König P, Utermann G (1996) Lipoprotein metabolism in renal replacement therapy: a review. *Israel Journal of Medical Sciences* 32:371–389.

24. Sakurai T, Oka T, Hasegawa H, Igaki N, Miki S, Goto T (1992) Comparison of lipids, apoproteins and associated enzyme activities between diabetic and nondiabetic end-stage renal disease. *Nephron* 61:409–414.
25. Monzani G, Bergesio F, Ciuti R, Rosati A, Frizzi V, Serruto A, *et al.* (1996) Lipoprotein abnormalities in chronic renal failure and dialysis patients. *Blood Purification* 14:262–272.
26. Bagdade JD, Albers JJ (1977) Plasma high-density lipoprotein concentrations in chronic hemodialysis and renal transplant patients. *New England Journal of Medicine* 296:1436–1439.
27. Dieplinger H, Lobentanz E-M, König P, Graf H, Sandholzer C, Matthys E, *et al.* (1992) Plasma apolipoprotein A-IV metabolism in patients with chronic renal disease. *European Journal of Clinical Investigation* 22:166–174.
28. Seishima M, Muto Y (1987) An increased apo A-IV serum concentration of patients with chronic renal failure on hemodialysis. *Clinica Chimica Acta* 167:303–311.
29. Steinmetz A, Utermann G (1985) Activation of lecithin:cholesterol acyltransferase by human apolipoprotein A-IV. *Journal of Biological Chemistry* 260:2258–2264.
30. Tenkanen H, Ehnholm C (1993) Molecular biology of apolipoprotein A-IV. *Current Opinion in Lipidology* 4:95–99.
31. Duverger N, Tremp G, Caillaud JM, Emmanuel F, Castro G, Fruchart JC, *et al.* (1996) Protection against atherogenesis in mice mediated by human apolipoprotein A-IV. *Science* 273:966–968.
32. Cohen RD, Castellani LW, Qiao JH, Van Lenten BJ, Lusis AJ, Reue K (1997) Reduced aortic lesions and elevated high density lipoprotein levels in transgenic mice overexpressing mouse apolipoprotein A-IV. *Journal of Clinical Investigation* 99:1906–1916.
33. Weintraub M, Burstein A, Rassin T, Liron M, Ringel Y, Cabili S, *et al.* (1992) Severe defect in clearing postprandial chylomicron remnants in dialysis patients. *Kidney International* 42:1247–1252.
34. Savdie E, Gibson JC, Crawford GA, Simons LA, Mahoney JF (1980) Impaired plasma triglyceride clearance as a feature of both uremic and post-transplant triglyceridemia. *Kidney International* 18:774–782.
35. Chan MK, Persaud J, Varghese Z, Moorhead JF (1984) Pathogenic roles of post-heparin lipases in lipid abnormalities in hemodialysis patients. *Kidney International* 25:812–818.
36. Arnadottir M, Nilsson-Ehle P (1994) Parathyroid hormone is not an inhibitor of lipoprotein lipase activity. *Nephrology, Dialysis, Transplantation* 9:1586–1589.
37. Arnadóttir M (1997) Pathogenesis of dyslipoproteinemia in renal insufficiency: The role of lipoprotein lipase and hepatic lipase. *Scandinavian Journal of Clinical and Laboratory Investigation* 57:1–11.
38. Cryer A (1981) Tissue lipoprotein lipase activity and its action in lipoprotein metabolism. *International Journal of Biochemistry* 13:525–541.
39. Bergesio F, Monzani G, Ciuti R, Serruto A, Benucci A, Frizzi V, *et al.* (1992) Lipids and apolipoproteins change during the progression of chronic renal failure. *Clinical Nephrology* 38:264–270.
40. Massry SG, Akmal M (1989) Lipid abnormalities, renal failure, and parathyroid hormone. *American Journal of Medicine* 87:5-42N–5-44N.
41. Vaziri ND, Wang XQ, Liang K (1997) Secondary hyperparathyroidism downregulates lipoprotein lipase expression in chronic renal failure. *American Journal of Physiology* 273:F925–F930.
42. Mak RHK (1998) 1,25-Dihydroxyvitamin D_3 corrects insulin and lipid abnormalities in uremia. *Kidney International* 53:1353–1357.
43. Vaziri ND, Liang K (1997) Down-regulation of VLDL receptor expression in chronic experimental renal failure. *Kidney International* 51:913–919.
44. Hörkkö S, Huttunen K, Kervinen K, Kesäniemi YA (1994) Decreased clearance of uraemic and mildly carbamylated low-density lipoprotein. *European Journal of Clinical Investigation* 24:105–113.
45. Hörkkö S, Huttunen K, Kesäniemi YA (1995) Decreased clearance of low-density lipoprotein in uremic patients under dialysis treatment. *Kidney International* 47:1732–1740.

46. Gonen B, Goldberg AP, Harter HR, Schonfeld G (1985) Abnormal cell-interactive properties of low-density lipoproteins isolated from patients with chronic renal failure. *Metabolism* 34:10–14.

47. Bucala R, Makita Z, Vega G, Grundy S, Koschinsky T, Cerami A, *et al.* (1994) Modification of low density lipoprotein by advanced glycation end products contributes to the dyslipidemia of diabetes and renal insufficiency. *Proceedings of the National Academy of Sciences of the USA* 91:9441–9445.

48. Vlassara H, Fuh H, Makita Z, Krungkrai S, Cerami A, Bucala R (1992) Exogenous advanced glycosylation end products induce complex vascular dysfunction in normal animals: a model for diabetic and aging complications. *Proceedings of the National Academy of Sciences of the USA* 89:12043–12047.

49. Makita Z, Bucala R, Rayfield EJ, Friedman EA, Kaufman AM, Korbet SM, *et al.* (1994) Reactive glycosylation endproducts in diabetic uraemia and treatment of renal failure. *Lancet* 343:1519–1522.

50. Wang X, Bucala R, Milne R (1998) Epitopes close to the apolipoprotein B low density lipoprotein receptor-binding site are modified by advanced glycation end products. *Proceedings of the National Academy of Sciences of the USA* 95:7643–7647.

51. O'Neal D, Lee P, Murphy B, Best J (1996) Low-density lipoprotein particle size distribution in end-stage renal disease treated with hemodialysis or peritoneal dialysis. *American Journal of Kidney Diseases* 27:84–91.

52. Rajman I, Harper L, McPake D, Kendall MJ, Wheeler DC (1998) Low-density lipoprotein subfraction profiles in chronic renal failure. *Nephrology, Dialysis, Transplantation* 13:2281–2287.

53. Aviram M, Lund-Katz S, Phillips MC, Chait A (1988) The influence of the triglyceride content of low density lipoprotein on the interaction of apolipoprotein B-100 with cells. *Journal of Biological Chemistry* 263:16842–16848.

54. Kleinman Y, Eisenberg S, Oschry Y, Gavish D, Stein O, Stein Y (1985) Defective metabolism of hypertriglyceridemic low density lipoprotein in cultured human skin fibroblasts. Normalization with bezafibrate therapy. *Journal of Clinical Investigation* 75:1796–1803.

55. Zechner R, Dieplinger H, Roscher A, Kostner GM (1984) The low-density-lipoprotein pathway of native and chemically modified low-density lipoproteins isolated from plasma incubated *in vitro*. *Biochemical Journal* 224:569–576.

56. Portman RJ, Scott RC III, Rogers DD, Loose-Mitchell DS, Lemire JM, Weinberg RB (1992) Decreased low-density lipoprotein receptor function and mRNA levels in lymphocytes from uremic patients. *Kidney International* 42:1238–1246.

57. Chapkin RS, Haberstroh B, Liu T, Holub BJ (1983) Characterization of the individual phospholipids and their fatty acids in serum and high-density lipoprotein of the renal patient on long-term maintenance hemodialysis. *J Lab Clin Med* 101:726–735.

58. Dasgupta A, Kenny MA, Ahmad S (1990) Abnormal fatty acid profile in chronic hemodialysis patients: possible deficiency of essential fatty acids. *Clin Physiol Biochem* 8:238–243.

59. Loscalzo J, Freedman J, Rudd MA, Barsky-Vasserman I, Vaughan DE (1987) Unsaturated fatty acids enhance low density lipoprotein uptake and degradation by peripheral blood mononuclear cells. *Arteriosclerosis* 7:450–455.

60. Kuo P, Weinfeld M, Loscalzo J (1990) Effect of membrane fatty acyl composition on LDL metabolism in Hep G2 hepatocytes. *Biochemistry* 29:6626–6632.

61. Fuh MMT, Lee C-M, Jeng C-Y, Shen D-C, Shieh S-M, Reaven GM, *et al.* (1990) Effect of chronic renal failure on high-density lipoprotein kinetics. *Kidney International* 37:1295–1300.

62. Brunzell JD, Albers JJ, Haas LB, Goldberg AP, Agadon L, Sherrard DJ (1977) Prevalence of serum lipid abnormalities in chronic hemodialysis. *Metabolism* 26:903–910.

63. Goldberg AP, Appelbaum-Bowden DM, Bierman EL, Hazzard WR, Haas LB, Sherrard DJ, *et al.* (1979) Increase in lipoprotein lipase during clofibrate treatment of hypertriglyceridemia in patients on hemodialysis. *New England Journal of Medicine* 301:1073–1076.

64. Atger V, Duval F, Frommherz K, Drüeke T, Lacour B (1988) Anomalies in composition of uremic lipoproteins isolated by gradient ultracentrifugation: relative enrichment of HDL in apolipoprotein C-III at the expense of apolipoprotein A-I. *Atherosclerosis* 74:75–83.

65. Shoji T, Nishizawa Y, Nishitani H, Yamakawa M, Morii H (1992) Impaired metabolism of high density lipoprotein in uremic patients. *Kidney International* 41:1653–1661.
66. Steinberg D, Parthasarathy S, Crew TE, Khoo JC, Witztum JL (1989) Beyond cholesterol. Modification of low density lipoprotein that increase its atherogenicity. *New England Journal of Medicine* 320:915–924.
67. Toborek M, Wasik T, Drózdz M, Klin M, Magner-Wróbel K, Kopieczna-Grzebieniak E (1992) Effect of hemodialysis on lipid peroxidation and antioxidant system in patients with chronic renal failure. *Metabolism* 41:1229–1232.
68. McEneny J, Loughrey CM, McNamee PT, Trimble ER, Young IS (1997) Susceptibility of VLDL to oxidation in patients on regular haemodialysis. *Atherosclerosis* 129:215–220.
69. Maggi E, Bellazzi R, Falaschi F, Frattoni A, Perani G, Finardi G, et al. (1994) Enhanced LDL oxidation in uremic patients: an additional mechanism for accelerated atherosclerosis? *Kidney International* 45:876–883.
70. Sutherland WHF, Walker RJ, Ball MJ, Stapley SA, Robertson MC (1995) Oxidation of low density lipoproteins from patients with renal failure or renal transplants. *Kidney International* 48:227–236.
71. Westhuyzen J, Saltissi D, Healy H (1997) Oxidation of low density lipoprotein in hemodialysis patients: effect of dialysis and comparison with matched controls. *Atherosclerosis* 129:199–205.
72. Itabe H, Yamamoto H, Imanaka T, Shimamura K, Uchiyama H, Kimura J, et al. (1996) Sensitive detection of oxidatively modified low density lipoprotein using a monoclonal antibody. *Journal of Lipid Research* 37:45–53.
73. Maggi E, Bellazzi R, Gazo A, Seccia M, Bellomo G (1994) Autoantibodies against oxidatively-modified LDL in uremic patients undergoing dialysis. *Kidney International* 46:869–876.
74. Liu G, Hultin M, Ostergaard P, Olivecrona T (1992) Interaction of size-fractionated heparins with lipoprotein lipase and hepatic lipase in the rat. *Biochemical Journal* 285:731–736.
75. Weintraub M, Rassin T, Eisenberg S, Ringel Y, Grosskopf I, Iaina A, et al. (1994) Continuous intravenous heparin administration in humans causes a decrease in serum lipolytic activity and accumulation of chylomicrons in circulation. *Journal of Lipid Research* 35:229–238.
76. Schrader J, Stibbe W, Armstrong VW, Kandt M, Muche R, Köstering H, et al. (1988) Comparison of low molecular weight heparin to standard heparin in hemodialysis/hemofiltration. *Kidney International* 33:890–896.
77. Deuber HJ, Schulz W (1991) Reduced lipid concentrations during four years of dialysis with low molecular weight heparin. *Kidney International* 40:496–500.
78. Nikolay J, Schulz E, Traut G, Nieth H, Biesel E, Zielke E (1990) The effect of anticoagulation with low-molecular-weight heparin upon increased triglyceride and cholesterol concentrations in chronic hemodialysis patients. *Nieren- und Hochdruckkrankheiten* 19:519–523.
79. Schmitt Y, Schneider H (1993) Low-molecular-weight heparin (LMWH) influence on blood lipids in patients on chronic haemodialysis. *Nephrology, Dialysis, Transplantation* 8:438–442.
80. Yang C, Wu T, Huang C (1998) Low molecular weight heparin reduces triglyceride, VLDL and cholesterol/HDL levels in hyperlipidemic diabetic patients on hemodialysis. *American Journal of Nephrology* 18:384–390.
81. Elisaf MS, Germanos NP, Bairaktari HT, Pappas MB, Koulouridis EI, Siamopoulos KC (1997) Effect of conventional vs. low-molecular-weight heparin on lipid profile in hemodialysis patients. *American Journal of Nephrology* 17:153–157.
82. Hombrouckx R, Devos JY, Larno L (1994) Standard heparin (SH) versus 3 low-molecular-weight heparins (LMWH) in chronic dialysis. Nephrology, Dialysis, *Transplantation* 9:988–988 (Abstract).
82a. Saltissi D, Morgan C, Westhuyzen J, Healy H (1999) Comparison of low-molecular-weight heparin (enoxaparin sodium) and standard unfractionated heparin for haemodialysis anticoagulation. *Nephrology, Dialysis, Transplantation* 14:269–2703.
83. Kronenberg F, König P, Lhotta K, Steinmetz A, Dieplinger H (1995) Low molecular weight heparin does not necessarily reduce lipids and lipoproteins in hemodialysis patients. *Clinical Nephrology* 43:399–404.

84. Kronenberg F, König P, Neyer U, Auinger M, Pribasnig A, Meisl T, *et al.* (1995) Influence of various heparin preparations on lipoproteins in hemodialysis patients: a multicentre study. *Thrombosis and Haemostasis* 74:1025–1028.

85. Spaia S, Pangidis P, Kanetidis D, Mavropoulou E, Vakaloudi A, Karagiannis A, *et al.* (1995) Longterm effects of low-molecular-weight heparin in hemodialyzed patients. *Hellenic Nephrology* 6:426–430.

86. Pollock CA, Wyndham R, Collett PV, Elder G, Field MJ, Kalowski S, *et al.* (1994) Effects of erythropoietin therapy on the lipid profile in end-stage renal failure. *Kidney International* 45:897–902.

87. Prata MM, Madeira C, Vicente O, Miguel MJ (1998) Lipid profile in haemodialysis patients treated with recombinant human erythropoietin. *Nephrology, Dialysis, Transplantation* 13:2345–2347.

88. Allegra V, Martimbianco L, Vasile A (1997) Lipid and apolipoprotein patterns during erythropoietin therapy: roles of erythropoietin, route of administration, and diet. *Nephrology, Dialysis, Transplantation* 12:924–932.

88a. Goto T, Saika H, Takahashi T, Maeda A, Mune M, Yukawa S (1999) Erythropoietin supplement increases plasma lipoprotein lipase and hepatic triglyceride lipase lveles in hemodialysis patients. *Kidney Int. Suppl.* 71:S213–S215.

89. Mak RH (1996) Effect of recombinant human erythropoietin on insulin, amino acid, and lipid metabolism in uremia. *Journal of Pediatrics* 129:97–104.

90. Kronenberg F, Trenkwalder E, Kronenberg MF, König P, Utermann G, Dieplinger H (1998) Influence of hematocrit on the measurement of lipoproteins demonstrated by the example of lipoprotein(a). *Kidney International* 54:1385–1389.

91. Donahoo WT, Kosmiski LA, Eckel RH (1998) Drugs causing dyslipoproteinemia. *Endocrinology and Metabolism Clinics of North America* 27:677–697.

92. Kasiske BL, Ma JZ, Kalil RS, Louis TA (1995) Effects of antihypertensive therapy on serum lipids. *Annals of Internal Medicine* 122:133–141.

93. Blankestijn PJ, Vos PF, Rabelink TJ, van Rijn HJ, Jansen H, Koomans HA (1995) High-flux dialysis membranes improve lipid profile in chronic hemodialysis patients. *Journal of the American Society of Nephrology* 5:1703–1708.

94. Seres DS, Strain GW, Hashim SA, Goldberg IJ, Levin NW (1993) Improvement of plasma lipoprotein profiles during high-flux dialysis. *Journal of the American Society of Nephrology* 3:1409–1415.

95. Ingram AJ, Parbtani A, Churchill DN (1998) Effects of two low-flux cellulose acetate dialysers on plasma lipids and lipoproteins—a cross-over trial. *Nephrology, Dialysis, Transplantation* 13:1452–1457.

96. Otsubo Y, Uchida Y, Yasumoto Y, Yamashita W, Arima T (1993) ApoCIII is a potent factor on lipid abnormalities in hemodialysis patients. *Journal of the American Society of Nephrology* 4:375–375 (Abstract).

97. Sperschneider H, Deppisch R, Beck W, Wolf H, Stein G (1997) Impact of membrane choice and blood flow pattern on coagulation and heparin requirement—potential consequences on lipid concentrations. *Nephrology, Dialysis, Transplantation* 12:2638–2646.

98. Fishbane S, Bucala R, Pereira BJG, Founds H, Vlassara H (1997) Reduction of plasma apolipoprotein-B by effective removal of circulating glycation derivatives in uremia. *Kidney International* 52:1645–1650.

99. Llopart R, Donate T, Oliva JA, Roda M, Rousaud F, Gonzalez-Sastre F, *et al.* (1995) Triglyceride-rich lipoprotein abnormalities in CAPD-treated patients. *Nephrology, Dialysis, Transplantation* 10:537–540.

100. Chan MK, Varghese Z, Persaud JW, Baillod RA, Moorhead JF (1982) Hyperlipidemia in patients on maintenance hemo- and peritoneal dialysis: the relative pathogenic roles of triglyceride production and removal. *Clinical Nephrology* 17:183–190.

101. Ramos JM, Heaton A, McGurk JG, Ward MK, Kerr DNS (1983) Sequential changes in serum lipids and their subfractions in patients receiving continuous ambulatory peritoneal dialysis. *Nephron* 35:20–23.

102. Lindholm B, Norbeck HE (1986) Serum lipids and lipoproteins during continuous ambulatory peritoneal dialysis. *Acta Medica Scandinavica* 220:143–151.
103. Shoji T, Nishizawa Y, Nishitani H, Yamakawa M, Morii H (1991) Roles of hypoalbuminemia and lipoprotein lipase on hyperlipoproteinemia in continuous ambulatory peritoneal dialysis. *Metabolism* 40:1002–1008.
104. Heaton A, Johnston DG, Burrin JM, Orskov H, Ward MK, Alberti KG, et al. (1983) Carbohydrate and lipid metabolism during continuous ambulatory peritoneal dialysis (CAPD): the effect of a single dialysis cycle. *Clinical Science* 65:539–545.
105. Blumenkrantz MJ, Gahl GM, Kopple JD, Kamdar AV, Jones MR, Kessel M, et al. (1981) Protein losses during peritoneal dialysis. *Kidney International* 19:593–602.
106. Kagan A, Bar-Khayim Y, Schafer Z, Fainaru M (1990) Kinetics of peritoneal protein loss during CAPD: II. Lipoprotein leakage and its impact on plasma lipid levels. *Kidney International* 37:980–990.
107. Appel GB, Blum CB, Chien S, Kunis CL, Appel AS (1985) The hyperlipidemia of nephrotic syndrome: relation to plasma albumin concentration, oncotic pressure and viscosity. *New England Journal of Medicine* 312:1544–1548.
108. McLean JW, Tomlinson JE, Kuang W-J, Eaton DL, Chen EY, Fless GM, et al. (1987) cDNA sequence of human apolipoprotein(a) is homologous to plasminogen. *Nature* 330:132–137.
109. Loscalzo J, Weinfeld M, Fless GM, Scanu AM (1990) Lipoprotein(a), fibrin binding, and plasminogen activation. *Arteriosclerosis* 10:240–245.
110. Kraft HG, Menzel HJ, Hoppichler F, Vogel W, Utermann G (1989) Changes of genetic apolipoprotein phenotypes caused by liver transplantation. Implications for apolipoprotein synthesis. *Journal of Clinical Investigation* 83:137–142.
111. Krempler F, Kostner GM, Bolzano K, Sandhofer F (1980) Turnover of lipoprotein(a) in man. *Journal of Clinical Investigation* 65:1483–1490.
112. Rader DJ, Cain W, Zech LA, Usher D, Brewer HB Jr (1993) Variation in lipoprotein(a) concentrations among individuals with the same apolipoprotein(a) isoform is determined by the rate of lipoprotein(a) production. *Journal of Clinical Investigation* 91:443–447.
113. Kronenberg F, Trenkwalder E, Lingenhel A, Friedrich G, Lhotta K, Schober M, et al. (1997) Renovascular arteriovenous differences in Lp(a) plasma concentrations suggest removal of Lp(a) from the renal circulation. *Journal of Lipid Research* 38:1755–1763.
114. Oida K, Takai H, Maeda H, Takahashi S, Shimada A, Suzuki J, et al. (1992) Apolipoprotein(a) is present in urine and its excretion is decreased in patients with renal failure. *Clinical Chemistry* 38:2244–2248.
115. Mooser V, Seabra MC, Abedin M, Landschulz KT, Marcovina S, Hobbs HH (1996) Apolipoprotein(a) kringle 4-containing fragments in urine. Relationship to plasma levels of lipoprotein(a). *Journal of Clinical Investigation* 97:858–864.
116. Kostner KM, Maurer G, Huber K, Stefenelli T, Dieplinger H, Steyrer E, et al. (1996) Urinary excretion of apo(a) fragments. Role in apo(a) catabolism. *Arteriosclerosis, Thrombosis and Vascular Biology* 16:905–911.
117. Mooser V, Marcovina SM, White AL, Hobbs HH (1996) Kringle-containing fragments of apolipoprotein(a) circulate in human plasma and are excreted into the urine. *Journal of Clinical Investigation* 98:2414–2424.
118. Utermann G (1989) The mysteries of lipoprotein(a). *Science* 246:904–910.
119. Utermann G, Menzel HJ, Kraft HG, Duba HC, Kemmler HG, Seitz C (1987) Lp(a) glycoprotein phenotypes: inheritance and relation to Lp(a)-lipoprotein concentrations in plasma. *Journal of Clinical Investigation* 80:458–465.
120. Kamboh MI, Ferrell RE, Kottke BA (1991) Expressed hypervariable polymorphism of apolipoprotein (a). *American Journal of Human Genetics* 49:1063–1074.
121. Marcovina SM, Zhang ZH, Gaur VP, Albers JJ (1993) Identification of 34 apolipoprotein(a) isoforms: differential expression of apolipoprotein(a) alleles between American blacks and whites. *Biochemical and Biophysical Research Communications* 191:1192–1196.

122. Kraft HG, Lingenhel A, Bader G, Kostner GM, Utermann G (1996) The relative electrophoretic mobility of apo(a) isoforms depends on the gel system: proposal of a nomenclature for apo(a) phenotypes. *Atherosclerosis* 125:53–61.

123. Lackner C, Boerwinkle E, Leffert CC, Rahmig T, Hobbs HH (1991) Molecular basis of apolipoprotein (a) isoform size heterogencity as revealed by pulsed-field gel electrophoresis. *Journal of Clinical Investigation* 87:2153–2161.

124. Kraft HG, Köchl S, Menzel HJ, Sandholzer C, Utermann G (1992) The apolipoprotein(a) gene: a transcribed hypervariable locus controlling plasma lipoprotein(a) concentration. *Human Genetics* 90:220–230.

125. Boerwinkle E, Menzel HJ, Kraft HG, Utermann G (1989) Genetics of the quantitative Lp(a) lipoprotein trait. III. Contribution of Lp(a) glycoprotein phenotypes to normal lipid variation. *Human Genetics* 82:73–78.

126. Utermann G. (1995) Lipoprotein(a). In: Scriver CR, Beaudet AL, Sly WS, Valle D, editors. The metabolic and molecular bases of inherited disease, pp. 1887–1912. McGraw-Hill.

127. Kronenberg F, Utermann G, Dieplinger H (1996) Lipoprotein(a) in renal disease. American *Journal of Kidney Diseases* 27:1–25.

128. Kronenberg F, Steinmetz A, Kostner GM, Dieplinger H (1996) Lipoprotein(a) in health and disease. *Critical Reviews in Clinical Laboratory Sciences* 33:495–543.

129. Armstrong VW, Cremer P, Eberle E, Manke A, Schulze F, Wieland H, *et al.* (1986) The association between serum Lp(a) concentrations and angiographically assessed coronary atherosclerosis: dependence on serum LDL levels. *Atherosclerosis* 62:249–257.

130. Hopkins PN, Wu LL, Hunt SC, James BC, Vincent GM, Williams RR (1997) Lipoprotein(a) interactions with lipid and nonlipid risk factors in early familial coronary artery disease. *Arteriosclerosis Thrombosis and Vascular Biology* 17:2783–2792.

131. Sandholzer C, Saha N, Kark JD, Rees A, Jaross W, Dieplinger H, *et al.* (1992) Apo(a) isoforms predict risk for coronary heart disease: a study in six populations. *Arteriosclerosis and Thrombosis* 12:1214–1226.

132. Wild SH, Fortmann SP, Marcovina SM (1997) A prospective case-control study of lipoprotein(a) levels and apo(a) size and risk of coronary heart disease in Stanford Five-City Project participants. *Arteriosclerosis Thrombosis and Vascular Biology* 17:239–245.

133. Klausen IC, Sjol A, Hansen PS, Gerdes LU, Moller L, Lemming L, *et al.* (1997) Apolipoprotein(a) isoforms and coronary heart disease in men—a nested case-control study. *Atherosclerosis* 132:77–84.

134. Grainger DJ, Kirschenlohr HL, Metcalfe JC, Weissberg PL, Wade DP, Lawn RM (1993) Proliferation of human smooth muscle cells promoted by lipoprotein(a). *Science* 260:1655–1658.

135. Grainger DJ, Kemp PR, Metcalfe JC, Liu AC, Lawn RM, Williams NR, *et al.* (1995) The serum concentration of active transforming growth factor-β is severely depressed in advanced atherosclerosis. *Nature Medicine* 1:74–79.

136. Galle J, Bengen J, Schollmeyer P, Wanner C (1995) Impairment of endothelium-dependent dilation in rabbit renal arteries by oxidized lipoprotein(a)—role of oxygen-derived radicals. *Circulation* 92:1582–1589.

137. Syrovets T, Thillet J, Chapman MJ, Simmet T (1997) Lipoprotein(a) is a potent chemoattractant for human peripheral monocytes. *Blood* 90:2027–2036.

138. Poon M, Zhang XX, Dunsky KG, Taubman MB, Harpel PC (1997) Apolipoprotein(a) induces monocyte chemotactic activity in human vascular endothelial cells. *Circulation* 96:2514–2519.

139. Takami S, Yamashita S, Kihara S, Ishigami M, Takemura K, Kume N, *et al.* (1998) Lipoprotein(a) enhances the expression of intercellular adhesion molecule-1 in cultured human umbilical vein endothelial cells. *Circulation* 97:721–728.

140. Rath M, Niendorf A, Reblin T, Dietel M, Krebber H-J, Beisiegel U (1989) Detection and quantification of lipoprotein(a) in the arterial wall of 107 coronary bypass patients. *Arteriosclerosis* 9:579–592.

141. Hervio L, Chapman MJ, Thillet J, Loyau S, Anglés-Cano E (1993) Does apolipoprotein(a) heterogeneity influence lipoprotein(a) effects on fibrinolysis. *Blood* 82:392–397.

142. Hervio L, Girard-Globa A, Durlach V, Anglés-Cano E (1996) The antifibrinolytic effect of lipoprotein(a) in heterozygous subjects is modulated by the relative concentration of each of the apolipoprotein(a) isoforms and their affinity for fibrin. *European Journal of Clinical Investigation* 26:411–417.

142a. Kronenberg F, Kronenberg MF, Kiechl S, Trenkwalder E, Santer P, Oberhollenzer F, *et al.* (1999) Role of lipoprotein(a) and apolipoprotein(a) phenotype in atherogenesis: prospective results from the Bruneck Study. *Circulation* 100:1154–1160.

143. Tate JR, Rifai N, Berg K, Couderc R, Dati F, Kostner GM, *et al.* (1998) International Federation of Clinical Chemistry standardization project for the measurement of lipoprotein(a). Phase I. Evaluation of the analytical performance of lipoprotein(a) assay systems and commercial calibrators. *Clinical Chemistry* 44:1629–1640.

144. Zimmermann J, Herrlinger S, Pruy A, Metzger T, Wanner C (1999) Inflammation enhances cardiovascular risk and mortality in hemodialysis patients. *Kidney International* 55:648–658.

145. Dieplinger H, Lackner C, Kronenberg F, Sandholzer C, Lhotta K, Hoppichler F, *et al.* (1993) Elevated plasma concentrations of lipoprotein(a) in patients with end-stage renal disease are not related to the size polymorphism of apolipoprotein(a). *Journal of Clinical Investigation* 91:397–401.

146. Hirata K, Kikuchi S, Saku K, Jimi S, Zhang B, Naito S, *et al.* (1993) Apolipoprotein(a) phenotypes and serum lipoprotein(a) levels in maintenance hemodialysis patients with/without diabetes mellitus. *Kidney International* 44:1062–1070.

147. Auguet T, Sentí M, Rubies-Prat J, Pelegrí A, Pedro-Botet J, Nogués X, *et al.* (1993) Serum lipoprotein(a) concentration in patients with chronic renal failure receiving haemodialysis: influence of apolipoprotein(a) genetic polymorphism. *Nephrology, Dialysis, Transplantation* 8:1099–1103.

148. Webb AT, Reaveley DA, O'Donnell M, O'Connor B, Seed M, Brown EA (1993) Lipoprotein(a) in patients on maintenance haemodialysis and continuous ambulatory peritoneal dialysis. *Nephrology, Dialysis, Transplantation* 8:609–613.

149. Barbagallo CM, Averna MR, Sparacino V, Galione A, Caputo F, Scafidi V, *et al.* (1993) Lipoprotein (a) levels in end-stage renal failure and renal transplantation. *Nephron* 64:560–564.

150. Fiorini F, Masturzo P, Mij M, Bertolini S (1995) Lipoprotein(a) levels in hemodialysis patients: relation to glucose intolerance and hemodialysis duration. *Nephron* 70:500–501.

151. Kronenberg F, König P, Lhotta K, Öfner D, Sandholzer C, Margreiter R, *et al.* (1994) Apolipoprotein(a) phenotype-associated decrease in lipoprotein(a) plasma concentrations after renal transplantation. *Arteriosclerosis and Thrombosis* 14:1399–1404.

152. Kerschdorfer L, König P, Neyer U, Bösmüller C, Lhotta K, Auinger M, *et al.* (1999) Lipoprotein(a) plasma concentrations after renal transplantation: a prospective evaluation after 4 years of follow-up. *Atherosclerosis* 144:38–391.

152a. Kronenberg F, Kuen E, Ritz E, Junker R, König P, Kraatz G, et al. (2000) Lipoprotein(a) serum concentrations and apolipoprotein(a) phenotypes in mild and moderate renal failure. *Journal of the American Society of Nephrology* 11:105–115.

153. Stenvinkel P, Berglund L, Heimbürger O, Pettersson E, Alvestrand A (1993) Lipoprotein(a) in nephrotic syndrome. *Kidney International* 44:1116–1123.

154. Gazzaruso C, Bonetti G, Garzaniti A, Pini G, Ragazzoni A, Bianchi C, *et al.* (1996) Increased plasma concentrations of lipoprotein(a) for every phenotype of apolipoprotein(a) in patients with chronic renal failure treated by hemodialysis. *Nutrition, Metabolism and Cardiovascular Disease* 6:203–210.

155. Kario K, Matsuo T, Kobayashi H, Matsuo M, Asada R, Koide M (1995) High lipoprotein (a) levels in chronic hemodialysis patients are closely related to the acute phase reaction. *Thrombosis and Haemostasis* 74:1020–1024.

156. Wade DP, Clarke JG, Lindahl GE, Liu AC, Zysow BR, Meer K, *et al.* (1993) 5′ control regions of the apolipoprotein(a) gene and members of the related plasminogen gene family. *Proceedings of the National Academy of Sciences of the USA* 90:1369–1373.

157. Maeda S, Abe A, Seishima M, Makino K, Noma A, Kawade M (1989) Transient changes of serum lipoprotein(a) as an acute phase protein. *Atherosclerosis* 78:145–150.
158. Slunga L, Johnson O, Dahlén GH, Eriksson S (1992) Lipoprotein(a) and acute-phase proteins in acute myocardial infarction. *Scandinavian Journal of Clinical and Laboratory Investigation* 52:95–101.
159. Trenkwalder E, Gruber A, König P, Dieplinger H, Kronenberg F (1997) Increased plasma concentrations of LDL-unbound apo(a) in patients with end-stage renal disease. *Kidney International* 52:1685–1692.
160. Heimbürger O, Stenvinkel P, Berglund L, Tranæus A, Lindholm B (1996) Increased plasma lipoprotein(a) in continuous ambulatory peritoneal dialysis is related to peritoneal transport of proteins and glucose. *Nephron* 72:135–144.
161. Yang WS, Min WK, Park JS, Kim SB (1997) Effect of increasing serum albumin on serum lipoprotein(a) concentration in patients receiving CAPD. *American Journal of Kidney Diseases* 30:507–513.
162. Black IW, Wilcken DEL (1992) Decreases in apolipoprotein(a) after renal transplantation: implications for lipoprotein(a) metabolism. *Clinical Chemistry* 38:353–357.
163. Segarra A, Chacón P, Martin M, Vilardell M, Vila J, Cotrina M, et al. (1995) Serum lipoprotein (a) levels in patients with chronic renal failure. Evolution after renal transplantation and relationship with other parameters of lipoprotein metabolism: a prospective study. *Nephron* 69:9–13.
164. Webb AT, Reaveley DA, O'Donnell M, O'Connor B, Seed M, Brown EA (1993) Does cyclosporin increase lipoprotein(a) concentrations in renal transplant recipients? *Lancet* 341:268–270.
165. Hunt BJ, Parratt R, Rose M, Yacoub M (1994) Does cyclosporin affect lipoprotein(a) concentrations? *Lancet* 343:119–120.
166. Sturrock NDC, Lang CC, MacFarlane LJ, Dockrell MEC, Ryan M, Webb DJ, et al. (1995) Serial changes in blood pressure, renal function, endothelin and lipoprotein (a) during the first 9 days of cyclosporin therapy in males. *Journal of Hypertension* 13:667–673.
167. Goldberg AP, Harter HR, Patsch W, Schechtman KB, Province M, Weerts C, et al. (1983) Racial differences in plasma high-density lipoproteins in patients receiving hemodialysis. A possible mechanism for accelerated atherosclerosis in white men *New England Journal of Medicine* 308:1245–1252.
168. Shoji T, Nishizawa Y, Kawagishi T, Kawasaki K, Taniwaki H, Tabata T, et al. (1998) Intermediate-density lipoprotein as an independent risk factor for aortic atherosclerosis in hemodialysis patients. *Journal of the American Society of Nephrology* 9:1277–1284.
169. Rostand SG, Kirk KA, Rutsky EA (1982) Relationship of coronary risk factors to hemodialysis-associated ischemic heart disease. *Kidney International* 22:304–308.
170. Koch M, Kutkuhn B, Grabensee B, Ritz E (1997) Apolipoprotein A, fibrinogen, age, and history of stroke are predictors of death in dialysed diabetic patients: a prospective study in 412 subjects. *Nephrology, Dialysis, Transplantation* 12:2603–2611.
171. Ritz E (1996) Why are lipids not predictive of cardiovascular death in the dialysis patient? *Mineral and Electrolyte Metabolism* 22:9–12.
172. Cressman MD, Heyka RJ, Paganini EP, O'Neil J, Skibinski CI, Hoff HF (1992) Lipoprotein(a) is an independent risk factor for cardiovascular disease in hemodialysis patients. *Circulation* 86:475–482.
173. Kronenberg F, Kathrein H, König P, Neyer U, Sturm W, Lhotta K, et al. (1994) Apolipoprotein(a) phenotypes predict the risk for carotid atherosclerosis in patients with end-stage renal disease. *Arteriosclerosis and Thrombosis* 14:1405–1411.
174. Wanner C, Bartens W, Walz G, Nauck M, Schollmeyer P (1995) Protein loss and genetic polymorphism of apolipoprotein(a) modulate serum lipoprotein(a) in CAPD patients. *Nephrology, Dialysis, Transplantation* 10:75–81.
175. Webb AT, Reaveley DA, O'Donnell M, O'Connor B, Seed M, Brown EA (1995) Lipids and lipoprotein(a) as risk factors for vascular disease in patients on renal replacement therapy. *Nephrology, Dialysis, Transplantation* 10:354–357.

176. Koch M, Kutkuhn B, Trenkwalder E, Bach D, Grabensee B, Dieplinger H, *et al.* (1997) Apolipoprotein B, fibrinogen, HDL cholesterol and apo(a) phenotypes predict coronary artery disease in hemodialysis patients. *Journal of the American Society of Nephrology* 8:1889–1898.

177. Kronenberg F, Neyer U, Lhotta K, Trenkwalder E, Auinger M, Pribasnig A, *et al.* (1999) The low molecular weight apo(a) phenotype is an independent predictor for coronary artery disease in hemodialysis patients: a prospective follow-up. *Journal of the American Society of Nephrology* 10:1027–1036.

178. Kraft HG, Lingenhel A, Köchl S, Hoppichler F, Kronenberg F, Abe A, *et al.* (1996) Apolipoprotein(a) Kringle IV repeat number predicts risk for coronary heart disease. *Arteriosclerosis, Thrombosis and Vascular Biology* 16:713–719.

179. Kronenberg F (1998) Homocysteine, lipoprotein(a) and fibrinogen: metabolic risk factors for cardiovascular complications of chronic renal disease. *Current Opinion in Nephrology and Hypertension* 7:271–278.

180. Levey AS, Beto JA, Coronado BE, Eknoyan G, Foley RN, Kasiske BL, *et al.* (1998) Controlling the epidemic of cardiovascular disease in chronic renal disease: what do we know? What do we need to learn? Where do we go from here? *American Journal of Kidney Diseases* 32:853–906.

181. Summary of the second report of the National Cholesterol Education Program (NCEP) Expert Panel on Detection, Evaluation, and Treatment of High Blood Cholesterol in Adults (Adult Treatment Panel II). (1993) *JAMA* 269:3015–3023.

182. London GM, Drüeke TB (1997) Atherosclerosis and arteriosclerosis in chronic renal failure. *Kidney International* 51:1678–1695.

183. Massy ZA, Ma JZ, Louis TA, Kasiske BL (1995) Lipid-lowering therapy in patients with renal disease. *Kidney International* 48:188–198.

184. Lowrie EG, Lew NL (1992) Commonly measured laboratory variables in hemodialysis patients: relationships among them and to death risk. *Seminars in Nephrology* 12:276–283.

184a. Chertow GM, Burke SK, Dillon MA, Slatopolsky E (1999) Long-term effects of sevelamer hydrochloride on the calcium x phosphate product and lipid profile of haemodialysis patients. *Nephrology, Dialysis, Transplantation* 14:2907–2914.

185. Berg AL, Nilsson-Ehle P (1996) ACTH lowers serum lipids in steroid-treated hyperlipemic patients with kidney disease. *Kidney International* 50:538–542.

186. Arnadottir M, Berg AL, Dallongeville J, Fruchart J-C, Nilsson-Ehle P (1997) Adrenocorticotropic hormone lowers serum Lp(a) and LDL cholesterol concentrations in hemodialysis patients. *Kidney International* 52:1651–1655.

187. Arnadottir M, Berg AL, Kronenberg F, Lingenhel A, Hugosson T, Hegbrandt J, *et al.* (1999) Corticotropin-induced reduction of plasma lipoprotein(a) concentrations in healthy individuals and hemodialysis patients: relation to apolipoprotein(a) size polymorphism. *Metabolism* 48:342–346.

188. Nakahama H, Nakanishi T, Uyama O, Sugita M, Miyazaki M, Yokokawa T, *et al.* (1993) Niceritrol reduces plasma lipoprotein(a) levels in patients undergoing maintenance hemodialysis. *Renal Failure* 15:189–193.

189. Mavromatidis K, Fitili C, Sombolos K (1998) Can acipimox reduce serum lipoprotein(a) levels in hemodialyzed patients? *Nephron* 78:489–489.

190. Bommer C, Werle E, Walter-Sack I, Keller C, Gehlen F, Wanner C, *et al.* (1998) D-Thyroxine reduces lipoprotein(a) serum concentration in dialysis patients. *Journal of the American Society of Nephrology* 9:90–96.

191. Utermann G, Hoppichler F, Dieplinger H, Seed M, Thompson G, Boerwinkle E (1989) Defects in the low density lipoprotein receptor gene affect lipoprotein (a) levels: multiplicative interaction of two gene loci associated with premature atherosclerosis. *Proceedings of the National Academy of Sciences of the USA* 86:4171–4174.

192. Kronenberg F (1995) Lipoprotein(a) in renal disease: what we have, what we need, what we can forget. *Nephrology, Dialysis, Transplantation* 10:766–769.

PART III
Clinical manifestations, diagnosis, and management

9

Hyperhomocysteinemia in chronic renal disease

Bruce F. Culleton and Andrew G. Bostom

Introduction

Cardiovascular disease (CVD) is the major cause of death both in the general population and in patients with end-stage renal failure (ESRF). CVD is responsible for about 40% of all deaths in both demographic groups.[1,2] Although the proportion of people dying of cardiovascular causes is similar, the risk of CVD is far greater for patients with ESRF. Even after stratification by age, gender, race, and presence of diabetes, CVD mortality in dialysis patients is 10–20 times higher than in the general population.[3] Renal transplant recipients (RTRs) experience at least twofold increases in the annual death rate from CVD, and fourfold increases in pooled non-fatal and fatal CVD incidence relative to population-based estimates[1,3–5] (Table 9.1). The excess risk of CVD in chronic renal disease is due, in part, to a higher prevalence of established arteriosclerotic risk factors, including hypertension, diabetes, dyslipidemia, and physical inactivity.[4,6–8] However, unique renal-related risk factors, including hemodynamic and metabolic factors characteristic of chronic renal disease, are also likely to contribute to this excess CVD risk.[4,6–8]

Prominent among these unique renal-related risk factors are elevated levels of the putatively atherothrombotic sulfur-containing amino acid homocysteine. Homozygous genetic disorders (i.e. the homocystinurias) result in marked hyperhomocysteinemia (total homocysteine (tHcy) levels of 100–500 μmol/L) and are clearly associated with precocious

Table 9.1 Arteriosclerotic cardiovascular disease (CVD) incidence after renal transplantation (from reference 7)

	Post-transplant incidence[a] (%) Patients without CVD pre-transplantation	All patients	Expected[b] CVD incidence (%)
1. Angina	6.4	10.3	2.3
2. Myocardial infarction	6.4	7.8	1.3
3. Transient ischemic attacks	3.7	4.5	–
4. Thrombotic strokes	3.3	3.7	0.6
5. Peripheral vascular disease	2.6	3.0	–
6. Coronary heart disease (1 and 2)	11.0	15.1	3.4
7. Cerebrovascular disease (3 and 4)	6.0	7.3	–
8. Total CVD (1–5)	15.8	21.3	4.7

[a]Based on a mean of 46 $\pm$ 36 months of follow-up.
[b]Framingham data.[98]

atherothrombotic events.[9] tHcy-lowering treatment reduces the incidence of such outcomes among these patients.[9,10] In addition, pooled observational studies suggest that mild to moderate hyperhomocysteinemia (tHcy levels of 12–99 μmol/L) is also a significant risk factor for arteriosclerotic CVD among the general population.[11–13] However, randomized, controlled clinical trial data confirming these reported associations are unavailable. Moreover, the impact of cereal grain flour fortification with folic acid[14,15] on plasma tHcy levels within the general population may obfuscate the results from any such future trials conducted in the United States. Chronic renal disease patients have an excess prevalence of mild to moderate hyperhomocysteinemia, which has been independently linked to their development of CVD outcomes in recent prospective observational studies.[16–19] Accordingly, lowering tHcy levels in patients with chronic renal disease may reduce the excess incidence of arteriosclerotic CVD outcomes.

The overall chronic renal disease population can be divided into four subgroups encompassing various stages, treatment modalities, and treatment settings. These include chronic renal insufficiency, defined as a reduction in glomerular filtration rate (GFR) due to chronic renal disease, generally manifest as an elevated serum creatinine; ESRF treated by hemodialysis; ESRF treated by peritoneal dialysis; and RTRs.[8] RTRs are considered to have chronic renal disease because, typically, GFR is reduced and declines progressively over time. Although the most common cause of progressive renal function decline in RTRs is chronic rejection, a number of non-immunological factors have been shown to be associated with chronic rejection, and commonly, such factors are identical to those associated with progressive renal disease in native kidneys.[8]

Renal transplant recipients comprise a unique subpopulation to test tHcy-lowering therapy for the reduction of CVD outcomes. In addition to the high rate of *de novo* and recurrent CVD events, RTRs have a high prevalence of hyperhomocysteinemia, which contrasts with other potential target populations with normal renal function.[20] Furthermore, tHcy levels can be 'normalized' safely and effectively with combined folic acid, vitamin B12, and vitamin B6 treatment.[21] In many ways the renal transplant population is representative of the larger population of patients with chronic renal disease who have not yet reached ESRF.[8] As such, should homocysteine-lowering by B-vitamin supplementation in RTRs reduce the rate of occurrence of CVD events, these findings could probably be generalized to the much more sizable population of patients with renal insufficiency progressing to ESRF. However, currently there are no data from randomized, controlled trials demonstrating that successful treatment of mild hyperhomocysteinemia actually reduces CVD outcomes. As such, we do not believe screening or treatment recommendations for mild hyperhomocysteinemia in this patient population can or should be provided.

Epidemiology: determinants of plasma/serum homocysteine levels, and the prevalence and etiology of hyperhomocysteinemia (Table 9.2)

General populations

Approximately 70–80% of circulating plasma/serum tHcy is bound to large proteins (e.g. albumin),[22] the remainder consisting of a 'free' acid-soluble fraction, i.e. reduced Hcy (<1%), homocystine (the homodisulfide), and the predominant non-protein-bound forms, homocysteine-mixed disulfides.[22] Folate, pyridoxal 5'-phosphate (PLP or 'active' vitamin B6), and vitamin B12 are the main vitamin cofactors/substrates for homocysteine metabo-

Table 9.2 Comparison of fasting plasma total homocysteine levels in population-based controls free of renal disease who were age-, gender-, and race-matched (one-to-one) to end-stage renal failure (ESRF) patients on maintenance dialysis, and children and young adults with homocystinuria

	Controls	ESRF patients	Homocystinurics
10th to 90th percentile range of tHcy (μmol/L)	7–14	12–39	50–300

Data from references 9, 10, 22, 34–36, 57, 84.

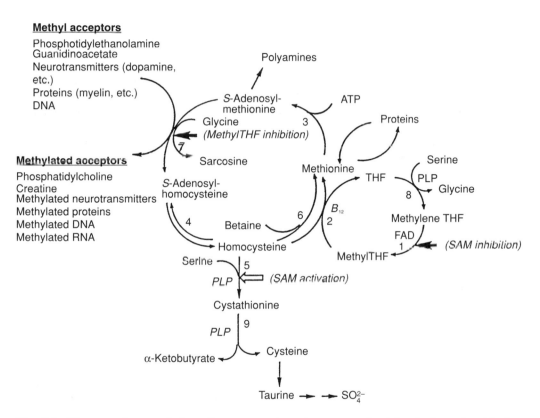

Fig. 9.1 Homocysteine metabolism. Enzyme reactions that are regulated by *S*-adenosylmethionine (SAM) and 5-methyltetrahydrofolate (MethylTHF) are indicated by large arrows. Open arrow indicates activation, closed arrows indicate inhibition. Enzymes: (1) 5,10-methylenetetrahydrofolate reductase; (2) methionine synthase; (3) *S*-adenosylmethionine synthase; (4) *S*-adenosylhomocysteine hydrolase; (5) cystathionine beta synthase; (6) betaine:homocysteine methyltransferase; (7) glycine N-methyltransferase; (8) serine hydroxymethylase; (9) cystathionase.

lism (Fig. 9.1). Vitamin B12 and folate play critical roles in the remethylation of homocysteine to methionine.[23] Betaine (trimethylglycine) is another substrate that participates in the remethylation of homocysteine to methionine via a B12/folate-independent reaction.[24]

Vitamin B6 (as PLP), conversely, has a minor role in the remethylation pathway, but is crucial for the irreversible transsulfuration of homocysteine to cystathionine, as well as the subsequent hydrolysis of cystathionine to cysteine and alpha-ketobutyrate.[24] Consistent with this underlying biochemistry, population-based data indicate that intake and plasma status of folate, vitamin B6, and vitamin B12 are important determinants of tHcy levels.[23] Mild, sub-clinical inherited defects in the key remethylation or transsulfuration pathway enzymes, alone or via interactions with B-vitamin status, may also influence tHcy levels in general populations.[23–25] Selhub and Miller[24] have hypothesized that two distinct forms of hyperho-mocysteinemia can result when normal *S*-adenosylmethionine (SAM)-regulated partitioning of homocysteine between the remethylation and transsulfuration pathways is disrupted. Impairment of the remethylation pathway due primarily (on a population basis) to inade-quate status of folate or vitamin B12 results in hyperhomocysteinemia under fasting condi-tions. Conversely, impairment of the transsulfuration pathway is associated with normal or only very mildly elevated tHcy levels under fasting conditions, but substantial elevations fol-lowing a methionine load. Both animal model findings[26,27] and clinical observations from humans[28–30] support this hypothesis. Finally, a randomized, placebo-controlled 2 × 2 factorial designed tHcy-lowering intervention study recently demonstrated that B6 treatment inde-pendently reduced the 2-hour post-methionine loading (PML) increase in tHcy levels among stable renal transplant recipients.[21]

Creatinine[31,32] and albumin[33] are two additional, independent determinants of tHcy levels in general populations, unrelated to B-vitamin status. The generation of *S*-adenosylhomocys-teine from *S*-adenosylmethionine is coupled to creatine–creatinine synthesis, which probably accounts for the direct association observed between creatinine and fasting tHcy levels in persons with normal renal function.[31,32] As noted earlier, 70–80% of serum/plasma tHcy is protein-bound, most probably to albumin,[22] which may account for the direct relationship between albumin and tHcy levels found in the general population.[33]

Severe cases of hyperhomocysteinemia, as in homocystinuria, may be due to rare homozy-gous defects in genes encoding for enzymes involved in either homocysteine remethylation or transsulfuration. The classic form of such a disorder is that caused by homozygosity for a defective gene encoding cystathionine beta synthase (CBS), a condition in which fasting plasma homocysteine concentrations can be as high as 400–500 μmol/L (~1 in 200 000 births).[34] Homozygous defects of other genes that lead to similar elevations in plasma homo-cysteine concentration include those encoding methylenetetrahydrofolate reductase (MTHFR)[35] or for any of the enzymes that participate in the synthesis of methylated vitamin B12.[36]

Populations with renal disease

It has been convincingly demonstrated that normal urinary excretion of homocysteine is trivial,[37,38] and plasma elimination of homocysteine in ESRF is grossly retarded.[39] However, the ultimate etiology of the mild hyperhomocysteinemia so consistently noted in renal insufficiency and ESRF (see below) remains unexplained. Despite *in vitro* studies demonstrat-ing renal tubular metabolism of homocysteine[40,41] and rat model evidence of significant *in vivo* renal homocysteine metabolism,[42] non-significant mean human renal arteriovenous differences for fasting (total and non-protein bound) homocysteine were recently reported.[43] These findings[43] have rekindled a search for 'uremia-induced' extrarenal (presumptively, hepatic defects) in homocysteine metabolism. It should be noted, however, that: (i) it may be haz-ardous to extrapolate findings regarding renal homocysteine metabolism from the fasting to non-fasting state; and (ii) mild decrements in GFR, determined either by direct measure-

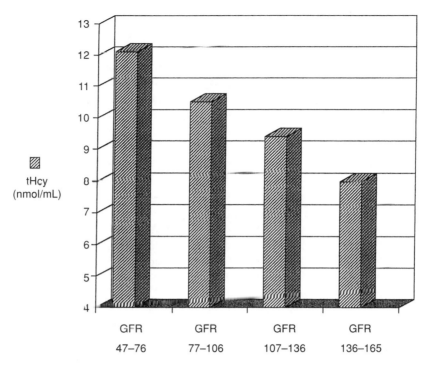

Fig. 9.2 Plasma total homocysteine (tHcy) in relation to glomerular filtration rate (GFR) (mL/min/m²) determined by Cr[51] EDTA clearance among 80 subjects with diabetes mellitus and serum creatinine values <115 μmol/L (<1.3 mg/dL) (modified from reference 45).

ment[44,45] or using a sensitive surrogate like cystatin C,[46] encompassing clearly non-uremic ranges of GFR are strongly and independently associated with (linear) increases in fasting tHcy levels. Indeed, evidence has been presented that 'hyperfiltrating' diabetic subjects with supernormal GFR may have 'subnormal' fasting tHcy levels[45] (Fig. 9.2).

In an early (i.e. pre-cyclosporin/tacrolimus era) study of 27 stable RTRs, Wilcken and colleagues[47] reported a significant association between creatinine and cysteine–homocysteine mixed disulfide concentrates within a serum creatinine range of ~100–500 μmol/L. In accord with these data, we found that renal function may be a particularly crucial determinant of tHcy levels in RTRs, both under fasting conditions and following a methionine load.[48] Although Arnadottir and colleagues[49,50] have contended that cyclosporin use exerts an 'independent' influence on fasting tHcy levels in these patients, both multivariable regression modeling[48] and matched analyses[38] have revealed that cyclosporin use is not an independent determinant of tHcy levels in RTRs after appropriate adjustment for renal function indices (in particular), age, and sex. Finally, although unadjusted correlations between fasting plasma tHcy and folate levels among RTRs have been reported,[38,47–49] multivariable modeling to determine the independent strength of this association (for example, relative to indices of renal function) was not performed in any of these studies.

Plasma or serum levels of free, protein-bound, and tHcy are elevated in patients with varying degrees of renal impairment.[19,47,49,51–56] Several reports[51,57] have documented the prevalence of mild to moderate hyperhomocysteinemia in dialysis patients relative to age-, gender-, and race-matched population-based controls free of clinical renal disease whose serum creatinine levels were 1.5 mg/dL or less. These data indicated that hyperhomocysteinemia (fasting tHcy levels >13.9 μmol/L, the 90th percentile control value) occurred in 83% of the dialysis patients, a 105-fold increased risk (matched prevalence odds) relative to the controls. This disparity exists despite higher folate levels in dialysis patients than in control subjects due to daily supplementation with multivitamins (usually containing 1–2 mg of folic acid, 10 mg of vitamin B6, and 12 μg of vitamin B12) in the hemodialysis population. Recently, prevalence data for fasting hyperhomocysteinemia in RTRs have been published.[48] These analyses provide the first documentation of an apparent excess prevalence of PML hyperhomocysteinemia (matched odds ratio 6.9) and combined fasting and PML hyperhomocysteinemia (matched odds ratio 18.0) in RTRs versus age- and gender-matched population-based controls with normative renal function.

The US Food and Drug Administration (FDA) published a regulation in early 1996[14,15] that all enriched flour breads, rice, pasta, cornmeal, and other cereal grain products would be required to contain 140 μg of folic acid per 100 g by January 1998. The goal of this fortification policy was to increase intake of folate by women of childbearing age to reduce the risk of neural tube defects. Cereal grain flour products fortified with 140 μg folic acid per 100 g flour began appearing voluntarily in the United States after March 1996.[15] The availability of such products was widespread in Southeast New England by July 1997 (J. Watson, President, Watson Foods, New Haven, CT, personal communication). Given that chronic renal disease renders individuals somewhat refractory to the effect of low-dose folic acid supplementation on fasting tHcy levels (see below), improved folate status secondary to the FDA-mandated cereal grain fortification policy[14,15] would be expected to have a much more limited impact on the prevalence of mild fasting hyperhomocysteinemia in renal transplant versus coronary artery disease patients.

To test this hypothesis, fasting tHcy levels were evaluated in a consecutive series of renal transplant and coronary artery disease patients living in the Providence, Rhode Island, metropolitan area.[20] Between October 1997 and late September 1998, fasting plasma tHcy, folate, and vitamin B12 levels were determined in a total of 86 RTRs with stable allograft function and 175 coronary artery disease patients whose serum creatinine was $\leq$1.4 mg/dL. All subjects were either non-users of any supplements containing folic acid, vitamins B6 or B12, or had refrained from using such supplements for $\geq$6 weeks, and were examined at least 3–4 months after the widespread availability of folic acid fortified cereal grain products in this region. Key results are summarized in Table 9.3. The prevalence of fasting tHcy levels $\geq$12 μmol/L (69.8% vs. 10.9%, $p < 0.001$) was markedly increased in the RTRs, despite a much younger mean age and a relative preponderance of women. The unadjusted odds ratio (95% confidence interval) for a tHcy level $\geq$12 μmol/L, comparing the renal transplant to coronary artery disease patients, was 25.5 (10.8–60.5), and adjustment for potential confounding by age, gender, albumin, and vitamin status did not appreciably attenuate this odds ratio: 20.3 (7.9–52.2). In the current era of folic acid fortified cereal grain flour, hyperhomocysteinemia is much more common in stable renal transplant versus coronary artery disease patients. As a result, RTRs may be a preferable, high risk target population for controlled trials conducted in the United States evaluating the tenable hypothesis that lowering total homocysteine levels will reduce cardiovascular disease outcomes.

Table 9.3 Comparison of plasma folate status and prevalence of fasting tHcy levels ≥12 in μmol/L among Rhode Island renal transplant recipients and coronary artery disease patients examined in the post-fortification period (from reference 20)

	Renal transplant recipients	Coronary artery disease patients	P-value[b]
N	86	175	–
Age (years; mean ± SD)	46 ±12	61 ± 9	<0.001
Sex (no./% men)	53 (61.6%)	140 (80.0%)	0.001
tHcy (μmol/L)	15.6[a]	8.3	<0.001
tHcy ≥ 12 μmol/L, %	69.8	10.9	<0.001
Folate < 3 ng/mL, %	3.5	1.1	0.194

[a]Geometric means.
[b]Based on unpaired *t*-test, analysis of covariance, or chi square test.

Homocysteine and arteriosclerosis: epidemiological evidence

General populations

In 1969, the seminal observations of McCully first linked marked hyperhomocysteinemia (i.e. equivalent to tHcy levels of 100–450 μmol/L by current assays) to precocious arteriosclerotic vascular disease in autopsied children who died from distinct metabolic forms of homocystinuria.[58] Nearly thirty years later, a burgeoning amount of observational evidence has accumulated indicating that mild to moderate fasting, non-fasting, or PML hyperhomocysteinemia (i.e. tHcy levels ≥12 μmol/L to ≤100 μmol/L fasting or non-fasting; or ≥50 μmol/L to ≤140 μmol/L 6-hours PML) is an independent risk factor for arteriosclerotic outcomes. A recent series of meta-analyses,[11 13] which has been updated through August 1998 has concluded that the best estimate for the increased risk of arteriosclerotic CVD morbidity and mortality comparing fasting and or non-fasting tHcy levels of ≥15 μmol/L to ≤10 μmol/L, after adjustment for the established CVD risk factors, was 1.4. This estimate is unaffected when only prospective studies are analyzed (7 studies, N ~ 1400 incident events), including the recently reported Atherosclerosis Risk in Communities[59] and British United Provident Association[60] cohort studies (Dr S.A.A. Beresford, personal communication). More recent prospective data not included in these meta-analyses from the Scottish Heart Health Study[61] indicates that tHcy levels were independently predictive of incident coronary heart disease in both Scottish women and men. Furthermore, two additional prospective studies also not included in these meta-analyses have examined the potential association between tHcy levels and CVD mortality. The first of these reports found a strong, independent link between tHcy levels and subsequent CVD death in patients with angiographically-confirmed coronary artery disease,[62] while the second study found a more modest, but significant, independent association between tHcy levels and CVD mortality in the elderly population-based Framingham cohort.[63] Finally a large, multicenter European case-control study has confirmed that PML hyperhomocysteinemia confers a risk for prevalent CVD equal in magnitude to, and independent of, fasting hyperhomocysteinemia.[64] Initial prospective follow-up (~4.5 years) of this cohort with prevalent CVD has revealed that post-load hyperhomocysteinemia may independently predict subsequent CVD death.[65]

It has been proposed that clinical or even subclinical arteriosclerosis itself somehow raises tHcy levels, resulting in a spurious association between mild hyperhomocysteinemia and clinical CVD due to reverse causality.[59,66] This hypothesis appears untenable in light of the pooled epidemiological evidence from all published observational studies (as opposed to the highly selective citation methods exercised in references 59 and 66) conducted in populations free of renal disease (reviewed above), the prospective data from renal disease populations[16–19] reviewed below, and the following published findings from additional human and animal studies:

1. Despite the absence of any traditional CVD risk factors, 50% of untreated children and young adults with homocystinuria due to cystathionine beta-synthase deficiency experience a major atherothrombotic event by age 30.[9] Furthermore, strategies designed solely to reduce tHcy levels in these patients have been shown to decrease atherothrombotic event rates.[9,10]

2. In adults ($n = 38$; mean age 58 ± 12 years) with mild hyperhomocysteinemia, tHcy-lowering treatment reduces the rate of progression of ultrasound-determined extracranial carotid artery plaque area.[67]

3. Young, healthy subjects, free of clinical arteriosclerosis or CVD risk factors, who have normal baseline flow-mediated brachial artery reactivity, experience a dramatic 'dose-response' reduction in their flow-mediated brachial artery reactivity following acute hyperhomocysteinemia produced by an oral L-methionine load.[68]

4. Randomized, controlled studies have revealed that mild, dietary-induced hyperhomocysteinemia resulted in abnormal vascular reactivity among non-human primates,[69] as well as increased arterial stiffness, and frank atherothrombotic sequelae, in minipigs.[70]

Indeed, a plausible alternative to the reverse causality hypothesis is quite possible. There is a well-established association between subclinical coronary artery disease or generalized arteriosclerosis and nephrosclerosis.[71,72] Bearing these data in mind, a strong, independent association (partial $r = 0.379$; $p < 0.001$) has been demonstrated between the serum levels of cystatin C, a more sensitive marker of mildly impaired GFR than serum creatinine, and plasma tHcy levels, in 164 consecutively examined coronary artery disease patients whose serum creatinine was ≤1.4 mg/dL.[73] Accordingly, subclinical renal impairment (secondary to nephrosclerosis) and resultant mild hyperhomocysteinemia may antedate, and hence contribute to, the development of clinical arteriosclerosis, including coronary artery disease.

Finally, although we do not believe the reverse causality hypothesis is tenable, we certainly agree that simultaneous pursuit of two related areas of investigation will be required to confirm a causal relationship between hyperhomocysteinemia and CVD: (i) randomized, placebo-controlled trials of the effect of tHcy-lowering on recurrent and *de novo* CVD outcomes; and (ii) elucidation of the basic biological mechanism linking hyperhomocysteinemia to arteriosclerosis.

Populations with ESRF

Intractable survivorship effects resulting from the excess yearly mortality in dialysis-dependent ESRF and the failure to establish whether or not arteriosclerotic outcomes antedated the development of ESRF render hazardous any inference about tHcy–CVD associations suggested by cross-sectional studies. The potential relationship between hyperhomocysteinemia

and arteriosclerotic outcomes in ESRF requires more rigorous validation via prospective observational studies and, ultimately, clinical tHcy-lowering intervention trials.

Recently, the results from a prospective study of the relationship between baseline fasting
tHcy levels and subsequent CVD occurrence in 73 dialysis-dependent ESRF patients were
reported.[17] After a median follow-up of 17 months, 16 individuals experienced non-fatal or
fatal CVD events. After adjusting for prevalent CVD, traditional arteriosclerotic risk factors,
serum creatinine, serum albumin, and dialysis adequacy, fasting hyperhomocysteinemia (i.e.
comparing the upper [tHcy $\geq$ 27 μmol/L] to lower three quartiles [tHcy < 27 μmol/L])
conferred an increased risk for CVD of ~7-fold for fatal events and ~3.5-fold for pooled
non-fatal and fatal events. The risk conferred by hyperhomocysteinemia was similar in
women and men. Moustapha *et al.*[16] reported that patients in the highest quartile of homocysteine levels had a 45% incidence of CVD compared with 29% in patients in the lower
three quartiles (p = 0.06). When homocysteine was examined as a continuous variable, the
effect was significant (p = 0.01) and independent of diabetes. Another study in pre-dialysis
ESRF patients[18] yielded similar results. Clarke and colleagues from the Homocysteine
Trialists Collaborative Group pooled the data from these three investigations (R. Clarke,
personal communication). The pooled relative risk estimate for incident (*de novo*) or recurrent CVD (n = 95 total events) conferred by mild to moderate hyperhomocysteinemia
(i.e. comparing the upper to the lowest tertile of fasting tHcy) in these three prospective
studies was 2.8 (95% confidence interval: 1.6–5.0).

More recently, using a prospective design,[74] the potential relationship between baseline
non-fasting, pre-dialysis plasma tHcy levels and vascular access-related morbidity was examined in a cohort of 84 hemodialysis patients with a fistula or prosthetic graft as their primary
hemodialysis access. Vascular access thrombotic episodes were recorded over an 18-month
follow-up period. Forty-seven patients (56% of the total) had at least one access thrombosis
during follow-up (median follow-up 13 months; rate = 0.6 events per patient-year of follow-
up). Proportional hazards modeling revealed that each 1 μmol/L increase in the tHcy level
was associated with a 4.0% increase in the risk of access thrombosis (95% confidence interval: 1.0–6.0%, p = 0.008). This association persisted after adjustment for type of access
(fistula vs. graft), age, sex, time on dialysis, diabetes, smoking, hypertension, nutritional
status, urea reduction ratio, dyslipidemia, and the presence of previous vascular disease. In
contrast, using a weaker study design, Tomura and colleagues failed to demonstrate any difference in plasma homocysteine levels between a thrombosis-prone group of hemodialysis
patients with frequent graft loss (n = 24) and an age-matched control group with prolonged
graft survival.[75]

The association between fasting tHcy levels and incident CVD has also been examined in
a preliminary, nested case-control study of 42 renal transplant recipients.[19] These pilot data
indicated that mildly elevated fasting tHcy levels (>14 μmol/L) at a baseline examination
were associated with the subsequent development of CVD outcomes in men but not in
women. Table 9.4 summarizes the prospective studies evaluating the relations between
homocysteine and incident CVD in patients with chronic renal disease.

Homocysteine and arteriosclerosis: experimental evidence

The pathological mechanisms by which homocysteine promotes arteriosclerosis remain
unclear. Experimental data support a range of possibilities, including endothelial cell
injury,[76,77] enhanced low-density lipoprotein oxidation,[78] increased thromboxane-mediated

Table 9.4 Summary of prospective studies evaluating homocysteine (in $\mu mol/L$) as a risk factor for cardiovascular disease (CVD) in chronic renal failure

Study	N (with CVD)	Modality	Type of CVD[a]	CVD	No CVD	P value	Odds ratio	Follow-up
Bostom et al.[17]	73 (16)	HD, PD	C, H, P	–	–	–	3.5	17 months
Jungers et al.[18]	93 (24)	CRF	C, H	20.7 ± 1.6	12.8 ± 0.5	0.0001	11.4	6 years
Massy et al.[19]	94 (18)	RTRs	C, H, P	18.6 ± 7.8	13.1 ± 3.4	0.06	–	6 months
Moustapha et al.[16]	176 (55)	HD, PD	C, H, P	43.4 ± 50.6	27.4 ± 14.9	0.03	–	17 months

[a]Evidence of CVD was defined differently in the studies—cerebrovascular (C), coronary artery (H), and/or peripheral vascular (P) disease HD, hemodialysis; PD, peritoneal dialysis; CRF, chronic renal failure not yet on dialysis.

platelet aggregation,[79] inhibition of cell-surface thrombomodulin expression and protein C activation,[80] enhancement of lipoprotein (a)–fibrin binding,[81] and promotion of smooth muscle cell proliferation.[82] The *in vivo* relevance of findings from such experimental studies, however, has been questioned[83] owing to their lack of specificity to Hcy versus other much more abundant plasma thiols, including cysteine, and the use of grossly supraphysiological concentrations or non-physiological forms (i.e. D-L as opposed to L) of reduced Hcy. The data of Mansoor and colleagues[84] provide the background appropriate for adequate under-standing of the specific criticism regarding grossly supraphysiological concentrations. These investigators assessed concentrations of reduced Hcy across the widest possible spectrum of tHcy concentrations. Their data revealed that at tHcy concentrations of up to 100 μmol/L, levels of reduced Hcy accounted for only 1% or less (i.e. <1 μmol/L) of plasma tHcy. When tHcy exceeded 100 μmol/L, reduced Hcy began to rise exponentially, probably due to saturation of plasma protein-binding sites.[84] However, the highest reduced Hcy value these authors documented was in a subject with homozygous homocystinuria who had a tHcy >350 μmol/L, but a reduced Hcy of <100 μmol/L.[84] When juxtaposed to the con-centrations of reduced Hcy used in experimental studies,[76–82] i.e. 1000–10 000 μmol/L, the findings of Mansoor and colleagues[84] illustrate the dubious clinical relevance of these pub-lished data. In contrast, physiological models of mild, dietary-induced hyperhomocysteine-mia (i.e. tHcy ≤ 15 μmol/L) causing subclinical or frank atherothrombotic sequelae have recently been described in animal models.[69,70] Follow-up investigations employing these models may elucidate the *in vivo* relevance of the putative pathological mechanisms cited above.[76–82]

Hyperhomocysteinemia: screening and treatment

General populations (with normative renal function)

The severe hyperhomocysteinemia found in homozygous CBS deficiency has been treated with methionine restriction and supraphysiological doses of vitamin B6, vitamin B12, folate, and betaine.[9,10] Such treatment lowers Hcy levels and, more importantly, reduces the inci-dence of atherothrombotic events and mortality in these patients.[9,10] Management of this severe form of hyperhomocysteinemia (i.e. tHcy levels of 100–400 μmol/L) is the paradigm for treatment of the more common mild to intermediate forms of hyperhomocysteinemia. With the exception of methionine restriction, all the major therapeutic approaches to lower-ing Hcy alluded to earlier have been applied to populations with moderate hyperhomocys-teinemia. Although a recent meta-analysis[85] has provided important placebo-controlled data on (primarily folic acid-based) treatment of fasting tHcy elevations, none of the trials for treatment of PML hyperhomocysteinemia reported in non-renal populations[28–30] was placebo-controlled. Given these caveats, some general conclusions can be drawn from this published data:

1. Folic acid at 0.5–5.0 mg/day can effectively reduce fasting Hcy levels in moderately hyperhomocysteinemic and normohomocysteinemic persons with or without CVD who are free of renal insufficiency and are not vitamin B12 deficient.

2. Vitamin B12 (0.4–2.0 mg/day orally) can effectively normalize fasting Hcy in vitamin B12-deficient persons who respond only marginally to folic acid supplementation.

3. Vitamin B6 at doses up to 240–250 mg/day has no lowering effect on fasting Hcy levels.

4. Vitamin B6 at 20–250 mg/day appears to reduce the absolute PML, or PML increase in Hcy levels, by ~15–50% in persons with or without CVD who have mild PML hyperhomocysteinemia.

5. Even at doses of 250 mg/day vitamin B6, combined with 5 mg/day folic acid, an effective fasting and/or PML Hcy-lowering response may not be achieved in some individuals until after 6–12 weeks of treatment.

Populations with ESRF

With a single exception,[86] all the published Hcy-lowering intervention studies conducted in pre-dialysis or maintenance dialysis ESRF patients were uncontrolled, open label investigations.[47,51,87–94] Bearing this important caveat in mind, the following conclusions can be drawn from these studies:

1. Folic acid-based B-vitamin regimens, including folic acid at doses of 5–10 mg/day, appear to lower fasting tHcy levels by ~30–50%.

2. The addition of folic acid at 15 mg/day, plus 1 mg/day of vitamin B12 and 100 mg/day of vitamin B6 (vs. additional placebo), to a baseline regimen including 1 mg/day of folic acid, 10 mg vitamin B6, and 12 μg/day vitamin B12 can reduce fasting tHcy levels by ~25–30%. As folate is a substrate for the remethylation of tHcy, very high doses of folate may increase the conversion of tHcy to methionine simply by driving the reaction to the right. In addition, or alternatively, pharmacological doses of B12 may be efficacious in lowering tHcy levels in (elderly) dialysis patient's who have food B12 malabsorption and/or atrophic gastritis.

3. Even when given a total dose of 16 mg/day of folic acid, two-thirds of maintenance dialysis patients whose baseline fasting or non-fasting tHcy levels are >15–16 μmol/L will continue to maintain tHcy levels at or above this value.

4. There are no data available on the independent effect of B12 on fasting tHcy levels.

5. In accord with findings from general populations, vitamin B6 at up to 300 mg/day has no apparent effect on fasting tHcy levels. There are no data on the independent effect of vitamin B6 on PML tHcy levels.

6. Neither serine at 3–4 g/day nor betaine at 6 g/day appears to have any effect on fasting tHcy levels.

7. Oral *N*-acetylcysteine (NAC) at 1.2 g/day subacutely lowers non-fasting pre-hemodialysis tHcy levels by ~16%. It is unknown by which mechanism NAC lowers tHcy. It is possible that liver uptake of NAC–homocysteine mixed disulfides occurs, perhaps via pathways normally used in the extensive hepatic metabolism of NAC.

8. Oral 5-methyltetrahydrofolate treatment may afford greater tHcy-lowering efficacy relative to folic acid, although no controlled, direct comparative data are currently available.

Furthermore, given that ESRF patients are at high risk for morbidity and mortality related to protein calorie malnutrition,[95] methionine restriction to lower homocysteine levels in these patients, as suggested elsewhere,[52] seems unwarranted.

 Open label findings from RTRs with much milder decrements in renal function[47,96] have suggested that these patients are also refractory to low-dose folic acid-based tHcy-lowering supplementation. Finally, a recent block-randomized, placebo-controlled, 2 × 2 factorial study of 29 clinically stable RTRs demonstrated that, in contrast to what was observed in their maintenance dialysis counterparts,[86] the mild hyperhomocysteinemia in RTRs is very amenable to high-dose combination B-vitamin therapy (folic acid 5.0 mg/day, vitamin B6 50 mg/day, and vitamin B12 0.4 mg/day). Treated patients experienced mean reductions of fasting and PML tHcy levels of at least 25% after only 6 weeks, with 75% achieving 'normalization' of their tHcy levels.[21]

Conclusion

There is considerable epidemiological evidence for a relationship between plasma homocysteine and CVD, including among patients with chronic renal disease. However, it is not known whether reduction of plasma homocysteine will reduce CVD risk. In the absence of any data from randomized, controlled trials demonstrating a reduction in CVD outcomes with successful treatment of hyperhomocysteinemia in patients with chronic renal disease, we do not believe screening and treatment recommendations for mild hyperhomocysteinemia in this patient population can or should be offered. This suggested 'policy' is concordant with the recently published American Heart Association Position Paper on Homocysteine,[97] which emphasized that screening and treatment recommendations for hyperhomocysteinemia in the general population were premature, and must await the results of clinical trials of tHcy-lowering for secondary or primary CVD outcome prevention.

References

1. *US Renal Data System (USRDS) (1997) Annual Data Report*. National Institutes of Health, National Institute of Diabetes and Digestive and Kidney Diseases. Bethesda, MD.
2. US Dept of Health and Human Services (1996) *Morbidity and mortality: chartbook on cardiovascular, lung, and blood diseases*. Bethesda, MD.
3. Foley RN, Parfrey PS, Sarnak MJ. (1998) Clinical epidemiology of cardiovascular disease in chronic renal disease. *American Journal of Kidney Disease* 32:S112–19.
4. Kasiske BL, Guijarro C, Massy ZA, Wiederkehr MR, Ma JZ. (1996) Cardiovascular disease after renal transplantation. *Journal of the American Society of Nephrology* 7:158–65.
5. Arend SM, Mallat MJ, Westendorp RJ, van der Woude FJ, van Es LA. (1997) Patient survival after renal transplantation, more than 25 years follow-up. *Nephrology Dialysis Transplantation* 12:1672–9.
6. Luke RG. (1998) Chronic renal failure—a vasculopathic state. *New England Journal of Medicine* 339:841–3.
7. Kasiske BL. (1988) Risk factors for accelerated atherosclerosis in renal transplant recipients. *American Journal of Medicine* 84:985–92.
8. Levey AS, Beto JA, Coronado BE, Eknoyan G, Foley RN, Kasiske BL, *et al.* (1998) Controlling the epidemic of cardiovascular disease in chronic renal disease: what do we know? What do we need to learn? Where do we go from here? *American Journal of Kidney Disease* 32:853–906.
9. Mudd SH, Skovby F, Levy HL, Pettigrew KD, Wilcken B, Pyeritz RE, *et al.* (1985) The natural history of homocystinuria due to cystathionine beta-synthase deficiency. *American Journal of Human Genetics* 37:1–31.
10. Wilcken DE, Wilcken B. (1997) The natural history of vascular disease in homocystinuria and the effects of treatment. *Journal of Inherited Metabolic Disease* 20:295–300.
11. Omenn GS, Beresford SA, Motulsky AG. (1998) Preventing coronary heart disease: B vitamins and homocysteine. *Circulation* 97:421–4.

12. Boushey CJ, Beresford SA, Omenn GS, Motulsky AG. (1995) A quantitative assessment of plasma homocysteine as a risk factor for vascular disease. Probable benefits of increasing folic acid intakes. *Journal of the American Medical Association* 274:1049–57.

13. Beresford SA. (1997) Homocysteine, folic acid, and cardiovascular disease risk. In: Boushey CJ. Bendich A, Deckelbaum RJ, editors. *Preventive nutrition: the comprehensive guide for health professionals*, pp. 193–224. Totowa, NJ: Humana Press.

14. Food standards: amendment of standards of identity for enriched grain products to require addition of folic acid. (1996) *Federal Register* 61:8781–97.

15. Folic acid content of some grain foods is mandated by the FDA. (1998) *Wall Street Journal*, May 1.

16. Moustapha A, Naso A, Nahlawi M, Gupta A, Arheart KL, Jacobsen DW, *et al.* (1998) Prospective study of hyperhomocysteinemia as an adverse cardiovascular risk factor in end-stage renal disease. *Circulation* 97:138–41.

17. Bostom AG, Shemin D, Verhoef P, Nadeau MR, Jacques PF, Selhub J, *et al.* (1997) Elevated fasting total plasma homocysteine levels and cardiovascular disease outcomes in maintenance dialysis patients. A prospective study. *Arteriosclerosis, Thrombosis, and Vascular Biology* 17:2554–8.

18. Jungers P, Chauveau P, Bandin O, Chadefaux B, Aupetit J, Labrunie M, *et al.* (1997) Hyperhomocysteinemia is associated with atherosclerotic occlusive arterial accidents in predialysis chronic renal failure patients. *Mineral and Electrolyte Metabolism* 23:170–3.

19. Massy ZA, Chadefaux-Vekemans B, Chevalier A, Bader CA, Drueke TB, Legendre C, *et al.* (1994) Hyperhomocysteinaemia: a significant risk factor for cardiovascular disease in renal transplant recipients. *Nephrology Dialysis Transplantation* 9:1103–8.

20. Bostom AG, Gohh RY, Liaugaudas G, Beaulieu AJ, Han H, Jacques PF, *et al.* (1999) Prevalence of mild fasting hyperhomocysteinemia in renal transplant versus coronary artery disease patients after fortification of cereal grain flour with folic acid. *Atherosclerosis* 145:221–224.

21. Bostom AG, Gohh RY, Beaulieu AJ, Nadeau MR, Hume AL, Jacques PF, *et al.* (1997) Treatment of hyperhomocysteinemia in renal transplant recipients. A randomized, placebo-controlled trial. *Annals of Internal Medicine* 127:1089–92.

22. Ueland PM, Refsum H, Stabler SP, Malinow MR, Andersson A, Allen RH. (1993) Total homocysteine in plasma or serum: methods and clinical applications. *Clinical Chemistry* 39:1764–79.

23. Selhub J, Jacques PF, Wilson PW, Rush D, Rosenberg IH. (1993) Vitamin status and intake as primary determinants of homocysteinemia in an elderly population. *Journal of the American Medical Association* 270:2693–8.

24. Selhub J, Miller JW. (1992) The pathogenesis of homocysteinemia: interruption of the coordinate regulation by *S*-adenosylmethionine of the remethylation and transsulfuration of homocysteine. *American Journal of Clinical Nutrition* 55:131–8.

25. Jacques PF, Bostom AG, Williams RR, Ellison RC, Eckfeldt JH, Rosenberg IH, *et al.* (1996) Relation between folate status, a common mutation in methylenetetrahydrofolate reductase, and plasma homocysteine concentrations. *Circulation* 93:7–9.

26. Miller JW, Nadeau MR, Smith D, Selhub J. (1994) Vitamin B-6 deficiency vs folate deficiency: comparison of responses to methionine loading in rats. *American Journal of Clinical Nutrition* 59:1033–9.

27. Miller JW, Nadeau MR, Smith J, Smith D, Selhub J. (1994) Folate-deficiency-induced homocysteinaemia in rats: disruption of *S*-adenosylmethionine's co-ordinate regulation of homocysteine metabolism. *Biochemical Journal* 298:415–19.

28. Brattstrom L, Israelsson B, Norrving B, Bergqvist D, Thorne J, Hultberg B, *et al.* (1990) Impaired homocysteine metabolism in early-onset cerebral and peripheral occlusive arterial disease. Effects of pyridoxine and folic acid treatment. *Atherosclerosis* 81:51–60.

29. Franken DG, Boers GH, Blom HJ, Trijbels JM. (1994) Effect of various regimens of vitamin B6 and folic acid on mild hyperhomocysteinaemia in vascular patients. *Journal of Inherited Metabolic Disease* 17:159–62.

30. Ubbink JB, van der Merwe A, Delport R, Allen RH, Stabler SP, Riezler R, *et al.* (1996) The effect of a subnormal vitamin B-6 status on homocysteine metabolism. *Journal of Clinical Investigation* 98:177–84.

31. Brattstrom L, Lindgren A, Israelsson B, Andersson A, Hultberg B. (1994) Homocysteine and cysteine: determinants of plasma levels in middle-aged and elderly subjects. *Journal of Internal Medicine* 236:633–41.

32. Wu LL, Wu J, Hunt SC, James BC, Vincent GM, Williams RR, *et al.* (1994) Plasma homocyst(e)ine as a risk factor for early familial coronary artery disease. *Clinical Chemistry* 40:552–61.

33. Lussier-Cacan S, Xhignesse M, Piolot A, Selhub J, Davignon J, Genest J Jr. (1996) Plasma total homocysteine in healthy subjects: sex-specific relation with biological traits. *American Journal of Clinical Nutrition* 64:587–93.

34. Mudd SH, Levy HL, Skovby F. (1989) Disorders of transsulfuration. In: Scriver CR, Beaudet AL, Sly WS, Valle D, editors. *Metabolic basis of inherited disease*, 6th edn. McGraw-Hill.

35. Rosenblatt DS. (1989) Inherited disorders of folate transport and metabolism. In: Scriver CR, Beaudet AL, Sly WS, Valle D, editors. *Metabolic basis of inherited disease*, 6th edn, pp. 2049–64. McGraw-Hill.

36. Linnel JC, Bhatt HR. (1995) Inherited disorders of cobalamin metabolism and their management. *Ballieres Cliniques de Haematologie* 8:567–601.

37. Guttormsen AB, Schneede J, Ueland PM, Refsum H. (1996) Kinetics of total plasma homocysteine in subjects with hyperhomocysteinemia due to folate or cobalamin deficiency. *American Journal of Clinical Nutrition* 63:194–202.

38. Ducloux D, Fournier V, Rebibou JM, Bresson-Vautrin C, Gibey R, Chalopin JM. (1998) Hyperhomocyst(e)inemia in renal transplant recipients with and without cyclosporin. *Clinical Nephrology* 49:232–5.

39. Guttormsen AB, Ueland PM, Svarstad E, Refsum H. (1997) Kinetic basis of hyperhomocysteinemia in patients with chronic renal failure. *Kidney International* 52:495–502.

40. House JD, Brosnan ME, Brosnan JT. (1997) Characterization of homocysteine metabolism in the rat kidney. *Biochemical Journal* 328:287–92.

41. Foreman JW, Wald H, Blumberg G, Pepe LM, Segal S. (1982) Homocystine uptake in isolated rat renal cortical tubules. *Metabolism* 31:613–19.

42. Bostom A, Brosnan JT, Hall B, Nadeau MR, Selhub J. (1995) Net uptake of plasma homocysteine by the rat kidney *in vivo. Atherosclerosis* 116:59–62.

43. van Guldener C, Donker AJ, Jakobs C, Teerlink T, de Meer K, Stehouwer CD. (1998) No net renal extraction of homocysteine in fasting humans. *Kidney International* 54:166–9.

44. Arnadottir M, Hultberg B, Nilsson-Ehle P, Thysell H. (1996) The effect of reduced glomerular filtration rate on plasma total homocysteine concentration. *Scandinavian Journal of Clinical and Laboratory Investigation* 56:41–6.

45. Wollesen F, Brattstrom L, Refsum H, Ueland PM, Berglund L, Berne C. (1999) Plasma total homocysteine and cysteine in relation to GFR in diabetes mellitus. *Kidney International* 55:1028–35.

46. Bostom AG, Gohh RY, Bausserman L, Hakas D, Jacques PF, Selhub J, *et al.* (1999) Serum cystatin C as a determinant of fasting total homocysteine levels in renal transplant recipients with a normal serum creatinine. *Journal of the American Society of Nephrology* 10:164–6.

47. Wilcken DE, Gupta VJ, Betts AK. (1981) Homocysteine in the plasma of renal transplant recipients: effects of cofactors for methionine metabolism. *Clinical Science* 61:743–9.

48. Bostom AG, Gohh RY, Tsai MY, Hopkins-Garcia BJ, Nadeau MR, Bianchi LA, *et al.* (1997) Excess prevalence of fasting and postmethionine-loading hyperhomocysteinemia in stable renal transplant recipients. *Arteriosclerosis, Thrombosis, and Vascular Biology* 17:1894–900.

49. Arnadottir M, Hultberg B, Vladov V, Nilsson-Ehle P, Thysell H. (1996) Hyperhomocysteinemia in cyclosporin-treated renal transplant recipients. *Transplantation* 61:509–12.

50. Arnadottir M, Hultberg B, Wahlberg J, Fellstrom B, Dimeny E. (1998) Serum total homocysteine concentration before and after renal transplantation. *Kidney International* 54:1380–4.
51. Bostom AG, Shemin D, Lapane KL, Miller JW, Sutherland P, Nadeau M, *et al.* (1995) Hyperhomocysteinemia and traditional cardiovascular disease risk factors in end-stage renal disease patients on dialysis: a case-control study. *Atherosclerosis* 114:93–103.
52. Robinson K, Gupta A, Dennis V, Arheart K, Chaudhary D, Green R, *et al.* (1996) Hyperhomocysteinemia confers an independent increased risk of atherosclerosis in end-stage renal disease and is closely linked to plasma folate and pyridoxine concentrations. *Circulation* 94:2743–8.
53. Bachmann J, Tepel M, Raidt H, Riezler R, Graefe U, Langer K, *et al.* (1995) Hyperhomocysteinemia and the risk for vascular disease in hemodialysis patients. *Journal of the American Society of Nephrology* 6:121–5.
54. Wilcken DE, Gupta VJ. (1979) Sulphur-containing amino acids in chronic renal failure with particular reference to homocystine and cysteine–homocysteine mixed disulphide. *European Journal of Clinical Investigation* 9:301–7.
55. Hultberg B, Andersson A, Sterner G. (1993) Plasma homocysteine in renal failure. *Clinical Nephrology* 40:230–5.
56. Lilien M, Duran M, Van Hoeck K, Poll-The BT, Schroder C. (1999) Hyperhomocyst(e)inaemia in children with chronic renal failure. *Nephrology Dialysis Transplantation* 14:366–8.
57. Bostom AG, Shemin D, Lapane KL, Sutherland P, Nadeau MR, Wilson PW, *et al.* (1996) Hyperhomocysteinemia, hyperfibrinogenemia, and lipoprotein (a) excess in maintenance dialysis patients: a matched case-control study. *Atherosclerosis* 125:91–101.
58. McCully KS. (1969) Vascular pathology of homocysteinemia: implications for the pathogenesis of arteriosclerosis. *American Journal of Pathology* 56:111–28.
59. Folsom AR, Nieto FJ, McGovern PG, Tsai MY, Malinow MR, Eckfeldt JH, *et al.* (1998) Prospective study of coronary heart disease incidence in relation to fasting total homocysteine, related genetic polymorphisms, and B vitamins: the Atherosclerosis Risk in Communities (ARIC) study. *Circulation* 98:204–10.
60. Wald NJ, Watt HC, Law MR, Weir DG, McPartlin J, Scott JM. (1998) Homocysteine and ischemic heart disease: results of a prospective study with implications regarding prevention. *Archives of Internal Medicine* 158:862–7.
61. A'Brook R, Tavendale R, Tunstall-Pedoe H. (1998) Homocysteine and coronary risk in the general population: analysis from the Scottish Heart Health Study and Scottish MONICA Surveys. *European Heart Journal* 19(Suppl):(Abstract) 8.
62. Nygard O, Nordrehaug JE, Refsum H, Ueland PM, Farstad M, Vollset SE. (1997) Plasma homocysteine levels and mortality in patients with coronary artery disease. *New England Journal of Medicine* 337:230–6.
63. Bostom AG, Silbershatz H, Rosenberg IH, Selhub J, D'Agostino RB, Wolf PA, *et al.* (1999) Nonfasting plasma total homocysteine levels and all-cause and cardiovascular disease mortality in elderly Framingham men and women. *Archives of Internal Medicine* 59:1077–80.
64. Graham IM, Daly LE, Refsum HM, Robinson K, Brattstrom LE, Ueland PM, *et al.* (1997) Plasma homocysteine as a risk factor for vascular disease. The European Concerted Action Project. *Journal of the American Medical Association* 277:1775–81.
65. Meleady R, Lindgren A, Boers GH, Reis R, Wautrecht JC, Medrano M-J, *et al.* (1998) Plasma homocysteine as a prognostic risk factor for vascular disease. *European Heart Journal* 19(Suppl):(Abstract) 8.
66. Evans RW, Shaten BJ, Hempel JD, Cutler JA, Kuller LH. (1997) Homocyst(e)ine and risk of cardiovascular disease in the Multiple Risk Factor Intervention Trial. *Arteriosclerosis, Thrombosis, and Vascular Biology* 17:1947–53.
67. Peterson JC, Spence JD. (1998) Vitamins and progression of atherosclerosis in hyperhomocyst(e)inaemia [letter]. *Lancet* 351:263.

68. Chambers JC, McGregor A, Jean-Marie J, Kooner JS. (1998) Acute hyperhomocysteinaemia and endothelial dysfunction [letter]. *Lancet* 351:36–7.

69. Lentz SR, Sobey CG, Piegors DJ, Bhopatkar MY, Faraci FM, Malinow MR, *et al.* (1996) Vascular dysfunction in monkeys with diet-induced hyperhomocyst(e)inemia. *Journal of Clinical Investigation* 98:24–9.

70. Rolland PH, Friggi A, Barlatier A, Piquet P, Latrille V, Faye MM, *et al.* (1995) Hyperhomocysteinemia-induced vascular damage in the minipig. Captopril–hydrochlorothiazide combination prevents elastic alterations. *Circulation* 91:1161–74.

71. Tracy RE, Strong JP, Newman WP III, Malcom GT, Oalmann MC, Guzman MA. (1996) Renovasculopathies of nephrosclerosis in relation to atherosclerosis at ages 25 to 54 years. *Kidney International* 49:564–70.

72. Kasiske BL. (1987) Relationship between vascular disease and age-associated changes in the human kidney. *Kidney International* 31:1153–9.

73. Bostom AG, Bausserman L, Jacques PF, Liaugaudas G, Selhub J, Rosenberg IH. (1999) Cystatin C as a determinant of fasting plasma total homocysteine levels in coronary artery disease patients with a normal serum creatinine. *Arteriosclerosis Thrombosis and Vascular Biology* 19:2241–44.

74. Shemin D, Lapane KL, Bausserman L, Kanaan E, Kahn SI, Dworkin L, *et al.* (1999) Plasma total homocysteine and hemodialysis access thrombosis: a prospective study. *Journal of the American Society of Nephrology* 10:1095–1099.

75. Tamura T, Bergman SM, Morgan SL. (1998) Homocysteine, B vitamins, and vascular-access thrombosis in patients treated with hemodialysis. *American Journal of Kidney Disease* 32:475–81.

76. Harker LA, Ross R, Slichter SJ, Scott CR. (1976) Homocystine-induced arteriosclerosis. The role of endothelial cell injury and platelet response in its genesis. *Journal of Clinical Investigation* 58:731–41.

77. Wall RT, Harlan JM, Harker LA, Striker GE. (1980) Homocysteine-induced endothelial cell injury *in vitro*: a model for the study of vascular injury. *Thrombosis Research* 18:113–21.

78. Heinecke JW, Rosen H, Suzuki LA, Chait A. (1987) The role of sulfur-containing amino acids in superoxide production and modification of low density lipoprotein by arterial smooth muscle cells. *Journal of Biological Chemistry* 262:10098–103.

79. Di Minno G, Davi G, Margaglione M, Cirillo F, Grandone E, Ciabattoni G, *et al.* (1993) Abnormally high thromboxane biosynthesis in homozygous homocystinuria. Evidence for platelet involvement and probucol-sensitive mechanism. *Journal of Clinical Investigation* 92:1400–6.

80. Lentz SR, Sadler JE. (1991) Inhibition of thrombomodulin surface expression and protein C activation by the thrombogenic agent homocysteine. *Journal of Clinical Investigation* 88:1906–14.

81. Harpel PC, Chang VT, Borth W. (1992) Homocysteine and other sulfhydryl compounds enhance the binding of lipoprotein(a) to fibrin: a potential biochemical link between thrombosis, atherogenesis, and sulfhydryl compound metabolism. *Proceedings of the National Academy of Sciences of the United States of America* 89:10193–7.

82. Tsai JC, Perrella MA, Yoshizumi M, Hsieh CM, Haber E, Schlegel R, *et al.* (1994) Promotion of vascular smooth muscle cell growth by homocysteine: a link to atherosclerosis. *Proceedings of the National Academy of Sciences of the United States of America* 91:6369–73.

83. Selhub J, D'Angelo A. (1997) Hyperhomocysteinemia and thrombosis: acquired conditions. *Thrombosis and Haemostasis* 78:527–31.

84. Mansoor MA, Ueland PM, Aarsland A, Svardal AM. (1993) Redox status and protein binding of plasma homocysteine and other aminothiols in patients with homocystinuria. *Metabolism* 42:1481–5.

85. Homocysteine Lowering Trialists' Collaboration. (1998) Lowering blood homocysteine with folic acid based supplements: meta-analysis of randomised trials. *British Medical Journal* 316:894–8.

86. Bostom AG, Shemin D, Lapane KL, Hume AL, Yoburn D, Nadeau MR, *et al.* (1996) High dose-B-vitamin treatment of hyperhomocysteinemia in dialysis patients. *Kidney International* 49:147–52.

87. Chauveau P, Chadefaux B, Coude M, Aupetit J, Kamoun P, Jungers P. (1996) Long-term folic acid (but not pyridoxine) supplementation lowers elevated plasma homocysteine level in chronic renal failure. *Mineral and Electrolyte Metabolism* 22:106–9.

88. Wilcken DE, Dudman NP, Tyrrell PA, Robertson MR. (1988) Folic acid lowers elevated plasma homocysteine in chronic renal insufficiency: possible implications for prevention of vascular disease. *Metabolism* 37:697–701.

89. Janssen MJ, van Guldener C, de Jong GM, van den Berg M, Stehouwer CD, Donker AJ. (1996) Folic acid treatment of hyperhomocysteinemia in dialysis patients. *Mineral and Electrolyte Metabolism* 22:110–4.

90. van Guldener C, Janssen MJ, Lambert J, ter Wee PM, Jakobs C, Donker AJ, *et al.* (1998) No change in impaired endothelial function after long-term folic acid therapy of hyperhomocysteinaemia in haemodialysis patients. *Nephrology Dialysis Transplantation* 13:106–12.

91. Arnadottir M, Brattstrom L, Simonsen O, Thysell H, Hultberg B, Andersson A, *et al.* (1993) The effect of high-dose pyridoxine and folic acid supplementation on serum lipid and plasma homocysteine concentrations in dialysis patients. *Clinical Nephrology* 40:236–40.

92. Bostom AG, Shemin D, Nadeau MR, Shih V, Stabler SP, Allen RH, *et al.* (1995) Short term betaine therapy fails to lower elevated fasting total plasma homocysteine concentrations in hemodialysis patients maintained on chronic folic acid supplementation [letter]. *Atherosclerosis* 113:129–32.

93. Hong SY, Yang DH, Chang SK. (1998) Plasma homocysteine, vitamin B6, vitamin B12 and folic acid in end-stage renal disease during low-dose supplementation with folic acid. *American Journal of Nephrology* 18:367–72.

94. Perna AF, Ingrosso D, De Santo NG, Galletti P, Brunone M, Zappia V. (1997) Metabolic consequences of folate-induced reduction of hyperhomocysteinemia in uremia. *Journal of the American Society of Nephrology* 8:1899–905.

95. Bergstrom J. (1995) Nutrition and mortality in hemodialysis [editorial]. *Journal of the American Society of Nephrology* 6:1329–41.

96. Arnadottir M, Hultberg B. (1997) Treatment with high-dose folic acid effectively lowers plasma homocysteine concentration in cyclosporin-treated renal transplant recipients. *Transplantation* 64:1087(Abstract).

97. Malinow MR, Bostom AG, Krauss RM. (1999) Homocyst(e)ine, diet, and cardiovascular diseases: a statement for healthcare professionals from the Nutrition Committee, American Heart Association. *Circulation* 99:178–82.

98. Kannel WB, Gordon T. (1977) *The Framingham Study: an epidemiological investigation of cardiovascular disease* (publication no. 77–1247), pp. 94–103. Washington, DC: Department of Health, Education, and Welfare.

10

Microalbuminuria and atherosclerotic vascular disease

Jong-Yoon Yi and George L. Bakris

Introduction

Microalbuminuria (MAU) is defined as the presence of albumin in the urine above the normal range (of less than 30 milligrams per day) but below the detectable range with the conventional dipstick methodology. Data from several pioneering studies over the last two decades demonstrate that MAU is not only a predictor of diabetic complications but also a powerful independent risk factor of cardiovascular disease (CVD).[1-4] Moreover, MAU predicts development of ischemic cardiovascular events related to development of atherosclerosis. Numerous clinical studies in persons with either Type 1 or Type 2 diabetes and MAU demonstrate a higher CVD mortality.[5-7] It should be noted, however, that while the contribution of MAU as a prognostic indicator of cardiovascular events in individuals with diabetes is clear, it is still debatable in non-diabetic populations.[8-10]

Newer research has focused on how MAU may contribute to the pathogenesis of CVD. This area of research has centered primarily on populations with essential hypertension with or without diabetes. Several pathophysiological mechanisms as to how MAU may contribute to the development of atherosclerotic vascular disease have been proposed. However, evidence to support one clear mechanism is not yet available. The currently proposed mechanisms mainly involve local injury to the vascular smooth muscle cells and endothelial cells in the vasculature leading to cell proliferation and increases in vascular permeability (Table 10.1). MAU has also been shown to affect renal tissue morphology in distinct ways (Table 10.1).

This chapter will define and review the role of MAU in the context of atherosclerotic vascular disease development. It will focus on clinical and epidemiological evidence as well as data from experimental studies to describe how MAU contributes to acceleration of the atherosclerotic disease process and its clinical implications.

Table 10.1 Pathophysiological processes associated with the microalbuminuria

Local	
	1. Increased intraglomerular capillary pressure
	2. Increased shunting of albumin through glomerular membrane pores
	3. Loss of glomerular membrane charge
Systemic	
	1. Activation of inflammatory mediators
	2. Increased transcapillary escape rate of albumin
	3. Vascular endothelial dysfunction

Definition and prevalence of MAU

A consensus conference in 1985 defined MAU in persons with diabetes as an abnormal urinary excretion rate of albumin between the range of 20–200 μg/min or 30–300 mg/day.[11] It is also important to note that the range for the urinary excretion rate of albumin is 25% lower during sleep than during awake hours (15–150 μg/min); this is still the definition used today and is applicable to all individuals regardless of associated pathological condition. The reason for defining MAU in this range, below detection by the routine urine dipstick, is that urinary albumin excretion in this range was associated with much higher cardiovascular mortality rates as well as nephropathy progression among individuals with Type 1 diabetes. It should also be noted that this higher incidence of cardiovascular mortality in not similar in the hypertensive non-diabetic populations.

A high prevalence of MAU has been noted in early studies[12–14] of persons with diabetes. Considerably lower percentages, however, have been noted in the more recent, larger clinical trials.[15–17] These variations are mostly due to patient selection or inclusion criteria biases such as the severity of hypertension, age, race, coexisting renal disease, techniques used for detection of MAU, sampling size of the cohort, and day-to-day variability of albumin excretion, which ranges from 31 to 52%.

The prevalence of MAU in individuals with Type 2 diabetes mellitus is about 20% (range 12–36%) and affects about 30% of individuals with Type 2 diabetes aged over 55 years.[12,18] The rate of progression to diabetic nephropathy in individuals affected with Type 2 diabetes is 5% per year and 7.5% per year for those affected with Type 1 diabetes.[3,4] Subsequent chronic renal failure occurs at 1% per year in Type 2 diabetes patients, and the risk for those with Type 1 diabetes approaches 75% after 10 years.[7,19]

The prevalence of MAU ranges from 5 to 40% among non-diabetic persons with essential hypertension. The reason for this high variability relates to both duration of blood pressure control and associated lipid abnormalities, especially low-density lipoprotein levels. A recent analysis of the baseline data from the African-American Study of Kidney (AASK) Disease Trial illustrates this point. In this trial of 1097 African-Americans with hypertension and no diabetes, the strongest predictor of albuminuria at baseline was the level of low-density lipoprotein (LDL) cholesterol.[20] Moreover, small clinical studies have documented decreases in MAU when 3-hydroxy-3-methylglutaryl–coenzyme A (HMG–CoA) reductase inhibitors are used to lower LDL levels. A second related predictor was the duration of hypertension.[20] In this way, MAU may be the 'HbA1C' of blood pressure control, since blood pressure control with all agents, except dihydropyridine calcium antagonists and central and peripheral sympathetic blockers, reduce albuminuria.[21]

Pathophysiology

The exact pathophysiology as to how MAU contributes to or accelerates the atherosclerotic process is uncertain. The current understanding, however, suggests that mechanisms of vascular injury associated with MAU are different between those with and without diabetes who also have hypertension.[19,22,23] People with MAU have an elevated transcapillary escape rate of albumin, regardless of whether they have Type 1 or Type 2 diabetes. These individuals also have clusters of other metabolic and non-metabolic risk factors associated with CVD development. These risk factors include an elevated blood pressure, dyslipidemia, and insulin resistance.[15,17,24,25] All of these factors contribute to the genesis of atherosclerosis.

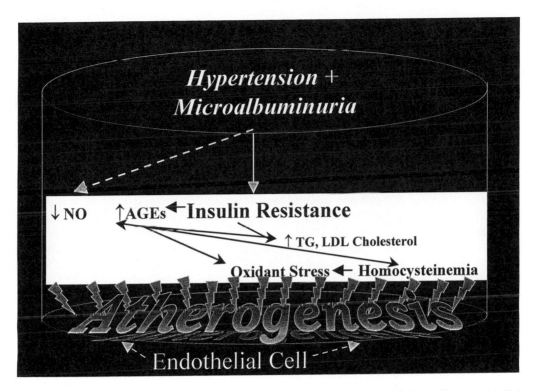

Fig. 10.1 Systemic effects of hypertension and microalbuminuria on the cellular milieu of epithelial and endothelial cells. NO, nitric oxide; AGEs, advanced glycation end-products; TG, triglycerides; LDL, low-density lipoprotein.

Collectively, these risk factors are called Syndrome X, as they frequently cluster in certain individuals. More recently, some authors have suggested that MAU should be added as a fifth element to the metabolic components of Syndrome X.[26]

In persons with MAU who do not have diabetes, generalized vascular leakiness is caused by alterations in the extracellular matrix. This contributes to the development of endothelial dysfunction, which ultimately promotes the atherosclerotic process.[19,27] Defective endothelial permeability permits lipid influx into the vessel wall causing atherosclerotic changes (Fig. 10.1). In many acute and chronic illnesses, MAU is associated with increased vascular permeability as the final common pathway through various mediators, including complement activation and macrophage, neutrophil, and endothelial activation from diverse inflammatory effectors.[22]

In addition to this systemic process, individuals with Type 2 diabetes manifest local injury at the level of the glomerular membrane that eventually leads to worsening of generalized vascular leakiness through increased albumin production secondary to renal losses.[19,28] There is probably a spectrum of local to generalized vascular dysfunction. However, it is difficult to predict which form of dysfunction individuals with Type 2 diabetes mellitus will manifest. This may explain the different course of diabetic renal diseases between the two types of diabetes. Individuals with either type of diabetes share early local structural changes in the kidney and vasculature, such as mesangial cellular hypertrophy and thickening of glomerular and tubular cells. Later, overt diabetic nephropathy occurs only among subjects who accumulate extracellular matrix in the mesangium, a process that correlates with increasing levels of MAU individuals with Type 1 diabetes. Continual accumulation of extracellular matrix over time causes defects in the glomerulus in general and in glomerular filtration rate.[27] In natural history studies, these decrements in glomerular filtration rate correlate with an increased incidence of ischemia-related cardiovascular events.

The single most significant determinant of development of diabetic vasculopathy as well as nephropathy is the resultant advanced glycosylation end-products and related moieties that accompany hyperglycemia.[8,27,28] Along with hyperglycemia, an increase in intraglomerular capillary pressure in the kidney and systemic hypertension are common in this setting. These abnormalities further contribute to renal and vascular dysfunction.

The role of albumin in the pathogenesis of vascular disease, however, may be quite different between the diabetic and non-diabetic hypertensive individual. First, albumin is present in a glycated state in diabetics. The glycation of albumin transforms it into an antigenic molecule that initiates a variety of cellular and immune reactions, such as activation of polymorphonuclear leukocytes. Second, direct injury of the glomerular membrane by advanced glycosylation end-products in diabetics results in a loss of glomerular membrane size selectivity.[8] This loss at the level of the cell membrane, in turn, contributes to increased leakiness of the cellular membrane and hence, increases albuminuria.

Additional studies provide evidence to support the concept that glycation of albumin generates a molecule that is associated with the generation of reactive oxygen species.[27,29] These oxygen-derived and hydroxyl radicals cause injury to epithelial cells (glomerular membrane), vascular smooth muscle cells, and mesangial cells. Advanced glycosylation end-products chelate with proteins on the glomerular membrane to neutralize the negative charge present. This induces a loss of charge selectivity and results in an increased leakiness of both vascular and renal cell membranes in diabetics. In the kidney this process not only affects the glomerular membrane but also mesangial matrix proteins.[30] These changes in membrane proteins subsequently contribute to increases in MAU over time, as well as development of nephropathy in diabetics.

MAU may not be a direct determinant of the genesis of non-diabetic hypertensive vascular or renal disease. This lack of pathogenicity may relate to the observation that the albumin moiety is not glycated. This could help to explain the disparate association between MAU and renal mortality.[8] Further evidence to demonstrate that albumin must be glycated to be pathogenic comes from studies in animal models. An interesting finding from these animal studies is that intermittent elevation of serum glucose induces similar changes in cell membranes to that seen in diabetics.[27] Hence, at the level of the vasculature, glycated albumin promotes an ideal environment for development of atherosclerosis.

Comorbid conditions associated with MAU

MAU reflects widespread vascular disease and is associated with the presence of an unfavorable risk profile and target organ damage, especially in diabetics. This section will cover the major risk factors for CVD in the context of MAU (see Table 10.2).

Hypertension

Several studies have shown that the amount of MAU present in a given individual is proportional to the systolic, diastolic, and mean blood pressure as measured by either clinic or

Table 10.2 Factors known to influence the development of microalbuminuria

---

1. Increased body mass index
2. Increased blood pressure (systolic, diastolic, mean)
3. Altered lipid levels
4. Insulin resistance (hyperinsulinemia)
5. Smoking
6. Salt sensitivity
7. Age
8. Endothelial dysfunction

24-hour ambulatory blood pressure monitoring.[24,31] This observation is further corroborated by the results of a recent clinical study of 787 untreated patients with MAU and essential hypertension. This study agreed with the findings of previous investigators and showed that patients with MAU had higher blood pressure levels.[15] An interesting finding in this study was that even borderline levels of MAU, those in the range of 28–30 mg/day, were associated with higher diastolic and mean blood pressure readings than normoalbuminuric hypertensive subjects. Another Italian population study with 1567 participants revealed an 18 mmHg higher systolic blood pressure in non-diabetics with MAU compared to those without MAU.[17] Moreover, the men with MAU in this trial showed a higher relative risk of having an elevated systolic blood pressure compare to the women with MAU.

Circadian blood pressure abnormalities, as seen in 'non-dippers' who are known to be at higher risk for CVD, have also been described in individuals with MAU.[32,33] Moreover, the timing of the development or worsening of hypertension in Type 1 or Type 2 diabetics with MAU is different.[19] Taken together, these studies all support the concept that the level of MAU reflects the duration of blood pressure control and lipid abnormalities, two major components of syndrome X. Hence, the degree of MAU may serve as an indicator of blood pressure and lipid control as does the HbA1c for glucose.

In Type 1 diabetes, hypertension is not a prominent clinical feature when MAU is present but becomes significant (both systolic blood pressure and diastolic blood pressure) when overt nephropathy develops. In contrast, blood pressure (mainly systolic blood pressure) is already elevated when MAU becomes manifest in Type 2 diabetes. Thus, MAU is not reflective of the duration of blood pressure control in diabetics.

Hyperinsulinemia

The term 'syndrome X' was coined by Reaven after he noted that insulin resistance and compensatory hyperinsulinemia form a common denominator between cardiovascular risk factors (hypertension, obesity, hyperinsulinemia, and glucose intolerance) and the development of CVD.[34] Recent data support the notion that MAU may represent an independent manifestation, possibly constituting the fifth element, of this cardio-metabolic syndrome.[10]

The defect in insulin action is linked to urinary albumin excretion in diabetics and in non-diabetics with hypertension. The mechanism underlying this link between insulin action and MAU, however, remains largely speculative.[24] Three hypotheses have been proposed: (1) the co-segregation theory, (2) the causal-relationship theory, and (3) the final-products-of-same-pathogenetic-factor theory.[31] A discussion of each of these hypotheses is beyond the scope of this chapter; the reader is referred to the cited reference for more information.[31]

Briefly, all these theories note that diabetics who have both hypertension and MAU show a greater abnormality of glucose intolerance and lipid metabolism. Both hyperinsulinemia and MAU have been shown to increase CVD risk in non-diabetics. Moreover, simultaneous occurrence of the aforementioned conditions in non-diabetic subjects identifies a group of individuals with an increased risk for CVD occurrence.[35]

Endothelial dysfunction

The endothelium produces components of the extracellular matrix and a variety of proteins that play an important role in vascular and renal function. An impairment of normal endothelial antithrombotic and vasodilatory properties is a main factor in atherogenesis.[28] Thus, it has been proposed that defective endothelial permeability may be the origin of MAU in the general population, in those with essential hypertension, and among those with diabetes.

Although endothelial dysfunction is not a discrete entity, several experiments and observations suggest that endothelial dysfunction may represent a common pathway for macro- and microvascular diseases.[22] Endothelial dysfunction seems to play a key role in (non-diabetic) glomerulosclerosis and atherosclerosis. Increased permeability of the endothelium allows atherosclerotic lipoprotein particles (oxidized LDL and others) to penetrate into the large vessel wall and promote the development of atherosclerotic plaques[23,28] (Fig. 10.1). This increase in vascular permeability coupled with beta-receptor hyporesponsiveness causes impaired insulin action by preventing insulin-mediated skeletal muscle vasodilation that compromises insulin-induced glucose uptake.

MAU is also associated with biochemical indices of endothelial dysfunction, such as increased plasma von Willebrand factor (vWF) and increased platelet adhesiveness. There are two ways to assess endothelial dysfunction in humans; one measures impaired endothelial-dependent vasodilation and the second uses elevated endothelial-dependent regulatory mediators.[28] vWF is the most extensively studied with regard to endothelial injury. Higher levels of vWF were found in individuals with MAU and a direct correlation between these two variables was described. A greater amount of MAU in subjects not only represents endothelial damage but is also associated with an adverse cardiovascular prognosis.[36] Other biochemical indices of endothelial dysfunction include elevations in the plasma levels of angiotensin II, tissue-type plasminogen activator (t-PA), and prothrombotic profile, including plasminogen activator inhibitor-1 (PAI-1) and endothelin.[28]

In conclusion, endothelial dysfunction seems to play a key role in (non-diabetic) glomerulosclerosis, MAU genesis, insulin sensitivity, and atherosclerosis. The relevance of these biochemical markers in the development of endothelial dysfunction requires further investigation. In this molecular area, endothelial cell dysfunction should be considered as 'micro' target organ damage rather than a marker of target organ damage or merely associated with target organ damage.

Dyslipidemia

Several studies have shown an increased association between patients with MAU and abnormalities in serum lipoproteins. These lipid abnormalities include a low level of high-density lipoprotein (HDL) as well as high levels of LDL, total triglycerides, and lipoprotein (a) [Lp (a)]. This observation is especially true in individuals with both essential hypertension and diabetes.[15,17,24,37] The most consistent association between lipoprotein abnormalities and

MAU rests with a low level of HDL. This supports the view that clearance of LDL cholesterol may be as important as lower levels of HDL to avoid vascular injury. It is of note, however, that a higher prevalence of MAU was not observed in homozygous familial hypercholesterolemics who develop severe, premature atherosclerosis and CVD.[38]

Associated clusters of other atherogenic risk factors with MAU may suggest atherogenic vascular damage. This association of MAU with an abnormal serum cholesterol profile may not be surprising since some conditions, such as endothelial dysfunction, are hypothesized as a common contributing factor in the pathogenesis of both MAU and atherosclerosis.[8,23] Dyslipidemia is evident at the onset of MAU in individuals with diabetes and accelerated nephropathies. Intervention to improve the abnormal lipid profiles delays or halts this atherosclerotic process.[39] Italian population data in 1567 participants showed a relative risk for the presence of MAU in men and women of 2.25 and 2.10, respectively, in those with a 1.0 mmol/L (40 mg/dL) higher plasma cholesterol level than normals.[17] However, the Copenhagen Heart Study did not reach the same conclusion.[16]

Genetic associations

Individuals with MAU are known to have an increased red-cell sodium–lithium countertransport and Lp(a) isoforms that are linked to atherosclerosis, nephropathy, and eventually to CVD.[40] Several genetic polymorphisms have also been examined in association with diabetic nephropathy and in people with essential hypertension.[41–43] The United Kingdom Prospective Diabetes Study (UKPDS) and others demonstrated that the ACE gene polymorphism is associated with MAU. Elevated activity of the renin–angiotensin system is an independent risk factor for CVD.[43] Increased albumin excretion rate has been observed in individuals with essential hypertension and diabetes with a DD ACE-genotype, but the debate as to whether or not this genotype causes MAU remains unsettled.[8]

Clinical applications

The presence of MAU may have limited diagnostic value since it represents a very sensitive, but disease-non-specific, manifestation of abnormal vascular permeability.[23] However, it has several applications in many other clinical situations. These applications include risk assessment, prognostic implications, and disease severity evaluation, and can be a marker of target organ damage from CVD (Table 10.3).

Vascular risk assessment

Since Yudkin *et al.*[1] reported that MAU was a predictor of vascular disease in non-diabetic subjects, several population-based studies have shown an association between increased

Table 10.3 Current clinical applications of microalbuminuria

1. Vascular risk assessment
2. Disease severity assessment
3. Prognostic implications
4. Marker of target organ damage

urinary albumin excretion and several established adverse cardiovascular risk profiles, such as increased serum lipid levels, body mass index, uric acid, blood pressure, insulin levels, smoking, male gender, and left ventricular mass.[15,17,44,45] It is very well established that people with MAU and Type 2 diabetes have much higher rates of atherosclerotic vascular disease than those without MAU.[19,46] Conversely, in populations of Type 1 diabetics, MAU heralds more rapid progression to end-stage renal failure with less atherosclerotic heart disease.[4,7]

Screening for MAU (spot urine for albumin/creatinine) is a relatively inexpensive procedure to identify patients who have target organ injury, endothelial injury, or CVD.[8–10] Routine assessment of MAU in diabetic patients is well advised, but in the general population and in those with hypertension without diabetes, its utility is still debatable. In part, this is due to the relatively low prevalence of MAU in the non-diabetic population and uncertainty of the significance of its modification in these groups.[10,26] However, targeting high-risk patients may be of greater value.

Prognostic implication

If MAU is associated with a higher risk of cardiovascular disease events and poorer prognostic value (or at least hypertensive target organ damage or diabetic complications), it should be more common in such subjects with diabetes and hypertension, respectively. Systematic overviews of the literature support the observation that MAU is more common in such groups.[12,15,17,26] MAU is a strong predictor of mortality (in both total and CVD-related) and CVD among Type 1 diabetics, Type 2 diabetics, and non-diabetic hypertensives.[5,6,25,35] In a recent meta-analysis, the overall odds ratio is 2.4 for total mortality and 2.0 for CVD morbidity and mortality in Type 2 diabetics with MAU.[12]

Other studies observed that subjects with MAU and Type 2 diabetes have annual approximated total mortality of 8% and CVD mortality of 4%. These values are up to four times higher compared to patients without MAU.[3,19] Total and cardiovascular mortality were twice as high in Type 1 diabetics who had MAU compared to those without MAU.[47]

MAU is not only a concomitant indicator of early target organ damage associated with CVD but is also associated with increased coronary morbidity and mortality in the non-diabetic population. Agrawal *et al.*[44] reported a significantly higher prevalence of coronary artery disease, stroke, and peripheral vascular disease among individuals with MAU. The prevalence of these disorders was 31%, 6%, and 7%, respectively, in non-diabetic hypertensive subjects with MAU compared to 22%, 4%, and 5% without MAU. However, others have failed to find this association of MAU with CVD mortality and target organ damage. In a prospective follow-up study of over 300 treated hypertensive men extending for an average of 3.3 years, Agewall *et al.*[48] showed no increased risk of CVD morbidity and mortality. These investigators did find, however, that although target organ damage was more common among patients with MAU than those without, macroalbuminuria and not MAU was the prognostic determinant.

Disease severity assessment

Measurement of urinary albumin excretion is a very sensitive tool in the presence of any inflammatory process including CVD. In many other acute inflammatory processes, such as trauma, sepsis, and surgery, the amount of MAU is proportional to the severity of the condition.[23] Ischemia and reperfusion are other conditions that follow this rule. MAU is also detected in the presence of an acute myocardial infarction or peripheral vascular disease; it is proportional to the severity of the infarct or claudication.[49,50]

There is a critical increase in vascular permeability just before organ failure starts. Early identification of MAU may influence the aggressiveness of management and ultimately the outcome of the diseases. This is also true in heart failure where MAU is known to increase as ejection fraction is reduced.

Marker of target organ damage

In several studies, patients with MAU had larger left ventricular mass and higher degrees of left ventricular hypertrophy than those without MAU.[15,51–53] This was documented by both electro- and echocardiographic criteria. However, this finding was not consistent in other populations who were relatively young (aged between 18 and 45) and had mild hypertension.[54] This association of MAU with left ventricular hypertrophy may be related to a higher blood pressure load.

The expression of atherosclerotic disease in the carotid artery, which is manifest as increase in intimal-media thickness, was also noted in both non–diabetic and diabetic subjects with MAU.[55,56] This vascular remodeling may be related to endothelial dysfunction whose role in atherogenesis was well described and discussed previously.

Vascular retinal changes and coronary artery disease are also more common among hypertensive patients with MAU than normoalbuminuric patients.[15,57] The incidence of hypertensive retinopathy is lower if MAU is reversible with treatment. MAU is also associated with a higher proportion of individuals developing macroalbuminuria.[57]

Therapeutic intervention

The merits of normalizing or reducing the level of MAU in diabetic subjects are unquestionable, but there are still several unanswered questions in non-diabetic patients.[10,58] There are well-proven renoprotective and cardiovasculo-protective effects of lowering MAU in diabetic patients with antihypertensive regimens containing either an angiotensin-converting enzyme (ACE) inhibitor or non-dihydropyridine calcium channel blockers. Low-protein diets and glycemic control also preserve renal function and prevent nephropathy in the very early stages of renal disease, but not once renal dysfunction is present, i.e. serum creatinine >1.3 mg/dL.[59–63] The effects of glucose control and low protein diet are partially independent of blood pressure reduction.

Some studies have also demonstrated the efficacy of treatment by reversal or reduction of urinary albumin loss in normotensives as well as in controlled hypertensive diabetics with MAU even without altering blood pressure or blood glucose control.[64] However, treatment of hypertension is very important for maintaining renal function among diabetics; this is probably best exemplified by the recently published UKPDS trial.[65] In this trial, blood pressure control yielded a relatively greater benefit over glucose control in Type 2 diabetics with nephropathy compared to those without nephropathy (Fig. 10.2).

The most effective and consistent results for preservation of renal function and reduction of cardiovascular events is treatment of blood pressure to levels below 130/85 mmHg in individuals with either renal insufficiency or diabetes.[62,66] The bulk of evidence supports the concept that an ACE inhibitor should be part of the antihypertensive cocktail used to lower pressure to

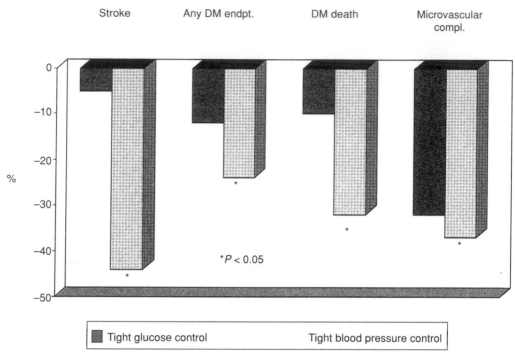

Fig. 10.2 Percentage reduction in cardiovascular events from the United Kingdom Prospective Study Group trial.[65] The relative benefit of tight glucose control versus tight blood pressure control. *P < 0.05 compared to tight glucose control. DM, Diabetes Mellitus; Microvascular compl, microvascular complications.

such levels in these populations. This primarily relates to the observations that ACE inhibitors markedly attenuate mesangial matrix expansion in models of diabetes and prevent development of atherosclerosis in cholesterol-fed rabbits. These agents also prevent glomerulosclerosis despite poor glucose control.[63] ACE inhibitors attenuate the rise in MAU as well as normalize kidney size and prevent renal death.[59,67] Therefore, this class of antihypertensive agents has compelling arguments for its use in the treatment of hypertension in individuals with diabetes and MAU.[58]

A long-term, randomized clinical trial is ongoing to assess some of the unanswered questions about ACE inhibitors for the prevention of diabetic nephropathy and CVD in patients with MAU and diabetes.[68] The importance of optimization of glucose control together with control and prevention of established CVD risk factors should not be discounted. A protein-restricted diet has been shown to be effective in delaying the development of diabetic nephropathy.[69] The current recommendation for daily protein intake from the American Diabetes Association is less than 0.8 g/kg of ideal body weight.[60] The efficacy and safety of a more stringent protein diet requires larger and long-term investigation.

It seems reasonable to consider that a decrease in MAU by non-diabetic hypertensive individuals should be beneficial. However, no specific treatment guidelines exist for non-diabetic hypertensive patients with MAU other than to lower blood pressure to less than 140/90 mmHg.[10] This is a higher value of blood pressure than that recommended for those with either diabetes or renal insufficiency, i.e. less than 130/85 mmHg.[70] No specific guidelines exist in this population for lowering MAU because the risk of developing renal failure

Table 10.4 Summary of our current state of knowledge regarding microalbuminuria

Hypertension
1. Microalbuminuria is not predictive of hypertensive renal disease development.
2. There are no data on the differential effects of antihypertensive drugs on microalbuminuria in the context of cardiovascular outcomes.
3. Microalbuminuria is indicative of a history of poor blood pressure control.

Diabetes
1. Microalbuminuria is predictive of a higher probability of cardiovascular morbidity and mortality.
2. Microalbuminuria is predictive of progressive renal disease.
3. Reduction of microalbuminuria after blood pressure normalization is predictive of a good renal outcome.

Questions still unanswered
1. What happens to cardiovascular outcome when microalbuminuria is treated in normotensives with diabetes?
2. Do the differential effects of antihypertensive drugs on microalbuminuria correspond with cardiovascular outcomes?

in this population is not known. Moreover, a debate still exists as to whether non-malignant hypertension affects renal function.[71] In addition, long-term prospective studies assessing the effect of antihypertensive treatment on renal protection or on modification of CVD risk and mortality are still unavailable.

Conclusion

Over the last few decades, our understanding of the epidemiology, pathophysiology, and clinical significance of MAU among diabetics, essential hypertensives, and the general population has deepened. MAU is associated with a higher prevalence of diabetic complications, metabolic and non-metabolic risk factors, and target organ damage, as well as adverse CVD events in both diabetic and non-diabetic individuals with essential hypertension. Many studies indicate that routine measurement and treatment for MAU should be employed in diabetic patients.[58] However, the long-term significance of MAU and the efficacy of specific treatment in non-diabetic hypertensives as well as the general population need further investigation before routine measurement of MAU can be advocated. Table 10.4 summarizes the current state of knowledge about MAU.

References

1. Yudkin JS, Forest RD, Jackson CA. (1988) Microalbuminuria as predictor of vascular disease in non-diabetic subjects: Islington Diabetes Survey. *Lancet* 2:530–533.
2. Damsgaard EM, Frøland A, Jørgensen OD, Mogensen CE. (1990) Microalbuminuria as predictor of increased mortality in elderly people. *British Medical Journal* 300:297–300.
3. Mogensen CE. (1984) Microalbuminuria predicts clinical proteinuria and early mortality in maturity-onset diabetes. *New England Journal of Medicine* 310:356–360.
4. Viberti GC, Jarrett RJ, Keen H. (1982) Microalbuminuria as prediction of nephropathy in diabetics. *Lancet* 2:611.

5. Viberti GC, Yip-Messent J, Morocutti A. (1992) Diabetic nephropathy. Future avenue. *Diabetes Care* 15:1216–1225.
6. Stephenson JM, Kenny S, Stevens LK, Fuller JH, Lee E. (1995) Proteinuria and mortality in diabetes: the WHO Multinational Study of Vascular Disease in Diabetes. *Diabetes Medicine* 12:149–155.
7. Mathiesen ER, Ronn B, Storm B, Foght H, Deckert T. (1995) The natural course of microalbuminuria in insulin-dependent diabetes: a 10-year prospective study. *Diabetes Medicine* 12:482–487.
8. Bakris GL. (1996) Microalbuminuria: prognostic implications. *Current Opinion in Nephrology and Hypertension* 5:219–223.
9. Gosling P. (1998) Microalbuminuria and cardiovascular risk: a word of caution. *Journal of Human Hypertension* 12:211–213.
10. Lydakis C, Efstratopoulos A, Lip GY. (1997) Microalbuminuria in hypertension: is it up to measure? *Journal of Human Hypertension* 11:695–697.
11. Mogensen CE, Chachati A, Christensen CK, Close, CF, Deckert T, Hommel E, *et al.* (1985–86) Microalbuminuria: an early marker of renal involvement in diabetes. *Uremia Investigation* 9:85–95.
12. Dinneen SF, Gerstein HC. (1997) The association of microalbuminuria and mortality in non-insulin-dependent diabetes mellitus: a systemic overview of the literature. *Archives of Internal Medicine* 157:1413–1418.
13. Bigazzi R, Bianchi S, Campese V, Baldari G. (1992) Prevalence of microalbuminuria in a large population of patients with mild to moderate essential hypertension. *Nephron* 61:94–97.
14. Mogensen CE, Poulsen PL. (1994) Epidemiology of microalbuminuria in diabetes and in the background population. *Current Opinion in Nephrology and Hypertension* 3:248–256.
15. Pontremoli R, Sofia A, Ravera M, Nicolella C, Viazzi F, Tirotta A, *et al.* (1997) Prevalence and clinical correlates of microalbuminuria in essential hypertension: the MAGIC (Microalbuminuria: A Genoa Investigation on Complications) study. *Hypertension* 30:1135–1143.
16. Jensen JS, Feldt-Rasmussen B, Borch-Johnsen K, Clausen P, Appleyard M, Jensen G. (1997) Microalbuminuria and its relation to cardiovascular disease and risk factors: a population-based study of 1254 hypertensive individuals. *Journal of Human Hypertension* 11:727–732.
17. Cirillo M, Senigalliese L, Laurenzi M, Alfieri R, Stamler J, Stamler R, *et al.* (1998) Microalbuminuria in nondiabetic adults: relation of blood pressure, body mass index, plasma cholesterol levels, and smoking: The Gubbio Population Study. *Archives of Internal Medicine* 158:1933–1939.
18. Mimran A, Ribstein J, Du Cailar G, Halimi JM. (1994) Albuminuria in normals and essential hypertension. *Journal of Diabetic Complications* 8150–8156.
19. Schmitz A. (1997) Microalbuminuria, blood pressure, metabolic control, and renal involvement: longitudinal studies in white non-insulin-dependent diabetic patients. *American Journal of Hypertension* 10:189S–197S.
20. Bakris GL, Randall O, Rahman M, Lea J, Ward H, Massry S, *et al.* (1998) for the African American Study of Kidney Disease (AASK) Study Group. Associations between cardiovascular risk factors and glomerular filtration rate at baseline in the AASK trial. *Journal of the American Society of Nephrology* 9:139(Abstract).
21. Tarif N, Bakris GL. (1997) Preservation of renal function: the spectrum of effects by calcium-channel blockers. *Nephrology, Dialysis and Transplantation* 12:2244–2250.
22. Gosling P. (1995) Microalbuminuria: a marker of systemic disease. *British Journal of Hospital Medicine* 54:285–290.
23. Jensen JS. (1995) Renal and systemic transvascular albumin leakage in severe atherosclerosis. *Arteriosclerosis, Thrombosis, and Vascular Biology* 15:1324–1329.
24. Bigazzi R, Bianchi S. (1995) Microalbuminuria as a marker of cardiovascular and renal disease in essential hypertension. *Nephrology, Dialysis and Transplantation* 10(Suppl 6):10–14.
25. Panayiotou BN. (1994) Microalbuminuria: pathogenesis, prognosis and management. *Journal of Internal Medicine Research* 22:181–201.

26. Alzaid AA. (1996) Microalbuminuria in patients with NIDDM: an overview. *Diabetes Care* 19:79–89.
27. Mogyorósi A, Ziyadeh FN. (1996) Update on pathogenesis, markers and management of diabetic nephropathy. *Current Opinion in Nephrology and Hypertension* 5:243–253.
28. Stehouwer CD, Lambet J, Donker AJ, van Hinsberg VW. (1997) Endothelial dysfunction and pathogenesis of diabetic angiopathy. *Cardiovascular Research* 34:55–68.
29. Yaqoob M, McClelland P, Patrick AW, Stevensen A, Mason H, White MC, *et al.* (1994) Evidence of oxidant injury and tubular damage in early diabetic nephropathy. *Quarterly Journal of Medicine* 87:601–607.
30. Shikata K, Makino H, Sugimoto H, Kushiro M, Ota K, Akijama K, *et al.* (1995) Localization of advanced glycation endproducts in the kidney of experimental diabetic rats. *Journal of Diabetes Complications* 9:269–271.
31. Pontremoli R. (1996) Microalbuminuria in essential hypertension—its relation to cardiovascular risk factors. *Nephrology, Dialysis and Transplantation* 11:2113–2135.
32. Bianchi S, Bigazzi R, Baldari G, Sgherri G, Campese VM. (1994) Diurnal variations of blood pressure and microalbuminuria in essential hypertension. *American Journal of Hypertension* 7:23–29.
33. Redon J, Liao Y, Lozano JV, Miralles A, Pascual JM, Cooper RS. (1994) Ambulatory blood pressure and microalbuminuria in essential hypertension: role of circadian variability. *Journal of Hypertension* 12:947–953.
34. Reaven GM. (1988) Banting lecture. Role of insulin resistance in human disease. *Diabetes* 37:1595–1607.
35. Kuusisto J, Mykkänen L, Pyörälä K, Laakso M. (1995) Hyperinsulinemic microalbuminuria. A new risk indicator for coronary heart disease. *Circulation* 91:831–837.
36. Stehouwer CD, Nauta JJ, Zeldenrust GC, Hackeng WH, Donker AJ, den Ottolander GJ. (1992) Urinary albumin excretion, cardiovascular disease, and endothelial dysfunction in non-insulin-dependent diabetes mellitus. *Lancet* 340:319–323.
37. Groop PH, Viberti GC, Elliot TG, Friedman R, Mackie A, Ehnholm C, *et al.* (1994) Lipoprotein(a) in type 1 diabetic patients with renal disease. *Diabetic Medicine* 11:961–967.
38. Zouvanis M, Raal FJ, Joffe BI, Seftel HC. (1995) Microalbuminuria is not associated with cardiovascular disease in patients with homozygous familial hypercholesterolemia. *Atherosclerosis* 113:289–292.
39. Keane WF. (1996) Lipids and progressive renal failure. *Wiener Klinische Wochenschrift* 108:420–424.
40. Yudkin JS. (1992) Microalbuminuria: a genetic link between diabetes and cardiovascular disease? *Annals of Medicine* 24:517–522.
41. Dudley CR, Keavney B, Straton IM, Turner RC, Ratcliffe PJ. (1995) UK Prospective Diabetes Study. XV: Relationship of renin–angiotensin system gene polymorphisms with microalbuminuria in NIDDM. *Kidney International* 48:1907–1911.
42. Marre M, Bernadet P, Gallois Y, Savagner F, Guyene TT, Hallab M, *et al.* (1994) Relationship between angiotensin I converting enzyme (ACE) gene polymorphism, plasma levels and diabetic retinal and renal complications. *Diabetes* 43:384–388.
43. Pontremoli R, Sofia A, Tirotta A, Ravera M, Nicolella C, Viazzi F, *et al.* (1996) The deletion polymorphism of the angiotensin I-converting enzyme gene is associated with target organ damage in essential hypertension. *Journal of the American Society of Nephrology* 7:2550–2558.
44. Agrawal B, Berger A, Wolf K, Luft FC. (1996) Microalbuminuria screening by reagent strip predicts cardiovascular risk in hypertension. *Journal of Hypertension* 14:223–228.
45. Winocour PH, Harland JO, Millar JP, Laker MF, Alberti KG. (1992) Microalbuminuria and associated cardiovascular risk factors in the community. *Atherosclerosis* 93:71–81.
46. Deckert T, Kofoed-Enevoldsen A, Norgaard K, Borch-Johnsen K, Feldt-Rasmussen B, Jensen T. (1992) Microalbuminuria. Implications for micro- and macrovascular disease. *Diabetes Care* 15:1181–1191.

47. Messent JW, Elliot TG, Hill RD, Jarrett RJ, Keen H, Viberti G. (1992) Prognostic significance of microalbuminuria in insulin-dependent diabetes mellitus: a twenty-three year follow-up study. *Kidney International* 41:836–839.

48. Agewall S, Wikstrand J, Ljungman S, Fagerberg B. (1997) Usefulness of microalbuminuria in predicting cardiovascular mortality in treated hypertensive men with and without diabetes mellitus. Risk Factor Intervention Study Group. *American Journal of Cardiology* 80:164–169.

49. Gosling P, Hughes EA, Reynolds TM, Fox JP. (1991) Microalbuminuria is an early response following acute myocardial infarction. *European Heart Journal* 12:508–513.

50. Hickey NC, Shearman CP, Gosling P, Simms MH. (1990) Assessment of intermittent claudication by quantitation of exercise-induced microalbuminuria. *European Journal of Vascular Surgery* 4:603–606.

51. Cerasola G, Cottone S, D'lgnoto G, Grasso L, Mangano MT, Carapelle E, *et al.* (1989) Microalbuminuria as a predictor of cardiovascular damage in essential hypertension. *Journal of Hypertension* 7(Suppl):S332–S333.

52. Pedrinelli R, Di Bello V, Catapano G, Talarico L, Materazzi F, Santoro G, *et al.* (1993) Microalbuminuria is a marker of left ventricular hypertrophy but not hyperinsulinemia in nondiabetic atherosclerotic patients. *Arteriosclerosis and Thrombosis* 13:900–906.

53. Redon J, Liao Y, Lozano JV, Miralles A, Baldo E, Cooper RS. (1994) Factors related to the presence of microalbuminuria in essential hypertension. *American Journal of Hypertension* 7:801–807.

54. Palatini P, Graniero GR, Mormino P, Mattarei M, Sanzuoul F, Cignacco GB, *et al.* (1996) Prevalence and clinical correlates of microalbuminuria in stage I hypertension: results from the Hypertension and Ambulatory Recording Venetian Study (HARVEST). *American Journal of Hypertension* 9:334–341.

55. Bigazzi R, Bianchi S, Nenci R, Baldari D, Campese VM. (1995) Increased thickness of the carotid artery in patients with essential hypertension and microalbuminuria. *Journal of Human Hypertension* 9:827–833.

56. Mykkanen L, Zaccaro DJ, O'Leary DH, Howard G, Robbins DC, Haffner SM. (1997) Microalbuminuria and carotid artery intima–media thickness in nondiabetic and NIDDM subjects. The Insulin Resistance Atherosclerosis Study (IRAS). *Stroke* 28:1710–1716.

57. Biesenbach G, Zazgornik J. (1994) High prevalence of hypertensive retinopathy and coronary heart disease in hypertensive patients with persistent microalbuminuria under short intensive therapy. *Clinical Nephrology* 41:211–218.

58. Bennett PH, Haffner S, Kasiske BL, Keane WF, Mogensen CE, Parving HH, *et al.* (1995) Screening and management of microalbuminuria in patients with diabetes mellitus: recommendations to the Scientific Advisory Board of the National Kidney Foundation from an ad hoc committee of the Council on Diabetes Mellitus of the National Kidney Foundation. *American Journal of Kidney Disease* 25:107–112.

59. Ravid M, Savin H, Jutrin I, Bentral T, Katz B, Lishner M. (1993) Long-term stabilizing effect of angiotensin converting enzyme inhibition on plasma creatinine and on proteinuria in normotensive type II diabetic patients. *Annals of Internal Medicine* 118:577–581.

60. American Diabetes Association, National Kidney Foundation Consensus (1994) Development conference on the diagnosis and management of nephropathy in patients with diabetes mellitus. *Diabetes Care* 17:1357–1361.

61. The Diabetes Control and Complications Trial Research Group (1993) The effect of intensive treatment of diabetes on the development and progression of long-term complications in insulin-dependent diabetes mellitus. *New England Journal of Medicine* 329:977–986.

62. Lewis EJ, Hunsicker LG, Bain RP, Rohde RD. (1993) The effect of angiotensin converting enzyme inhibition on diabetic nephropathy. *New England Journal of Medicine* 329:1456–1462.

63. Bakris GL, Williams B. (1995) ACE inhibitors and calcium antagonists alone or combined: does the progression of diabetic renal disease differ? *Journal of Hypertension* 13(Suppl):95–101.

64. Sano T, Kawamura T, Matsumae H, Sasaki H, Nakayama M, Hara T, *et al.* (1994) Effects of long-term enalapril treatment on persistent micro-albuminuria in well controlled hypertensive and normotensive NIDDM patients. *Diabetes Care* 17:420–424.
65. UK Prospective Diabetes Study Group (1998) Tight blood pressure control and risk of macrovascular and microvascular complications in type 2 diabetes: UKPDS 38. *British Medical Journal* 317:703–713.
66. Viberti G, Mogensen CE, Groop LC, Pauls JF. (1994) The effect of captopril on progression to clinical proteinuria in patients with insulin-dependent diabetes mellitus and microalbuminuria. European Microalbuminuria Captopril Study Group. *Journal of the American Medical Association* 271:275–279.
67. Bakris GL, Slataper R, Vicknair N, Sadler R. (1994) ACE inhibitor mediated reductions in renal size and microalbuminuria in normotensive, diabetic subjects. *Journal of Diabetic Complications* 8:2–6.
68. Gerstein HC, Bosch J, Pogue J, Taylor DW, Zinman B, Yusuf S. (1996) Rationale and design of a large study to evaluate the renal and cardiovascular effects of an ACE inhibitor and vitamin E in high-risk patients with diabetes. The MICRO-HOPE Study. *Diabetes Care* 19:1225–1228.
69. Zeller K, Whittaker E, Sullivan L, Raskin P, Jacobson HR. (1991) Effect of restricting dietary protein on the progression of renal failure in patients with insulin-dependent diabetes mellitus. *New England Journal of Medicine* 324:78–84.
70. The sixth report of the Joint National Committee on prevention, detection, evaluation and treatment of high blood pressure (1997) *Archives of Internal Medicine* 157:2413–2446.
71. Beevers DG, Lip GY. (1996) Does non-malignant essential hypertension cause renal damage? A clinician's view. *Journal of Human Hypertension* 10:695–699.

11

Oxidative stress and cardiovascular disease in end-stage renal failure

Béatrice Descamps-Latscha, Thao Nguyen Khoa, Véronique Witko-Sarsat, Ziad A. Massy, and Tilman L. B. Drüeke

Introduction

Atherosclerotic vascular disease remains the most frequent complication in uremic patients undergoing maintenance hemodialysis, accounting for approximately half of the deaths in these patients.[1-4] Although the prevalence of cardiovascular-related deaths in the end-stage renal failure (ESRF) population is highest in the elderly (approximately 150 cardiovascular-related deaths per 1000 patient-years at risk), it is still substantial (40 cardiovascular deaths per 1000 patient-years at risk) in the age group 20–40 years. Thus, as a percentage of total deaths, cardiovascular deaths are approximately equivalent across all age groups.[4] Interestingly, the high prevalence of atherosclerotic cardiovascular complications also found in uremic patients not yet on dialysis suggests that uremia-related factors *per se* can contribute to the genesis of atherosclerotic vascular lesions.[5]

Attention has recently been directed toward the role of inflammation,[6] as one of the prominent factors known to increase the incidence of atherosclerosis. In this connection, the concept that reactive oxygen species generated by activated macrophages infiltrating the vessel wall play a significant role in the pathogenesis of atherosclerosis is of increasing interest.[7-9] In particular, oxidative damage to low-density lipoproteins (LDLs) and endothelial cells is thought to be of prime importance in the development of fatty streaks, the early lesion in atherogenesis.[10] As a result, there is a growing interest in the development of adequate indices of oxidative stress, as well as of therapeutic strategies that could counteract the deleterious effects of oxidants and potentially decrease the incidence of cardiovascular complications in these patients.

This chapter investigates the potential role of oxidative stress in cardiovascular complications and considers: the agonists of oxidative stress, defined as an imbalance between pro- and antioxidant systems, and its relevant biological markers; the biochemical evidence for oxidative stress in ESRF patients; and the oxidative pathways in atheromatous lesions and the potential role of oxidative stress in the cardiovascular disease observed in ESRF patients.

Agonists and selective markers of oxidative stress

Oxidative stress is usually defined as a perturbation in the pro-oxidant–antioxidant balance leading to potential vascular dysfunction damage.[8] Such a definition incorporates damage products as indicators of oxidative stress and, accordingly, this area has been the subject of research with lipid peroxidation products, oxidized DNA bases, and, more recently, protein oxidation products being examined as indicators of oxidative stress.[11–13] Hence, both oxidant-generating systems and antioxidant activities need to be investigated to determine their respective contributions to oxidative stress.

Oxidant-generating systems

Generation of reactive oxygen species by the phagocyte NADPH oxidase

It is now well documented that following appropriate stimulation, both polymorphonuclear phagocytes (mainly neutrophils) and mononuclear phagocytes (monocytes and macrophages) develop a so-called respiratory burst that leads to the production of highly reactive oxygen species (ROS) that play a key role in host defense against pathogens and tumor cells but may also damage normal structures. At the molecular level, stimulation of the respiratory burst involves activation of an electron transfer chain, the NADPH–oxidase complex, which is dormant in the resting phagocyte but, following activation, becomes capable of reducing molecular oxygen in the presence of NADPH.

The NADPH–oxidase complex   The NADPH–oxidase enzyme complex involves both membrane and cytoplasmic components.[14] The former consists principally of a b-type cytochrome designated cytochrome b_{558}, characterized by a weak reducing potential at -245 mV and composed of two subunits, an α-subunit (p21-*phox*, for phagocyte oxidase) and a β-subunit (gp91-*phox*). The cytoplasmic components of NADPH–oxidase comprise p47-*phox*, which binds to gp91-*phox* after phosphorylation by protein kinase C, p67-*phox*, and a protein linked with GTP, rac-1 or rac-2, which hydrolyses GTP to GDP and thus facilitates the dissociation of the active complex.

Activation of NADPH–oxidase can be triggered by particulate agents, e.g. bacteria or yeasts, and by soluble agents, including phorbol esters, chemotactic peptides, or more physiological compounds, e.g. antibodies, activated complement components, or cytokines. This activation sets in motion classic cellular transduction pathways, notably activation and translocation of protein kinase C, phosphorylation of tyrosine kinases, activation of proteins linked to GTP, modulation of calcium flux, and the release of molecules derived from the phospholipid membrane due to the action of phospholipases A_2 and D. This results in the assembly and grouping in the membrane of components of NADPH–oxidase, giving them access to the substrate on both sides of the membrane and allowing univalent oxygen reduction into the superoxide anion at the expense of NADPH.

Reactive oxygen species (ROS)   The sequence of reactions leading to the production of ROS (reviewed in reference 15) is as follows: as soon as the superoxide anion ($O_2^{\cdot-}$) is formed, it is converted by superoxide dismutase (SOD) into hydrogen peroxide (H_2O_2) which, in the presence of iron, results in the production of singlet oxygen ($^1O_2^{\cdot}$) and hydroxyl radicals (OH$^{\cdot}$). Superoxide anion and hydrogen peroxide are themselves not particularly efficacious at killing microorganisms but are utilized by phagocytes as precursors for the production of more powerful oxidants. For example, superoxide anion interacts with nitric oxide (NO) to form highly toxic nitrogen derivatives (peroxynitrite), whilst hydrogen peroxide, which is able to cross plasma membranes, reacts with intracellular iron to form hydroxyl radicals by a series of interactions termed the Haber–Weiss cycle. Hydroxyl radicals are responsible for a number of toxic effects that have in the past been wrongly attributed to hydrogen peroxide.

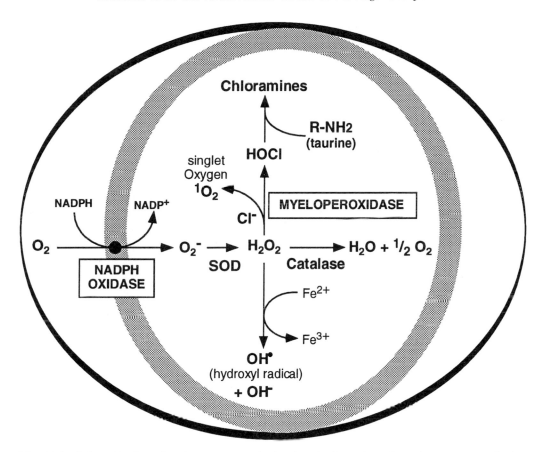

Fig. 11.1 Schematic view of a phagocyte vacuole showing the formation of reactive oxygen species by the NADPH/oxidase complex and the generation of chlorinated oxidants by the myeloperoxidase system.

Their spectrum of toxicity is vast, affecting most cellular components. In particular, they trigger peroxidation of cell membrane lipids,[16] promote protein aggregation,[11] and cause damage leading to mutation and/or cleavage of DNA.[17]

Formation of chlorinated oxidants by the phagocyte myeloperoxidase (MPO)

In addition to the formation of metabolites secondary to univalent oxygen reduction, phagocytic cells have the capacity to produce chlorinated oxidants due to MPO which, in the presence of chloride ions, converts hydrogen peroxide into hypochlorous acid (HOCl) (Fig. 11.1).

The MPO system In man, MPO is the sole enzyme capable of generating chlorinated oxidants.[18] It comprises two subunits linked by a disulfide bridge, a 57.5-kDa heavy chain and a 14-kDa light chain, as well as a heme group. The MPO gene has been cloned, and the existence of mRNA coding for a 90-kDa precursor, which can be cleaved to give the heavy and light chain of the mature protein, has been demonstrated.[19]

Although MPO can catalyze the oxidation of halides like bromide and iodide, chloride remains the main substrate as it is more readily available under physiological conditions.

Interestingly, chloride acts both as a substrate and as an inhibitor, each of these functions corresponding to a binding site on the MPO molecule. In order to be active, the inhibitory site requires protonation. This explains a maximal inhibition in acidic conditions, while the substrate binding site is not affected by the pH. The role of the superoxide anion in the modulation of MPO activity has also been proposed.[20]

Chlorinated oxidants Hypochlorous acid (OCl^-) is the most toxic and the most reactive species formed by phagocytic cells.[18] Its toxic effect is exerted not only towards microorganisms but also against normal or tumor cells. OCl^- can oxidize a number of molecules, such as lipids, proteoglycans, and other membrane or intracellular constituents necessary for the metabolism of the cell. Its selective targets remain membrane proteins and, notably, their thiol groups. Oxidation of intracellular enzymes, nucleotides, and cytochromes by OCl^- leads to inhibition of essential processes such as the respiratory chain. Finally, singlet oxygen ($^1O_2^\bullet$), formed by the reaction of OCl^- with H_2O_2, might also contribute to the toxicity of activate phagocytes.[20]

In addition, OCl^- can react with endogenous amines ($R-NH_2$) to generate chloramines ($RNH-Cl$), termed 'long-lived oxidants' in order to distinguish them from oxygen-free radicals whose lifespan is extremely short.[21] The great majority of chloramines is formed from taurine, a β-amino acid present in high amounts in leukocytes and considered as a selective scavenger of OCl^-.

Despite abundant literature on the toxic power of OCl^-, only a few studies have been undertaken to determine the role of chloramines in the toxicity of neutrophils. However, in contrast to other reactive oxygen species, the relative stability of chloramines allows them to accumulate at inflammatory sites despite the presence of marked concentrations of antioxidants at those sites. For example, in cystic fibrosis-associated lung inflammation, we demonstrated the presence of high concentrations of chloramines in the sputum of these patients which, interestingly enough, were closely correlated with the clinical scores in favor of good respiratory function.[22]

Antioxidant systems

Natural protection against oxidants involves distinct mechanisms requiring a large variety of enzymes capable of transforming or detoxifying oxidants (superoxide dismutase, catalase, and peroxidase), small molecules able to scavenge oxyradicals (α-tocopherol, ascorbic acid, carotenoids, and glutathione), or proteins able to sequestrate transition metal ions (lactoferrin, ceruloplasmin, and transferrin).[23]

Antioxidant enzymatic systems

Superoxide dismutase (SOD) represents the first line of defense against oxidative attack by accelerating the dismutation rate of the superoxide anion into hydrogen peroxide by approximately 1000-fold. This mechanism is of particular advantage for cell energy stores as it does not require or consume any cofactor. SOD is a metalloenzyme that is expressed as two molecular species in mammalians: a copper/zinc SOD (32 kDa) localized in the cytosol and a manganese SOD (40 kDa) localized in the mitochondrial matrix.

Catalase is responsible for the reduction of hydrogen peroxide to water. It is expressed in most cells, organs, and tissues, and is present at high concentrations in liver and erythrocytes. Within the cell, catalase is mainly located in peroxisomes. It comprises four protein subunits, each having a heme group bound to its active site.

Glutathione peroxidase belongs, like catalase, to the second line of defense by reducing the hydrogen peroxide and, in general, all organic lipid hydroperoxides. There are four isoforms in this family and each comprises four subunits which are identical and each bears one atom of selenium. Glutathione peroxidase requires a hydrogen donor: reduced glutathione. Contrary to SOD activity (which is electronically neutral), glutathione peroxidase activity is metabolically costly. In fact, the regeneration of reduced glutathione, the pool of which is limited within the cell, is achieved at the expense of glucose 6-phosphate by directing this compound towards the pentose–phosphate shunt.

Antioxidant non-enzymatic systems

Several antioxidant mechanisms have evolved to combat the potential threat of damage to vital biological structures from the aforementioned sources. Antioxidant molecules without enzymatic activities, which are also called scavengers, comprise:

Glutathione, a sulfide-containing tripeptide, present in all cell types and scavenging H_2O_2, $OH^{\cdot}$, $^1O_2^{\cdot}$, and chlorinated oxidants. Its major role in the control of the level of cell oxidation implicates glutathione in numerous cell functions, in particular the regulation of cell cycle and the formation of microtubules. Glutathione exerts a critical role in the regulation of lymphocyte functions, in particular, proliferation,[24] immunoglobulin production,[25] and cytokine synthesis.[26]

α-Tocopherol or vitamin E, which is localized mainly in the cell membrane in a strategic position for protecting it from lipid peroxidation. It interrupts the radical cascade by forming, via its hydroxyl group, a vitamin of low reactivity which does not attack lipid substrates.

Ascorbic acid or vitamin C, widely distributed in both intra- and extracellular media, directly scavenges $O_2^{\cdot-}$ and $OH^{\cdot}$ by forming semi-deshydro-ascorbic acid, which is itself scavenged by glutathione.

Cysteine, taurine, and methionine, which selectively scavenge hypochlorous acid and chloramines.

Uric acid, glucose, and mannitol, which also retain the capacity to neutralize some oxidants. Moreover, ferritin, transferrin, ceruloplasmin, and even albumin also exert antioxidant effects by sequestrating transition metal ions, thus limiting the formation of $OH^{\cdot}$ via the Haber–Weiss cycle.

Antioxidant protection against lipid peroxidation

Antioxidant protection against lipid peroxidation can be achieved through four different mechanisms: (1) via the action of SOD, catalase, and glutathione peroxidase that catalyse the breakdown of oxidants generated *in situ* by cellular metabolism; (2) via antioxidant proteins such as ceruloplasmin, transferrin, and albumin that sequester free transition metals ions which would facilitate the production of $OH^{\cdot}$; (3) via the action of water-soluble chain-breaking antioxidants such as ascorbate (which may also function as an oxidant as has been shown recently) and lipid-soluble chain-breaking antioxidants such as α-tocopherol, ubiquinone, vitamin A (retinol), and carotenoids that prevent the propagation phase of lipid peroxidation; and (4) via the action of high-density lipoprotein (HDL) enzymes such as paraoxonase and platelet-activating factor acetyl hydrolase that cause the destruction of oxidized lipids.

Oxidative stress markers

Lipid oxidation products

Polyunsaturated fatty acids (PUFAs), found in phospholipids, glycolipids, triglycerides, and cholesteryl esters, are among the most susceptible molecules to oxidative degradation in living tissues. The susceptibility to peroxidation of membrane or circulating lipids is largely influenced by their degree of unsaturation. The principal PUFAs in mammalian tissue are linoleic acid (18:2), arachidonic acid (20:4), and docosahexaenoic acid (22:6).

Lipid hydroperoxides are considered the major and primary products of lipid peroxidation. Formation of lipid hydroperoxides such as hydroxyoctadecadienoic acid (HODE) results from peroxyl radical-dependent chain reactions among unsaturated fatty acyl moieties. Since lipid hydroperoxides are peroxidation products, they could also initiate peroxidative products via their decomposition. Hydroperoxides are unstable and break down to smaller and more stable compounds such as aldehydes. Upon homolytic scission of hydroperoxides, a complex pattern of aldehydes (e.g. acrolein, 4-hydroxynonenal (4-HNE), and malondialdehyde (MDA)) result. A widely used index of lipid peroxidation is the measurement of MDA and reactives aldehydes by the thiobarbituric acid reactive substances (TBARS) assay.

More recently, other products of lipid oxidation have received considerable attention. Phospholipid oxidation products were grouped in four classes: (1) phospholipids in which the unsaturated fatty acid has additional oxygens, e.g. isoprostanes and hydroxy fatty acids; (2) phospholipids in which the fatty acid is fragmented but remains attached to the glycerol backbone; (3) liberated free fatty acid fragments that occur as a result of fragmentation (e.g. MDA) and free oxygenated fatty acids that are formed by hydrolysis of the phospholipids; and (4) lysophosphatidylcholine, the hydrolytic product of the phospholipid backbone.

Isoprostanes are prostaglandin isomers that are primarily products of arachidonic acid oxidation resulting from free-radical attack of cell membrane phospholipids[27] or circulating LDLs.[28] Isoprostanes are emerging as a new class of biologically active products of arachidonic acid metabolism of potential relevance to human vascular disease. Enhanced urinary excretion of F_2-isoprostane 8-iso-$PGF_2\alpha$ has been described in association with cardiac reperfusion injury and cardiovascular risk factors, including cigarette smoking, diabetes mellitus, and hypercholesterolemia.[29] F_2-isoprostanes are also found in atherosclerotic lesions.[30,31] Gas chromatography/mass spectrometry and immunoassays for F_2-isoprostanes have been developed.

Free radical-induced oxidation of LDL generates two major reactive aldehydes, MDA and 4-HNE, which interact with lysine residues in apolipoprotein B (apoB), the protein moiety of LDL. These protein adducts were found to be present in oxidized LDL (oxLDL) as well as in atherosclerotic lesions using immunochemical techniques. Phospholipid endoperoxides such as levuglandin E_2 can also form protein adducts.[32]

Protein oxidation products

In contrast to lipids, the reactions of proteins with various oxidants have not been studied extensively *ex vivo*, and it has been assumed that proteins are not particularly susceptible to free radical damage. However, in *in vitro* studies, it has been well established that proteins represent elective targets of oxidant mediated injury[11] (and revised in reference 33).

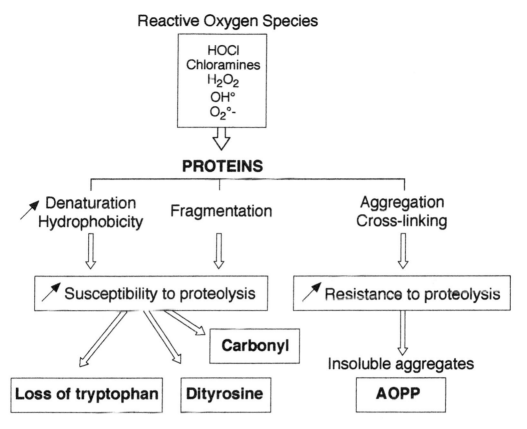

Fig. 11.2 Schematic representation of the various pathways leading to oxidative modifications of proteins.

Similarly, it has well documented that biochemical and structural modifications of proteins induced by oxidative attack can lead to functional alterations and, in particular, to the progressive loss of their metabolic, enzymatic, or immunological properties.

As schematically illustrated in Fig. 11.2, *in vitro* exposure of proteins to oxidants can lead to alterations in their primary, secondary, or tertiary structure, which vary depending on the type of oxidant. For a given oxidant, depending on the intensity of the oxidative attack, these modifications may go from the oxidation of a single amino acid residue to the fragmentation or complete denaturation of the protein across intermediary steps of increased hydrophobicity, augmented susceptibility, or resistance to proteolysis. This latter aspect well illustrates the complexity of the mechanisms and of the pathophysiological aspects of oxidative stress. Whereas moderate oxidation of proteins leads to augmentation of hydrophobicity and favors their catabolism by the multicatalytic or proteasome complex, intense oxidation generates insoluble products which resist proteolysis.[34,35]

Another aspect of the oxidative attack of proteins is the formation of covalent binding links between two tyrosine residues, leading to the generation of dityrosine.[36,37] The formation of carbonyls represents another early marker of protein oxidation.

The inactivation of enzymes represents an important consequence of this type of protein oxidation involving the catalytic effect of metals. The absence of major biochemical alterations suggests that minor modifications are sufficient to induce this inactivation. Besides these enzymes, inactivation of proteins such as the elastase inhibitor (α_1-proteinase inhibitor) can be induced by the oxidation of a methionine residue. Interestingly, radicals produced during lipid peroxidation may also exert an inhibitory effect on proteinases by methionine oxidation.

Our previous study, analyzing the structural modifications of β_2-microglobuline (β_2m) induced by reactive oxygen species generated by water pulse radiolysis,[38] clearly illustrates the selectivity of the protein damage depending on the type of oxidant. Whereas the hydroxyl radical alone induces aggregation and conformational changes of β_2m, the combination of hydroxyl radical with equimolar concentrations of superoxide anion induces fragmentation of β_2m. The loss of tryptophan and the production of dityrosine follow these structural modifications of β_2m induced by reactive oxygen species in a dose-dependent manner.

More recently, we described a novel protein oxidation marker, referred to as an advanced oxidation protein product (AOPP), in the plasma of uremic patients. Biochemical characterization of AOPP revealed that two distinct peaks at 670 kDa and approximately 70 kDa account for the total AOPP level in plasma. Protein electrophoresis showed that the high-molecular-weight AOPP peak is due mostly to albumin, which appears to form aggregates probably resulting from disulfide bridges and/or dityrosine cross-linking. The low-molecular-weight AOPP peak also contains albumin in its monomeric form. By contrast, we provided evidence that oxidatively modified albumin leads to AOPP formation *in vitro*. In order to determine the spectral characteristics of AOPP, UV absorbance and fluorescence emission spectra of native human serum albumin (HSA) and HSA treated with chlorinated oxidants (HSA–AOPP) were analyzed and compared with those of purified dityrosine. This led us to conclude that dityrosine effectively represents the main chromophore of AOPP with an absorption at 315 nm and an emission band at 410 nm (after excitation at 315 nm).

Study of the potential biological relevance of AOPP showed that AOPP can induce macrophage activation[39] and, therefore, may be considered not only as a measure of oxidative stress but also as a potent mediator of inflammation.[40]

In addition, advanced glycation end-products (AGEs) formed during Maillard reaction by non-enzymatic glycation can also be formed by oxidation. We have shown recently that there is a close relation between AGE and AOPP.[13] Other authors have also demonstrated the implication of increased oxidative stress in the formation of AGEs.[41]

Oxidative stress associated with ESRF

Conditions for the generation of oxidative stress are generally present in the uremic patient on maintenance hemodialysis in whom intermittent generation of oxidants recurs at each dialysis session, and in whom chronic antioxidant deficiency exists (Fig. 11.3).

Increased generation of oxidants in ESRF

The production of ROS by phagocytic cells can be easily quantified directly within whole blood by chemiluminescence (CL). Depending on the luminescent probe used, one may quantify either NADPH oxidase activity alone, i.e. the production of superoxide anion (as measured by lucigenin-amplified CL), or the intracellular production of hydrogen peroxide and MPO-dependent formation of chlorinated oxidants (as measured by luminol-amplified CL).[39,42]

In dialysis patients, we previously reported that each dialysis session triggers a significant increase in the basal whole blood luminol-amplified CL production, depending

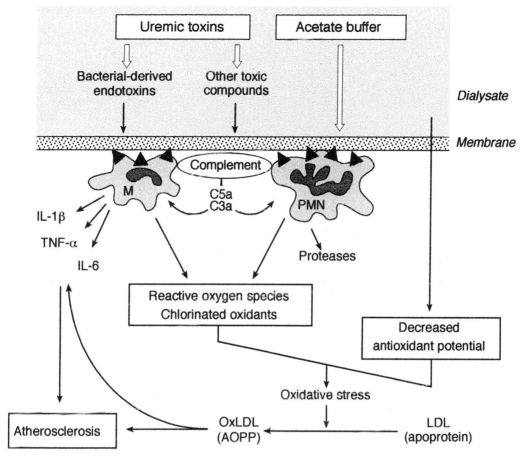

Fig. 11.3 Influence of chronic renal failure and dialysis treatment on phagocyte activation and subsequent oxidative stress-induced atherosclerosis.

strictly on the cellulosic nature of the dialysis membrane[43] and closely related to the amount of C5a and C3a generation.[44] More recently, we also observed that basal whole blood lucigenin-amplified CL production is increased at each dialysis session (B. Descamps-Latscha *et al.*, unpublished results). Other authors using flow cytometry also reported the increased generation of intracellular ROS in both monocytes and polymorphonuclear (PMN) cells during dialysis sessions simultaneously with leukopenia, and closely related to the membrane biocompatibility.[45–47] It has also been reported that dialysis performed with bioreactive membranes, such as cuprophane, increases expression by PMN cells and monocytes of CD11b, an adhesive molecule, which could contribute to the leukopenia observed 15 min after the start of the dialysis session. However, dialysis using biocompatible membranes, such as polysulfone membrane, also slightly increases CD11b monocyte expression, suggesting that the biocompatible membranes were not totally inert.[47]

The repetitive enhancement of ROS production associated with complement activation and overexpression of adhesive molecules in circulating leukocytes could promote endothelial cell membrane lipid peroxidation, thus leading to endothelial dysfunction and initiating vascular lesions, the first step in dialysis-induced atherosclerosis.

It is generally thought that such a repetitive activation of phagocytic cells induces a down-regulation of complement receptors and a decreased capacity to mount opsonin receptor-mediated oxidative responses, contributing to a reduction in the host defense mechanism of dialysis patients.[48]

Antioxidant deficiency in ESRF

Profound deficiencies in the activity of the glutathione system[49,50] and in selenium have been reported in dialysis patients.[51–53] In our own study, we were able to show that glutathione peroxidase activity is significantly altered, beginning at the early stages of chronic renal failure (CRF), regularly decreases with the progression of uremia, and is dramatically reduced in the dialysis patient in whom it is associated with a markedly reduced level of glutathione.[52] Importantly, the deficit of hexose monophosphate shunt pathway activity may cause a reduction in antioxidant reserve in uremic patients, since NADPH is a cofactor required to recycle oxidized glutathione back to the effective reduced form. More conflicting data have been reported in the literature regarding the levels and/or the activities of SOD, trace elements, e.g. copper and zinc, and other oxidant-scavenging molecules, such as ceruloplasmin and transferrin, in CRF patients. In fact, endogenous antioxidant activities may be low in dialysis patients owing to diminished oral intake, dietary restrictions, dialytic clearance, or as a result of increased degradation. Moreover, serum albumin, which can bind copper and scavenge HOCl, is frequently decreased in some CRF patients, especially in those who suffer from malnutrition.

Vitamin C deficiency, observed in CRF patients, can be caused by dietary restriction of fresh fruit and vegetables to avoid hyperkalemia, and to vitamin C loss during dialysis. However, others have reported plasma vitamin C concentrations within the normal range in the absence of any supplementation. Whether vitamin C by itself exerts a pro-oxidant[54] or an antioxidant effect[55] remains a matter of debate. Since vitamin C plays a key role in recycling α-tocopherol at the aqueous lipid interface, depletion of vitamin C in uremic patients is, therefore, likely to lead to rapid loss of LDL α-tocopherol in an oxidizing environment.

Plasma vitamin E concentrations in CRF patients have been shown to be usually normal, whereas erythrocyte and mononuclear cell concentrations appear to be decreased.[56] Vitamin E appears to be an important molecule in the protection against free radical-induced oxidative damage of LDL and biological membranes. The reported inefficiency of vitamin E to protect LDL particles against oxidation in CRF patients, despite a normal level, may be due to an alteration of its function resulting from vitamin C deficiency. Nevertheless, vitamin E oral supplementation[57] or dialysis with vitamin E-modified membrane[58] was shown to protect against oxidative stress during hemodialysis.

High plasma, liver, and skin concentrations of retinol occur in CRF patients and probably result from the elevated concentrations of retinol-binding protein, which accumulates in CRF, and from reduced urinary excretion of polar vitamin A metabolites. Normal plasma α- and β-carotene status has been reported for CRF patients. However, in one study a significant deficiency of plasma lycopene, which is the most reactive antioxidant carotenoid found in physiological amounts in humans, was observed in such patients.

Oxidative stress markers in ESRF patients

Lipid oxidation products

Until recently, biological evidence for *in vivo* oxidative stress in the dialysis patient relied almost solely on the measurement of lipid peroxidation by-products such as MDA and TBARS[49,59] or, more recently, 4-HNE[60] and F_2-isoprostanes[31,61] which, in general, poorly reflect the intensity of the oxidative stress.

As described below, the presence of oxidized LDL, which would represent an accurate means of evaluating oxidative stress in more direct association with atherosclerosis,[9,62] has also been demonstrated in these patients.[59,63–65]

Protein oxidation products

AOPPs are present at high concentrations in the plasma of uremic patients and closely correlate with dityrosine[13] and carbonyls[66] as other markers of protein oxidation. We also found that AOPP levels are elevated in non-dialyzed uremic patients and increase regularly with the progression of CRF (Fig. 11.4). Interestingly, in these latter patients, AOPP levels were closely related with those of the monocyte activation marker neopterin (Fig. 11.5) but not with T-cell or B-cell activation markers. Interestingly, a similar pattern of correlation was observed with pentosidine level as a marker of AGEs (Fig. 11.5) which, like AOPPs, are cross-linked protein products.[67] The hypothesis that protein oxidation might contribute to the effects attributed so far to AGE has been suggested.[41] The close correlation we found between plasma concentrations of AOPP and AGE–pentosidine and (carboxymethyl)lysine in both hemodialyzed[13] and non-dialyzed uremic patients[68] also supports this hypothesis (Fig. 11.6). In non-dialyzed uremic patients, this correlation remains significant after adjustment of AOPP and AGE values

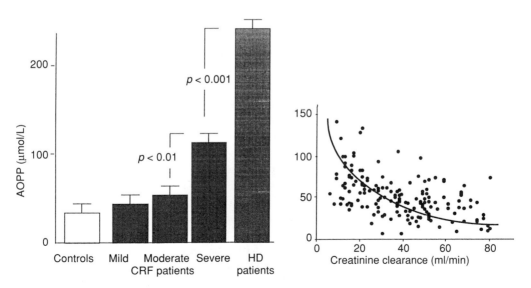

Fig. 11.4 Influence of chronic renal failure (CRF) and hemodialysis (HD) on advanced oxidation protein product (AOPP) plasma level. (Adapted from references 13 and 66.)

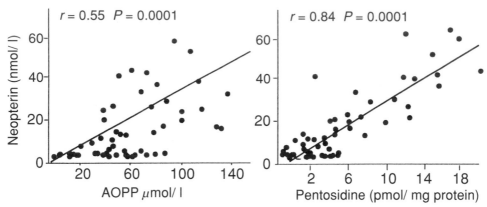

Fig. 11.5 Relationship between monocyte activation, the advanced oxidation protein product (AOPP), the advanced glycation protein end-product (AGE), and pentosidine.[66] Both AOPP and AGE are closely related to neopterin, a monocyte activation marker.

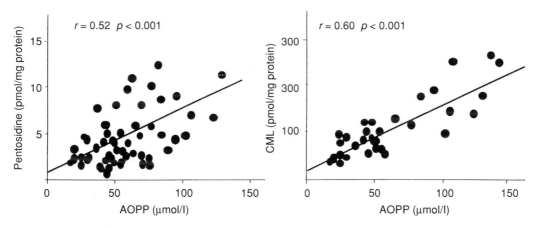

Fig. 11.6 Relationship between the advanced oxidation protein product (AOPP) and the advanced glycation protein end-product (AGE), pentosidine, and (carboxymethyl)lysine (CML).[66]

on creatinine clearance, strongly suggesting that the accumulation of AGE and AOPP in CRF is not solely a passive phenomenon, and implying a common pathophysiological mechanism.

Given the highly probable structural analogy between AGE and AOPP, it appeared to us essential to evaluate the biological actions of AOPP on monocytes/macrophages. Indeed, AGE exerts numerous biological activities, in particular pro-inflammatory actions such as increased expression of adhesion molecules[69] or cytokines, e.g. IL-6.[70] Recent *in vitro* studies in our laboratory have also shown that like HSA–AGE, HSA–AOPP is capable of triggering the respiratory burst of monocytes in normal subjects, and that the intensity of the response is proportional to the level of HSA–AOPP oxidation.[66]

Oxidative pathways in atheromatous lesions: potential role in cardiovascular disease of ESRF

Atherosclerosis and inflammation

Evidence has been steadily accumulating in recent years in favor of the hypothesis that inflammatory and immunological processes are involved in the pathogenesis of atherosclerosis, in addition to numerous other factors such as disturbances of lipoprotein metabolism, diabetes mellitus, arterial hypertension, and cigarette consumption. A major element underlying this hypothesis is the observation that the characteristic lesions of atherosclerosis represent different stages of a chronic inflammatory process in the artery wall.[6,71] The inflammation-induced activation of aortic smooth muscle cells can be considered a hallmark of atherosclerosis.[72] The mechanisms of this activation are progressively becoming clear and involve the generation of numerous inflammatory cytokines, the activation of nuclear factor-κB (NF-κB) signalling pathway, and the enhancement of COX-2 gene transcription.[71,73,74] This proinflammatory cascade is opposed by the activation of peroxisome proliferator-activated receptor alpha (PPARα) and its activators gemfibrozil, fenofibrate, and Wy14643.[75]

Key role of oxidized lipoproteins in atherosclerosis

Oxidation of lipids and lipoproteins such as LDL (oxLDL) has long been recognized as a key event in the atherogenic process via the induction of vessel wall inflammation.[76] Oxidatively modified compounds enter the vascular subendothelial space and can cause

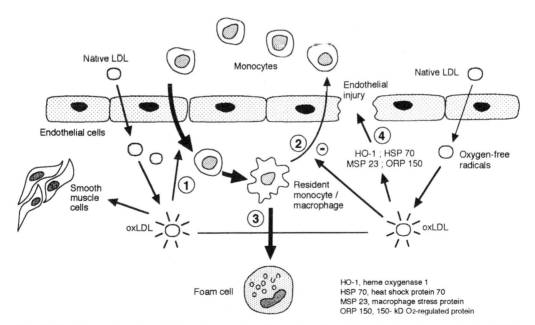

Fig. 11.7 Schematic view of the atherogenic effect of oxidized low-density lipoprotein (oxLDL) within the arterial vessel wall: monocyte recruitment and transformation into foam cells, endothelial injury, and smooth muscle cell proliferation.

injury, especially in the setting of reduced antioxidant defense, to both endothelial and underlying smooth muscle cells (Fig. 11.7).[77,78] Whereas only a small fraction of circulating LDLs display the chemical and immunological characteristics of minimally modified LDL, heavily oxidized lipids, including oxLDL, oxidized sterols, isoprostanes (see below), and products of the lipoxygenase pathway, are mainly found in atherosclerotic lesions.[76]

Mechanisms of oxLDL formation

Enhanced oxidant production and increased lipid peroxidation are generally associated with increased serum levels of cholesterol.[79–81] The oxidative modification of LDL in the arterial wall presumably begins with an oxidative attack of the surface polyunsaturated fatty acids, which includes arachidonic acid. Once initiated, non-enzymatic free radical-catalyzed mechanisms can lead to modifications of all the components of LDL and initiate modifications of surrounding cells and structures as well.[76] As mentioned above, a widely used index of lipid peroxidation is the measurement of MDA and reactives aldehydes by the TBARS assay. Although plasma MDA is not specific for the oxidation of LDL, it may reflect the intensity of lipid moiety oxidation in oxLDL (Fig. 11.8).

Another pathway of LDL modification is enzyme-mediated oxidation, through the generation of superoxide anion radicals by macrophage 15-lipoxygenase and NADPH oxidase[82] or by endothelial nitric oxide synthase (eNOS).[83] Under oxidative stress, NADPH oxidase activity is required for macrophage-dependent oxidation of LDL.[84] Charged superoxide anion not only oxidizes lipids directly, but can also inactivate antioxidants, such as catalase or α-tocopherol,[85,86] and thus can permit subsequent lipid peroxidation. Interestingly, eNOS-induced superoxide generation is Ca^{2+}/calmodulin-dependent and regulated primarily by tetrahydrobiopterin rather than L-arginine.[83] eNOS mRNA and protein expression were increased in experimental models of atherosclerosis in the rabbit despite impaired endothelium-dependent vascular relaxation.[87] However, eNOS protein expression and NO release subsequently were found to be decreased in human atherosclerosis.[88] It is possible that these

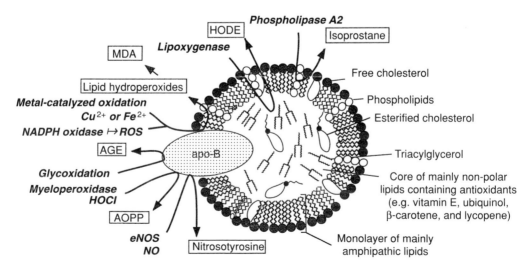

Fig. 11.8   Impact of the various oxidative pathways involved in the oxidation of low-density lipoprotein lipid and protein moieties.

apparently discrepant findings correspond to different stages of the atherosclerotic process. Thus, eNOS activity may be enhanced in initial stages, but reduced in more advanced stages, of arterial vessel damage. Whatever the precise explanation, the normal equilibrium between NO formation and reactive oxygen species appears to be perturbed in the process of atherosclerotic plaque formation.[80,89] The complexity of the situation is further exemplified by the demonstration that, on the one hand, NO is a scavenger molecule for superoxide anion but, on the other hand, it reacts with the latter to form peroxynitrite, another reactive oxygen species with highly cytotoxic effects.[80] When the balance between NO and superoxide anions is disturbed by lowering antioxidant protection through the induction of a vitamin-E deprived state, the relative excess of superoxide anions inhibits the vasorelaxant effect of NO, possibly via increased destruction of NO.[90]

LDL cholesterol oxidation may also occur via the enzyme MPO, a heme protein secreted by activated phagocytes present in human atherosclerotic lesions.[91] Molecular chlorine derived from hypochlorous acid has been shown to be the chlorinating intermediate in this oxidative process.[92]

In addition to the oxidation of the lipid moiety of LDL, oxidation of the protein moiety also occurs, i.e. of its major apolipoprotein, apoB (Fig. 11.9). This can occur through the generation of lipid hydroperoxides, followed by their breakdown and release of aldehydes and ketones, such as MDA and 4-HNE, which can modify lysine residues on apoB. Another pathway is via the activation of MPO, which uses H_2O_2 as an oxidizing substrate to generate a ferryl p-cation radical complex, which can be reduced to the native state by halide and other compounds (Fig. 11.10).[93] One substrate is L-tyrosine, which is converted to the tyrosyl radical.[37] The tyrosyl radical generated by MPO initiates LDL lipid peroxidation and generates o,o′-dityrosine cross-links in proteins.[37,94] Protein-bound dityrosine levels are markedly increased in human atherosclerotic lesions,[95] suggesting that the tyrosyl radical may play a role in LDL oxidation *in vivo*.

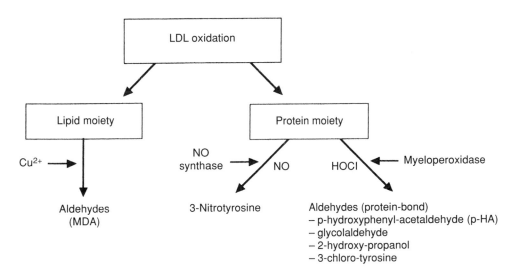

Fig. 11.9 Oxidative pathways leading to modifications of lipid and protein moieties of low–density lipoprotein (LDL).

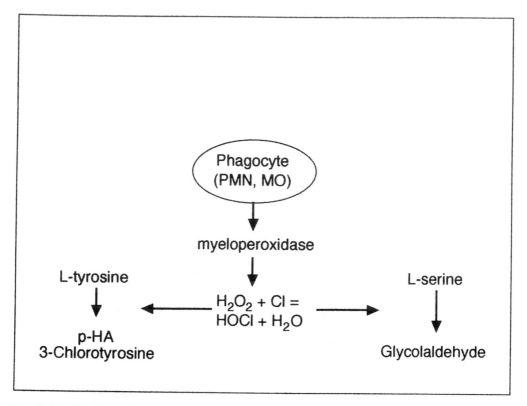

Fig. 11.10 Myeloperoxidase-induced generation of amino acid oxidation products in atherosclerotic lesions.

Enzymatically active MPO, as well as lipoproteins and other proteins oxidatively modified by the action of MPO, has been identified in human atherosclerotic vascular lesions. Moreover, oxLDL isolated from atherosclerotic tissue in such patients is not enriched in lipid oxidation products characteristically induced by the action of free metal ions, indicating the importance of amino acid–derived aldehydes generated by MPO in the formation of atherosclerosis. Thus hypochlorite-modified proteins, including oxLDL, which might correspond to AOPP have been shown to be present in human atherosclerotic lesions.[96]

In diabetes, auto–oxidation of carbohydrates, lipids, and ascorbate leads to AGEs or glycoxidation products. Both lipid peroxidation and glycoxidation favor the formation of protein carbonyls, which have been identified in the thickened intima of arterial walls and may play a role in atherogenesis.[97]

Preliminary reports have shown a decrease in plasma ubiquinone (CoQ_{10}) levels in CRF patients. Extracellular CoQ_{10} is incorporated into and transported within lipoprotein particles, particularly LDL. Ubiquinone has been found to inhibit the initiation and propagation of lipid peroxidation. It is possible that the decreased plasma CoQ_{10} levels in CRF patients are due to increased consumption of CoQ_{10} by free radicals.

Another mechanism which could contribute to increased lipoprotein oxidation in CRF patients is the reduction in paraoxonase activity, before as well as after the initiation of dialysis treatment.[98] Paraoxonase is an HDL-associated enzyme capable of hydrolyzing lipid peroxides.

There has been substantial interest in the vascular expression of SOD in the general population. Whereas either no change or an increase in total SOD was observed in athero-sclerotic vessels in previous studies,[99–101] the authors of a recent study identified a novel form of extracellular SOD (ecSOD) whose expression was increased in such vessels.[102] The source of this ecSOD was probably the lipid-laden macrophage. It is not yet well established whether the increase in ecSOD expression essentially represents a compensatory adaptive function in response to the oxidative environment, reducing, for example, LDL oxidation by endothelial cells.[101] Alternatively, it could contribute to aggravate atherogenesis by catalyzing the nitration of tyrosines by peroxynitrite,[102] which is produced by activated macrophages.[103,104]

Atherogenic effects of oxLDL on the vessel wall

OxLDL interacts with monocytes and macrophages via class A and class B scavenger recep-tors (MSR-A and MSR-B). MSR-A is a homotrimeric protein. There are two forms of MSR-A, type I containing a carboxy-terminal cysteine-rich domain which is not present in the type II receptor. Macrophages also express MSR-B. MSR-Bs comprise a heterogeneous family of proteins that includes collagen receptor CD36. CD36 was initially described as an 88-kDa membrane glycoprotein expressed by platelets, monocytes, and some endothelial cells to serve as an adhesion receptor for thrombospondin and collagen. Studies revealed that 50% of the oxLDL, but not acetylated LDL, accumulated by human monocytes is taken up by CD36, rendering it at least as important as the type A scavenger receptor.[105] Thus, CD36 might be a key factor in monocyte adhesion and foam cell formation. Lovastatin has been shown to increase CD36 expression by retarding the receptor internalization rate in proliferating lymphocytes.[106]

After oxLDL particles have been incorporated into macrophages, they induce the forma-tion of lipid peroxides and the accumulation of cholesteryl esters, resulting in the formation of foam cells (Fig. 11.7). The uptake of modified LDL particles by the macrophage is consid-ered to be an important defense step in the protection of the vessel wall against the inflammatory response induced by these active compounds.[107,108] However, oxLDL present in excess in the vessel wall induces focal inflammation by causing cell injury and attracting other monocytes via enhanced gene expression in endothelial cells of macrophage colony-stimulat-ing factor (M-CSF) and monocyte chemoattractant protein-1 (MCP-1).[109–111] This, in turn, leads to increased binding of oxLDL particles to their scavenger receptor, which is upregu-lated in vascular endothelial and smooth muscle cells, and an enhanced uptake of these oxi-dized particles by these cells. Interestingly, macrophage MCP-1 expression can be reduced by the hydroxymethylglutaryl–coenzyme A (HMG–CoA) reductase inhibitor lovastatin.[111]

Another recently suggested pathway in the induction and maintenance of endothelial dys-function, subsequent vessel wall remodeling, and, possibly, atherosclerosis is the enhanced secretion by vascular smooth muscle cells of vascular endothelial growth factor (VEGF), a potent and specific angiogenic factor with mitogenic activation restricted to endothelial cells, in response to increased oxidative stress.[113–114]

The transformation of the macrophage into a foam cell by internalized oxLDL, as well as the further recruitment of monocytes and their differentiation to macrophages, is mediated by two major oxidized lipid components of oxLDL, 9-HODE and 13-HODE, which activate the nuclear receptor PPARγ.[115,116] This suggests an unexpected role for PPARγ in atherogenesis.

The cell injury caused by oxLDL and lysophosphatidylcholine, one of its major components, eventually leads to a dose-dependent enhancement of endothelial cell apoptosis by sensitizing the endothelium to Fas–Fas ligand-promoted death signals to which it is normally resistant.[117] Moreover, oxLDL downregulates FLICE-inhibitory protein (FLIP), an intracellular caspase inhibitor.[118]

The inflammatory response itself can have a profound effect on lipoprotein movement within the artery wall.[6] Specifically, mediators of inflammation, such as tumor necrosis factor-α, interleukin-1, and M-CSF, increase binding of LDL to endothelium and smooth muscle and increase the transcription of the LDL-receptor gene.[119] After binding to scavenger receptors *in vitro*, modified LDL initiates a series of intracellular events that include the induction of urokinase-3 and inflammatory cytokines, such as interleukin-1.[120,121] Thus, a vicious circle of inflammation, modification of lipoproteins, and further inflammation can be maintained in the artery.

Another role of LDL present in arterial tissue might be to provide increased amounts of 'PUFA' substrate, accelerating non-enzymatic lipid peroxidation of various compounds such as lysophosphatidylcholine, oxidized phospholipids, hydroxy fatty acids, and isoprostanes. The latter group represents a novel family of prostaglandin-like isomers, termed more precisely F_2-isoprostanes, which result from free radical attack of cell membrane phospholipids.[61] They are formed by the oxidation of arachidonic acid esterified to phospholipids in cellular membranes. They can also form when LDL particles undergo either cell- or copper-mediated oxidation.[28,122] Elevated levels of F_2-isoprostanes in plasma and urine in animals and humans are observed in a variety of conditions, including vitamin E- or selenium-deficient rats, in chronic smokers, and the association with other cardiovascular risk factors, such as both type 1 and type 2 diabetes and hypercholesterolemia.[30,31] Increased F_2-isoprostane concentrations have also been found in atherosclerotic lesions where they localize to foam cells and extracellular matrix.[31] Interestingly, isoprostane generation can be suppressed and atherosclerosis reduced by vitamin E administration to apoE-deficient mice.[123] This finding strongly supports the hypothesis that oxidative stress is increased in this experimental model of atherosclerotic vessel disease, and that isoprostanes may be involved in its pathogenesis.

Potential role of oxidative stress in the accelerated atherosclerosis of ESRF

In CRF patients, several qualitative lipoprotein changes have been shown to occur, including increased carbamylation, transformation by AGE, and oxidation, which all favor, at least theoretically, the development of atherosclerosis.[124] The evidence that excessive oxidation of lipoproteins occurs includes: (1) the demonstration of an increase in plasma lipid peroxidation markers such as MDA and conjugated diene concentrations (although not in all reports[125,126]), particularly in lipoproteins, peripheral blood cells, and adipose tissue;[65,127] and (2) the observation of an increase in plasma oxLDL levels,[128] as well as in circulating reactive antibodies directed against them.[63,128,130] However, there has been no demonstration to date by immunohistochemistry or other methods that atherosclerotic lesions in CRF patients contain materials reactive with antibodies generated against oxLDL, as has been shown in the general population. Although longitudinal studies in non-renal patients have shown that circulating antibody titers directed against oxLDL were an independent cardiovascular risk factor for atherosclerosis progression,[131] this has not yet been demonstrated in uremic patients.

Studies in CRF patients have assessed the susceptibility of LDL to undergo oxidation *in vitro* and yielded conflicting results.[63,64,120,132] This discrepancy is probably caused by several factors influencing the duration of the lag-phase, which was used in these studies to measure the resistance of LDL to oxidation. As it is difficult to reconstitute the complexity of all interactive factors *in vitro*, this may explain why *in vitro* conditions do not necessarily reflect the *in vivo* situation.[133]

The uptake of oxLDL by phagocytes may be greater in uremic patients than in healthy subjects because of increased expression of type I scavenger receptors.[134] An increased formation of atheromatous lesions ensues.

Few data are available concerning MPO activity and related oxidation products in the plasma and the arterial wall of CRF patients. It is highly probable that the presence of high circulating levels of AOPP, which are mainly produced following reactions between circulating proteins and chlorinated oxidants,[13,66] might reflect increased MPO activity, and such an increase has been reported recently.[135] The presence of HOCl-modified lipoproteins and other proteins has also been demonstrated in diseased kidney tissue, including vascular structures.[136]

As mentioned above, oxidative stress may also be at the origin of enhanced AGE formation of proteins in non-diabetic uremic patients.[13] AGE formation involves oxidative modification of fructolysine (a compound containing a ketoamine link) and the formation of (carboxymethyl)lysine and pentosidine (Fig. 11.6). Elevated AGE levels lead, in turn, to the generation of reactive oxygen intermediates. In CRF patients, there is an increased rate of LDL modification by AGE, independent of glucose level. AGE moieties are present on both the apoB and the lipid components of LDL in such patients. Experimental data suggest that circulating AGE peptides can impair plasma clearance kinetics of native LDL, and may increase the susceptibility of LDL to oxidative changes. AGE-transformed proteins favor the development and progression of atheromatous lesions in diabetes via their endothelial receptor RAGE,[69] and atherosclerotic lesions in diabetic, apoE-deficient mice can be suppressed by the administration of soluble RAGE.[137] A similar noxious effect on the vessel wall has been shown to occur in CRF patients with high AGE levels, even in the absence of diabetes.[132]

In contrast to several recent studies showing the presence of oxidized lipoproteins, sterols, isoprostanes and products of the lipoxygenase pathways in atheromatous lesions of the general population, no such studies have been reported for arterial structures samples from uremic patients.

Conclusion

Oxidative stress is thought to play a major role in the pathogenesis of uremia- and/or dialysis-induced inflammatory complications. We propose that it contributes largely to the accelerated atherosclerotic process observed in ESRF patients and, thereby, to the high incidence of cardiovascular complications. This opens new stimulating avenues for the development of therapeutic strategies with antioxidant molecules to prevent or treat such life-threatening complications.

References

1. Lindner A., Charra B., Sherrard D.J., and Scribner B.H. (1974). Accelerated atherosclerosis in prolonged maintenance hemodialysis. *New England Journal of Medicine*, **290**, 697–701.
2. Ritz E., Deppisch R., Stier E., and Hansch G. (1994). Atherogenesis and cardiac death: are they related to dialysis procedure and biocompatibility? *Nephrology Dialysis Transplantation*, **9**, 165–172.

3. Jungers P., Nguyen Khoa T., Massy Z.A., Zingraff J., Labrunie M., Descamps-Latscha B., *et al.* (1999). Incidence of atherosclerotic arterial occlusive accidents in predialysis and dialysis patients: a multicentric study in the Ile de France district. *Nephrology Dialysis Transplantation*, **14**, 898–902.

4. Becker B.N., Himmelfarb J., Henrich W.L., and Hakim R.M. (1997). Reassessing the cardiac risk profile in chronic hemodialysis patients—a hypothesis on the role of oxidant stress and other non-traditional cardiac risk factors. *Journal of the American Society of Nephrology*, 8, 475–486.

5. Jungers P., Massy Z.A., Nguyen-Khoa T., Fumeron C., Labrunie M., Lacour B., *et al.* (1997). Incidence and risk factors of atherosclerotic cardiovascular accidents in predialysis chronic renal failure patients: a prospective study. *Nephrology Dialysis Transplantation*, 12, 2597–2602.

6. Ross R. (1999). Atherosclerosis—an inflammatory disease. *New England Journal of Medicine*, **340**, 115–126.

7. Sies H. (1997). Oxidative stress: oxidants and antioxidants. *Experimental Physiology*, 82, 291–295.

8. Halliwell B., Gutteridge J.M., and Cross C.E. (1992). Free radicals, antioxidants, and human disease: where are we now? *Journal of Laboratory and Clinical Medicine*, 119, 598–620.

9. Heinecke J.W. (1996). Atherosclerosis: cell biology and lipoproteins. *Current Opinion in Lipidology*, 7, U131–U136.

10. Steinberg D., Parthasarathy S., Carew T.E., Khoo J.C., and Witztum J.L. (1989). Beyond cholesterol. Modifications of low-density lipoprotein that increase its atherogenicity. *New England Journal of Medicine*, **320**, 916–924.

11. Davies K.J. (1987). Protein damage and degradation by oxygen radicals. I. General aspects. *Journal of Biological Chemistry*, **262**, 9895–9901.

12. Pryor W.A., and Godber S.S. (1991). Noninvasive measures of oxidative stress status in humans. *Free Radical Biology and Medicine*, **10**, 177–184.

13. Witko-Sarsat V., Friedlander M., Capeillere-Blandin C., Nguyen-Khoa T., Nguyen A.T., Zingraff J., *et al.* (1996). Advanced oxidation protein products as a novel marker of oxidative stress in uremia. *Kidney International*, **49**, 1304–1313.

14. Segal A.W., and Abo A. (1993). The biochemical basis of the NADPH oxidase of phagocytes. *Trends Biochemical Sciences*, **18**, 43–47.

15. Halliwell B., and Gutteridge J.M. (1989). Protection against oxidants in biological systems: the superoxide theory of oxygen toxicity. In: Halliwell B., and Gutteridge J.M., eds. *Free radicals in biology and medicine.* Clarendon Press, Oxford, pp. 86–179.

16. Wolff S.P., Garner A., and Dean R.T. (1986). Free radicals, lipids and protein degradation. *Trends Biochemical Sciences*, **11**, 27–31.

17. Imlay J.A., and Linn S. (1988). DNA damage and oxygen radical toxicity. *Science*, **240**, 1302–1309.

18. Klebanoff S.J. (1992) Oxygen metabolites from phagocytes. In: Gallin J.I., Goldstein I.M., and Snyderman R., eds. *Inflammation: basic principles and clinical correlates.* Raven Press, New York, pp. 541–589.

19. Nauseef W.M., McCormick S., and Yi H. (1992). Roles of heme insertion and the mannose-6-phosphate receptor in processing of the human myeloid lysosomal enzyme, myeloperoxidase. *Blood*, **80**, 2622–2633.

20. Allen R.C., Yevich S.J., Orth R.W., and Steele R.H. (1974). The superoxide anion and singlet molecular oxygen: their role in the microbicidal activity of the polymorphonuclear leukocyte. *Biochemical Biophysical Research Communications*, **60**, 909–917.

21. Weiss S.J., Lampert M.B., and Test S.T. (1983). Long-lived oxidants generated by human neutrophils: characterization and bioactivity. *Science*, **222**, 625–628.

22. Witko-Sarsat V., Delacourt C., Rabier D., Bardet J., Nguyen A.T., and Descamps-Latscha B. (1995). Neutrophil-derived long-lived oxidants in cystic fibrosis sputum. *American Journal of Respiratory Critical Care Medicine*, **152**, 1910–1916.

23. Halliwell B., and Gutteridge J.M. (1990). The antioxidants of human extracellular fluids. *Archives of Biochemistry and Biophysics*, **280**, 1–8.
24. Witko-Sarsat V., Nguyen A.T., and Descamps-Latscha B. (1993). Immunomodulatory role of phagocyte-derived chloramines involving lymphocyte glutathione. *Mediators of Inflammation*, **2**, 235–241.
25. Farber C.M., Liebes L.F., Kanganis D.N., and Silber R. (1984). Human B lymphocytes show greater susceptibility to H_2O_2 toxicity than T lymphocytes. *Journal of Immunology*, **132**, 2543–2546.
26. Liang C.M., Lee N., Cattell D., and Liang S.M. (1989). Glutathione regulates interleukin-2 activity on cytotoxic T-cells. *Journal of Biological Chemistry*, **264**, 13519–13523.
27. Morrow J.D., Frei B., Longmire A.W., Gaziano J.M., Lynch S.M., Shyr Y., *et al.* (1995). Increase in circulating products of lipid peroxidation (F2-isoprostanes) in smokers. Smoking as a cause of oxidative damage. *New England Journal of Medicine*, **332**, 1198–1203.
28. Lynch S.M., Morrow J.D., Roberts L.J., and Frei B. (1994). Formation of non-cyclooxygenase-derived prostanoids (F2-isoprostanes) in plasma and low-density lipoprotein exposed to oxidative stress *in vitro*. *Journal of Clinical Investigation*, **93**, 998–1004.
29. Reilly M., Delanty N., Lawson J.A., and FitzGerald G.A. (1996). Modulation of oxidant stress *in vivo* in chronic cigarette smokers. *Circulation*, **94**, 19–25.
30. Gniwotta C., Morrow J.D., Roberts L.J., and Kuhn H. (1997). Prostaglandin F2-like compounds, F2-isoprostanes, are present in increased amounts in human atherosclerotic lesions. *Arteriosclerosis Thrombosis and Vascular Biology*, **17**, 3236–3241.
31. Pratico D., Iuliano L., Mauriello A., Spagnoli L., Lawson J.A., MacLouf J., *et al.* (1997). Localization of distinct F2-isoprostanes in human atherosclerotic lesions. *Journal of Clinical Investigation*, **100**, 2028–2034.
32. Hoppe G., Subbanagounder G., Oneil J., Salomon R.G., and Hoff H.F. (1997). Macrophage recognition of LDL modified by levuglandin E(2), an oxidation product of arachidonic acid. *Biochemical Biophysical Acta*, **1344**, 1–5.
33. Dean T.R., Fu S., Stocker R., and Davies M.J. (1997). Biochemistry and pathology of radical-mediated protein oxidation. *Biochemical Journal*, **324**, 1–18.
34. Pacifici R.F., Kono Y., and Davies K.J. (1993). Hydrophobicity as the signal for selective degradation of hydroxyl radical-modified hemoglobin by the multicatalytic proteinase complex, proteasome. *Journal of Biological Chemistry*, **268**, 15405–15411.
35. Giulivi C., and Davies K.J. (1993). Dityrosine and tyrosine oxidation products are endogenous markers for the selective proteolysis of oxidatively modified red blood cell hemoglobin by (the 19S) proteasome. *Journal of Biological Chemistry*, **268**, 8752–8759.
36. Gross A.J., and Sizer I.W. (1959). The oxidation of tyramine, tyrosine and related compounds by peroxidase. *Journal of Biological Chemistry*, **234**, 1611–1616.
37. Heinecke J.W., Li W., Daehnke H.D., and Goldstein J.A. (1993). Dityrosine, a specific marker of oxidation, is synthesized by the myeloperoxidase–hydrogen peroxide system of human neutrophils and macrophages. *Journal of Biological Chemistry*, **268**, 4069–4077.
38. Capeillere-Blandin C., Delaveau T., and Descamps-Latscha B. (1991). Structural modifications of human beta 2 microglobulin treated with oxygen-derived radicals. *Biochemical Journal*, **277**, 175–182.
39. Witko-Sarsat V., Nguyen-Khoa T., Canteloup S., Nguyen A.T., Jungers P., Drüeke T., *et al.* (1997). Advanced oxidation protein products (AOPP) as novel mediators between activated neutrophils and monocytes in chronic renal failure (CRF). *Journal of the American Society of Nephrology*, **8**, 488A.
40. Witko-Sarsat V., and Descamps-Latscha B. (1997). Advanced oxidation protein products: novel uraemic toxins and pro-inflammatory mediators in chronic renal failure? *Nephrology Dialysis Transplantation*, **12**, 1310–1312.

41. Miyata T., Wada Y., Cai Z., Iida Y., Horie K., Yasuda Y., *et al.* (1997). Implication of an increased oxidative stress in the formation of advanced glycation end products in patients with end-stage renal failure. *Kidney International*, **51**, 1170–1181.

42. Allen R.C. (1986). Phagocytic leukocyte oxygenation activities and chemiluminescence: a kinetic approach to analysis. *Methods in Enzymology*, **133**, 449–493.

43. Nguyen A.T., Lethias C., Zingraff J., Herbelin A., Naret C., and Descamps-Latscha B. (1985). Hemodialysis membrane-induced activation of phagocyte oxidative metabolism detected *in vivo* and *in vitro* within microamounts of whole blood. *Kidney International*, **28**, 158–167.

44. Descamps-Latscha B., Goldfarb B., Nguyen A.T., Landais P., London G., Haeffner-Cavaillon N., *et al.* (1991). Establishing the relationship between complement activation and stimulation of phagocyte oxidative metabolism in hemodialyzed patients: a randomized prospective study. *Nephron*, **59**, 279–285.

45. Dinarello C.A. (1983). The biology of interleukin 1 and its relevance to haemodialysis. *Blood Purification*, **1**, 197–224.

46. Himmelfarb J., Lazarus J.M., and Hakim R. (1991). Reactive oxygen species production by monocytes and polymorphonuclear leukocytes during dialysis. *American Journal of Kidney Diseases*, **17**, 271–276.

47. Cristol J.P., Canaud B., Rabesandratana H., Gaillard I., Serre A., and Mion C. (1994). Enhancement of reactive oxygen species production and cell surface markers expression due to haemodialysis. *Nephrology Dialysis Transplantation*, **9**, 389–394.

48. Vanholder R., Ringoir S., Dhondt A., and Hakim R.M. (1991). Phagocytosis in uremic and hemodialysis patients: a prospective and cross sectional study. *Kidney International*, **39**, 320.

49. Richard M.J., Arnaud J., Jurkovitz C., Hachache T., Meftahi H., Laporte F., *et al.* (1991). Trace elements and lipid peroxidation abnormalities in patients with chronic renal failure. *Nephron*, **57**, 10–15.

50. Mimic-Oka J., Simic T., Ekmescic V., and Dragicevik P. (1995). Erythrocyte glutathione peroxidase and superoxide dismutase activities in different stages of chronic renal failure. *Clinical Nephrology*, **44**, 44–48.

51. Saint-Georges M.D., Bonnefont D.J., Bourely B.A., Jaudon M.C., Cereze P., Chaumeil P., *et al.* (1989). Correction of selenium deficiency in hemodialyzed patients. *Kidney International*, **27**, S274–S277.

52. Céballos-Picot I., Witko-Sarsat V., Merad-Boudia M., Nguyen A.T., Thévenin M., Jaudon M.C., *et al.* (1996). Glutathione antioxidant system as a marker of oxidative stress in chronic renal failure. *Free Radical Biology and Medicine*, **21**, 845–853.

53. Ross E.A. (1997). Low whole blood and erythrocyte levels of glutathione in hemodialysis and peritoneal dialysis patients. *American Journal of Kidney Diseases*, **30**, 489–494.

54. Podmore I.D., Griffiths H.R., Herbert K.E., Mistry N., Mistry P., and Lunec J. (1998). Vitamin C exhibits pro-oxidant properties. *Nature*, **392**, 559.

55. Levine M., Daruwala R.C., Park J.B., Rumsey S.C., and Wang Y. (1998). Does vitamin C have a pro-oxidant effect? *Nature*, **395**, 231.

56. Peuchant E., Delmas-Beauvieux M.C., Dubourg L., Thomas M.J., Perromat A., Aparicio M., *et al.* (1997). Antioxidant effects of a supplemented very low protein diet in chronic renal failure. *Free Radical Biology and Medicine*, **22**, 313–20.

57. Cristol J.P., Bosc J.Y., Badiou S., Leblanc M., Lorrho R., Descomps B., *et al.* (1997). Erythropoietin and oxidative stress in hemodialysis: beneficial effects of vitamin E supplementation. *Nephrology Dialysis Transplantation*, **12**(11), 2312–2317.

58. Galli F., Rovidati S., Chiarantini L., Campus G., Canestrari F., and Buoncristiani U. (1998). Bioreactivity and biocompatibility of a vitamin E-modified multi-layer hemodialysis filter. *Kidney International*, **54**, 580–589.

59. Paul J.L., Sall N.D., Soni T., Poignet J.L., Lindenbaum A., Man N.K., *et al.* (1993). Lipid peroxidation abnormalities in hemodialyzed patients. *Nephron*, **64**, 106–109.

60. Esterbauer H., Schaur R.J., and Zollner H. (1991). Chemistry and biochemistry of 4-hydrox-ynonenal, malonaldehyde and related aldehydes. *Free Radical Biology and Medicine*, 11, 81–128.

61. Morrow J., Awad J., Boss H., Blair I., and Jackson R. (1992). Non-cyclooxygenase-derived prostanoids (F2-isoprostanes) are formed in situ on phospholipids. *Proceedings of the National Academy of Sciences of the USA*, 89, 10721–10725.

62. Stocker R. (1994). Lipoprotein oxidation: mechanistic aspects, methodological approaches and clinical relevance. *Current Opinion Lipidology*, 5, 422–433.

63. Maggi E., Bellazzi R., Falaschi F., Frattoni A., Perani G., Finardi G., *et al.* (1994). Enhanced LDL oxidation in uremic patients: an additional mechanism for accelerated atherosclerosis? *Kidney International*, 45, 876–883.

64. Sutherland W.H., Walker R.J., Ball M.J., Stapley S.A., and Robertson M.C. (1995). Oxidation of low density lipoproteins from patients with renal failure or renal transplants. *Kidney International*, 48, 227–236.

65. Daschner M., Lenhartz H., Botticher D., Schaefer F., Wollschlager M., Mehls O., *et al.* (1996). Influence of dialysis on plasma lipid peroxidation products and antioxidant levels. *Kidney International*, 50, 1268–1272.

66. Witko-Sarsat V., Friedlander M., Nguyen-Khoa T., Capeillere-Blandin C., Nguyen A.T., Canteloup S., *et al.* (1998). Advanced oxidation protein products as novel mediators of inflammation and monocyte activation in chronic renal failure. *Journal of Immunology*, 161, 2524–2532.

67. Baynes J.W. (1991). Role of oxidative stress in development of complications in diabetes. *Diabetes*, 40, 405–412.

68. Friedlander M.A., Witko-Sarsat V., Nguyen A.T., Wu Y.C., Labrunie M., Verger C., *et al.* (1996). The advanced glycation endproduct pentosidine and monocyte activation in uremia. *Clinical Nephrology*, 45, 379–382.

69. Schmidt A.M., Hori O., Chen J.X., Li J.F., Crandall J., Zhang J., *et al.* (1995). Advanced glycation endproducts interacting with their endothelial receptor induce expression of vascular cell adhesion molecule-1 (VCAM-1) in cultured human endothelial cells and in mice. A potential mechanism for the accelerated vasculopathy of diabetes. *Journal of Clinical Investigation*, 96, 1395–1403.

70. Morohoshi M., Fujisawa K., Uchimura I., and Numano F. (1995). The effect of glucose and advanced glycosylation end products on IL-6 production by human monocytes. *Annals of the New York Academy of Sciences*, 748, 562–570.

71. Koenig W., Sund M., Frohlich M., Fischer H.G., Lowel H., Doring A., *et al.* (1999). C-Reactive protein, a sensitive marker of inflammation, predicts future risk of coronary heart disease in initially healthy middle-aged men: results from the MONICA (Monitoring Trends and Determinants in Cardiovascular Disease). Angsburg Cohort Study, 1984–1992. *Circulation*, 99, 237–242.

72. Ross R. (1993). The pathogenesis of atherosclerosis: a perspective for the 1990s. *Nature*, 362, 801–809.

73. Yamamoto K., Arakawa T., Ueda N., and Yamamoto S. (1995). Transcriptional roles of nuclear factor κB and nuclear factor-interleukin-6 in the tumor necrosis factor α-dependent induction of cylooxygenase-2 in MC3T3-E1 cells. *Journal of Biological Chemistry*, 270, 31315–31320.

74. Newton R., Kuitert L.M., Bergman M., Adcock I.M., and Barnes P.J. (1997). Evidence for involvement of NF-κB in the transcriptional control of COX-2 gene expression by IL-1β. *Biochemical Biophysical Research Communications*, 237, 28–32.

75. Forman B.M., Chen J., and Evans R.M. (1997). Hypolipidemic drugs, polyunsaturated fatty acids, and eicosanoids are ligands for peroxisome proliferator-activated receptor α and δ. *Proceedings of the National Academy of Sciences of the USA*, 94, 4312–4317.

76. Witztum J.L. (1998). To E or not to E—how do we tell? *Circulation*, 98, 2785–2787.

77. Navab M., Hamalevy S., Vanlenten B.J., Fonarow G.C., Cardinez C.J., Castellani L.W., *et al.* (1997). Mildly oxidized LDL induces an increased apolipoprotein J/paraoxonase ratio. *Journal of Clinical Investigation*, 99, 2005–2019.

268 *Cardiovascular disease in end-stage renal failure*

78. Steinberg D. (1997). Low density lipoprotein oxidation and its pathobiological significance. *Journal of Biological Chemistry*, **272**, 20963–20966.
79. Lavi A., Brook G.J., Dankner G., BenAmotz A., and Aviram M. (1991). Enhanced *in vitro* oxidation of plasma lipoproteins derived from hypercholesterolemic patients. *Metabolism*, **40**, 794–799.
80. Harrison D.G. (1997). Cellular and molecular mechanisms of endothelial cell dysfunction. *Journal of Clinical Investigation*, **100**, 2153–2157.
81. Kurose I., Wolf R.E., Grisham M.B., and Granger D.N. (1998). Hypercholesterolemia enhances oxidant production in mesenteric venules exposed to ischemia/reperfusion. *Arteriosclerosis Thrombosis and Vascular Biology*, **18**, 1583–1588.
82. Heinecke J.W., Kawamura A., Suzuki L., and Chait, A. (1993). Oxidation of low-density lipoprotein by thiols: superoxide-dependent and independent mechanisms. *Journal of Lipid Research*, **34**, 2051–2061.
83. Xia Y., Tsai A.L., Berka V., and Zweier J.L. (1998). Superoxide generation from endothelial nitric-oxide synthase. A Ca^{2+}/calmodulin-dependent and tetrahydrobiopterin regulatory process. *Journal of Biological Chemistry*, **273**, 25804–25808.
84. Aviram M., Rosenblatt M., Etzioni A., and Levy R. (1996). Activation of NADPH oxidase is required for macrophage-mediated oxidation of low-density lipoprotein. *Metabolism*, **45**, 1069–1079.
85. Kono Y., and Fridovich I. (1982). Superoxide radical inhibits catalase. *Journal of Biological Chemistry*, **257**, 5751–5754.
86. Fukuzawa K., and Gebicki J.M. (1983). Oxidation of α-tocopherol in micelles and liposomes by the hydroxyl, perhydroxyl, and superoxide free radicals. *Archives of Biochemistry and Biophysics*, **226**, 242–251.
87. Kanazawa K., Kawashima S., Mikami S., Miwa Y., Hirata K., Suematsu M., *et al.* (1996). Endothelial constitutive nitric oxide synthase protein and mRNA increased in rabbit atherosclerotic aorta despite impaired endothelium-dependent vascular relaxation. *American Journal of Pathology*, **148**, 1949–1956.
88. Oemar B.S., Tschudi M.R., Godoy N., Brovkovich V., Malinski T., and Lüscher T.F. (1998). Reduced endothelial nitric oxide synthase expression and production in human atherosclerosis. *Circulation*, **97**, 2494–2498.
89. Cooke J.P., and Dzau V.J. (1997). Nitric oxide synthase: role in the genesis of vascular disease. *Annual Review of Medicine*, **48**, 489–509.
90. Davidge S.T., Ojimba J., and McLaughlin M.K. (1998). Vascular function in the vitamin E-deprived rat: an interaction between nitric oxide and superoxide anions. *Hypertension*, **31**, 830–835.
91. Heinecke J.W. (1997). Mechanisms of oxidative damage of low density lipoprotein in human atherosclerosis. *Current Opinion in Lipidology*, **8**, 268–274.
92. Hazen S.L., Hsu F.F., Duffin K., and Heinecke J.W. (1996). Molecular chlorine generated by the myeloperoxidase–hydrogen peroxide–chloride system of phagocytes converts low density lipoprotein cholesterol into a family of chlorinated sterols. *Journal of Biological Chemistry*, **271**, 23080–23088.
93. Hurst J.K., and Barette W.C. (1989). Leukocytic oxygen activation and microbicidal oxidative toxins. *Critical Review of Biochemical Molecular Biology*, **24**, 271–328.
94. Francis G.A., Mendez A.J., Bierman E.L., and Heinecke J.W. (1993). Oxidative tyrosylation of high density lipoprotein by peroxidase enhances cholesterol removal from cultured fibroblasts and macrophage foam cells. *Proceedings of the National Academy of Sciences of the USA*, **90**, 6631–6635.
95. Jacobs J.S., Cistola D.P., Hsu F.F., Muzaffar S., Mueller D.M., Hazen S.L., *et al.* (1996). Human phagocytes employ the myeloperoxidase–hydrogen peroxide system to synthesize dityrosine, trityrosine, pulcherosine, and isodityrosine by a tyrosyl radical-dependent pathway. *Journal of Biological Chemistry*, **271**, 19950–19956.

96. Hazell L.J., Arnold L., Flowers D., Waeg G., Malle E., and Stocker R. (1996). Presence of hypochlorite-modified proteins in human atherosclerotic lesions. *Journal of Clinical Investigation*, **97**, 1535–1544.

97. Miyata T., Inagi R., Asahi K., Yamada Y., Horie K., and Sakai H. (1998). Generation of protein carbonyls by glycoxidation and lipoxidation reactions with autoxidation products of ascorbic acid and polyunsaturated fatty acids. *FEBS Letters*, **437**, 24–28.

98. Dantoine T.F., Debord J., Charmes J.P., Merle L., Marquet P., Lachatre G., *et al.* (1998). Decrease in serum paraoxonase activity in chronic renal failure. *Journal of the American Society of Nephrology*, **9**, 2082–2088.

99. Del Boccio G., Lapenna D., Porreca E., Pennelli A., Savini F., and Feliciani P. (1990). Aortic antioxidant defense mechanisms: time-related changes in cholesterol-fed rabbits. *Atherosclerosis*, **81**, 127–135.

100. Sharma R.C., Crawford D.W., Kramsch D.M., Sevenian A., and Jiao Q. (1992). Immunolocalization of native antioxidant scavenger enzymes in early hypertensive and atherosclerotic arteries. Role of oxygen free radicals. *Arteriosclerosis Thrombosis and Vascular Biology*, **12**, 403–415.

101. Fang X., Weintraub N.L., Rios C.D., Chappell D.A., Zwacka R.M., Engelhardt J.F., *et al.* (1998). Overexpression of human superoxide dismutase inhibits oxidation of low-density lipoprotein by endothelial cells. *Circulation Research*, **82**, 1289–1297.

102. Fukai T., Galis Z.S., Meng X.P., Parthasarathy S., and Harrison D.G. (1998). Vascular expression of extracellular superoxide dismutase in atherosclerosis. *Journal of Clinical Investigation*, **101**, 2101–2111.

103. Beckman J.S., Ischiropoulos H., Zhu L., van der Woerd M., Smith C., and Chen J. (1992). Kinetics of superoxide dismutase- and iron-catalyzed nitration of phenolics by peroxynitrite. *Archives of Biochemical Biophysics*, **298**, 438–445.

104. Ischiropoulos H., Zhu L., Chen J., Tsai M., Martin J.C., and Smith C.D. (1992). Peroxynitrite-mediated tyrosine nitration catalyzed by superoxide dismutase. *Archives of Biochemical Biophysics*, **298**, 431–437.

105. Endemann G., Stanton L.W., Madden K.S., Bryant C.M., White R.T., and Protter A.A. (1993). CD36 is a receptor for oxidized low density lipoprotein. *Journal of Biological Chemistry*, **268**, 11811–11814.

106. Chan P.C., Lafreniere R., and Parsons H.G. (1997). Lovastatin increases surface low density lipoprotein receptor expression by retarding the receptor internalization rate in proliferating lymphocytes. *Biochemical Biophysical Research Communications*, **235**, 117–122.

107. Diaz M.N., Frei B., Vita J.A., and Keaney J.F.J. (1997). Antioxidants and atherosclerotic heart disease [Review]. *New England Journal of Medicine*, **337**, 408–416.

108. Han J., Hajjar D.P., Febbraio M., and Nicholson A.C. (1997). Native and modified low density lipoproteins increase the functional expression of the macrophage class B scavenger receptor, CD36. *Journal of Biological Chemistry*, **272**, 21654–21659.

109. Leonard E.J., and Yoshimura T. (1990). Human monocyte chemoattractant protein-1 (MCP-1). *Immunology Today*, **11**, 97–101.

110. Rajavashisth T.B., Andalibi A., Territo M.C., Berliner J.A., Navab M., Fogelman A.M., *et al.* (1990). Induction of endothelial cell expression of granulocyte and macrophage colony-stimulating factors by modified low-density lipoproteins. *Nature*, **344**, 254–257.

111. Boring L., Gosling I., Chensue S.W., Kunkel S.L., Farese R.V.J., and Broxmeyer H.E. (1997). Impaired monocyte migration and reduced type 1 (Th1) cytokine responses in C-C chemokine receptor 2 knockout mice. *Journal of Clinical Investigation*, **100**, 2552–2561.

112. Park Y.S., Guijarro C., Kim Y., Massy Z.A., Kasiske B.L., Keane W.F., *et al.* (1998). Lovastatin reduces glomerular macrophage influx and expression of monocyte chemoattractant protein-1-mRNA in nephrotic rats. *American Journal of Kidney Diseases*, **31**, 190–194.

113. Kuroki M., Voest E.E., Amano S., Beerepoot L.V., Takashima S., Tolentino M., *et al.* (1996). Reactive oxygen intermediates increase vascular endothelial growth factor expression *in vitro* and *in vivo*. *Journal of Clinical Investigation*, **98**, 1667–1675.

114. Ruef J., Hu Z.Y., Yin L.Y., Wu H., Hanson S.R., and Kelly A.B. (1997). Induction of vascular endothelial growth factor in balloon-injuried baboon arteries. A novel role for reactive oxygen species in atherosclerosis. *Circulation Research*, **81**, 24–33.

115. Tontonoz P., Nagy L., Alvarez J.G., Thomazy V.A., and Evans R.M. (1998). PPAR gamma promotes monocyte/macrophage differentiation and uptake of oxidized LDL. *Cell*, **93**, 241–252.

116. Nagy L., Tontonoz P., Alvarez J.G., Chen H., and Evans R.M. (1998). Oxidized LDL regulates macrophage gene expression through ligand activation of PPAR gamma. *Cell*, **93**, 229–240.

117. Sata M., and Walsh K. (1998). Oxidized LDL activates Fas-mediated endothelial cell apoptosis. *Journal of Clinical Investigation*, **102**, 1682–1689.

118. Sata M., and Walsh K. (1998). Endothelial cell apoptosis induced by oxidized LDL is associated with the down-regulation of the cellular caspase FLIP. *Journal of Biological Chemistry*, **273**, 33103–33106.

119. Hajjar D.P., and Haberland M.E. (1997). Lipoprotein trafficking in vascular cells: molecular Trojan horses and cellular saboteurs. *Journal of Biological Chemistry*, **272**, 22975–22978.

120. Palkama T., Matikainen S., and Hurme M. (1993). Tyrosine kinase activity is involved in the protein kinase C induced expression of interleukin-1 beta gene in monocytic cells. *FEBS Letters*, **319**, 100–104.

121. Geng Y.J., and Libby P. (1995). Evidence for apoptosis in advanced human atheroma: colocalization with interleukin-1 beta-converting enzyme. *American Journal of Pathology*, **147**, 251–266.

122. Pratico D., and FitzGerald G.A. (1996). Generation of 8-epiprostaglandin F$_2$alpha by human monocytes. Discriminate production by reactive oxygen species and prostaglandin endoperoxidase synthase-2. *Journal of Biological Chemistry*, **271**, 8919–8924.

123. Pratico D., Tangirala R.K., Rader D.J., Rokach J., and FitzGerald G.A. (1998). Vitamin E suppresses isoprostane generation *in vivo* and reduces atherosclerosis in ApoE-deficient mice. *Nature Medicine*, **4**, 1189–1192.

124. London G.M., and Drüeke T.B. (1997). Atherosclerosis and arteriosclerosis in chronic renal failure (Editorial Review). *Kidney International*, **51**, 1678–1695.

125. Taccone-Gallucci M., Lubrano R., Belli A., Citti G., Morosetti M., Meloni C., *et al.* (1989). Lack of oxidative damage in serum polyunsaturated fatty acids before and after dialysis in chronic uremic patients. *International Journal of Artificial Organs*, **12**, 515–518.

126. Schulz T., and Schiffl H. (1995). Preserved antioxidative defense of lipoproteins in renal failure and during hemodialysis. *American Journal of Kidney Diseases*, **25**, 564–571.

127. Hultqvist M., Hegbrant J., Nilsson-Thorell C., Lindholm T., Nilsson P., Linden T., *et al.* (1997). Plasma concentrations of vitamin C, vitamin E and/or malondialdehyde as markers of oxygen free radical production during hemodialysis. *Clinical Nephrology*, **47**, 37–46.

128. Maggi E., Bellazzi R., Gazo A., Seccia M., and Bellomo G. (1994). Autoantibodies against oxidatively-modified LDL in uremic patients undergoing dialysis. *Kidney International*, **46**, 869–876.

129. Itabe H., Yamamoto H., Imanaka T., Shimamura K., Uchiyama H., Kimura J., *et al.* (1996). Sensitive detection of oxidatively modified low density lipoprotein using a monoclonal antibody. *Journal of Lipid Research*, **37**, 45–53.

130. Holvoet P., Donck J., Landeloos M., Brouwers E., Luijtens K., Arnout J., *et al.* (1996). Correlation between oxidized low density lipoproteins and von Willebrand factor in chronic renal failure. *Thrombosis Haemostasis*, **76**, 663–669.

131. Salonen J.T., Ylä-Herttuala S., Yamamoto R., Butler S., Korpela H., Salonen R., *et al.* (1992). Autoantibody against oxidised LDL and progression of carotid atherosclerosis. *Lancet*, **339**, 883–887.

132. Jackson P., Loughrey C.M., Lightbody J.H., McNamee P.T., and Young I.S. (1995). Effect of hemodialysis on total antioxidant capacity and serum antioxidants in patients with chronic renal failure. *Clinical Chemistry*, **41**, 1135–1138.

133. Carbonneau M.A., Peuchant E., Sess D., Canioni P., and Clerc M. (1991). Free and bound malonaldehyde measured as thiobarbituric acid adduct by HPLC in serum and plasma. *Clinical Chemistry*, **37**, 1423–1429.

134. Ando M., Lundkvist I., Bergstrom J., and Lindholm B. (1996). Enhanced scavenger receptor expression in monocyte-macrophages in dialysis patients. *Kidney International*, **49**, 773–780.

135. Gündüz Z., Dusunsel R., Kose K., Utas C., and Dogan P. (1996). The effects of dialyzer reuse on plasma antioxidative mechanisms in patients on regular hemodialysis treatment. *Free Radical Biology and Medicine*, **21**, 225–231.

136. Malle E., Woenckhaus C., Waeg G., Esterbauer H., Grone E.F., and Grone H.J. (1997). Immunological evidence for hypochlorite-modified proteins in human kidney. *American Journal of Pathology*, **150**, 603–615.

137. Park L., Raman K.G., Lee K.J., Lu Y., Ferran L.J., Chow W.S., *et al.* (1998). Suppression of accelerated diabetic atherosclerosis by the soluble receptor for advanced glycation endproducts. *Nature Medicine*, **4**, 1025–1031.

138. Takayama F., Aoyama I., Tsukushi S., Miyazaki T., Miyazaki S., Morita T., *et al.* (1998). Immunohistochemical detection of imidazolone and N(epsilon)-(carboxymethyl)lysine in aortas of hemodialysis patients. *Cellular and Molecular Biology*, **44**, 1101–1109.

12

Hypertension in end-stage renal failure

Jean Ribstein, Georges Mourad, Angel Argiles, and Albert Mimran

Introduction

Hypertension can cause or promote renal failure. In most cases, the process of renal deterioration is quite slow, and coronary or cerebrovascular events occur beforehand as indirect complications of the hypertensive process. In recent years, a decrease in cerebrovascular and coronary mortality has been observed in several (but not all) countries, whereas the prevalence of end-stage renal failure (ESRF), as well as congestive heart failure, has increased.[1] The follow-up of large cohorts within a substantial number of years has indicated that hypertension is an independent risk factor for ESRF, particularly in African-Americans.[2] Finally, the latest North American and European reports indicate that the incidence of ESRF caused by hypertension continues to increase more rapidly than ESRF secondary to other major causes except diabetes mellitus (DM).[3] Whether ESRF attributed to hypertension results primarily from nephroangiosclerosis, atheromatous renal vascular disease, cholesterol crystal embolism, or other atherosclerosis-associated forms of renal injury should be a reason for thorough investigation in patients presenting with advanced renal deterioration. Special attention should be paid to renovascular disease since it is a potentially reversible cause of ESRF (see Table 12.1), even in some dialysis-dependent patients.[4,5]

Chronic parenchymal renal disease is the most common cause of secondary hypertension, accounting for approximately 5% of all cases, and the clinician should measure indices of renal function (i.e. proteinuria, altered urinary sediment, increased serum creatinine) in a newly diagnosed patient with hypertension. Arterial hypertension is present in only a

Table 12.1

Why to search for ischemic nephropathy
Renovascular disease is found in 16% of new ESRF cases
Critical renovascular disease is noted in 22% of patients aged more than 50 years starting renal replacement therapy
Hemodialysis is discontinued after revascularization in 80% of patients already on dialysis for 1–9 months

When to search for ischemic nephropathy in ESRF patients
Age > 50 years
Multiple atheromatous lesions
Recent and rapid deterioration in renal function
Acute renal failure induced by administration of angiotensin-converting enzyme inhibitors or angiotensin receptor antagonists

fraction of such patients when serum creatinine is normal; however, its prevalence progressively increases with the degree of deterioration of renal function, and reaches 80–90% in patients entering dialysis programs.[6] Although several studies have suggested that in patients with renal parenchymal disease, 'adequate' control of blood pressure will decrease the number of cardiovascular complications, reduce the incidence of malignant nephrosclerosis, and slow the progression of renal failure, the level of arterial pressure that needs to be achieved still remains a subject of debate.[7,8]

As emphasized in the opening chapters of this book, cardiovascular disease is recognized as the leading cause of death in patients with chronic renal failure and patients on renal replacement therapy. More than two decades ago, aggregation of several risk factors was thought to accelerate the atherosclerotic process in the dialysis patient.[9] Of note, patients who now enter dialysis programs are older, and present with significantly more comorbid risk factors than in previous years. Since it is a major risk factor contributing to cerebrovascular disease, congestive heart failure, and coronary heart disease in the renal as well as in the general population, hypertension is a potent determinant of survival in ESRF.[10,11] Although most studies have demonstrated that outcome is related to hypertension,[12–15] several surveys indicate that hypertension is not 'adequately' controlled in a number of dialysis patients.[16,17]

The present review will analyze known mechanisms of hypertension in chronic renal failure and ESRD (Fig. 12.1) and subsequently deal with some therapeutic proposals derived from these mechanisms. It is presumed that an increase in extracellular fluid volume is the major factor in the prevalence of hypertension and that its control during the first month of dialysis causes a substantial reduction of this prevalence. However, several other factors probably contribute to the maintenance of the hypertensive state, including activation of the

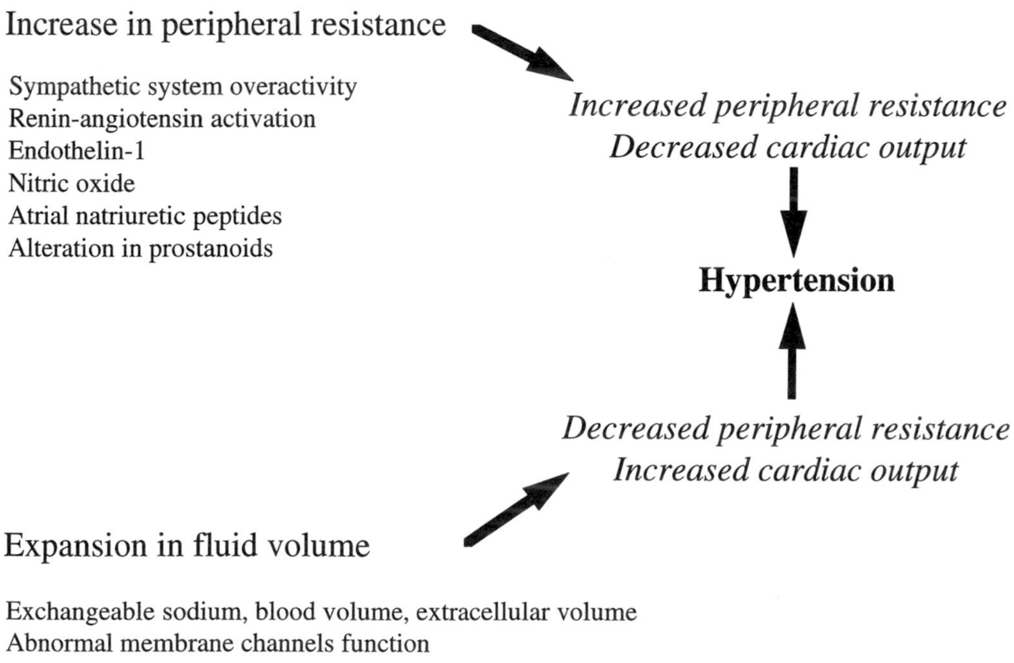

Increase in peripheral resistance

Sympathetic system overactivity
Renin-angiotensin activation
Endothelin-1
Nitric oxide
Atrial natriuretic peptides
Alteration in prostanoids

Increased peripheral resistance
Decreased cardiac output

Hypertension

Decreased peripheral resistance
Increased cardiac output

Expansion in fluid volume

Exchangeable sodium, blood volume, extracellular volume
Abnormal membrane channels function

Fig. 12.1 Pathogenetic factors in ESRF-induced hypertension.

renin–angiotensin axis, sympathetic overactivity, altered balance between endothelium-derived vasoconstrictors and vasodilators, use of erythropoietin, hyperparathyroidism, and pre-existing (essential) hypertension. It must be recognized that many uncertainties remain in this area, and an in-depth review of the literature recently led an ad hoc committee to conclude that not enough data were available to submit an evidence-based clinical practice guideline for these patients.[18] However, the interest and time spent in controlling blood pressure in dialysis patients should not be neglected in the absence of such guidelines.[19]

Hemodynamics of hypertension in ESRF

Patients with advanced renal failure usually have a significantly higher cardiac index than non-uremic controls, a difference mainly accounted for by an increased heart rate.[20] Plasma volume is higher than normal, whether its estimate is related to actual body weight or lean body mass.[21] Extracellular fluid volume and total body sodium content, measured as exchangeable sodium with a sodium isotope or as total body sodium using neutron activation analysis, are usually increased.[22] Water compartments and total body sodium content are indeed increased during the early stages of renal failure in a number of patients,[23] with blood pressure in chronic renal failure being correlated with extracellular fluid volume and exchangeable sodium.[23,24] In addition, it was shown that oral sodium loading results in an increase in blood pressure, whereas elimination of sodium and volume overload by diuretics or dialysis returned blood pressure to normal.[22,25]

It is of interest that in patients with advanced renal failure, correction of anemia by serial transfusion was associated with a progressive decrease in cardiac output and an increase in both total peripheral resistance and mean arterial pressure.[20] Most likely, increased hematocrit alleviated peripheral vasodilation due to inadequate oxygen delivery to tissues and increased blood viscosity. Moreover, when 52 hypertensive and 23 normotensive uremic patients were compared, cardiac output was similar in both groups, whereas total peripheral resistance was higher in the hypertensives, thus suggesting that hypertension was sustained by a high total peripheral resistance.[20] Hemodynamic studies were also performed in 12 patients with ESRF and severe but non-malignant hypertension, and in 8 patients with ESRF and no history of hypertension who underwent bilateral nephrectomy. Bilateral nephrectomy resulted in a significant reduction in blood pressure in all hypertensives, and no change in normotensive subjects. In the hypertensive subgroup, no change in heart rate or stroke index, but a reduction in total peripheral resistance, occurred in every case, thus suggesting the role of a vasopressor substance(s) of renal origin in the maintenance of hypertension.[20] Nevertheless, hypertension is still observed in a small number of anephric patients with no sodium–volume overload, an observation consistent with the possible role of a defect in vasodilator substance(s) of renal origin.

Sodium and volume excess in ESRF

As glomerular filtration rate decreases, the fractional excretion of sodium increases proportionately, resulting in an increase in the average rate of sodium excretion per remaining functioning nephron. In the patient with advanced renal insufficiency, sodium balance is usually maintained on unrestricted salt intake, and the mechanism accounting for this adaptive process is described as the 'magnification phenomenon'.[26] The ability to maintain sodium balance in response to the ingestion of a fixed amount of sodium when renal function progressively fails probably requires an increase in the release of a 'transmitter'(on the detector side of the system controlling body sodium), and/or an increase in the sensitivity of the remaining functional nephrons to the 'transmitter'(on the effector side of the control system). Based on a series of animal experiments with reduced renal mass and exposure to salt loading, it was proposed that an expanded sodium space and intravascular volume would be associated with an initial increase in cardiac output, followed by a return to normal cardiac output and an increase in total peripheral resistance underlying a sustained increase in blood pressure, the so-called 'whole body autoregulation' phenomenon.[27]

Such a sequence of hemodynamic events was demonstrated in some,[28] but not all,[29,30] series of nephrectomized patients. In six anephric patients who had been normotensive before nephrectomy, salt and water loading led to increased body sodium and hypervolemia, but no hypertension.[20] Arterial pressure increased when sodium intake was raised from 20 to 120 mmol/day in 10 patients with advanced renal failure (creatinine clearance approximately 10 ml/min), whereas it remained constant in eight normal subjects ingesting 20, 120, and more than 1100 mmol/day of sodium (in order to obtain similar sodium loads per unit glomerular filtration rate).[31] In fact, patients with preterminal renal failure are exquisitely 'salt-sensitive', thus resulting in hypertension even when maintained on a normal sodium intake.[23]

One (or more) of the saliuretic substances released in response to expansion of extracellular volume might cause a rise in arterial pressure by inhibiting the Na–K ATPase in the smooth muscle cells of the arterial wall, as it does putatively in the tubular cells, its prime target.[32] One such substance—probably secreted in the anterior hypothalamic area—inhibits the sodium pump, and secondarily raises the calcium content of the vascular smooth muscle cell. Several groups have reported the presence of sodium-pump inhibitors in uremia,[33] but a causal relation between such substances and high blood pressure has not been convincingly established thus far. Of note, sodium excess may interfere with several other mechanisms bearing on vasomotor tone and stiffness, including 'waterlogging,' thickening of the muscular component or alteration in the protein matrix, and potentiation of the noradrenergic control system.

Interestingly, fluid removal cured malignant hypertension in the first reported long-term survivor of uremia.[34] Also in the 1960s, Vertes and colleagues observed that blood pressure became normal when 'dry-weight' was reduced by dialysis in 35 of 40 ESRF hypertensive patients.[25] In the five patients in whom blood pressure remained high despite fluid removal, plasma renin activity was 10 times higher than in the volume-responsive group.[25] These observations led to the individualization of the so-called 'volume-dependent' and 'renin-dependent' types of hypertension. Hypertension in dialysis patients thus consists primarily of extracellular fluid overload and an increase in peripheral resistance.

Increased vascular resistance in ESRF

The renin–angiotensin system

Plasma renin levels tend to be higher in patients with vascular alterations (renal artery stenosis, nephroangiosclerosis, polyarteritis) or glomerulonephritis than in those with primary tubulo-interstitial diseases, and are not suppressed when renal function is impaired progressively.[35] Ischemia of the juxtaglomerular apparatus, or interference with an inhibitory feedback on this structure, were suggested to explain increased renin release. Although the 'inappropriate' maintenance of renin activation in the presence of sodium overload parallels the difference in prevalence of hypertension associated with these nephropathies, the role of the renin system remains controversial. A correlation between renin and blood pressure was found by some[25] but not all[21] groups. When compared with normal subjects, renin levels of hypertensive patients with terminal renal failure were approximately double for a given sodium/volume state.[24,35] Moreover, in such patients, blood pressure correlated more closely with both plasma renin and volume (or exchangeable sodium) than with any of these parameters considered individually.[24] In addition, suppressed levels of circulating renin activity in chronic renal disease do coexist with an activated renal renin system, and inhibition of angiotensin II attenuates the progression of several experimental and clinical renal diseases.[36]

The important role of the renin–angiotensin system in dialysis-resistant hypertensive patients was confirmed by normalization of blood pressure following the administration of the angiotensin antagonist saralasin.[37] Similar results were subsequently obtained with the angiotensin-converting enzyme inhibitor captopril.[38] Following salt removal by dialysis, blockade of the renin system was able to normalize blood pressure in most dialysis patients.

The sympathetic nervous system

Increased sympathetic activity was shown in ESRF patients with intact native kidneys, but not in anephric patients.[39] It is postulated that renal chemoreceptors might be sensitive to uremic toxins, and that the afferent limb may, in turn, stimulate central sympathetic outflow. Experimental evidence also showed that neural fibers originating in the kidney can be activated by changes in renal blood flow, changes in pressure in the renal artery, renal vein, and ureter, or changes in the urinary tonicity or sodium content in the renal pelvis.

The sympathetic nervous system is activated in chronic renal failure, as demonstrated by increased circulating norepinephrine levels, an increased rate of sympathetic nerve discharge (estimated by the highly reliable technique of microneurographic recording of peroneal nerve sympathetic activity), and the positive effect of the sympatholytic agent clonidine.[40] In addition, a relationship between sympathetic activity and the renin–angiotensin system was suggested by the simultaneous fall in arterial pressure and sympathetic activity during long-term treatment with the angiotensin-converting enzyme inhibitor enalapril.[40]

Other vasoactive factors

In addition to renin, various substances synthesized mainly by the kidney or vascular structures may play either a vasoconstrictor, pro-hypertensive role or a vasodepressor, antihypertensive role. It was reported that chronic renal failure was associated with low levels of serum prostaglandins or urinary kallikrein. Whereas it was known for some time that renomedullary interstitial cells, the source of neutral and polar lipids potentially active as vasodilators, were altered in renal parenchymal diseases, no data on renomedullary lipids are available in patients with ESRF.

ESRF patients were shown to have elevated circulating levels of endothelin-1,[41] which has been associated with elevated blood pressure. The future use of endothelin receptor blockers in man may help to clarify this issue.[42] In addition, uremia is associated with the accumulation of substances, such as asymmetrical dimethylarginine, that act as endogenous inhibitors of nitric oxide synthesis from L-arginine, and infusion of an excess of L-arginine has been shown to lower arterial pressure in uremia.[43]

Hyperparathyroidism, which is a common complication of chronic renal failure and ESRF, is associated with an increase in vascular tone via a rise in intracellular calcium.[44] Parathyroid hormone (PTH) may have a direct effect on renin secretion, as well as on sensitization of vascular smooth muscle to vasopressors. It has also been reported that a vasopressor factor different from PTH could be isolated from the parathyroid glands of patients with tertiary hyperparathyroidism.

General principles of managing hypertension in ESRF

How to assess hypertension

Based on available information, it is unclear which blood pressure reading should be used for diagnosing hypertension and monitoring antihypertensive treatment.

Measurements of blood pressure before and after dialysis

Cyclic changes in blood pressure are observed in dialysis patients, owing to cyclic changes in hydration status. When comparing predialysis, postdialysis, and basal (days without dialysis) blood pressure, it was observed that both predialysis and postdialysis blood pressures were strongly related to basal blood pressure, although the levels are different. Generally, predialysis blood pressure overestimates, whereas postdialysis underestimates, average blood pressure. The decrease in blood pressure observed after hemodialysis is less marked in hypertensive patients. Postdialysis blood pressure is usually more closely correlated with basal interdialysis blood pressure.[45]

Ambulatory monitoring of blood pressure

Studies using 24- to 48-hour blood pressure monitoring generally confirm the above-mentioned observations. They also indicate that a substantial number of ESRF patients have lost the normal diurnal variation in blood pressure: in over 70% of patients, night-time blood pressure decreases by less than 15–20%.[46] Interestingly, the prevalence of abnormal rhythm is similar in hemodialysis and peritoneal dialysis patients and remains at about 60–70% in renal transplant recipients.[47] The loss of the nocturnal decline in blood pressure may be related to the lack of sleep, lack of physical activity, overhydration, or autonomic neuropathy. It was demonstrated that the best blood pressure predictor of left ventricular hypertrophy was nocturnal systolic blood pressure.[48] This implies that even mildly elevated blood pressure during the day might be associated with a significant global burden on the cardiovascular system,[49] and that blood pressure should be measured over 24 hours in patients with left ventricular hypertrophy despite apparently normal blood pressure. It may be postulated that diagnosis and treatment of nocturnal hypertension (by administering antihypertensive medications at night, reducing dry weight, profiling low-sodium status and long-duration hemodialysis) may decrease the incidence of death due to cardiovascular disease in these patients.

Self-measurement of blood pressure

This method is increasingly popular in the general hypertensive population, but it is unknown whether it can be used in place of 24-hour or ambulatory monitoring blood pressure as a more cost-effective tool in the measurement of blood pressure in dialysis patients.

Echocardiography

Echocardiography, which is much more sensitive than other techniques (such as fundoscopy) with regard to end-organ damage, was proposed as a means of early diagnosis and follow-up monitoring. Increased cardiac afterload due to hypertension usually results in concentric left ventricular hypertrophy. Left ventricular hypertrophy may be present at the start of dialysis treatment and its prevalence remains very high among dialysis patients. However, reversal of left ventricular hypertrophy in dialysis patients was reported with good blood pressure control.[50] Poor tolerance to ultrafiltration, congestive heart failure, arrhythmia, angina pectoris, and myocardial infarction, which contribute to the two- to threefold increase in cardiovascular mortality in dialysis patients, are direct consequences of left ventricular hypertrophy.

What is the optimal blood pressure in patients with ESRF?

The Joint National Committee on Prevention, Evaluation, and Treatment of High Blood Pressure[1] recommends a target blood pressure of less than 125/75 mmHg in patients with chronic renal insufficiency, based on the outcome of proteinuric subjects in the Modification of Diet and Renal Disease (MDRD) study. Whether these values are reasonable in dialysis patients is unknown, especially in view of the increasing prevalence of hypertension in an aging renal failure population with diabetes mellitus and atheromatous disease. In fact, lowering blood pressure too rapidly or too much may be hazardous in these patients, particularly in those with cerebrovascular disease. Others have advised that blood pressure should be maintained below 135/85 mmHg by day and below 120/80 mmHg by night.[18] Overall, the clinician should tailor the target blood pressure individually, after a comprehensive evaluation of all cardiovascular risk factors.

Treatment

Salt and volume reduction

Since no doubt remains that salt retention and sodium-fluid volume expansion is a dominant mechanism in ESRF-associated hypertension, salt and volume reduction is advocated as the cornerstone of antihypertensive therapy in such patients. Whereas a modest restriction of salt intake (approximately 5 g/day of sodium chloride) may suffice in mild renal failure, very rigid restriction or the use of diuretics (sometimes in large doses) combined with avoidance of excessive intake is mandatory in the majority of patients when glomerular filtration rate approaches 10 ml/min. Thiazide diuretics are ineffective whenever the glomerular filtration rate falls below 25 ml/min, except when used to reinforce the effects of loop diuretics. Potassium-sparing agents must be avoided altogether in almost all patients with advanced renal insufficiency, and even quite early in patients prone to hyporeninemic hypoaldosteronism—i.e. aging, diabetes mellitus, or obstructive uropathy. Most side-effects, including worsening of renal function, can be avoided by a prudent depletion combined with an adequate diet in a fraction (as yet unquantified in large trials) of patients with terminal renal failure.

Hemodialysis sessions produce cyclic changes in total body sodium and water content that are related to blood pressure. Fluid removal to achieve fluid balance is an important target of dialysis. Usually, dialysis treatments include a prescription for fluid removal until the patient's 'dry weight' is achieved at the end of the dialysis session. Dry weight is a clinically-derived value, which reflects the lowest weight a patient can tolerate without intradialytic symptoms (cramps, hypotension, etc.) and without hypertension or signs of fluid overload before the next dialysis session. As the determination of dry weight is imprecise and may not account for changes in nutritional status and lean body mass, inaccurate assessment of dry weight is a common problem. Recently, biochemical markers of volume overload (i.e. atrial natriuretic peptide, circulating cyclic GMP), echocardiographic examination of the inferior vena cava diameter and bioimpedance spectroscopy have been proposed to monitor dry weight in dialysis patients. The clinical utility of these methods is still under investigation.[51]

Reaching dry weight is an important component of dialysis adequacy. Not only is hypertension corrected in 70–80% of patients set at their correct dry weight but also the efficacy of antihypertensive agents is potentiated. Careful evaluation should be performed periodically to ensure that the prescribed dry weight is appropriate.

Factors facilitating extracellular volume control in ESRF patients

The first factor is dialysis time. In contrast to most other reports, the experience of Charra *et al.*[52] showed that long dialysis is associated with better control of blood pressure than short dialysis. Whether normotension in long dialysis schedules is achieved because of adequate extracellular volume alone or along with other factors has not been elucidated. We observed an increase in blood pressure when reducing dialysis time in a longitudinal study involving 24 patients sequentially treated with long and short dialysis. This increase in blood pressure was correlated to an increase in estimated body weight, suggesting that the rise in blood pressure was due to volume overload. Recently, a multicenter study assessing the differences in fluid status and blood pressure in two groups of patients receiving long or short dialysis showed that normotension can be achieved regardless of dialysis duration and dose when postdialysis extracellular volume is adequate.[53] However, these authors also found a group of 14 patients treated with long dialysis with increased extracellular volume and normotension, suggesting that long dialysis provides something more than simply controlling body weight.

Interdialytic weight gain should be limited in order to attenuate the interdialytic increase in blood pressure. To allow adequate fluid removal, the dialytic procedure may include the use of ultrafiltration controllers, a bicarbonate bath, manipulation of the dialysate sodium content, and the use of isolated ultrafiltration in order to prevent hypotension and cramps, the most common limiting factors for fluid removal. Of note, correction of the extracellular volume by adapting the estimated weight of the dialysis patients is a difficult, time-consuming task that is poorly accepted by the patient and frequently neglected by the clinician.

Reduction of the ultrafiltration rate during dialysis (weight loss/unit time) frequently obviates hypotensive episodes. However, reduction of the ultrafiltration rate is only allowed in those patients with limited fluid intake and small total volume excess, as well as when it is associated with an increase in dialysis time. Reduction in ultrafiltration rate in any other situation will protract increasing volume overload resulting in resistant hypertension. Increase in dialysate sodium also improves cardiovascular stability during dialysis. Thirst induction and increase in fluid intake between dialysis sessions are limiting factors.

Changes in serum calcium level may influence cardiovascular stability during dialysis. It has been suggested that lowering dialysate calcium concentration results in a decrease in

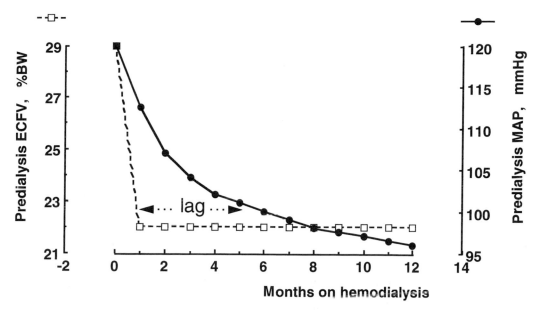

Fig. 12.2 Schematic evolution of blood pressure in relation to dry weight during the first year of hemodialysis. Blood pressure (—●—, predialysis mean arterial pressure, MAP) decreases progressively after targeted dry weight (--□--, expressed as percentage body weight, %BW) is obtained (the 'lag phenomenon'). ECFV, extracellular fluid volume. (Taken from reference 56 with permission.)

blood pressure. In a prospective study of stepwise lowering dialysate calcium concentration, we found a statistically significant decrease in diastolic blood pressure and heart rate after 1 year using a low dialysate calcium concentration (1.25 mmol/l), but no difference in hypotensive episodes during dialysis.[54] Recently, the absence of a blood pressure decrease during dialysis with low dialysate calcium concentration was confirmed, and it was observed that high dialysate calcium concentration results in impaired cardiac relaxation, suggesting that positive calcium balance during dialysis may be harmful for cardiac function.[55]

Finally, another factor limiting control of volume overload in dialysis patients has been denoted the lag phenomenon and concerns dialysis prescription (Fig. 12.2).[56] It has been demonstrated that blood pressure decreases in a sequential manner after reaching dry weight (no volume overload). The delay in normalizing blood pressure after reaching proper control of volume overload has been termed the lag phenomenon and may last weeks or months. This delay may lead the patient and the physician to conclude that resistant hypertension is not volume-dependent and modify the estimated dry weight, re-introducing an extracellular volume overload which will hinder blood pressure control.

The supposed advantages of using high flux hemodialysis or convective techniques like hemodiafiltration and hemofiltration have not been demonstrated. Although we found better blood pressure stability in a group of patients with high cardiovascular risk,[57] this difference did not appear when analyzing the complete population over a 2-year period.[58]

It has been suggested, but is not universally admitted, that continuous ambulatory peritoneal dialysis may have a better effect on blood pressure control than hemodialysis because of smoother volume removal and more sustained control of fluid balance.[59,60]

Antihypertensive drugs

In those patients in whom ultrafiltration and maintenance of an appropriate dry weight do not adequately control hypertension, antihypertensive medications are indicated. Most drugs increase vascular instability and may cause frequent and profound hypotensive episodes during dialysis. Thus, dosage and schedule must be arranged in order to decrease the action of these drugs during dialysis session.

Because centrally-acting drugs are felt to be safe and effective, these drugs have been used widely in the treatment of ESRF hypertensives. Alpha-methyldopa, clonidine, and newer imidazoline derivatives were shown to spare (or slightly improve) renal blood flow (and sometimes glomerular filtration rate) in patients with chronic renal parenchymal disease. Dose reduction (or increase in time between doses) of these drugs is recommended; however, this does not always attenuate the prevalence or the degree of side-effects, such as dry mouth or postural hypotension and the rebound phenomenon with clonidine.

Beta-blockers are generally well tolerated in uremic patients, and initial reports on an adverse effect on renal function were not confirmed. Some beta-blockers (including atenolol, bisoprolol, acebutolol) are excreted mainly by the kidney, thus requiring dosage adjustments in uremic patients, whereas others (including metoprolol, propranolol, labetalol) need only slight reduction in ESRF. Their preferential use, or disuse, will depend mainly on associated diseases; thus, beta-blockers are the treatment of choice in patients with coronary heart disease.

In addition to blood pressure reduction, calcium antagonists theoretically possess a number of properties that may contribute to a favorable effect against progression of renal injury under diverse experimental conditions and perhaps in clinical disorders (i.e. reduction in mitogenic effects of growth factors, attenuation of trafficking of macromolecules and uremic calcinosis, blockade of pressure-induced calcium entry, decreased free radical formation), but discrepancies were observed between trials. Opposite effects also occurred at other levels of the cardiovascular system, thus explaining the recent controversies over the use of short-acting dihydropyridines (which activate the adrenergic nervous system and may precipitate rapid falls in blood pressure) in patients at risk of coronary heart disease.

Calcium-channel blockers are not the only direct vasodilators available, and one should not forget that minoxidil (almost always combined with a beta-blocker and a diuretic in the non-dialyzed uremic patient) is a very potent antihypertensive drug, most notably in the renal patient.

In patients with chronic renal failure, angiotensin-converting enzyme inhibitors (ACEIs), and more recently angiotensin I (AT$_1$) receptor blockers, are effective antihypertensive agents. ACEIs are indicated particularly in cases of congestive heart failure; however, the dialysis population exhibits specific side-effects of ACEIs such as worsening of anemia and risk of anaphylactoid reaction to polyacrylonitrile membranes. Thus far, these side-effects as well as chronic cough have not been described with AT$_1$ receptor blockers.

Bilateral nephrectomy was advocated in the past to obtain a prompt control of hypertension (particularly malignant hypertension). Availability of new drugs and new dialysis techniques, and elimination of anemia, increased transfusion requirements, attenuated loss of residual renal function, and potential permanent hypotension make the use of nephrectomy no longer necessary for the treatment of hypertension or in preparation for renal transplantation.

Special situations

Hypertension in the diabetic patient

The number of dialysis patients suffering diabetes mellitus is increasing rapidly. These patients are generally hypertensive, but frequently experience orthostatic hypotension and peridialysis hypotension with severe symptoms, rendering the management of hypertension particularly difficult.

Since exchangeable sodium is increased in the diabetic patient, reduction of sodium intake and administration of diuretic drugs (when residual diuresis persists) are particularly suitable approaches in such patients. It is also important to reach the target dry weight at each dialysis session. Long dialysis, with slow ultrafiltration rate and glucose-containing dialysate, may help to avoid the risk of severe hypotension.

In addition to decreasing blood pressure, ACEIs may prevent end-organ vascular disease in diabetics. It is reasonable to assume that angiotensin receptor blockers will have similar efficacy, but confirmation of this assumption is still pending. Calcium-channel blockers are effective in reducing hypertension in dialysis patients but may result in severe hypotensive episodes. Beta-blockers are avoided by some physicians in diabetic patients because of their side-effects (absence of hypoglycemic symptoms). However, it was recently suggested that cardiac death rates in non-insulin dependent diabetes mellitus (NIDDM) patients on dialysis not receiving beta-blockers approaches 30%, and that the cardiac benefit derived from beta-blockade is particularly significant in NIDDM patients.[61]

In practice, diabetic patients must be at their dry weight before starting antihypertensive treatment. Atherosclerotic cerebrovascular disease should be excluded by ultrasound-Doppler echography, as cerebral autoregulation is impaired and rapid lowering of blood pressure may result in cerebral hypoperfusion and cerebrovascular accidents. Initial doses of antihypertensive medications must be decreased, and, if needed, gradually increased. ACEI is the first line therapy, followed by beta-blockers and calcium-channel blockers if necessary.

As coronary artery disease is frequent in DM, some physicians fear the development of cardiac ischemia when lowering blood pressure below 85 mmHg ('J-curve' phenomenon). In the MDRD study, no evidence of a J-curve phenomenon was found.[62] In fact, a low systolic blood pressure is a marker of severe cardiac disease rather than a cause of cardiac death. Nevertheless, diabetic patients should be monitored carefully when initiating antihypertensive treatment as cardiac ischemia may develop in some cases.

Finally, owing to autonomic neuropathy, severe orthostatic hypotension (which is associated with increased mortality) may be observed in diabetic patients. It is advisable to avoid hypovolemia and administer the maximum of antihypertensive medications at bedtime to avoid nocturnal hypertension and severe standing hypotension.

Erythropoietin-associated hypertension

Erythropoietin (rhEpo) treatment is a major advance which has provided substantial improvements in clinical well-being, myocardial function, and lipid profiles in dialysis patients. Treatment of anemia with rhEpo results in a reduction of heart rate, cardiac contractility, and left ventricular hypertrophy, and a small increase (10 mmHg) in blood pressure. Hypertension is the most frequent side-effect of rhEpo therapy (30% of patients) and usually appears during the first 3 months of treatment. It may present as

Table 12.2 Practical recommendations for treatment of erythropoietin (rhEpo)-induced hypertension

---

Try to decrease the actual dry weight
Decrease doses or interrupt treatment and reintroduce later at lower dosage
Introduce or increase antihypertensive medications (beta-blockers, calcium channel blockers, or angiotensin-converting enzyme inhibitors)
Discontinue rhEpo and give IV antihypertensive drugs in cases of malignant hypertension
Bleeding and hemodilution in cases of severe hypertension associated with rapid increase in hematocrit

---

de novo hypertension in a previously normotensive patient or as worsening of existing hypertension. The precise cause of rhEpo-associated hypertension is not totally understood, but factors such as an increase in plasma viscosity and augmentation of peripheral vascular resistances have been implicated. Moreover, rhEpo may bind directly to endothelial cell surface receptors, resulting in smooth muscle contraction. Finally, it was suggested that rhEpo-induced hypertension is hematocrit-independent and associated with elevated cytosolic calcium and attenuated activity of the nitric oxide pathway. These abnormalities may be reversed by calcium channel blockade.[63] A history of hypertension, elevated dry weight, rapid correction of anemia (≤ weeks), and high target hemoglobin levels (≥12 g/dl) are associated with increased risk of rhEpo-induced hypertension. Practical recommendations for treatment of rhEpo-associated hypertension are summarized in Table 12.2.

Refractory hypertension

Despite volume control and antihypertensive medications, some dialysis patients remain hypertensive. When faced with this problem, clinicians should first suspect an overestimation of the 'dry weight'. In fact, measurement of vasopressin levels suggested the presence of water excess in the majority of patients with refractory hypertension. Second, one should also exclude renovascular hypertension, expanding cysts in polycystic disease, and the use of over-the-counter vasculative medications. In addition to the combination of salt depletion and blockade of the renin system, it was reported that the association of minoxidil and beta-blockade may be useful in this situation.

Conclusion

Hypertension is both a cause—of apparently increasing incidence—and a complication—of persisting importance—of ESRF. Simply put, hypertension is a potent determinant of survival in ESRF patients. Sodium/volume excess is the dominant mechanism underlying the rise in blood pressure in ESRF. Up to 90% of patients entering dialysis programs are hypertensive, whereas less than 10% may require antihypertensive therapy when 'dry weight' is maintained over the long-term through longer dialysis sessions combined with a low-salt diet. A number of antihypertensive drugs may help to correct the other mechanisms of hypertension in the hypertensive dialysis patient, but the interplay of comorbid risk factors and situations may make the maintenance of optimal blood pressure difficult.

References

1. The sixth report of the Joint National Committee on prevention, detection, evaluation, and treatment of high blood pressure (1997) *Archives of Internal Medicine* 157:2413–46
2. Klag MJ, Whelton PK, Randall BL, Neaton JD, Brancati FL, Stamler J. (1997) End-stage renal disease in African-American and white men: 16-year MRFIT findings. *Journal of the American Medical Association* 277:1293–8
3. Valderràbano F, Gòmez-Campderà F, Jones EH. (1998) Hypertension as cause of end-stage renal disease: lessons from international registries. *Kidney International* 68:s60–6
4. Kaylor WM, Novick AC, Ziegelbaum M, Vidt DG. (1989) Reversal of end-stage renal failure with surgical revascularization in patients with atherosclerotic renal artery stenosis. *Journal of Urology* 141:486–8
5. Hansen KJ, Thomason RB, Craven TE, Fuller SB, Keith DR, Appel RG, et al. (1995) Surgical management of dialysis-dependent ischemic nephropathy. *Journal of Vascular Surgery* 21:197–211
6. Brown JJ, Düsterdieck G, Fraser F, Lever AF, Robertson JI, Tree M, et al. (1971) Hypertension and chronic renal failure. *British Medical Bulletin* 27:128–135.
7. Mimran A, Ribstein J. (1992) Antihypertensive therapy in renal disease and transplantation. *Journal of Hypertension* 10(Suppl 5):s79–85
8. Klahr S, Levey AS, Beck GJ, Caggiula AW, Hunsicker L, Kusek JW, et al. (1994) The effects of dietary protein restriction and blood-pressure control on the progression of chronic renal disease. Modification of Diet in Renal Disease Study Group. *New England Journal of Medicine* 330:877–84
9. Lindner A, Charra B, Sherrard DJ, Scribner BH. (1974) Accelerated atherosclerosis in prolonged maintenance hemodialysis. *New England Journal of Medicine* 290:697–701
10. Degoulet P, Legrain M, Reach I, Aime F, Devries C, Rojas P, et al. (1982) Mortality risk factors in patients treated by chronic hemodialysis. Report of the Diaphane Collaborative Study. *Nephron* 31:103–10
11. Charra B, Calemard E, Cuche M, Laurent G. (1983) Control of hypertension and prolonged survival on maintenance hemodialysis. *Nephron* 33:96–9
12. Rostand SG, Brunzell JD, Cannon RO III, Victor RG. (1991) Cardiovascular complications in renal failure *Journal of the American Society of Nephrology* 2:1053–62
13. Salem MM. (1995) Hypertension in the hemodialysis population: a survey of 649 patients. *American Journal of Kidney Diseases* 26:461–8
14. Kimura G, Tomita J, Nakamura S, Uzu T, Inenaga T. (1996) Interaction between hypertension and other cardiovascular risk factors in survival of hemodialyzed patients. *American Journal of Hypertension* 9:1006–12
15. Foley RN, Parfrey PS, Harnett JD, Kent GM, Murray DC, Barre PE. (1996) Impact of hypertension of cardiomyopathy, morbidity and mortality in end-stage renal disease. *Kidney International* 49:1379–85
16. Cheigh JS, Milite C, Sullivan SF, Rubin A, Stenzel KH. (1992) Hypertension is not adequately controlled in hemodialysis patients. *American Journal of Kidney Diseases* 19:453–9
17. Cheigh JS, Serur D, Paguirigan M, Stenzel KH, Rubin A. (1994) How well is hypertension controlled in CAPD patients? *Advances in Peritoneal Dialysis* 10:55–8
18. Mailloux LU, Haley WE. (1998) Hypertension in the ESRD patient: pathophysiology, therapy, outcomes, and future directions. *American Journal of Kidney Diseases* 32:705–19
19. Dorhout Mees EJ. (1999) Hypertension in haemodialysis patients: who cares? *Nephrology, Dialysis, and Transplantation* 14:28–30
20. Kim KE, Swartz C. (1993) Cardiovascular complications of end-stage renal disease. In: Schrier RW, Gottschalk CW, editors. *Diseases of the kidney*, pp. 2817–44. Boston: Little Brown & Co.
21. Cangiano JL, Ramirez-Muxo O, Ramirez-Gonzales R, Trevino A, Campos JA. (1976) Normal renin uremic hypertension: study of cardiac hemodynamics, plasma volume, extracellular fluid volume, and the renin angiotensin system. *Archives of Internal Medicine* 136:17–23

22. Blumberg A, Nelp WB, Hegstrom RM, Scribner BH. (1967) Extracellular volume in patients with chronic renal disease treated for hypertension by sodium restriction. *The Lancet* 2:69–73

23. Weidmann P. (1984) Pathogenesis of hypertension associated with chronic renal failure. *Contributions to Nephrology* 41:47–65

24. Safar ME, London GM, Weiss YA, Milliez PL. (1975) Overhydration and renin in hypertensive patients with terminal renal failure: a hemodynamic study. *Clinical Nephrology* 4:183–8

25. Vertes V, Cangiano JL, Berman LB, Gould A. (1969) Hypertension in end-stage renal disease. *New England Journal of Medicine* 280:978–81

26. Bricker NS, Fine LG, Kaplan M, Epstein M, Bourgoignie JJ, Light A. (1978) 'Magnification phenomenon' in chronic renal disease. *New England Journal of Medicine* 299:1287–93

27. Guyton AC. (1987) Renal function curve: a key to understanding the pathogenesis of hypertension. *Hypertension* 10:1–6

28. Coleman TG, Bower JD, Langford HG, Guyton AC. (1970) Regulation of arterial pressure in the anephric state. *Circulation* 42:509–14

29. Merrill JP, Giordano C, Heetderky DR. (1961) The role of the kidney in human hypertension. I. Failure of hypertension to develop in the renoprival subjects. *American Journal of Medicine* 31:931–40

30. Tarazi RC, Dustan HP, Frohlich ED, Gifford RW Jr, Hoffman GC. (1970) Plasma volume and chronic hypertension. Relationship to arterial pressure levels in different hypertensive disease. *Archives of Internal Medicine* 125:835–42

31. Koomans HA, Roos JC, Dorhout Mees EJ, Delawi IM. (1985) Sodium balance in renal failure. A comparison of patients with normal subjects under extremes of sodium intake. *Hypertension* 7:714–21

32. De Wardener HE, MacGregor GA. (1980) Dahl's hypothesis that a saluretic substance may be responsible for sustained rise in arterial pressure: its possible role in essential hypertension. *Kidney International* 18:1–9

33. Kelly RA, O'Hara DS, Mitch WE, Steinman TI, Goldszer RC, Somomon HS, *et al.* (1986) Endogenous digitalis-like factors in hypertension and chronic renal insufficiency. *Kidney International* 30:723–9

34. Scribner BH. (1960) The treatment of chronic uremia by means of intermittent hemodialysis. A preliminary report. *Transactions of the American Society of Artificial Organs* 7:136–49

35. Weidmann P, Maxwell MH. (1975) The renin–angiotensin–aldosterone system in terminal renal failure. *Kidney International* 8 (Suppl 1):s219–34

36. Rosenberg ME, Smith LJ, Correa-Rotter R, Hostetter TH. (1994) The paradox of the renin–angiotensin system in chronic renal disease. *Kidney International* 45:403–10

37. Mimran A, Shaldon S, Barjon P, Mion CM. (1978) The effect of an angiotensin antagonist (saralasin) on arterial pressure and plasma aldosterone in hemodialysis-resistant hypertensive patients. *Clinical Nephrology* 9:63–7

38. Wauters JP, Waeber B, Brunner HR, Guignard JP, Turini GA, Gavras H. (1981) Uncontrollable hypertension in patients on hemodialysis: long-term treatment with captopril and salt subtraction. *Clinical Nephrology* 16:86–92

39. Converse RL Jr, Jacobsen TN, Toto RD, Jost CM, Cosentino F, Fouad-Tarazi F, *et al.* (1992) Sympathetic overactivity in patients with chronic renal failure. *New England Journal of Medicine* 327:1912–18

40. Ligtenberg G, Blankestijn PJ, Oey DL, Klein IH, Dijkhorst-Oei LT, Boomsma F, *et al.* (1999) Reduction of sympathetic hyperactivity by enalapril in patients with chronic renal failure. *New England Journal of Medicine* 340:1321–8

41. Koyama H, Tabata T, Nishizawa Y, Inoue T, Morii H, Yamaji T. (1989) Plasma endothelin levels in patients with uremia. *The Lancet* 1:991–2

42. Hand MF, Haynes WG, Webb DJ. (1999) Reduced endogenous endothelin-1-mediated vascular tone in chronic renal failure. *Kidney International* 55:613–20

43. Vallance P, Leone A, Calver A, Collier J, Moncada S. (1992) Accumulation of an endogenous inhibitor of nitric oxide synthesis in chronic renal failure. *The Lancet* 339:572–5
44. Raine AE, Bedford L, Simpson AW, Ashley CC, Brown R, Woodhead JS, *et al.* (1993) Hyperparathyroidism, platelet intracellular free calcium and hypertension in chronic renal failure. *Kidney International* 43:700–5
45. Lopez-Gomez JM, Verde E, Perez-Garcia R. (1998) Blood pressure, left ventricular hypertrophy and long-term prognosis in hemodialysis patients. *Kidney International* 68:s92–8
46. Farmer CK, Goldsmith DJ, Cox J, Dallyn P, Kingswood JC, Sharpstone P. (1997) An investigation of the effect of advancing uremia, renal replacement therapy, and renal transplantation on blood pressure diurnal variability. *Nephrology, Dialysis, and Transplantation* 12:2301–7
47. Farmer CK, Goldsmith DJ. (1998) Nocturnal hypertension in dialysis patients. *Seminars in Dialysis* 11:261–3
48. Tucker B, Fabbian F, Giles M, Thuraisingham RC, Raine AE, Baker LR. (1997) Left ventricular hypertrophy and ambulatory blood pressure monitoring in chronic renal failure. *Nephrology, Dialysis, and Transplantation* 12:724–8
49. Amar J, Vernier I, Rossignol E, Lenfant V, Conte JJ, Chamontin B. (1997) Influence of nycthemeral blood pressure pattern in treated hypertensive patients on hemodialysis. *Kidney International* 51:1863–6
50. Cannella G, Paoletti E, Delfino R, Peloso G, Molinari S, Traverso GB. (1993) Regression of left ventricular hypertrophy in hypertensive dialyzed uremic patients on long-term antihypertensive therapy. *Kidney International* 44:881–6
51. Jaeger JQ, Mehta RL. (1999) Assessment of dry weight in hemodialysis: an overview. *Journal of the American Society of Nephrology* 10:392–403
52. Charra B, Calemard E, Ruffet M, Chazot C, Terrat J-C, Vanel T, *et al.* (1992) Survival as an index of adequacy of dialysis. *Kidney International* 41:1286–91
53. Katzarski KS, Charra B, Luik AJ, Nisell J, Divino Filho JC, Leypoldt JK, *et al.* (1999) Fluid state and blood pressure control in patients treated with long and short haemodialysis. *Nephrology, Dialysis, and Transplantation* 14:369–75
54. Argilès A, Kerr PG, Canaud B, Flavier JL, Mion CM. (1993) Calcium kinetics and the long-term effects of lowering dialysate calcium concentration. *Kidney International* 43:630–40
55. Näppi SE, Saha HH, Virtanen VK, Mustonen JT, Pasternack AI. (1999) Hemodialysis with high-calcium dialysate impairs cardiac relaxation. *Kidney International* 55:1091–6
56. Charra B, Bergström J, Scribner BH. (1998) Blood pressure control in dialysis patients: importance of the lag phenomenon. *American Journal of Kidney Diseases* 32:720–4
57. Mion M, Kerr PG, Argilès A, Canaud B, Flavier JL, Mion CM. (1992) Haemofiltration in high-cardiovascular risk patients. *Nephrology, Dialysis, and Transplantation* 7:453–4
58. Kerr PG, Argilès A, Flavier JL, Canaud B, Mion CM. (1992) Comparison of hemodialysis and hemodiafiltration: a long-term longitudinal study. *Kidney International* 41:1035–40
59. Saldanha LF, Weiler EW, Gonick HC. (1993) Effect of continuous ambulatory peritoneal dialysis on blood pressure control. *American Journal of Kidney Diseases* 21:184–8
60. Rocco MV, Flanigan MJ, Beaver S, Frederick P, Gentile DE, McClellan WM, *et al.* (1996) Core Indicators for Peritoneal Dialysis Study Group. *American Journal of Kidney Diseases* 30:165–73
61. Koch M, Thomas B, Tschope W, Ritz E. (1993) Survival and predictors of death in dialysed diabetic patients. *Diabetologia* 36:1113–7
62. Klahr S. (1996) Role of dietary protein and blood pressure in the progression of renal disease (abstract). *Kidney International* 49:179
63. Ni Z, Wang XQ, Vaziri ND. (1998) Nitric oxide metabollism in erythropoietin-induced hypertension: effect of calcium channel blockade. *Hypertension* 32:724–9.

13

Congestive heart failure and its management in end-stage renal failure

Liam F. Casserly and Michael M. Givertz

Introduction

Despite advances in the fields of dialysis and renal transplantation, morbidity and mortality remain high in patients with end-stage renal failure (ESRF). Although an overall reduction in crude death rate has been reported in the United States ESRF population since 1988, cardiovascular disease remains the most common cause of mortality. Cardiac arrest and acute myocardial infarction account for the majority of cardiac deaths, but congestive heart failure (CHF) contributes significantly to all other cardiovascular mortality.[1]

Epidemiology

Incidence and prevalence

CHF is present in approximately 40% of patients at initiation of dialysis. Of 220 patients starting dialysis in Canada between 1970 and 1975, 45% reported a history of CHF.[2] Similarly, 41% of incident patients in the United States Renal Data System (USRDS) and 31% of patients who survived 6 months in a prospective, multicenter, Canadian study of chronic renal failure had CHF at initiation of dialysis.[3] Despite improvement in the medical management of ESRF over the past two decades (biocompatible membranes, bicarbonate-based dialysate, and superior dialysis technology), CHF remains a common clinical entity, especially in older patients.

In addition to contributing to the burden of disease at initiation of dialysis, CHF accounts for a significant number of hospitalizations in patients on chronic renal replacement therapy. Fifty-six percent of patients with CHF at baseline developed recurrent CHF during follow-up on dialysis compared to only 25% of patients without CHF at baseline.[3] Overall, the rate of hospitalization for CHF in the cohort followed by Harnett and colleagues was 7% per year. Similar findings have been reported in the Canadian Hemodialysis Morbidity Study.[4]

Prognosis

CHF is a strong independent predictor of death in patients with ESRF. Hutchinson and colleagues[2] reported a doubling in the relative risk of death in uremic patients with CHF prior to initiation of dialysis compared to ESRF patients without CHF. This increase in mortality occurred during the first 6 months of dialysis. In a subsequent study, CHF was a

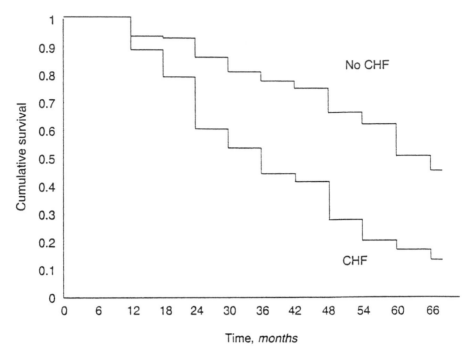

Fig. 13.1 Unadjusted survival curves demonstrating the increase in mortality in ESRF patients with congestive heart failure (CHF) at the time of initiation of dialysis compared to patients without CHF ($p < 0.001$). Adapted from Harnett and colleagues,[3] with permission.

strong predictor of mortality in ESRF for all modalities of treatment.[3] The median survival of patients with CHF at baseline was 36 months compared to 62 months in those without CHF (Fig. 13.1). The prognosis was worse for patients with CHF at baseline who had recurrent CHF during follow-up, with a median survival of only 18 months. The adverse prognosis attributed to CHF appears to be independent of age, diabetes, and ischemic heart disease.

Myocardial abnormalities alter survival directly in patients with ESRF. Using echocardiography to follow changes in ventricular size and function, Foley and colleagues[5] performed a large, prospective, observational study in 432 patients with ESRF. At initiation of dialysis, left ventricular hypertrophy (LVH), dilatation, and systolic dysfunction were present in 74%, 36%, and 15% of patients, respectively. While older age, diabetes, CHF, peripheral vascular disease, and systolic dysfunction predicted death at all times, increased LV volume and mass were the strongest independent predictors of late mortality (i.e. after 2 years). Patients with abnormal echocardiograms at initiation of dialysis had decreased survival, independent of age, gender, and diabetes.

Pathophysiology

Congestive heart failure is a clinical syndrome characterized by signs and symptoms of volume overload and/or reduced cardiac output. In pathophysiological terms, heart failure occurs when the heart fails to pump blood at a rate sufficient to meet the metabolic needs of

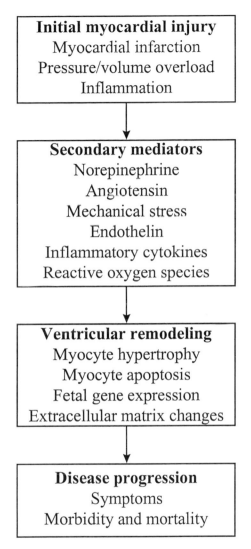

Fig. 13.2 Proposed sequence of events in the progression of myocardial failure. After an initial injury, various secondary mediators such as norepinephrine, angiotensin, and mechanical stress act on the myocardium to cause ventricular remodeling. Recent studies suggest that additional mediators, including endothelin, cytokines, and reactive oxygen species, are upregulated in human heart failure. As these factors have the ability to cause growth and apoptosis in cardiac myocytes, and alter the extracellular matrix, they may also play an important role in remodeling. Adapted from Colucci,[109] with permission.

the body or when it does so only with an elevated filling pressure. Over the past two decades, our understanding of the pathophysiology of CHF has changed considerably. It is now recognized that many acute adaptations to cardiac injury become maladaptive over time. Neurohormonal activation, for example, which initially helps to maintain blood pressure and cardiac output, may promote ventricular remodeling and contribute to disease progression in heart failure (Fig. 13.2). In the setting of ESRF, pressure and volume overload,

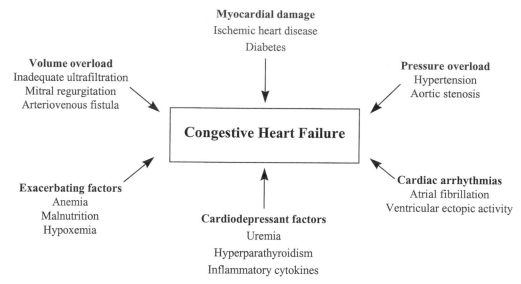

Fig. 13.3 Factors contributing to the development of congestive heart failure in patients with ESRF. Adapted from Leier and Boudoulas,[110] with permission.

ischemic and valvular heart disease, arrhythmias, malnutrition, and cardiodepressant factors accelerate disease progression (Fig. 13.3).

Systolic vs. diastolic dysfunction

Most commonly, heart failure reflects an abnormality of ventricular contractile function. End-systolic volume, end-diastolic volume, and end-diastolic pressure are increased, and stroke volume falls. Symptoms of reduced cardiac output and systemic and pulmonary congestion develop. Systolic dysfunction may result from loss of myocytes (e.g. myocardial infarction), chronic volume overload, or dilated cardiomyopathy, and is characterized clinically by cardiomegaly and low ejection fraction. More than one-third of patients with CHF have preserved LV systolic function, with diastolic dysfunction causing impairment in ventricular filling. In patients with diastolic heart failure, LV end-diastolic pressures are elevated, and pulmonary vascular congestion develops. Common causes of diastolic heart failure include ischemia and LVH. A major cause of heart failure in ESRF, that due to coronary artery disease, often reflects a combination of systolic and diastolic dysfunction: systolic dysfunction due to prior infarction and ischemia-induced decrease in contractility, and diastolic dysfunction due to replacement fibrosis and ischemia-induced decrease in distensibility.

Neurohormonal activation

Reduced cardiac output and increased filling pressures cause activation of the sympathetic nervous system and renin–angiotensin system.[6] Primary consequences of neurohormonal activation include an increase in systemic vascular resistance and sodium and water retention. Following a primary myocardial injury, elevated circulating catecholamines help to maintain cardiac output, blood pressure, and vital organ perfusion. The long-term effects of sympathetic overactivity, however, are deleterious and include myocardial hypertrophy and fibrosis, beta-receptor downregulation, a proarrhythmic state, impaired baroreceptor function, and peripheral vascular endothelial dysfunction.[7] Like norepinephrine, angiotensin II is upregulated in heart failure and results in systemic vasoconstriction and intravascular volume expansion. In the myocardium, stimulation of angiotensin receptors causes hypertrophy and fibrosis.

Whereas systemic vasoconstriction and volume retention contribute to the progression of LV failure, increased pulmonary vascular tone may contribute to right ventricular failure and reduced exercise tolerance. Endothelin (ET)-1 is a potent vasoconstrictor peptide with growth-promoting effects that may play an important role in the systemic and pulmonary vasoconstriction in patients with heart failure.[8] ET-1 also mediates hypertrophy and fibrosis in failing myocardium.[9] Plasma ET-1 levels are elevated in ESRF and are associated with the development of LVH.[10] Other potential mediators of LV failure include aldosterone, inflammatory cytokines, and reactive oxygen species.[11]

Ventricular hypertrophy and remodeling

Increased ventricular wall stress due to LV dilatation or increased afterload stimulates myocardial hypertrophy. The resultant increase in wall thickness normalizes wall stress and maintains contractility. At the cellular level, increases in myocyte size, mitochondrial and myofibrillar mass, and interstitial collagen content occur. Molecular events include reappearance of fetal gene expression and the production of abnormal proteins.[7] If additional chamber dilatation occurs or the increase in wall thickness is insufficient, systolic and diastolic wall stresses remain abnormally elevated. Further remodeling may occur, resulting in hemodynamic failure.

Volume overload and pulmonary edema

Increased total body volume is the most common precipitant of acute pulmonary edema in patients with ESRF. Once an acute ischemic event has been excluded, ultrafiltration alone may be sufficient to treat left-sided congestion. In one study, 70% of patients presenting to the emergency room with pulmonary edema were discharged following ultrafiltration without untoward consequences.[12] From a pathophysiological perspective, volume removal shifts a patient along the LV function curve to a point where he or she is asymptomatic with preserved cardiac output (Fig. 13.4). Thus, establishing an accurate dry weight in the ESRF patient is central to achieving the goal of adequate ultrafiltration.

Dry weight is defined as the weight below which hypotension and/or muscle cramps develop. In ESRF patients with systolic dysfunction, pulmonary edema is often heralded by excessive weight gain. In patients with predominant diastolic dysfunction, minimal weight gain does not exclude volume overload as the cause of pulmonary edema. Several investigators have been unable to demonstrate a difference in interdialytic weight gain between patients who develop CHF and those who do not. The difference could come from a difference in the basal hydration state: overhydration in those who develop CHF versus euvolaemic state in those who are free of CHF.

The pulmonary capillary bed may contribute to the development of pulmonary edema in patients with ESRF. In the setting of normal pulmonary artery pressures, capillary hydraulic pressure is low, and capillaries are more permeable than other tissues to albumin.[13] These factors might be expected to protect the lungs from edema formation in the setting of mild to moderate hypoalbuminemia, which is common in ESRF. However, older studies have

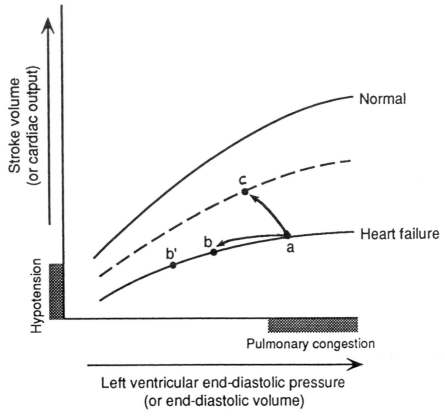

Fig. 13.4 The effects of ultrafiltration and vasodilator therapy on the left ventricular (LV) function curve in a patient with ESRF and chronic heart failure. Point a represents the failing heart on an LV function curve that has been shifted downward compared to normal. Stroke volume (SV) is reduced and LV end-diastolic pressure (LVEDP) is increased resulting in pulmonary congestion. Ultrafiltration (moving from point a to point b) reduces LV pressure without a significant change in stroke volume. Excessive ultrafiltration (moving to point b') results in a fall in SV and hypotension. Balanced vasodilation with an angiotensin-converting enzyme inhibitor (moving to point c) augments SV and reduces LVEDP. Adapted from Frankel and Fifer,[111] with permission.

suggested that reversible capillary permeability to sodium in the uremic environment may contribute to the development of pulmonary edema.[14,15]

Pathogenesis and etiology

Acute heart failure

In general, the clinical manifestations of heart failure depend on the rate at which the syndrome develops (i.e. whether enough time has elapsed for compensatory mechanisms to become operative and interstitial fluid to accumulate). Acute heart failure can occur in a number of settings in the ESRF patient (Table 13.1). The most common precipitant of acute heart failure is volume overload usually due to inadequate ultrafiltration or patient non-compliance with fluid and sodium restriction. Acute infective endocarditis secondary to

Table 13.1 Etiology of heart failure in ESRF

Acute	Volume overload
	Infective endocarditis
	Sepsis
	Pericardial tamponade
	Myocardial infarction
	Atrial arrhythmias
Chronic	Volume overload
	Hypertension
	Ischemic heart disease
	Valvular heart disease (e.g. aortic stenosis, mitral regurgitation)
	Constrictive pericarditis
	ESRF-specific factors (e.g. arteriovenous fistula, anemia, cardiodepressant factors)
	Sleep apnea
	Malnutrition
	Systemic disease with cardiac and renal involvement (e.g. sarcoidosis)

infection of a central catheter or synthetic vascular graft can result in severe aortic and/or mitral regurgitation with or without valve rupture. In this setting, acute heart failure is an indication for urgent surgical repair and prolonged treatment with parenteral antibiotics. Valvular calcification in ESRF makes patients more susceptible to the development of endocarditis. Sepsis without valvular involvement is also common in this patient population and may be related to indwelling grafts or catheters, and underlying diabetes. The sepsis syndrome is associated with marked activation of inflammatory cytokines that can exert direct negative inotropic effects and precipitate heart failure. Pericarditis leading to large pericardial effusions has been reported in ESRF, and pericardial tamponade may occur following ultrafiltration. Myocardial infarction is the single most common non-fatal cardiac complication in the ESRF patient. A high degree of suspicion for an acute ischemic event should prevail when a uremic patient presents with new onset heart failure, even in the absence of chest pain. Finally, the acute onset of atrial fibrillation or flutter during or immediately following dialysis may precipitate heart failure. Atrial arrhythmias often occur in ESRF patients with hypertension and LVH as a result of acute fluid and electrolyte shifts. Pericarditis has been a frequent cause of acute heart failure in the early days of renal replacement therapy when dialysis treatment was initiated relatively late in the course of chronic renal failure. It still occurs occasionally at present, most often due to underdialysis, for example in the case of insufficient a-v fistula blood flow.

Chronic heart failure

Non-invasive techniques have been used to demonstrate ventricular remodeling in patients with ESRF. Parfrey and colleagues[16] obtained serial echocardiograms in 275 of 432 uremic patients followed in a prospective observational study. At a mean follow-up of 17 months, 8% of patients with LVH at baseline and 22% of patients with LV dilatation developed systolic dysfunction defined as a fractional shortening less than or equal to 25%. Conversely, 11% and 7% of patients with LVH and LV dilatation, respectively, normalized their echocardiographic abnormalities. Patients with progressive dilatation and impairment of systolic function had gradual lowering of blood pressure. Time on dialysis appears to corre-late with the reduction in ejection fraction.[17] The mechanisms responsible for ventricular remodeling in ESRF are incompletely understood, but are most likely to involve a chronic interplay between prevalent cardiovascular disease states (e.g. hypertension, coronary artery disease) and ESRF-specific factors (e.g. anemia, uremia).

Hypertension

In the non-ESRF population, hypertension is a well-established risk factor for the develop-ment of LVH and dilated cardiomyopathy.[18] Likewise, in ESRF, hypertension appears to play an important contributory role in the development of heart failure.[16,17] Cardiac hyper-trophy and hypertension in ESRF are discussed in detail in Chapters 7 and 12, respectively.

Ischemic heart disease

Most commonly, ischemia-induced heart failure in patients with ESRF is due to obstructive coronary artery disease. In uremic patients with LVH, ischemia may occur in the absence of significant coronary artery disease as a result of abnormal coronary vasodilator reserve, altered myocardial oxygen delivery, and small vessel disease.[19,20] Calcification of small blood vessels due to a high calcium-phosphorus product appears to contribute to reduced myocar-dial blood flow under conditions of stress. Myocardial capillary density may also be decreased in hypertensive renal failure.[21] Ischemic heart disease in ESRF is discussed in detail in Chapters 3 and 14.

Valvular heart disease

Valvular disease is common in ESRF, although the extent to which it contributes to CHF is not known (see Chapter 16). In uremic patients, calcific lesions of the mitral and aortic valves tend to occur approximately 20 years earlier than in the general population.[22] Aortic calcification is present in 30–50% of patients, while hemodynamically significant aortic stenosis occurs in only a minority (i.e. 3–14% of all dialysis patients).[23] Risk factors for the development of aortic calcification include increasing age, length of time on dialysis, and increased calcium-phosphorus product. Mitral calcification with associated regurgitation is also a common echocardiographic finding.[24] In one study, intensive ultrafiltration resulted in a marked decrease in mitral and tricuspid regurgitation,[25] suggesting that valvular insufficiency may be secondary to increased preload rather than intrinsic valvular disease. Rapid calcification of bioprosthetic valves has also been reported.

Pericardial disease

Uremic pericarditis and asymptomatic pericardial effusions are common in patients with ESRF. Repeated episodes of pericarditis may lead to asymptomatic thickening of the pericardium. Chronic constrictive pericarditis is a rare complication of uremia-associated pericardial disease.[26]

Ventricular arrythmias

Ventricular ectopic activity (VEA) is common in ESRF, occurring in 18–56% of patients depending on the population studied.[27] As assessed by 24-hour Holter monitoring, VEA occurs predominantly during, and for 4 hours following, dialysis. Ventricular arrhythmias in ESRF have been associated with increased LV mass and dimensions, regional wall motion abnormalities, and reduced fractional shortening.[27,28] VEA is more common with hemodialysis than peritoneal dialysis,[29] and may be precipitated by potassium shifts or increased calcium-phosphorus product. The incidence of sudden cardiac death in ESRF patients with heart failure has not been well defined.

Nocturnal hypoxemia

Sleep apnea is common in ESRF patients,[30] and repeated episodes of nocturnal hypoxemia may contribute to hypertension and the development of LVH and cardiomyopathy.[31] While supplemental oxygen and continuous positive airway pressure have been shown to have beneficial effects in non-uremic heart failure patients with sleep-disordered breathing,[32] their therapeutic role in ESRF has not been tested.

ESRF-specific factors

Several factors common to patients with ESRF predispose to the development of CHF and cardiomyopathy. These include arteriovenous fistulae, chronic anemia, nutritional deficiencies, and 'cardiodepressant' factors associated with uremia.

Arteriovenous fistulae   In healthy dialysis patients, occlusion of an arteriovenous fistula results in a significant reduction in cardiac output. Rarely, a large arteriovenous fistula carrying blood flows of up to 2.5 l/min can lead to high-output cardiac failure.[33] This problem may go unrecognized for long periods, but when diagnosed is correctable by surgical ligation. In dialysis patients, an a-v fistula blood flow of more than 1000 to 1500 ml/min may contribute or even cause high-output cardiac failure, that is at a flow rate much lower than in non-uraemic patients. This is probably due to concomitant factors such as anaemia and hypertension.

Anemia   Chronic anemia may contribute to the progression of heart failure in ESRF. Each 1 g/dl decrease in hemoglobin level is independently associated with the development of LV dilatation and of *de novo* and recurrent heart failure.[34] Recombinant human erythropoietin, now used routinely in the treatment of the anemia of renal disease, may alter cardiovascular structure and function. Partial correction of anemia with erythropoietin leads to regression of LVH,[35] and attenuates the hyperdynamic circulation associated with ESRF.[36] However, complete normalization of hematocrit in ESRF patients with heart failure may increase mortality.[37]

Malnutrition   It is estimated that 30–60% of dialysis patients are malnourished, and serum albumin is a strong independent predictor of mortality in this population.[38] A dialysis patient with a serum albumin < 2.5 g/dl has a threefold increased risk of mortality compared with a dialysis patient with a history of myocardial infarction (a risk equaled only by a history of acquired immune deficiency syndrome (AIDS) or metastatic cancer).[39] Hypoalbuminemia is also a risk factor for the development of heart failure in ESRF. Both the Canadian Hemodialysis Morbidity Study[4] and Foley and colleagues[40] found that a serum albumin less than 3.0 g/dl was associated with a greater likelihood of developing *de novo* and recurrent CHF.

The syndrome of cardiac cachexia is well recognized in non-ESRF patients with CHF and is associated with an adverse prognosis. Several metabolic pathways that cause catabolic/anabolic imbalance have been implicated in this syndrome, including the growth hormone-insulin-like growth factor-1 system and the pituitary–thyroid hormone axis. In 1990, Levine and colleagues[41] demonstrated increased circulating levels of tumor necrosis

Table 13.2   Potential cardiodepressant factors in ESRF

Urea
Creatinine
Secondary hyperparathyroidism
Hypocalcemia
Hypophosphatemia
Increased calcium-phosphorus product
Inflammatory cytokines
Acetate buffer
Acidosis
Hypoxemia

---

factor (TNF)-α in patients with severe chronic heart failure and cardiac cachexia. Subsequent studies have confirmed that plasma concentrations of inflammatory cytokines are increased in patients with symptomatic heart failure, and predict a worse prognosis.[42] *In vitro* studies demonstrate that inflammatory cytokines are expressed in failing human myocardium, can depress myocardial function through the generation of nitric oxide, and may contribute to ventricular remodeling by stimulating myocyte apoptosis.[11]

Inflammatory cytokines may also contribute to myocardial failure and negative protein catabolism in ESRF. TNF-α, interleukin (IL)-1β, and IL-6 are increased in patients with ESRF, partly as a consequence of blood–dialysis membrane interaction.[43] In addition to cytokine activation, other mechanisms that may contribute to heart failure in malnourished ESRF patients include selenium and carnitine deficiencies, altered lipoprotein profile, and hypercoagulability.

Cardiodepressant factors   Although a single myocardial toxin has not been identified, several humoral factors have been implicated in cardiac dysfunction associated with ESRF (Table 13.2).[44]

Uremic serum   In 1944, Raab reported variable toxic effects of human ESRF serum on isolated frog and intact rabbit hearts. Uremic serum caused an increase in myocardial contractility in some preparations and bradycardia with standstill in others.[45] Subsequent studies have shown dose-dependent negative inotropic and chronotropic effects, and arrhythmogenic effects of urea and creatinine in cultured myocytes.[46] In isolated guinea pig hearts, urea reduced mechanical activity, increased myocardial oxygen consumption, and attenuated the positive inotropic response to norepinephrine.[47] These toxic effects were not seen with creatinine or guanidinosuccinic acid. Reports of marked improvement in systolic function following initiation of dialysis or renal transplantation provide indirect clinical evidence for the reversible cardiodepressant effect of uremia.

Calcium-phosphate homeostasis   Patients with ESRF develop secondary hyperparathyroidism, and parathyroid hormone (PTH) may play a role in the pathogenesis of cardiovascular disease.[44] Myocardial PTH receptors mediate an increase in intracellular calcium via voltage-dependent calcium channels. Whereas acute exposure to PTH causes positive inotropic and chronotropic effects, chronic exposure may increase basal intracellular calcium and inhibit cardiocyte metabolism and function.[48,49] PTH has also been linked to the development of LVH and cardiac fibrosis.

There have been several case reports of cardiomyopathy related to hypocalcemia and hypophosphatemia. In ESRF, elevated phosphorus and calcium-phosphorus product are associated with an increased risk of mortality that is independent of medical comorbidities, adequacy of dialysis, nutrition, and markers of compliance.[50] Increased myocardial calcium content in ESRF may also contribute to the development of heart failure. In one study, myocardial calcium content was associated with LV dilatation and impaired systolic function, and correlated with the calcium-phosphorus product.[51] Patients in this study all had evidence of advanced secondary hyperparathyroidism.

Acetate buffer   Acetate buffer in the dialysate may cause hemodynamic instability, but is rarely used today.

Systemic disease with cardiac and renal involvement

In patients presenting with ESRF and non-ischemic cardiomyopathy not related to diabetes or hypertension, a few uncommon systemic diseases should be considered in the differential diagnosis. Amyloidosis refers to a group of diseases that share a common pathological process: extracellular deposition of insoluble fibrillar proteins in the kidney, heart, and other organ systems.[52] AL amyloidosis, a plasma cell dyscrasia related to multiple myeloma, is the most common of these diseases with approximately 1275–3200 new cases per year in the US.[53] Renal involvement in AL amyloidosis usually presents as proteinuria, often resulting in the nephrotic syndrome, but rarely progresses to ESRF. Cardiac involvement is common and manifests as a restrictive cardiomyopathy with rapidly progressive heart failure, atrial arrhythmias, and thromboembolism. Postural hypotension secondary to autonomic neuropathy complicates pharmacological management. Symptomatic heart failure is associated with a median survival of 6 months.[52]

Sarcoidosis is a chronic systemic disease that may rarely present with ESRF and CHF. Pathologically, sarcoidosis is characterized by accumulation of helper T cells and mononuclear phagocytes, formation of non-caseating granulomas, and derangement of normal tissue architecture.[54] Primary renal involvement is characterized by interstitial nephritis, as well as chronic hypercalciuria causing nephrocalcinosis and obstructive uropathy. Approximately 5% of patients with sarcoidosis have cardiac involvement manifesting as left and/or right ventricular systolic dysfunction, conduction system disease, and arrhythmias.[55] Other multisystem diseases associated with cardiac and renal failure include human immunodeficiency virus (HIV)/AIDS, scleroderma, systemic lupus erythematosis, and primary oxalosis.

Diagnosis of CHF in ESRF

Patient evaluation

The assessment of chronic heart failure offers a particular challenge to clinicians due to the poor correlation between physical signs and symptoms, and cardiac function. In patients with dilated cardiomyopathy, several studies have demonstrated the limited reliability of the medical history, physical examination, and chest X-ray in diagnosing heart failure.[56] Conflicting test results may lead to under-diagnosis and inadequate therapy. This situation may arise in patients with ESRF in whom the absence of interdialytic weight gain does not rule out heart failure.

Symptoms

As in non-uremic patients, the symptoms of CHF in ESRF may be classified as left-sided or right-sided. Breathlessness is the cardinal symptom of left-sided heart failure and may progress from exertional dyspnea to orthopnea and paroxysmal nocturnal dyspnea. Pulmonary venous congestion, the primary mechanism responsible for breathlessness, leads to decreased lung compliance, hypoxemia, and ventilation–perfusion mismatch. Other common symptoms of left-sided heart failure include fatigue and mental dullness resulting from reduced cardiac output. Symptoms of right-sided heart failure are less common in ESRF since routine dialysis limits volume overload, and weight is followed closely. Elevated systemic venous pressures may result in edema of the gastrointestinal tract manifesting as right upper abdominal discomfort, nausea, bloating, and anorexia. These symptoms may also be related to uremia or digoxin toxicity. Lower extremity edema, another common manifestation of right-sided failure, may be exacerbated by hypoalbuminemia.

Physical signs

Patients with ESRF and compensated heart failure may appear adequately nourished and comfortable at rest, while patients with chronic decompensated heart failure may appear anxious, pale, and malnourished. Other findings that suggest severe LV failure include cool extremities and cyanosis.

Vital signs

Sinus tachycardia may be present due to increased sympathetic activity. The pulse may be irregular if atrial fibrillation is present or alternately strong and weak (pulsus alternans) with severe LV dysfunction. Tachypnea may be present in patients with marked elevation of left-sided filling pressures or pleural effusions. The blood pressure may be high (in diastolic heart failure), normal (in compensated heart failure), or low (in end-stage heart failure). Narrow pulse pressure suggests a critical reduction in cardiac output.[56]

Left-sided signs

Most commonly, ESRF patients with heart failure present with left-sided findings only. Examination of the lungs may reveal rales, rhonchi, or wheezing due to pulmonary congestion. The left ventricular apex may be laterally displaced in dilated cardiomyopathy or sustained in patients with long-standing hypertension. An S4 gallop due to reduced ventricular compliance is common in patients with diastolic heart failure while an S3 gallop is a relatively specific but insensitive finding in LV systolic failure. A holosystolic murmur of mitral regurgitation may be heard at the apex and may be due to ischemic, calcific, or infective mitral valve disease, or may be secondary to LV dilatation. A pericardial rub may be present with uremic pericarditis.

Right-sided signs

Jugular venous distention may be present in ESRF patients with elevated systemic venous pressure due to right ventricular failure, constrictive pericarditis, or pericardial tamponade. Other signs of right-heart failure in ESRF patients who are inadequately ultrafiltered include tender hepatomegaly, ascites, and lower extremity edema. Examination of the lungs may reveal dullness at the bases owing to the presence of chronic pleural effusions. Tricuspid regurgitation manifests as a holosystolic murmur at the left sternal border, prominent v waves in the jugular venous pulse, and a pulsatile liver.

Non-invasive testing

Echocardiography

The use of doppler and two-dimensional echocardiography has become routine in the evaluation of ESRF patients with known or suspected heart failure. Owing to the high prevalence of cardiac disease, it is recommended that any patient who develops pulmonary edema should be evaluated with an echocardiogram. Because ventricular dimensions and LV mass index are preload-dependent measures, it is recommended that echocardiography be performed following dialysis when the patient is within 1 kg of dry weight and fluid and electrolytes have equilibrated. In patients with large pericardial effusions, echocardiography immediately following dialysis may show tamponade physiology despite hemodynamic stability, and, therefore, serial studies are recommended.

Echocardiography provides an accurate and rapid determination of LV dimensions, mass and systolic function (including details of regional wall motion), assessment of valvular morphology and function, and detection of intracavitary thrombi and pericardial effusions. Important hemodynamic information, such as cardiac output, pulmonary artery pressures, and valve areas, may be obtained. The use of echocardiography to evaluate diastolic function is problematic in normal subjects and ESRF patients. Traditional measures of LV relaxation, including the early-to-late atrial filling wave (E/A) ratio and isovolumic relaxation time (IVRT), are load-dependent and must be interpreted cautiously in the context of the patient's volume status, heart rate, and blood pressure. Several authors have demonstrated that volume removal accounts for the observed impairment in diastolic function following dialysis.[57] Recently, newer echocardiographic techniques such as color M-mode and tissue doppler have been shown to provide accurate, load-independent measures of LV relaxation.[58] E/A ratio and IVRT may now be combined with measures of color M-mode propagation and peak early myocardial diastolic velocity to quantify diastolic function.

In patients with poor echocardiographic windows (e.g. due to chronic obstructive pulmonary disease or chest wall abnormalities), radionuclide ventriculography (RVG) or cardiac magnetic resonance imaging (MRI) may be used to assess ventricular performance. RVG provides a reliable quantification of right and left ventricular ejection fraction and volumes, at rest or with exercise. Recently, cardiac MRI has emerged as a highly accurate and quantitative tool for the evaluation of ventricular function and myocardial mass.[59] Serial MRI studies may be used to assess ventricular remodeling in response to pharmacological or surgical therapy for heart failure.

Other non-invasive tools to assess preload

Most non-invasive techniques are limited in their ability to diagnose volume overload in dialysis patients with myocardial dysfunction. Given the significant mortality risk associated with the development of pulmonary edema, and the availability of effective therapy to treat systolic or diastolic failure, the importance of detecting pulmonary congestion cannot be underestimated. The following non-invasive tools have been evaluated in ESRF.

Hematocrit and serum albumin measurement   The continuous measurement of hematocrit during dialysis may be used to determine the rate and quantity of fluid ultrafiltered, but does not reflect intravascular volume status. Likewise, changes in serum albumin concentration correlate with changes in blood volume, but do not indicate total body volume. The timing of these tests influences the interpretation of results since plasma refilling levels off within 2 hours following dialysis.[60]

Inferior vena cava (IVC) diameter measurement   The antero-posterior diameter of the IVC may be measured below the diaphragm in the hepatic segment to reflect volume status. In ESRF, IVC diameter has been shown to correlate with right atrial pressure, blood volume, atrial natriuretic peptide (ANP) levels before dialysis, and the change in ANP levels with dialysis.[61] In addition, the change in IVC diameter with dialysis correlates with changes in intracardiac filling pressures. There are several limitations in the use of IVC diameter to assess volume status, including wide interpatient variability, the need for patient compliance with respiratory maneuvers, and the confounding effects of tricuspid regurgitation.

Investigational device for non-invasive measurement of pulmonary capillary wedge pressure   The bedside Valsalva maneuver can be performed in patients with heart failure to determine both the presence and severity of LV dysfunction. McIntyre and colleagues[62] developed a pressurized, finger pulse detector to transmit continuous arterial waveforms during the Valsalva maneuver to a personal computer for analysis of pulmonary capillary wedge pressure (PCWP) (VeriCor®, CVP Diagnostics, Inc., Boston, MA, USA). In the cardiac catheterization laboratory, the VeriCor® device has been shown to provide an accurate measurement of PCWP in control subjects and in patients with symptomatic heart failure.[62] Preliminary data from ESRF patients undergoing dialysis have also demonstrated that the device is sensitive to acute changes in preload (Fig. 13.5) and, thus, may be useful in guiding ultrafiltration.

Cardiopulmonary exercise testing

Treadmill or bicycle exercise testing with continuous gas-exchange analysis provides a safe, objective, and reproducible measurement of functional capacity in patients with symptomatic LV failure.[63] Numerous studies have demonstrated the prognostic significance of peak oxygen consumption which is used routinely to decide on the timing of cardiac transplantation. Cardiopulmonary exercise testing may be of particular use in patients with ESRF and exertional breathlessness to help differentiate cardiac from pulmonary causes of dyspnea. In addition, cardiopulmonary exercise testing may be used to monitor recovery of cardiovascular function following renal or combined cardiac and renal transplantation.

Non-invasive detection of coronary artery disease in ESRF

Cardiac risk factors such as hypertension and diabetes contribute to the high prevalence of atherosclerotic coronary artery disease in patients with ESRF (see Chapters 3 and 14). In turn, ischemic heart disease is responsible for a high incidence of CHF and cardiovascular mortality.[64] In ESRF patients with a history of CHF or cardiomyopathy being considered for renal transplant, the preoperative detection of significant coronary artery disease and subsequent revascularization may reduce the risk of a perioperative cardiac event and graft failure. Pharmacological stress imaging with dipyridamole-thallium or dobutamine stress echocardiography has been recommended for risk stratification. While these tests may provide an accurate method for detecting coronary stenoses and for predicting future coro-

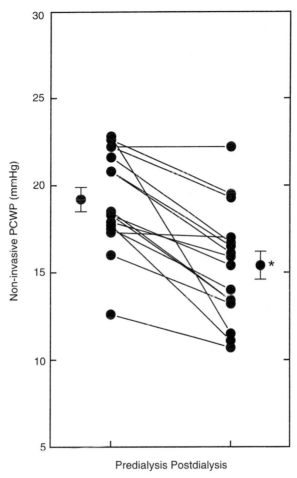

Fig. 13.5 Change in pulmonary capillary wedge pressure (PCWP) as measured by a novel non-invasive Valsalva response recorder[62] in 16 patients with ESRF undergoing routine hemodialysis (*p < 0.001).

nary events in ESRF, suboptimal sensitivity and specificity have been reported.[65] Normal dobutamine stress echocardiography can identify a low-risk population.[66]

Invasive testing

Right and left heart catheterization

In hospitalized patients with ESRF and CHF, assessment of volume status and/or cardiac output may be necessary for managing hemodynamic instability. The gold standard for evaluating cardiac hemodynamics is right heart catheterization using a balloon-tipped flotation catheter. This invasive but relatively safe procedure may be performed at the bedside or in the cardiac catheterization laboratory under fluoroscopic guidance. Fluoroscopy may be particularly useful in patients with pulmonary hypertension and tricuspid regurgitation in whom the Swan–Ganz catheter may coil in the right atrium. Simultaneous measurement of right- and left-sided cardiac filling pressures is used to diagnose constrictive pericarditis or pericardial tamponade. In addition, invasive hemodynamics can provide an accurate determination of the severity of valvular stenosis. Although a recent report suggested that the pulmonary artery catheter may increase mortality in critically ill patients,[67] the study was methodologically flawed, and in the subgroup of patients with CHF the relative hazard of death was 1.

Coronary angiography

In ESRF patients with CHF, coronary angiography should be performed prior to renal transplant when cardiac risk factors are present or when the patient has a history of angina or prior myocardial infarction. If left main or multivessel coronary artery disease is found, surgical revascularization may be indicated to reduce the risk of subsequent cardiac events. Complications associated with routine coronary angiography in patients with ESRF and atherosclerosis include pulmonary edema, cholesterol embolization, and local vascular complications.

Endomyocardial biopsy

The role of right ventricular endomyocardial biopsy in patients with dilated cardiomyopathy remains controversial. Proposed clinical indications include detection and monitoring of myocarditis, diagnosis of secondary cardiomyopathy, and differentiation of restrictive cardiomyopathy from constrictive pericarditis.[68] In ESRF patients with CHF, endomyocardial biopsy may be used to diagnose a systemic disease such as amyloidosis or sarcoidosis that carries important prognostic and therapeutic implications. In patients with HIV nephropathy and cardiomyopathy, endomyocardial biopsy may detect a treatable infectious myocarditis (e.g. due to aspergillus or toxoplasma). Although the overall complication rate from endomyocardial biopsy is low (i.e. 2–6%), cardiac perforation and mortality may occur rarely.[69]

Table 13.3　Treatment of heart failure in ESRF

Acute	Reduce preload	Emergent ultrafiltration
		Nitroglycerin, nitroprusside
	Correct reversible factors	PTCA for unstable angina
		Cardioversion of AF
Chronic	Optimize preload and afterload	Ultrafilter to dry weight
		Treat hypertension
	Correct reversible factors	PTCA or CABG for ischemia
		Surgical correction of valvular disease
	Improve exacerbating conditions	Partial correction of anemia
		Optimize calcium–phosphorus product
		Ligation of arteriovenous fistula
		Nutritional supplementation (?)
	Pharmacological therapy	ACE inhibitors and other vasodilators
		Digoxin
		Beta-blockers
	Uremic therapy	Dialysis
		Renal transplantation
	Treat systemic disease	Immunosuppression for sarcoidosis

PTCA, percutaneous transluminal coronary angioplasty; CABG, coronary artery bypass grafting; AF, atrial fibrillation; ACE, angiotensin-converting enzyme.

Therapy

General goals

The general goals of therapy in treating ESRF patients with CHF include relief of symptoms, improved quality of life, and prolonged survival. Achieving these goals requires an integrated approach, provided by an experienced team of physicians, nurse specialists, a nutritionist, and a social worker. The approach is outlined in Table 13.3, and includes optimization of loading conditions, correction of reversible or exacerbating factors, and use of pharmacological and/or surgical therapy with proven beneficial effects in non-ESRF patients with heart failure.

Optimize preload and afterload

Paramount in the treatment and prevention of heart failure in patients with ESRF is the attainment of dry weight via ultrafiltration and dietary fluid and sodium restriction. Effective volume control reduces the risk of developing pulmonary edema acutely, and has been shown to have long-term beneficial effects on the prevalence and complications of hypertension.[70] In one study, aggressive ultrafiltration with extended dialysis times over 1 month led to the withdrawal of antihypertensive medications in 84% of patients.[71] Retrospective, uncontrolled data suggest that intensive ultrafiltration and sodium restriction may cause regression of LVH.[72]

In the ESRF patient with CHF, hypertension that is not correctable with ultrafiltration should be managed with antihypertensive medications. ACE inhibitors are the mainstay of drug therapy (see below). Alternative or adjunctive agents include hydralazine, nitrates, beta-adrenergic antagonists, angiotensin receptor antagonists, and second-generation dihydropyridine calcium-channel antagonists. As in the general population, secondary (reversible) causes of hypertension should be considered in ESRF patients with episodic or severe elevations in blood pressure despite the use of three or more antihypertensive agents. The effects of antihypertensive therapy on cardiovascular morbidity and mortality in ESRF are unknown.

Correct reversible factors

Ischemia may precipitate or worsen heart failure in patients with ESRF. While the management of ischemic heart disease in the ESRF population is beyond the scope of this chapter (see Chapters 3 and 14), a few general recommendations can be made. Ischemia in the absence of epicardial coronary artery disease may occur in patients with LVH and diastolic dysfunction. Management strategies in these patients should focus on volume and blood pressure control, correction of anemia, and prevention of atrial arrhythmias. In ESRF patients with CHF and ischemia secondary to epicardial coronary stenoses, beta-blockers and nitrates are effective anti-ischemic therapy. In addition, percutaneous or surgical revascularization should be considered even though the risks of percutaneous transluminal coronary angioplasty (PTCA) and coronary artery bypass grafting (CABG) are higher than in the non-ESRF population.[73] As in the general population, the most significant predictor of early and late mortality following CABG in ESRF patients is a history of CHF.[74]

Improve exacerbating conditions

Metabolic, hormonal, and nutritional factors that are specific to ESRF and may exacerbate CHF should be identified and treated.

Anemia   The anemia of chronic renal disease is correctable with recombinant human erythropoietin and iron supplements. Small, uncontrolled studies suggest that correcting anemia in patients with ESRF causes regression of left ventricular hypertrophy and dilatation.[35] However, the effects of partial versus complete correction of anemia on cardiovascular morbidity and mortality are not completely known. A recent study randomized 1233 patients with CHF or ischemic heart disease undergoing hemodialysis to receive erythropoietin sufficient to maintain a hematocrit of 42% versus 30%.[37] After two and a half years of follow-up, there was a trend towards an increased risk of death or non-fatal myocardial infarction in the 'normal' hematocrit group compared to the 'low' hematocrit group (relative risk 1.3, 95% confidence interval 0.9–1.9). Current guidelines recommend achieving a hematocrit in the range of 33–36%.

Calcium-phosphate homeostasis   Recent trends in the management of ESRF have emphasized the importance of controlling hyperparathyroidism. Phosphorus levels should be maintained below 6.5 mg/dl while maintaining calcium levels sufficient to suppress PTH. In order to prevent calcification of cardiac valves and epicardial and intramyocardial blood vessels, hyperphosphatemia should be controlled prior to the initiation of vitamin D therapy. When the calcium-phosphorus product is elevated, calcium-containing phosphate binders are contraindicated.

The effect of surgical or medical reduction of PTH levels on LV mass and function in ESRF has been evaluated. Some studies have demonstrated improvement in systolic function in patients with mild systolic failure and severe secondary hyperparathyroidism following parathyroidectomy[75] or vitamin D therapy,[76] while others have shown no benefit. Fellner and colleagues[77] reported a case series of seven ESRF patients without evidence of heart disease who underwent parathyroidectomy. After controlling for ionized calcium, heart rate, preload, and afterload, PTH did not appear to have a direct effect on cardiac contractility. In non-ESRF patients with primary hyperparathyroidism and normal cardiac function, parathyroidectomy may cause regression of LVH.[78]

Arteriovenous fistulae   In rare cases, high output cardiac failure is due to an arteriovenous fistula, and may be treated by surgical ligation of the fistula. If there is diagnostic uncertainty as to the hemodynamic significance of the fistula, echocardiography or right heart catheterization may be used to assess the change in cardiac output with fistula compression.

Malnutrition   The effect of nutritional supplementation on the development or progression of heart failure or cardiomyopathy in patients with ESRF is unknown.

Pharmacological therapy

In general, the beneficial effects of pharmacological agents in the treatment of ESRF patients with heart failure must be inferred from large, prospective trials that routinely excluded ESRF patients.

ACE inhibitors and other vasodilators

One of the most important advances in the treatment of heart failure was the recognition that pump function is critically dependent on afterload.[79] Arterial vasodilators shift the ventricular function curve upward and to the left, resulting in an increase in cardiac output (Fig. 13.4), while venodilators redistribute central blood volume to the periphery, thereby decreasing the signs and symptoms of elevated cardiac filling pressures. In patients with CHF, ACE inhibitors exert a balanced dilator effect on the arterial and venous system, and may attenuate the chronic effects of neurohormonal activation.

Several large, prospective, controlled studies have demonstrated the beneficial effects of ACE inhibitors on clinical signs and symptoms, exercise tolerance, quality of life, hospitalizations, and survival in non-ESRF patients with chronic heart failure. ACE inhibitors are indicated for the treatment of patients with asymptomatic or symptomatic LV systolic dysfunction, of either ischemic or non-ischemic etiology. Similar benefits are seen with several ACE inhibitors,[80] and high-dose therapy appears to be more effective than low-dose.[81] In patients with ESRF, ACE inhibitors have been shown to reduce left ventricular hypertrophy[82] and mass,[83] and decrease arterial wave reflections[84] independent of their antihypertensive effects. Uncontrolled data suggest that ACE inhibitors may impair erythropoiesis in patients with ESRF. However, a recent retrospective study was unable to demonstrate a difference in hematocrit between dialysis patients treated with or without an ACE inhibitor.[85] The role of ACE inhibitors in the treatment of patients with diastolic heart failure remains unknown.

Approximately 10% of non-ESRF patients do not tolerate ACE inhibitors because of hypotension, cough, azotemia, hyperkalemia, or angioedema. In ESRF patients who are intolerant of ACE inhibitors, alternative vasodilator therapy should be considered. The first Veterans Administration Heart Failure Trial (V-HeFT I) demonstrated a survival benefit of hydralazine plus isosorbide-dinitrate compared to placebo,[86] although this combination was less effective than enalapril in V-HeFT II.[87] Amlodipine may be used safely to reduce blood pressure in patients with severe chronic heart failure on ACE inhibitors, but has not been shown to reduce cardiovascular morbidity or mortality.[88] The effect of angiotensin receptor antagonists on survival in heart failure is unknown. Several large, randomized trials are currently underway to test whether ACE inhibition, angiotensin receptor blockade, or the combination is more effective at slowing disease progression.

Digoxin

Clinical trials have shown that digoxin increases left ventricular ejection fraction (LVEF) and exercise tolerance, and decreases symptoms in patients with chronic heart failure. Withdrawal of digoxin leads to worsening of symptoms and increased hospitalization.[89] The Digitalis Investigation Group trial[90] randomized 6800 patients with an LVEF less than or equal to 45% receiving an ACE inhibitor and diuretic to digoxin or placebo and showed no difference in overall survival. While there were fewer deaths due to heart failure in the digoxin-treated group, these were offset by an excess of arrhythmic deaths. In ESRF patients with systolic heart failure, digoxin is recommended as adjunctive therapy for patients who remain symptomatic on ACE inhibitors. Digoxin may also be used to control ventricular response in atrial fibrillation. The dose of digoxin may need to be decreased by 75% in patients on dialysis.

Beta-adrenergic antagonists

Historically, beta-blockers were contraindicated in the treatment of chronic heart failure because of concern for negative inotropic effects precipitating clinical deterioration. It is now recognized that chronic overactivity of the sympathetic nervous system plays an important role in the pathophysiology of heart failure, and drugs that interfere with this system can prevent disease progression. In the 1970s and early 1980s, small uncontrolled trials suggested beneficial effects of beta-blockers in dilated cardiomyopathy. An increasing body of evidence now indicates that beta-blockers improve LV function, reduce hospitalizations, and prolong survival in patients with chronic systolic heart failure.[91] Carvedilol, a combination alpha- and beta-blocker with *in vitro* antioxidant properties, has recently been approved for the treatment of mild to moderate heart failure.[92] Large, prospective trials of bisoprolol (CIBIS II) and metoprolol (MERIT-HF) were stopped recently due to a 32–35% reduction in all-cause mortality.[93] New consensus guidelines for the management of heart failure recommend beta-blockers, in addition to ACE inhibitors and diuretics, for the long-term management of patients with mild to moderate CHF.[91]

Beta-blockers may have variable actions related in part to their non-beta-blocking effects (e.g. direct vasodilation) and must be titrated slowly in symptomatic patients. Adverse effects include lightheadedness, worsening heart failure, and bradycardia or heart block. In ESRF patients with CHF of ischemic etiology, beta-blockers may also be used to treat hypertension, prevent myocardial infarction, and control ventricular response in atrial fibrillation.

Uremic therapy

Ultrafiltration

The importance of volume control in dialysis patients is well established. In pre-ESRF patients with chronic heart failure refractory to diuretic therapy, ultrafiltration without hemodialysis may be indicated for volume removal. In some cases, the need for ultrafiltration may be temporary, and several reports have demonstrated sustained beneficial effects of isolated ultrafiltration in patients with moderate to severe heart failure. In one study, 36 non-ESRF patients with NYHA functional class II to III heart failure were assigned randomly to a single session of ultrafiltration (mean ultrafiltrate, 1.8 liters) or standard medical therapy. Ultrafiltration caused significant reductions in right- and left-sided cardiac filling pressures and extravascular lung water, and improved functional capacity at 6 months.[94] The improvement in peak oxygen consumption appears to be inversely related to baseline cardiac and pulmonary function.[95] Elevated plasma norepinephrine levels may also be decreased by ultrafiltration.[96]

Dialysis

Timely initiation and adequacy of dialysis are critical in the management of ESRF patients with CHF. Gradual achievement of dry weight helps to control blood pressure and relieves symptoms of pulmonary and systemic congestion, while avoiding dialysis-associated hypotension and subsequent ischemia. In addition, dialysis may favorably affect ventricular structure and function in patients with heart failure.

Mode of dialysis   The most effective mode of dialysis for patients with cardiovascular disease is unknown. In a study of 432 Canadian dialysis patients, there was no difference in cardiac morbidity and mortality between patients treated with hemodialysis and peritoneal dialysis.[16] Retrospective analysis of the USRDS revealed a small excess of cardiovascular mortality in diabetic patients treated with peritoneal dialysis,[97] but a more recent analysis which included both prevalent and incident cases found no difference.[98] Currently, the choice of dialysis mode is dependent primarily on patient preference, as well as the general belief that heart failure symptoms are better managed with the gradual ultrafiltration of peritoneal dialysis.

Advances in dialysis technology In the past, acetate dialysate was associated with hemodynamic instability and decreased patient tolerability; it has since been replaced by dialysate buffered with bicarbonate. Excessive generation of inflammatory cytokines, specifically TNF-α, IL-1β, and IL-6, may occur with exposure of blood to dialysis membranes and may contribute to dialysis-associated malnutrition and heart failure.[43] Use of biocompatible synthetic membranes may reduce cytokine activation. Other dialysis techniques that may favorably affect ESRF patients with heart failure include high flux dialyzers,[99] increased calcium dialysate,[100] and longer dialysis times.[70]

Impact of dialysis on heart failure and prognosis Bailey and colleagues were the first to report reversible cardiomyopathy with dialysis.[101] Four patients with serum blood urea nitrogen (BUN) ranging from 126 to 172 mg/dl, radiographic cardiomegaly, and symptomatic heart failure had marked improvement in symptoms and normalization of heart size on chest X-ray following the initiation of dialysis. An increase in ejection fraction has been reported in patients with dilated cardiomyopathy following a single dialysis with continued improvement with chronic renal replacement therapy.[102]

In the National Cooperative Dialysis Study, CHF occurred more frequently in patients with greater azotemia and shorter dialysis. Others have demonstrated significant associations between uremic symptoms and subsequent risk of cardiac events[103] and mortality,[2] although these associations were less significant when corrected for age, duration of diabetes, and heart failure. Subsequent retrospective studies in larger numbers of patients have confirmed the relationship between adequacy of dialysis and survival.[104] A large on-going prospective trial is aimed at determining the impact of 'standard' vs. 'high-dose' dialysis on clinical outcomes and survival.[105]

Renal transplant

While there is little direct evidence that uremia itself causes cardiomyopathy in humans, reports of improvement in myocardial structure and function following renal transplantation provide strong indirect support for this hypothesis. Parfrey and colleagues[106] reviewed the clinical course and echocardiograms of 102 patients with ESRF who underwent successful renal transplantation. One year after transplantation, fractional shortening had normalized in all patients with baseline systolic dysfunction. In addition, significant reductions in LV mass and volume were demonstrated. This study confirmed earlier case reports of improved LVEF after renal transplant,[107] and has suggested that LV dysfunction should not be considered a contraindication to transplantation. For selected patients with end-stage cardiac and renal failure, combined heart and kidney transplantation may be an effective therapeutic option.[108]

References

1. Anonymous. (1997). Patient mortality and survival. USRDS. United States Renal Data System. *American Journal of Kidney Diseases*, **30**, S86–106.
2. Hutchinson, T.A., Thomas, D.C., and MacGibbon, B. (1982). Predicting survival in adults with end-stage renal disease: an age equivalence index. *Annals of Internal Medicine*, **96**, 417–23.
3. Harnett, J.D., Foley, R.N., Kent, G.M., Barre, P.E., Murray, D., and Parfrey, P.S. (1995). Congestive heart failure in dialysis patients: prevalence, incidence, prognosis and risk factors. *Kidney International*, **47**, 884–90.

4. Churchill, D.N., Taylor, D.W., Cook, R.J., LaPlante, P., Barre, P., Cartier, P., *et al.* (1992). Canadian Hemodialysis Morbidity Study. *American Journal of Kidney Diseases*, **19**, 214–34.
5. Foley, R.N., Parfrey, P.S., Harnett, J.D., Kent, G.M., Murray, D.C., and Barre, P.E. (1995). The prognostic importance of left ventricular geometry in uremic cardiomyopathy. *Journal of the American Society of Nephrology*, **5**, 2024–31.
6. Francis, G.S., Benedict, C., Johnstone, D.E., Kirlin, P.C., Nicklas, J., Liang, C.S., *et al.* (1990). Comparison of neuroendocrine activation in patients with left ventricular dysfunction with and without congestive heart failure. A substudy of the Studies of Left Ventricular Dysfunction (SOLVD). *Circulation*, **82**, 1724–9.
7. Colucci, W.S., and Braunwald, E. (1997). Pathophysiology of heart failure. In *Heart Disease: A Textbook of Cardiovascular Medicine*. 5th edition. E. Braunwald, editor. W.B. Saunders Company, Philadelphia, 394–420.
8. Cody, R.J., Haas, G.J., Binkley, P.F., Capers, Q., and Kelley, R. (1992). Plasma endothelin correlates with the extent of pulmonary hypertension in patients with chronic congestive heart failure. *Circulation*, **85**, 504–9.
9. Colucci, W.S. (1996). Myocardial endothelin. Does it play a role in myocardial failure? *Circulation*, **93**, 1069–72.
10. Demuth, K., Blacher, J., Guerin, A.P., Benoit, M.O., Moatti, N., Safar, M.E., *et al.* (1998). Endothelin and cardiovascular remodeling in end-stage renal disease. *Nephrology, Dialysis, Transplantation*, **13**, 375–83.
11. Givertz, M.M., and Colucci, W.S. (1998). New targets for heart-failure therapy: endothelin, inflammatory cytokines, and oxidative stress. *Lancet*, **352**, SI34–8.
12. Sacchetti, A., McCabe, J., Torres, M., and Harris, R.L. (1993). ED management of acute congestive heart failure in renal dialysis patients. *American Journal of Emergency Medicine*, **11**, 644–7.
13. Rose, B.D. (1994). The total body water and the plasma sodium concentration. In *Clinical Physiology of Acid–Base and Electrolyte Disorders*. 4th edition. B.D. Rose, editor. McGraw-Hill, New York, 219–34.
14. Gibson, D.G. (1966). Haemodynamic factors in the development of acute pulmonary edema in renal failure. *Lancet*, **2**, 1217–20.
15. Crosbie, W.A., Snowden, S., and Parsons, V. (1972). Changes in lung capillary permeability in renal failure. *British Medical Journal*, **4**, 388–90.
16. Parfrey, P.S., Foley, R.N., Harnett, J.D., Kent, G.M., Murray, D.C., and Barre, P.E. (1996). Outcome and risk factors for left ventricular disorders in chronic uraemia. *Nephrology, Dialysis, Transplantation*, **11**, 1277–85.
17. London, G.M., and Parfrey, P.S. (1997). Cardiac disease in chronic uremia: pathogenesis. *Advances in Renal Replacement Therapy*, **4**, 194–211.
18. Levy, D., Larson, M.G., Vasan, R.S., Kannel, W.B., and Ho, K.K. (1996). The progression from hypertension to congestive heart failure. *JAMA*, **275**, 1557–62.
19. Rostand, S.G., Kirk, K.A., and Rutsky, E.A. (1984). Dialysis-associated ischemic heart disease: insights from coronary angiography. *Kidney International*, **25**, 653–9.
20. Roig, E., Betriu, A., Castaner, A., Magrina, J., Sanz, G., and Navarro-Lopez, F. (1981). Disabling angina pectoris with normal coronary arteries in patients undergoing long-term hemodialysis. *American Journal of Medicine*, **71**, 431–4.
21. Amann, K., Wiest, G., Zimmer, G., Gretz, N., Ritz, E., and Mall, G. (1992). Reduced capillary density in the myocardium of uremic rats–a stereological study. *Kidney International*, **42**, 1079–85.
22. Maher, E.R., Young, G., Smyth-Walsh, B., Pugh, S., and Curtis, J.R. (1987). Aortic and mitral valve calcification in patients with end-stage renal disease. *Lancet*, **2**, 875–7.
23. Malergue, M.C., Urena, P., Prieur, P., Guedon-Rapoud, C., and Petrover, M. (1997). Incidence and development of aortic stenosis in chronic hemodialysis. An ultrasonographic and biological study of 112 patients. *Archives des Maladies du Coeur et des Vaisseaux*, **90**, 1595–601.

24. Straumann, E., Meyer, B., Misteli, M., Blumberg, A., and Jenzer, H.R. (1992). Aortic and mitral valve disease in patients with end stage renal failure on long-term haemodialysis. *British Heart Journal*, **67**, 236–9.

25. Cirit, M., Ozkahya, M., Cinar, C.S., Ok, E., Aydin, S., Akcicek, F., *et al.* (1998). Disappearance of mitral and tricuspid regurgitation in haemodialysis patients after ultrafiltration. *Nephrology, Dialysis, Transplantation*, **13**, 389–92.

26. Renfrew, R., Buselmeier, T.J., and Kjellstrand, C.M. (1980). Pericarditis and renal failure. *Annual Review of Medicine*, **31**, 345–60.

27. Kimura, K., Tabei, K., Asano, Y., and Hosoda, S. (1989). Cardiac arrhythmias in hemodialysis patients. A study of incidence and contributory factors. *Nephron*, **53**, 201–7.

28. Tamura, K., Tsuji, H., Nishiue, T., Tokunaga, S., Yajima, I., Higashi, T., *et al.* (1998). Determinants of ventricular arrhythmias in hemodialysis patients. Evaluation of the effect of arrhythmogenic substrate and autonomic imbalance. *American Journal of Nephrology*, **18**, 280–4.

29. Canziani, M.E., Cendoroglo Neto, M., Saragoca, M.A., Cassiolato, J.L., Ramos, O.L., Ajzen, H., *et al.* (1995). Hemodialysis versus continuous ambulatory peritoneal dialysis: effects on the heart. *Artificial Organs*, **19**, 241–4.

30. Kimmel, P.L., Miller, G., and Mendelson, W.B. (1989). Sleep apnea syndrome in chronic renal disease. *American Journal of Medicine*, **86**, 308–14.

31. Zoccali, C., Benedetto, F.A., Tripepi, G., Cambareri, F., Panuccio, V., Candela, V., *et al.* (1998). Nocturnal hypoxemia, night–day arterial pressure changes and left ventricular geometry in dialysis patients. *Kidney International*, **53**, 1078–84.

32. Tkacova, R., Rankin, F., Fitzgerald, F.S., Floras, J.S., and Bradley, T.D. (1998). Effects of continuous positive airway pressure on obstructive sleep apnea and left ventricular afterload in patients with heart failure. *Circulation*, **98**, 2269–75.

33. Engelberts, I., Tordoir, J.H., Boon, E.S., and Schreij, G. (1995). High-output cardiac failure due to excessive shunting in a hemodialysis access fistula: an easily overlooked diagnosis. *American Journal of Nephrology*, **15**, 323–6.

34. Foley, R.N., Parfrey, P.S., Harnett, J.D., Kent, G.M., Murray, D.C., and Barre, P.E. (1996). The impact of anemia on cardiomyopathy, morbidity, and mortality in end-stage renal disease. *American Journal of Kidney Diseases*, **28**, 53–61.

35. Pascual, J., Teruel, J.L., Moya, J.L., Liano, F., Jimenez-Mena, M., and Ortuno, J. (1991). Regression of left ventricular hypertrophy after partial correction of anemia with erythropoietin in patients on hemodialysis: a prospective study. *Clinical Nephrology*, **35**, 280–7.

36. Fellner, S.K., Lang, R.M., Neumann, A., Korcarz, C., and Borow, K.M. (1993). Cardiovascular consequences of correction of the anemia of renal failure with erythropoietin. *Kidney International*, **44**, 1309–15.

37. Besarab, A., Bolton, W.K., Browne, J.K., Egrie, J.C., Nissenson, A.R., Okamoto, D.M., *et al.* (1998). The effects of normal as compared with low hematocrit values in patients with cardiac disease who are receiving hemodialysis and epoetin. *New England Journal of Medicine*, **339**, 584–90.

38. Bergstrom, J., and Lindholm, B. (1998). Malnutrition, cardiac disease, and mortality: an integrated point of view. *American Journal of Kidney Diseases*, **32**, 834–41.

39. Mesler, D.E., McCarthy, E.P., Byrne-Logan, S., Ash, A.S., and Moskowitz, M.A. (1999). Does the survival advantage of non-white dialysis patients persist after case mix adjustment? *American Journal of Medicine*, 106;300–06.

40. Foley, R.N., Parfrey, P.S., Harnett, J.D., Kent, G.M., Murray, D.C., and Barre, P.E. (1996). Hypoalbuminemia, cardiac morbidity, and mortality in end-stage renal disease. *Journal of the American Society of Nephrology*, **7**, 728–36.

41. Levine, B., Kalman, J., Mayer, L., Fillit, H.M., and Packer, M. (1990). Elevated circulating levels of tumor necrosis factor in severe chronic heart failure. *New England Journal of Medicine*, **323**, 236–41.

42. Torre-Amione, G., Kapadia, S., Benedict, C., Oral, H., Young, J.B., and Mann, D.L. (1996). Proinflammatory cytokine levels in patients with depressed left ventricular ejection fraction: a report from the studies of left ventricular dysfunction (SOLVD). *Journal of the American College of Cardiology*, **27**, 1201–6.

43. Herbelin, A., Urena, P., Nguyen, A.T., Zingraff, J., and Descamps-Latscha, B. (1991). Influence of first and long-term dialysis on uraemia-associated increased basal production of interleukin-1 and tumour necrosis factor alpha by circulating monocytes. *Nephrology, Dialysis, Transplantation*, **6**, 349–57.

44. Horl, W.H., and Riegel, W. (1993). Cardiac depressant factors in renal disease. *Circulation*, **87**, IV-77–82.

45. Raab, W. (1944). Cardiotoxic substances in the blood and heart muscle in uremia (their nature and action). *Journal of Laboratory and Clinical Medicine*, **1**, 715–34.

46. Weisensee, D., Low-Friedrich, I., Riehle, M., Bereiter-Hahn, J., and Schoeppe, W. (1993). *In vitro* approach to 'uremic cardiomyopathy'. *Nephron*, **65**, 392–400.

47. Kersting, F., Brass, H., and Heintz, R. (1978). Uremic cardiomyopathy: studies on cardiac function in the guinea pig. *Clinical Nephrology*, **10**, 109–13.

48. Bogin, E., Levi, J., Harary, I., and Massry, S.G. (1982). Effects of parathyroid hormone on oxidative phosphorylation of heart mitochondria. *Mineral and Electrolyte Metabolism*, **7**, 151–6.

49. Smogorzewski, M., Perna, A.F., Borum, P.R., and Massry, S.G. (1988). Fatty acid oxidation in the myocardium: effects of parathyroid hormone and CRF. *Kidney International*, **34**, 797–803.

50. Block, G.A., Hulbert-Shearon, T.E., Levin, N.W., and Port, F.K. (1998). Association of serum phosphorus and calcium x phosphate product with mortality risk in chronic hemodialysis patients: a national study. *American Journal of Kidney Diseases*, **31**, 607–17.

51. Rostand, S.G., Sanders, C., Kirk, K.A., Rutsky, E.A., and Fraser, R.G. (1988). Myocardial calcification and cardiac dysfunction in chronic renal failure. *American Journal of Medicine*, **85**, 651–7.

52. Falk, R.H., Comenzo, R.L., and Skinner, M. (1997). The systemic amyloidoses. *New England Journal of Medicine*, **337**, 898–909.

53. Kyle, R.A., Linos, A., Beard, C.M., Linke, R.P., Gertz, M.A., O'Fallon, W.M., et al. (1992). Incidence and natural history of primary systemic amyloidosis in Olmsted County, Minnesota, 1950 through 1989. *Blood*, **79**, 1817–22.

54. Crystal, R.G. (1998). Sarcoidosis. In *Harrison's Principles of Internal Medicine*. 14th edition. A.S. Fauci, E. Braunwald, K.J. Isselbacher, J.D. Wilson, J.B. Martin, D.L. Kasper, et al., editors. McGraw-Hill, New York, 1922–8.

55. Sharma, O.P., Maheshwari, A., and Thaker, K. (1993). Myocardial sarcoidosis. *Chest*, **103**, 253–8.

56. Stevenson, L.W., and Perloff, J.K. (1989). The limited reliability of physical signs for estimating hemodynamics in chronic heart failure. *JAMA*, **261**, 884–8.

57. Chakko, S., Girgis, I., Contreras, G., Perez, G., Kessler, K.M., and Myerburg, R.J. (1997). Effects of hemodialysis on left ventricular diastolic filling. *American Journal of Cardiology*, **79**, 106–8.

58. Garcia, M.J., Thomas, J.D., and Klein, A.L. (1998). New Doppler echocardiographic applications for the study of diastolic function. *Journal of the American College Cardiology*, **32**, 865–75.

59. Peshock, R.M., Willett, D.L., Sayad, D.E., Hundley, W.G., Chwialkowski, M.C., Clarke, G.D., et al. (1996). Quantitative MR imaging of the heart. *Magnetic Resonance Imaging Clinics of North America*, **4**, 287–305.

60. Koomans, H.A., Geers, A.B., and Mees, E.J. (1984). Plasma volume recovery after ultrafiltration in patients with chronic renal failure. *Kidney International*, **26**, 848–54.

61. Leunissen, K.M., Kouw, P., Kooman, J.P., Cheriex, E.C., deVries, P.M., Donker, A.J., et al. (1993). New techniques to determine fluid status in hemodialyzed patients. *Kidney International*, **41**(Suppl.), S50–6.

62. McIntyre, K.M., Vita, J.A., Lambrew, C.T., Freeman, J., and Loscalzo, J. (1992). A noninvasive method of predicting pulmonary-capillary wedge pressure. *New England Journal of Medicine*, **327**, 1715–20.

63. Myers, J., and Gullestad, L. (1998). The role of exercise testing and gas-exchange measurement in the prognostic assessment of patients with heart failure. *Current Opinions in Cardiology*, **13**, 145–55.

64. de Lemos, J.A., and Hillis, L.D. (1996). Diagnosis and management of coronary artery disease in patients with end-stage renal disease on hemodialysis. *Journal of the American Society of Nephrology*, **7**, 2044–54.

65. Boudreau, R.J., Strony, J.T., duCret, R.P., Kuni, C.C., Wang, Y., Wilson, R.F., *et al.* (1990). Perfusion thallium imaging of type I diabetes patients with end stage renal disease: comparison of oral and intravenous dipyridamole administration. *Radiology*, **175**, 103–5.

66. Reis, G., Marcovitz, P.A., Leichtman, A.B., Merion, R.M., Fay, W.P., Werns, S.W., *et al.* (1995). Usefulness of dobutamine stress echocardiography in detecting coronary artery disease in end-stage renal disease. *American Journal of Cardiology*, **75**, 707–10.

67. Connors, A.F., Jr., Speroff, T., Dawson, N.V., Thomas, C., Harrell, F.E., Jr., Wagner, D., *et al.* (1996). The effectiveness of right heart catheterization in the initial care of critically ill patients. SUPPORT Investigators. *JAMA*, **276**, 889–97.

68 Levine, M.J., and Baim, D.S. (1991). Endomyocardial Biopsy. In *Cardiac Catheterization, Angiography and Intervention*. 4th edition. W. Grossman and D.S. Baim, editors. Lea and Febiger, Philadelphia, 383–95.

69. Deckers, J.W., Hare, J.M., and Baughman, K.L. (1992). Complications of transvenous right ventricular endomyocardial biopsy in adult patients with cardiomyopathy: a seven-year survey of 546 consecutive diagnostic procedures in a tertiary referral center. *Journal of the American College of Cardiology*, **19**, 43–7.

70. Charra, B., Calemard, M., and Laurent, G. (1996). Importance of treatment time and blood pressure control in achieving long-term survival on dialysis. *American Journal of Nephrology*, **16**, 35–44.

71. Charra, B., Bergstrom, J., and Scribner, B.H. (1998). Blood pressure control in dialysis patients: importance of the lag phenomenon. *American Journal of Kidney Diseases*, **32**, 720–4.

72. Ozkahya, M., Ok, E., Cirit, M., Aydin, S., Akcicek, F., Basci, A., *et al.* (1998). Regression of left ventricular hypertrophy in haemodialysis patients by ultrafiltration and reduced salt intake without antihypertensive drugs. *Nephrology, Dialysis, Transplantation*, **13**, 1489–93.

73. Herzog, C.A. (1997). Diagnosis and treatment of ischemic heart disease in dialysis patients. *Current Opinion in Nephrology and Hypertension*, **6**, 558–65.

74. Kaul, T.K., Fields, B.L., Reddy, M.A., and Kahn, D.R. (1994). Cardiac operations in patients with end-stage renal disease. *Annals of Thoracic Surgery*, **57**, 691–6.

75. Drueke, T., Fauchet, M., Fleury, J., Lesourd, P., Toure, Y., Le Pailleur, C., *et al.* (1980). Effect of parathyroidectomy on left-ventricular function in haemodialysis patients. *Lancet*, **1**, 112–4.

76. McGonigle, R.J., Fowler, M.B., Timmis, A.B., Weston, M.J., and Parsons, V. (1984). Uremic cardiomyopathy: potential role of vitamin D and parathyroid hormone. *Nephron*, **36**, 94–100.

77. Fellner, S.K., Lang, R.M., Neumann, A., Bushinsky, D.A., and Borow, K.M. (1991). Parathyroid hormone and myocardial performance in dialysis patients. *American Journal of Kidney Diseases*, **18**, 320–5.

78. Stefenelli, T., Mayr, H., Bergler-Klein, J., Globits, S., Woloszczuk, W., and Niederle, B. (1993). Primary hyperparathyroidism: incidence of cardiac abnormalities and partial reversibility after successful parathyroidectomy. *American Journal of Medicine*, **95**, 197–202.

79. Cohn, J.N., and Franciosa, J.A. (1977). Vasodilator therapy of cardiac failure. *New England Journal of Medicine*, **297**, 27–31.

80. Garg, R., and Yusuf, S. (1995). Overview of randomized trials of angiotensin-converting enzyme inhibitors on mortality and morbidity in patients with heart failure. Collaborative Group on ACE Inhibitor Trials. *JAMA*, **273**, 1450–6.

81. Packer, M. Poole-Wilson, P. A., Armstrong, P. W., Cleland, P. G., Horowitz. J. D., Massie, R. M., *et al.* (1999). Comparative effects of low and high doses of the angiotensin-converting enzyme inhibitor, lisinopril, on morbidity and mortality in chronic heart failure. *Circulation*, **100**, 2312–8

82. Cannella, G., Paoletti, E., Delfino, R., Peloso, G., Rolla, D., and Molinari, S. (1997). Prolonged therapy with ACE inhibitors induces a regression of left ventricular hypertrophy of dialyzed uremic patients independently from hypotensive effects. *American Journal of Kidney Diseases*, **30**, 659–64.

83. London, G.M., Pannier, B., Guerin, A.P., Marchais, S.J., Safar, M.E., and Cuche, J.L. (1994). Cardiac hypertrophy, aortic compliance, peripheral resistance, and wave reflection in end-stage renal disease. Comparative effects of ACE inhibition and calcium channel blockade. *Circulation*, **90**, 2786–96.

84. London, G.M., Pannier, B., Vicaut, E., Guerin, A.P., Marchais, S.J., Safar, M.E., *et al.* (1996). Antihypertensive effects and arterial haemodynamic alterations during angiotensin converting enzyme inhibition. *Journal of Hypertension*, **14**, 1139–46.

85. Cruz, D.N., Perazella, M.A., Abu-Alfa, A.K., and Mahnensmith, R.L. (1996). Angiotensin-converting enzyme inhibitor therapy in chronic hemodialysis patients: any evidence of erythropoietin resistance? *American Journal of Kidney Diseases*, **28**, 535–40.

86. Cohn, J.N., Archibald, D.G., Ziesche, S., Franciosa, J.A., Harston, W.E., Tristani, F.E., *et al.* (1986). Effect of vasodilator therapy on mortality in chronic congestive heart failure. Results of a Veterans Administration Cooperative Study. *New England Journal of Medicine*, **314**, 1547–52.

87. Cohn, J.N., Johnson, G., Ziesche, S., Cobb, F., Francis, G., Tristani, F., *et al.* (1991). A comparison of enalapril with hydralazine-isosorbide dinitrate in the treatment of chronic congestive heart failure. *New England Journal of Medicine*, **325**, 303–10.

88 Packer, M., O'Connor, C.M., Ghali, J.K., Pressler, M.L., Carson, P.E., Belkin, R.N., *et al.* (1996). Effect of amlodipine on morbidity and mortality in severe chronic heart failure. Prospective Randomized Amlodipine Survival Evaluation Study Group. *New England Journal of Medicine*, **335**, 1107–14.

89. Packer, M., Gheorghiade, M., Young, J.B., Costantini, P.J., Adams, K.F., Cody, R.J., *et al.* (1993). Withdrawal of digoxin from patients with chronic heart failure treated with angiotensin-converting-enzyme inhibitors. RADIANCE Study. *New England Journal of Medicine*, **329**, 1–7.

90. The Digitalis Investigation Group. (1997). The effect of digoxin on mortality and morbidity in patients with heart failure. *New England Journal of Medicine*, **336**, 525–33.

91. Packer, M., and Cohn, J.N. (1999). Consensus recommendations for the management of chronic heart failure. *American Journal of Cardiology*, **83**, 1A–38A.

92. Packer, M., Bristow, M.R., Cohn, J.N., Colucci, W.S., Fowler, M.B., Gilbert, E.M., *et al.* (1996). The effect of carvedilol on morbidity and mortality in patients with chronic heart failure. US Carvedilol Heart Failure Study Group. *New England Journal of Medicine*, **334**, 1349–55.

93. CIBIS II Investigators and Committees. (1999). The Cardiac Insufficiency and Bisoprolol Study (CIBIS II): a randomized trial. *Lancet*, **353**, 9–13.

94. Agostoni, P.G., Marenzi, G.C., Pepi, M., Doria, E., Salvioni, A., Perego, G., *et al.* (1993). Isolated ultrafiltration in moderate congestive heart failure. *Journal of the American College of Cardiology*, **21**, 424–31.

95. Marenzi, G.C., Lauri, G., Guazzi, M., Perego, G.B., and Agostoni, P.G. (1995). Ultrafiltration in moderate heart failure. Exercise oxygen uptake as a predictor of the clinical benefits. *Chest*, **108**, 94–8.

96. Agostoni, P.G., Marenzi, G.C., Sganzerla, P., Assanelli, E., Guazzi, M., Perego, G.B., *et al.* (1995). Lung–heart interaction as a substrate for the improvement in exercise capacity after body

fluid volume depletion in moderate congestive heart failure. *American Journal of Cardiology*, **76**, 793–8.

97. Bloembergen, W.F., Port, F.K., Mauger, E.A., and Wolfe, R.A. (1995). A comparison of mortality between patients treated with hemodialysis and peritoneal dialysis. *Journal of the American Society of Nephrology*, **6**, 177–83.

98. Vonesh, E.F., and Moran, J. (1999). Mortality in end-stage renal disease: a reassessment of differences between patients treated with hemodialysis and peritoneal dialysis. *Journal of the American Society of Nephrology*, **10**, 354–65.

99. Churchill, D.N., Taylor, D.W., Tomlinson, C.W., Beecroft, M.L., Gorman, J., and Stanton, E. (1993). Effect of high-flux hemodialysis on cardiac structure and function among patients with end-stage renal failure. *Nephron*, **65**, 573–7.

100. Henrich, W.L., Hunt, J.M., and Nixon, J.V. (1984). Increased ionized calcium and left ventricular contractility during hemodialysis. *New England Journal of Medicine*, **310**, 19–23.

101. Bailey, G.L., Hampers, C.L., and Merrill, J.P. (1967). Reversible cardiomyopathy in uremia. *Transactions American Society for Artificial Internal Organs*, **13**, 263–70.

102. Hung, J., Harris, P.J., Uren, R.F., Tiller, D.J., and Kelly, D.T. (1980). Uremic cardiomyopathy—effect of hemodialysis on left ventricular function in end-stage renal failure. *New England Journal of Medicine*, **302**, 547–51.

103. Fernandez, J.M., Carbonell, M.E., Mazzuchi, N., and Petruccelli, D. (1992). Simultaneous analysis of morbidity and mortality factors in chronic hemodialysis patients. *Kidney International*, **41**, 1029–34.

104. Held, P.J., Port, F.K., Wolfe, R.A., Stannard, D.C., Carroll, C.E., Daugirdas, J.T., *et al.* (1996). The dose of hemodialysis and patient mortality. *Kidney International*, **50**, 550–6.

105. Depner, T., Beck, G., Daugirdas, J., Kusek, J., and Eknoyan, G. (1999). Lessons from the Hemodialysis (HEMO) Study: an improved measure of the actual hemodialysis dose. *American Journal of Kidney Diseases*, **33**, 142–9.

106. Parfrey, P.S., Harnett, J.D., Foley, R.N., Kent, G.M., Murray, D.C., Barre, P.E., *et al.* (1995). Impact of renal transplantation on uremic cardiomyopathy. *Transplantation*, **60**, 908–14.

107. Burt, R.K., Gupta-Burt, S., Suki, W.N., Barcenas, C.G., Ferguson, J.J., and Van Buren, C.T. (1989). Reversal of left ventricular dysfunction after renal transplantation. *Annals of Internal Medicine*, **111**, 635–40.

108. Laufer, G., Kocher, A., Grabenwoger, M., Berlakovich, G.A., Zuckermann, A., Ofner, P., *et al.* (1997). Simultaneous heart and kidney transplantation as treatment for end-stage heart and kidney failure. *Transplantation*, **64**, 1129–34.

109. Colucci, W.S. (1997). Molecular and cellular mechanisms of myocardial failure. *American Journal of Cardiology*, **80**, 15L–25L.

110. Leier, C.V., and Boudoulas, H. (1997). Renal disorders and heart disease. In *Heart Disease: A Textbook of Cardiovascular Medicine*. 5th edition. E. Braunwald, editor. W.B. Saunders Company, Philadelphia, 1914–38.

111. Frankel, S.K., and Fifer, M.A. (1998). Heart failure. In *Pathophysiology of Heart Disease*. 2nd edition. L.S. Lilly, editor. Williams & Wilkins, Baltimore, 193–216.

14

Diagnosis and management of ischaemic heart disease in end-stage renal failure

Alistair M.S. Chesser and Tessa Savage

Introduction

Despite advances in dialysis and transplantation therapy, the prognosis of patients with end-stage renal failure (ESRF) remains poor. Data from the United States Renal Data System[1] reveal that the 5-year survival of all patients commencing dialysis is 29.4%. Of these deaths, 47.2% are of cardiac origin. Acute myocardial infarction is the cause of death in 10.5% of all ESRF patients, and 'cardiac arrest' the cause of death in 20.2%. The prognosis for diabetic patients is less good still. Twenty-seven per cent of diabetic patients commencing dialysis treatment fail to survive 1 year.[1] Irrespective of transplantation status, 44.5% of all deaths in diabetic patients with ESRF are secondary to cardiac causes. The recognition of ischaemic heart disease in ESRF patients is, therefore, of paramount importance but is complicated by the fact that many of these patients are asymptomatic.[2,3] The aim is to identify the patient with significant coronary artery disease before significant morbidity occurs, and especially before the patient is put forward for transplantation, as there is increasing evidence that if these patients are not recognized and treated, morbidity and mortality following transplantation are increased.[4] Revascularization, risk factor modifications, and attention to the dialysis prescription may be required.

In this chapter we will discuss which patients should be considered most at risk of ischaemic heart disease, how patients with significant coronary disease can be identified, and how such patients should be managed.

Non-invasive assessment of cardiac function

Patients may present with classical symptoms of angina: central crushing chest pain, with radiation to one or both arms or the jaw, brought on or exacerbated by exertion, cold, or after meals. The pain may be relieved by rest or by administration of nitrates. However, many ESRF patients do not have such typical symptoms. Atypical chest pain, otherwise unexplained cardiac failure, arrhythmias, hypotensive episodes while on dialysis, or collapse may all reflect underlying ischaemic heart disease, and such symptoms usually warrant further investigation. Furthermore, ischaemic heart disease is often asymptomatic in these patients, even when severe. Physical examination should enable the detection of valve defects or obstructive cardiomyopathy, which can present in similar ways to ischaemic heart disease.

The resting electrocardiogram (ECG) is usually the first line of investigation in the assessment of suspected ischaemic heart disease. In the normal population, its sensitivity is poor: in the absence of symptoms at the time of recording, the resting ECG is normal in one-third to one-half of all patients with ischaemic heart disease. The ECG can be normal in uraemic patients with ischaemic heart disease, as well. A more common problem is the fact that the resting ECG in ESRF patients is often abnormal even in the absence of ischaemic heart disease. Repolarization abnormalities are common, and the changes associated with hypertension and/or left ventricular hypertrophy may mask changes caused by ischaemia. Nevertheless, typical Q-waves or loss of R-wave progression remain reliable indicators of previous myocardial infarction: Morrow and colleagues[5] studied the ECGs of 85 insulin-dependent diabetics with ESRF. Twenty-four out of 85 patients had evidence on the resting ECG of 'previous myocardial infarction or ischaemic changes'. Thirteen of these patients (54%) had a subsequent cardiovascular event over a mean follow-up period of 30 months.

Echocardiography is non-invasive and widely available. It is able reliably to exclude significant valve lesions, can detect regional wall motion abnormalities which often reflect underlying ischaemic heart disease, and enables an assessment to be made of left ventricular function. This may be of particular use in dialysis patients in whom clinical findings and the chest X-ray usually cannot always distinguish between fluid overload and impaired cardiac function. The most common cause of poor left ventricular function in ESRF patients is coronary artery disease.[6] Reduced ejection fraction in the context of coronary artery disease is associated with a poor prognosis.[7] Such patients might benefit from early revascularization and from angiotensin-converting enzyme inhibitor treatment. In addition, these patients need careful volume restriction, and may require shorter interdialytic intervals.

While the ECG may provide evidence suggestive of ischaemic heart disease and the echocardiogram will provide an assessment of left ventricular function, only coronary angiography can delineate the extent and severity of coronary artery disease. Although angina can occur in ESRF patients with normal coronary arteries,[8] angiography remains the gold standard test and is an essential prerequisite if revascularization is being considered. Angiography defines the coronary anatomy, and enables the physician to define the cardiac prognosis. However, angiography is invasive, is relatively expensive, and can cause complications. For these reasons it is not an ideal screening test, and should only be performed on those with a relatively high probability of ischaemic heart disease.

Which patients should receive coronary angiography?

Dialysis patients considered unsuitable for transplantation

Patients considered to be unfit for transplantation for medical reasons have a poor prognosis, irrespective of whether cardiac intervention occurs or not. Most authors recommend that angiography be reserved for those patients who have incapacitating anginal symptoms despite maximal medical treatment.[9] In this situation, if the patient is considered fit enough to undergo the procedure, revascularization may be appropriate.

Dialysis patients awaiting transplantation

This is a large and important group of patients. Transplantation in patients with coronary disease is associated with a higher incidence of graft loss, perioperative morbidity, and long-term mortality.[2,4,10] In a survey of US transplantation centres, Ramos and colleagues[11] found that 83% of centres performed some sort of screening procedure for coronary disease.

Angiography is usually reserved for those patients with positive thallium scintigraphy, the role of which is discussed below, although 15% of centres perform angiography routinely on all diabetics considered for transplantation. In patients commencing dialysis therapy, there is an early risk of myocardial infarction, with 29% of infarctions occurring within 1 year and 52% occurring within 2 years.[12] Thus, screening should be carried out when appropriate as early as possible after the initiation of dialysis.

Diabetic patients

In the US, 26% of all renal transplants performed are carried out on diabetic patients.[1] These patients are at high risk of coronary disease and death. Philipson and colleagues[10] found that overall mortality following transplantation was 5.4% in those insulin-dependent diabetic patients without coronary artery disease, 20% in those with 'moderate' coronary artery disease, and 62% in those with 'severe' coronary disease (i.e. triple vessel disease, left main stem disease and/or severe left ventricular dysfunction). Similarly, Weinrauch and co-workers[13] found in a group of diabetics on dialysis that 2-year survival was 88% in those with no coronary artery disease and 22% in those with coronary artery disease. Sixty-two per cent of the deaths in the group with coronary disease were secondary to cardiac causes. Braun and co-workers[6] found that only 44% of 25 insulin-dependent diabetics with significant coronary disease remained alive after 2 years of follow-up.

The rationale for screening these patients for ischaemic heart disease prior to transplantation is that there is some evidence that revascularization can improve the prognosis, especially in asymptomatic diabetic patients. Manske and co-workers[14] reported a study in which 26 insulin-dependent diabetics with no symptoms suggestive of ischaemic heart disease and with normal left ventricular function were found at screening angiography to have significant ischaemic heart disease. Thirteen patients were assigned to receive revascularization (either coronary artery bypass surgery (CABG) or percutaneous transluminal coronary angioplasty (PTCA)), and 13 patients were assigned to medical management (the combination of aspirin and a calcium channel blocking drug). The study was discontinued early when an interim analysis revealed that the revascularized group experienced significantly fewer cardiac events (Fig. 14.1). The results of this trial, by the authors' own admission, need to be interpreted with caution: it was aborted prior to the planned date, the numbers of patients are small, and the patients assigned to 'medical' treatment did not receive as intensive treatment as might have been possible. Nevertheless, it does lend significant weight to the argument that revascularization improves the prognosis of diabetic patients with significant ischaemic heart disease undergoing transplantation.

Do all diabetic patients require screening?

Attempts have been made to identify a 'low risk' subgroup of diabetic patients who do not require screening. Manske and co-workers[15] concluded after a retrospective analysis that diabetics under the age of 45, with less than a 5-pack-year history of smoking, a duration of diabetes of less than 25 years, and a normal ECG (excluding changes caused by left ventricular hypertrophy) have a very low risk of having coronary artery disease. They prospectively examined 26 such patients and found these factors together have a sensitivity of 97% and a specificity of 96% in the exclusion of significant ischaemic heart disease.

Diabetics who do not fulfil all of these criteria require screening for the presence of ischaemic heart disease. Those with clear symptoms of angina, a history or ECG changes

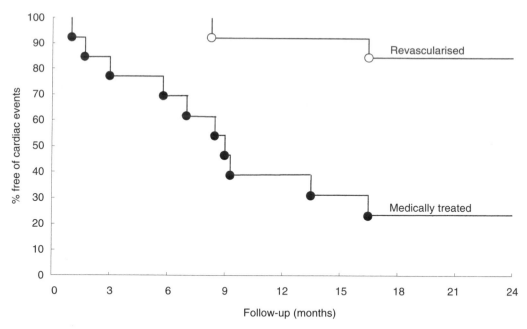

Fig. 14.1 Fewer cardiac events in revascularized asymptomatic diabetic patients following transplantation when compared with medically treated patients. (From Manske *et al.*[14].)

consistent with myocardial infarction, or poor left ventricular function are at very high risk, and most centres proceed directly to angiography. For other diabetics underlying ischaemic heart disease remains possible. For these patients, coronary angiography is not an ideal screening test, as discussed above, and, therefore, attempts have been made to identify a less invasive but still reliable substitute. The exercise ECG stress test is rarely of use in these circumstances. Abnormalities of the resting ECG may make the interpretation of an exercise ECG stress test impossible. In addition to this, many ESRF patients have poor exercise tolerance and are unable to achieve the heart rates necessary for an exercise test. Autonomic neuropathy may also affect the ability to achieve the desired heart rate.[16] While more than 80% of non-renal patients with significant ischaemic heart disease can be identified by exercise ECG stress testing, only a small percentage of ESRF patients have diagnostic tests.

The role of thallium scintigraphy

A reduction in myocardial perfusion is the earliest event in the development of myocardial ischaemia. In non-renal patients, the use of isotope-labelled perfusion tracers and scintigraphic imaging to demonstrate areas of decreased perfusion is a sensitive and specific method of detecting coronary artery disease.[17-19] Cardiovascular stress can be provoked by exercise (either using a treadmill or an exercise bicycle) or by pharmacological means. Drugs used to provoke stress are either inotropes, e.g. dobutamine, or vasodilators, e.g. dipyridamole or adenosine. The isotope used is usually thallium-201 or technetium-99m. The isotope is injected at peak exercise and a gamma camera is placed over the heart. Images obtained are compared with rest images. In order to try and improve sensitivity, single photon emission computerized tomography (SPECT) can be used. Areas of ischaemia have reduced isotope uptake: these may be fixed defects (reduced uptake on both resting and stress images) or reversible defects (reduced uptake on the stress images; restored uptake on the rest images).

Thallium scintigraphy is established as a screening test in detecting ischaemic heart disease in patients preparing to undergo vascular surgery.[20] Several studies have attempted to examine whether thallium testing is valid as a screening test in ESRF, particularly in diabetic patients being considered as candidates for renal transplantation. The accuracy of exercise thallium scintigraphy depends heavily on whether the patient is able to achieve the desired heart rate (usually considered to be 85% of the predicted maximum rate adjusted for age). Studies in diabetic patients with ESRF disease suggest that if this rate is achieved, and the result of the test is unequivocally negative, then the probability of a future cardiac event is low. Philipson and colleagues[10] found no subsequent cardiac complications in such patients, although only 7 out of 60 diabetic patients in this study fulfilled these criteria for a negative test. Holley and co-workers[21] obtained negative tests in 64 of the 180 patients they studied, and of the 48 of these patients who went on to be transplanted, only one developed a cardiac complication. Derfler and co-workers[22] obtained similar results, with only 1.9% of those patients with a negative test developing cardiac complications during the follow-up period. If a heart rate of 85% of the predicted maximum is not reached, a negative test becomes much less reliable in predicting no future cardiac complications, as demonstrated by Morrow and co-workers[5] in whose study 22 out of 67 patients with a 'negative' test had a subsequent cardiac event. Only six patients in this study, however, actually achieved a heart rate of 85% of the predicted maximum.

Studies using pharmacological stress show similar results. Camp and colleagues,[23] Brown and co-workers[24] and Le and colleagues[25] all studied diabetic patients, and found that those with normal thallium scintigraphy had a very low incidence of cardiac complications over their study periods. None of these studies included angiography, but those studies which have done so reveal that normal thallium scintigraphy results can be obtained even in the presence of significant coronary lesions. Boudreau and co-workers[26] performed thallium scintigraphy and coronary angiography on 80 diabetic ESRF patients. Six of these patients had a normal thallium test and evidence of significant ischaemic heart disease at angiography. Marwick and colleagues[27] performed dipyridamole SPECT thallium scintigraphy and angiography on 45 ESRF patients. All of their patients were at 'high risk' of having coronary disease, being either diabetic, over the age of 40, or with a history of chest pain. Twelve of 31 patients (38.7%) with negative thallium studies had significant coronary disease at angiography. Five of the six patients who died from cardiac causes over the subsequent 26 months of follow-up had had a negative thallium study.

What conclusions can be drawn from these apparently conflicting results? Biases in patient selection and referral patterns, differences in the study protocols, and different end-points in study designs may account for many of the differences in the results among these trials. However, we agree with the conclusion of Manske and co-workers[15] that diabetic transplant candidates who do not fall into the 'low risk' subgroup as defined by Manske and colleagues should all receive coronary angiography prior to transplantation. The prevalence of significant ischaemic heart disease is so high in this group of patients that the reliability of thallium scintigraphy is not sufficiently great to justify risking the overlooking of significant coronary disease which might benefit from intervention prior to transplantation. Future research may refine these criteria, and enable other groups of patients to avoid angiography with relative safety.

Non-diabetic candidates for transplantation

Symptomatic patients

Patients known to have ischaemic heart disease, i.e. those with angina, a history of myocardial infarction, or typical ECG changes of myocardial infarction, are likely to have a positive stress thallium study, and even if they do not, this test is unlikely to make any contribution to the management of these patients. Angiography is recommended as it enables the anatomy and severity of the coronary artery disease to be assessed. Patients with extensive (i.e. triple vessel or left main stem) disease are likely to benefit from revascularization, as discussed below.

Patients with impaired left ventricular function should also receive coronary angiography. Poor left ventricular function is often associated with severe coronary disease in these patients. In non-renal patients it is the patients with impaired left ventricular function who benefit the most from revascularization,[28] although these patients also have a higher perioperative morbidity. Studies intended specifically to demonstrate that such patients in the ESRF population also benefit from revascularization have not been performed, although this is likely to be the case.

Asymptomatic patients

Asymptomatic non-diabetic patients with no evidence of ischaemic heart disease on the ECG are the least likely candidates for transplantation to have significant ischaemic heart disease. Younger patients in this group in particular are at particularly low risk, and are unlikely to require screening.

The study of Le and colleagues[25] used a 'two-tiered' risk stratification. Patients under the age of 50, with no history of angina or insulin-dependent diabetes or congestive cardiac failure, and with normal resting ECGs were considered at low risk of cardiac events and received no further cardiac evaluation. All other patients were considered to be at higher risk and underwent exercise stress thallium scintigraphy (or dipyridamole thallium scintigraphy if they were unable to exercise). In the follow-up period (mean 46 months) only one cardiac death occurred in the 'low risk' group of 94 patients. In the high risk group (excluding the diabetic patients), two cardiac deaths occurred in the 17 patients with a 'normal' thallium study, although it should be noted that on average only 77% of the maximal predicted heart rate was achieved in these patients. Five of the 21 patients with abnormal thallium tests had subsequent cardiac events. The results of this study suggest that younger patients with no risk factors do not require screening. Older patients, those with left ventricular impairment or a history of angina with negative thallium scintigraphy are at lower risk of future cardiac complications compared with those with positive tests.

Dobutamine stress echocardiography

The combination of echocardiography with stress (either exercise or pharmacological stress) has now become established as an alternative method for the diagnosis of coronary artery disease in the non-renal population. Studies using dobutamine stress echocardiography[29–31] have shown sensitivities of 72–82%, specificities of 77–83%, and positive predictive accuracies of 76–82%, comparable to dipyridamole stress echocardiography.[32] One study of dobutamine stress echocardiography in ESRF patients[33] examined 97 patients who were awaiting renal transplantation. They report a sensitivity of 95% and a specificity of 86% for predicting death or cardiovascular events over the subsequent 12 months. This was a small study,

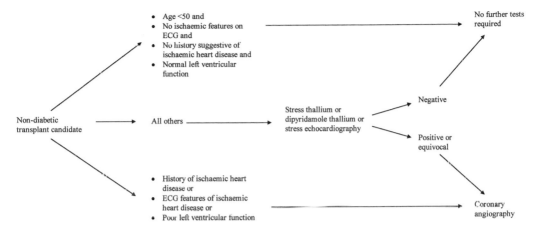

Fig. 14.2   Possible strategy for the pre-transplant assessment of the non-diabetic patient.

with only a short follow-up period, and only 30% of the patients were transplanted within the confines of the study. Further studies are needed to confirm these encouraging results.

Strategy for the management of the transplant candidate

There is no universal agreement on the optimal management strategy for the patient await-ing transplantation. Ramos and colleagues[11] found that 21% of US centres have no specific policy on the exclusion of patients for transplantation based on cardiac problems. Undoubtedly, this is in part because the published studies often do not agree. Larger studies are required, with more patients and longer follow-up periods, to enable decisions to be made on which patients should be excluded and which will benefit the most from screening, angiography, and revascularization.

At present, in non-diabetic patients, there is evidence to support the view that patients under the age of 50, with no ischaemic features on the ECG, with no history suggestive of ischaemic heart disease, and with normal left ventricular function do not require further investigation (see Fig. 14.2).

At the opposite end of the spectrum, those with clear clinical or electrocardiographic evi-dence of ischaemic heart disease or those with poor left ventricular function should receive angiography. Other patients, at moderate risk, should receive either stress thallium (if they are able to achieve the target heart rate), dipyridamole thallium scintigraphy, or stress echocardio-graphy. Which of these tests is most appropriate will depend on the condition of the patient as well as on local expertise in performing and interpreting the results of the investigations. If the result of this investigation is normal, further investigation is not required. If it is abnormal or equivocal, angiography should be performed. Diabetics under the age of 45 who have had dia-betes for less than 25 years, with less than a 5-pack-year history of smoking and with no clini-cal, electrocardiographic, or echocardiographic evidence of ischaemic heart disease or left ventricular dysfunction do not require further investigation. All other diabetics should receive angiography (see Fig. 14.3). If angiography reveals significant disease, then revascularization and/or exclusion of the patient as a transplant candidate may be considered.

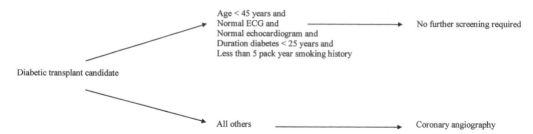

Fig. 14.3 Possible strategy for the pre-transplant assessment of the diabetic patient.

If thallium scintigraphy and/or angiography are normal, it is rational for the patient to be further assessed after a suitable time interval to ensure that coronary disease has not progressed. There are currently no data to determine what a suitable time interval should be, and studies addressing this important question are needed.

Transplant recipients

The receipt of a transplant does not appear to provide protection against the progression of cardiovascular disease. The risk of coronary events is as high post-transplantation as it is in comparable dialysis patients. Cardiovascular causes are responsible for 29.6% of the deaths of transplant patients, and 36.6% of these deaths are secondary to myocardial infarction.[1] The cardiovascular death rate is highest in the first year after transplantation, and thereafter increases linearly with a constant annual mortality rate.[34]

The inexactitude of exercise and thallium testing which complicates investigation of coronary disease in the pre-transplant patient remains a problem in the transplant recipient. There should, therefore, be a low threshold for angiography. Any patient with limiting angina despite optimal anti-anginal treatment, with chronic stable angina and evidence of ischaemia at low workload, or with angina following a myocardial infarction should be referred for angiography. A few patients may require angiography in order to make the diagnosis of ischaemic heart disease, where non-invasive testing has provided undiagnostic results.

Medical management of ischaemic heart disease in renal patients

Acute myocardial infarction

Acute myocardial infarction is ascribed as the immediate cause of death in 10.5% of all ESRF patients.[1] Overall mortality following myocardial infarction is 59.3% at 1 year and 89.9% at 5 years.[12] Cardiac mortality is 40.8% at 1 year and 70.2% at 5 years. Mortality figures have not improved since the introduction of thrombolysis therapy, although there has been a small improvement in survival if adjustment is made for comorbidity and age. The survival of patients with ESRF after myocardial infarction is significantly worse than that of patients without ESRF and with myocardial infarction. The figures for transplant patients are better than those for dialysis patients, although still worse than those for non-renal patients.

It is not clear why ESRF patients fare so poorly after myocardial infarction, and there have been few published trials to guide the management of these patients. There are no published data on the survival of ESRF patients who receive reperfusion therapy, and therefore most centres use the same criteria for administration of thrombolysis as for non-renal patients. The effect of aspirin in myocardial infarction in these patients has also not been studied. In the absence of data, these patients are usually managed using protocols drawn up for non-renal patients. Similarly, the protective role of angiotensin-converting enzyme inhibitors following myocardial infarction in patients with impaired left ventricular function[35] in the non-renal population is presumed, in the absence of clinical trials, to extend to patients with ESRF.

Anaemia

The management of anaemia in ESRF has been transformed in recent years by the use of erythropoietin. Target haemoglobin levels vary between centres, although National Kidney Foundation guidelines in the US recommend a target haematocrit of 33–36%.[36] In patients with ischaemic heart disease it is important to keep the haemoglobin within the desired range. Besarab and colleagues[37] showed a 30% decrease in the incidence of death or primary cardiac event for each 10% rise in haematocrit up to 45%. Too low a level will also predispose to anginal symptoms and the worsening of left ventricular hypertrophy. Too high a level may increase the risk of thrombosis occurring, and there remains concern over the morbidity associated with infections related to iron usage.[38] High levels of iron stores have also been reported to be associated with increased risk of cardiovascular disease,[39] although a subsequent study which measured transferrin saturation rather than serum ferritin levels failed to replicate these results.[40]

Anti-anginal therapy

Beta blockers, calcium channel blockers, and nitrates are all used in patients with ESRF and can provide symptomatic benefit. Beta blockers may exacerbate the problems of fluid overload, particularly in those with markedly impaired left ventricular function. The doses of those drugs which are normally excreted by the kidneys, e.g. atenolol, may require reduction. Although symptomatic improvement is often self-evident, no trials have studied the impact of anti-anginal drugs on survival in patients with ESRF.

Aspirin

Several randomized trials in non-renal patients have shown that aspirin given to high risk patients with known vascular disease significantly reduces the risk of myocardial infarction, stroke, and cardiovascular death.[41] It is not yet clear whether this benefit extends to ESRF patients. Although the risk of vascular thrombotic events is high, platelet function is impaired in uraemia and these patients also have an increased risk of bleeding complications such as gastrointestinal and intracerebral haemorrhage. One small trial of aspirin in dialysis patients failed to demonstrate an increase in bleeding complications, but also failed to demonstrate a decrease in thrombotic events.[42] A large controlled trial is needed to evaluate the benefits of aspirin in ESRF patients.

Risk factor modification

The control of hypertension, hyperparathyroidism, obesity, and lifestyle changes (dietary modification, stopping smoking, and increasing exercise activity) are all fundamental to the management of ischaemic heart disease, especially in the ESRF population. Aggressive control of lipid abnormalities is required. These aspects are covered in detail in other chapters.

Dialysis prescription

It is desirable to minimize rapid fluid shifts and changes in blood pressure during dialysis in patients with coronary artery disease and for this reason continuous ambulatory peritoneal dialysis (CAPD) is often the dialysis modality of choice, especially if left ventricular function is poor.[43] CAPD also has the advantage that an arteriovenous fistula, with its additional blood flow increasing the demands on the heart, is not required. If haemodialysis is required, care must be taken to avoid hypotension during dialysis sessions. This may be worsened by large interdialytic weight gains, necessitating rapid removal of fluid. The use of bicarbonate rather than acetate in the dialysate may lessen this risk,[44,45] and there is some evidence that the use of biocompatible membranes may also be of benefit.[46] Hyper- and hypokalaemia should be avoided to minimize the risk of arrhythmias.

Revascularization in patients with ESRF

Results in the non-renal population

Coronary artery bypass surgery (CABG) has been shown to produce clear benefits in long-term mortality and cardiac morbidity in certain patient groups.[47–49] The greatest benefit is gained by those with the highest preoperative risk, especially those patients with left ventricular dysfunction. When compared to medical management, improvements in long-term survival have been shown in patients with triple vessel disease, with or without left ventricular dysfunction, although with the greatest benefit for those with left ventricular dysfunction. Mortality is also improved in those patients with significant left main stem or proximal left anterior descending artery disease. However, no survival benefit has been demonstrated in patients with single-vessel disease and normal left ventricular function. Many of these studies were performed before the widespread use of internal mammary artery grafting, which has been shown to be associated with prolonged graft survival.[50] In addition to this, the recognition of the benefits of aspirin and the introduction of aggressive lipid-lowering strategies have occurred since the time of many of these trials.

   Percutaneous transluminal coronary angioplasty (PTCA) has developed rapidly over recent years. Studies have shown that when compared with medical treatment in single-vessel disease, symptom control and hospital readmission rates are improved in PTCA-treated patients.[51] A number of trials have compared PTCA with CABG. There have been many differences in study design between these trials, making direct comparison difficult. A meta-analysis of all the early trials[52] showed that there was no difference in infarct rate or medium term survival between the two techniques. However, the need for subsequent revascularization is consistently greater in PTCA-treated patients. In the first year of follow-up, 33.7% of PTCA-treated patients required another revascularization procedure compared with 3.3% of CABG-treated patients. In the longer term, the need for revascularization remains higher in PTCA treated patients (4.5 versus 1.8 per 100 patient-years). Similar results were obtained in the BARI trial.[53] This has been the only study, with 5 years of follow-up data, with the power to detect differences in mortality. Overall survival rates were not different between the CABG- and PTCA-treated groups, but there were significantly fewer subsequent revascularization procedures in the CABG-treated group (5% versus 52%). Most of these repeat procedures occurred during the first year, when the risk of restenosis is the most high. Diabetics were analysed as a subgroup in this study: in these patients long-term survival was significantly better with CABG than with PTCA (81% versus 65%). The poor outcome of diabetics who undergo PTCA has also been demonstrated by other studies.[54]

Techniques have improved even since the publication of these studies, and it is likely that in time the rates of restenosis, currently the limiting factor in the long-term success of the procedure, will be reduced. The introduction and refinement of the use of intra-coronary stents[55,56] has reduced rates of restenosis and limited the morbidity of acute dissection during the procedure itself. Versaci *et al.*[57] studied 120 patients with isolated stenosis of the proximal left anterior descending artery. Those patients assigned to stenting with PTCA had a higher rate of event free survival and lower rate of restenosis at 12 months compared with those patients assigned to PTCA alone. This and the development of more effective anti-platelet agents such as ticlopidine[58] and blockade of the platelet glycoprotein IIb/IIIa receptor[59] and of other techniques such as laser angioplasty and atherectomy mean that results with percutaneous coronary revascularization are likely to continue to improve.

Revascularization in the renal population

CABG

In patients with ESRF, the enormous fluid shifts which occur during cardiopulmonary bypass are more difficult to manage than in patients with normal renal function. This, the timing and route of perioperative dialysis, and the increased bleeding and infective complications of these patients led to reluctance initially amongst surgeons to accept ESRF patients for grafting. Gradually, however, as experience built up, it has become clear that CABG can be carried out in these patients. The perioperative mortality is higher than in the general population, ranging from 0 to 20% in published series (see Table 14.1). The wide discrepancies in perioperative mortality probably relate to differences in patient selection criteria, comorbidity, and the urgency of the cardiac surgery.

The long-term prognosis, however, appears to be relatively good. Symptomatic improvement and reduced need for anti-anginal medication is reported universally. Only a few of the published studies have examined long-term survival. Opsahl and colleagues[60] experienced a perioperative mortality of 3%, but after 2 years of follow-up 92% of their study patients remained alive. A comparable group of ESRF patients who received medical management for their coronary artery disease had a 2-year survival of 51%. Batiuk and co-workers[61] report a 2-year survival of 77%, while Sauve and co-workers[62] report a 2-year survival of 63%. These figures are similar to those in unselected dialysis patients (many of whom do not have coronary artery disease), if actuarial survival is corrected from the time when dialysis was commenced,[34] and they are better than those reported for dialysis patients with coronary artery disease treated medically.[63]

Table 14.1 Perioperative death rates in studies of CABG in ESRF patients (only studies with five or more patients are included)

	Perioperative mortality	% Perioperative mortality
Francis et al.[69]	1/8	12.5
Monson et al. [70]	2/14	14.3
Laws et al. [71]	1/9	11.1
Marshall et al.[72]	1/12	8.3
Albert et al.[73]	0/11	0
Opsahl et al. [60]	1/39	2.6
Peper et al.[74]	1/31	3.2
Rostand et al.[75]	4/20	20
Blakeman et al.[76]	1/16	6.3
Deutsch et al.[77]	1/16	6.3
Batiuk et al.[61]	4/25	16.0
De Meyer et al.[67]	2/18	11.1
Ko et al.[78]	3/16	18.8
Rinehart et al.[68]	2/60	3.3
Total	24/295	8.1

PTCA

Studies using PTCA in patients with ESRF have been much less encouraging, tending to demonstrate high rates of procedural morbidity and of restenosis. In the study of Reusser and colleagues,[64] 38% of ESRF patients subjected to PTCA experienced a problem around the time of the procedure, compared with 0% in non-renal control patients. During the follow-up period, 50% of renal patients compared with 15% of controls had a cardiac event. Two-thirds of the study patients who underwent repeat angiography had restenosis of their lesions. Results similar have been obtained by other investigators.[65,66] De Meyer and colleagues[67] report 'restenosis' in only one of 10 patients within 6 months of PTCA, although in this study recurrent angina was used as a surrogate end-point for restenosis and the actual rate was probably higher. Rinehart and colleagues[68] compared CABG with PTCA in a total of 84 ESRF patients. PTCA was associated with an increased risk of recurrent angina and combined cardiovascular events (Fig. 14.4). All-cause mortality was not significantly different between groups, although there was a trend towards higher cardiovascular mortality in the PTCA-treated group. Again, angina was used as a surrogate end-point for restenosis in this study, although there was a 69% restenosis rate in the 13 patients with recurrent angina who were studied with repeat angiography.

In conclusion, in patients with ESRF, PTCA is associated with a high rate of restenosis. With the rapidly improving techniques and results in PTCA, the introduction of intracoronary stents and improvements in anti-platelet medication, it is likely that a role for the technique in ESRF patients will soon be found. Until future studies have demonstrated this, CABG remains the revascularization procedure of choice in most ESRF patients. A limited role exists for PTCA for those patients with persistent symptoms despite medical therapy with single- or two-vessel disease and favourable anatomy, with the proviso that restenosis is common and repeat procedures may be necessary. Stenting is likely to prove beneficial, although no evidence in renal patients yet exists to support this assertion.

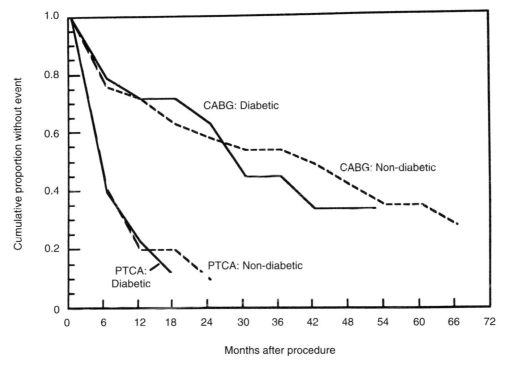

Fig. 14.4 Coronary artery bypass surgery (CABG) is associated with fewer post-procedure cardiac events than percutaneous transluminal coronary angioplasty (PTCA) in ESRF patients. (From Rinehart *et al.*[68].)

Conclusions

Properly designed multicentre prospective controlled studies are required to evaluate which interventions are appropriate to alleviate the burden of cardiovascular disease in the dialysis and transplant population. Until the results of such trials are available, management has to be based on the results of the small trials which have been conducted on the ESRF population and by extrapolation (which may or may not be valid) from larger studies in non-renal patients.

Nevertheless, it is clear that coronary artery disease is a major cause of death and of morbidity in patients with ESRF. Revascularization is recommended for patients with multivessel disease, especially if left ventricular function is impaired. Single-vessel disease is usually best managed medically. CABG, although associated with a higher perioperative mortality than in the non-renal population, is the preferred method of revascularization, as PTCA in these patients has an unacceptably high risk of restenosis. Nevertheless, PTCA may be of use in the control of symptoms in the patient with single-vessel or two-vessel disease who fails to respond to medical treatment, or in the control of symptoms in any patient considered too high risk for CABG. The benefits of intracoronary stenting and of newer antiplatelet agents in the non-renal population have not yet been proven to extend to the ESRF population, although this is likely to be the case.

The high mortality associated with coronary artery disease in this population dictates that all patients with a history of ischaemic heart disease or abnormalities on the ECG suggestive of ischaemic heart disease should receive angiography prior to transplantation, so that revascularization can be carried out if necessary. Asymptomatic coronary disease is common in ESRF patients, particularly in those with diabetes. Myocardial infarction often occurs soon after the commencement of renal replacement therapy and carries a poor prognosis. Thus screening where appropriate should be carried out as soon as possible after the initiation of dialysis. There is no screening test for coronary artery disease which is totally satisfactory in patients with ESRF, and for this reason many centres recommend coronary angiography be performed on all diabetic patients considered for transplantation unless they are under the age of 45 and have no other risk factors. Asymptomatic coronary artery disease also occurs in non-diabetic ESRF patients, although less commonly. Screening of older patients in this group with thallium scintigraphy or dobutamine stress echocardiography is recommended, and any patient who has a normal or equivocal test should receive angiography prior to transplantation.

Aspirin is probably beneficial in ESRF patients with ischaemic heart disease, and dialysis prescriptions should be crafted to minimize the risk of hypotensive episodes. Finally, the importance of risk factor modification cannot be overemphasized. Coronary artery disease is a diffuse process, and only if there is aggressive treatment of risk factors such as lipid abnormalities, hypertension, hyperparathyroidism, and smoking will the most benefit be obtained. These interventions often need to be targeted early in the course of chronic renal failure, so as to minimize the progression of coronary disease.

References

1. United States Renal Data System: USRDS (1997). *Annual Data Report*. The National Institutes of Health, National Institute of Diabetes and Digestive and Kidney Diseases, Bethesda, MD.
2. Bennett W.M., Kloster F., Rosch J., Barry J., Porter G.A. (1978). Natural history of asymptomatic coronary arteriographic lesions in diabetic patients with end-stage renal disease. *American Journal of Medicine*, 65, 779–784.
3. Weinrauch L., D'Elia J.A., Healy R.W., Gleason R.E., Christlieb R., Leland O.S. (1978). Asymptomatic coronary artery disease: angiographic assessment of diabetics evaluated for renal transplantation. *Circulation*, 58, 1184–1190.
4. Weinrauch L.A., D'Elia J.A., Healy R.W., Gleason R.E., Takacs F.J., Libertino J.A., *et al*. (1978). Asymptomatic coronary artery disease: angiography in diabetic patients before renal transplantation. Relation of findings to postoperative survival. *Annals of Internal Medicine*, 88, 346–348.
5. Morrow C.E., Schwartz J.S., Sutherland D.E.R., Simmons R.L., Ferguson R.M., Kjellstrand C.M., *et al*. (1983). Predictive value of thallium stress testing for coronary and cardiovascular events in uremic diabetic patients before renal transplantation. *American Journal of Surgery*, 146, 331–335.
6. Braun W.E., Phillips D., Vidt D.G., Novick A.C., Nakamoto S., Popowniak K.L., *et al*. (1981). Coronary arteriography and coronary artery disease in 99 diabetic and nondiabetic patients on chronic hemodialysis or renal transplantation programs. *Transplant Proceedings*, 13, 128–135.
7. Franciosa J.A., Wilen M., Ziesche S., Cohn J.N. (1983). Survival in men with severe chronic left ventricular failure due to either coronary heart disease or idiopathic dilated cardiomyopathy. *American Journal of Cardiology*, 51, 831–836.
8. Rostand S.G., Kirk K.A., Rutsky E.A. (1984). Dialysis-associated ischemic heart disease: insights from coronary angiography. *Kidney International*, 25, 653–659.
9. De Lemos J.A., Hillis L.D. (1996). Diagnosis and management of coronary artery disease in patients with end-stage renal disease on hemodialysis. *Journal of the American Society of Nephrology*, 7, 2044–2054.

10. Philipson J.D., Carpenter B.J., Itzkoff J., Hakala T.R., Rosenthal J.T., Taylor R.J., *et al.* (1986). Evaluation of cardiovascular risk for renal transplantation in diabetic patients. *American Journal of Medicine*, 81, 630–634.

11. Ramos E.L., Kasiske B.L., Alexander S.R., Danovitch G.M., Harmon W.E., Kahana L., *et al.* (1994). The evaluation of candidates for renal transplantation. *Transplantation*, 57, 490–497.

12. Herzog C.A., Ma J.Z., Collins A.J. (1998). Poor long-term survival after acute myocardial infarction among patients on long-term dialysis. *New England Journal of Medicine*, 339, 799–805.

13. Weinrauch L.A., D'Elia J.A., Monaco A.P., Gleason R.E., Welty F., Nishan P., *et al.* (1992). Preoperative evaluation for diabetic renal transplantation: impact of clinical, laboratory, and echocardiographic parameters on patient and allograft survival. *American Journal of Medicine*, 93, 19–28.

14. Manske C.L., Wang Y., Rector T., Wilson R.F., White C.W. (1992). Coronary revascularisation in insulin-dependent diabetic patients with chronic renal failure. *Lancet*, 340, 998–1002.

15. Manske C.L., Thomas W., Wang Y., Wilson R.F. (1993). Screening diabetic transplant candidates for coronary artery disease: identification of a low risk subgroup. *Kidney International*, 44, 617–621.

16. Radice M., Rocca A., Bedon E., Musaccio N., Morabito A., Segalini G. (1996). Abnormal response to exercise in middle-aged NIDDM patients with and without autonomic neuropathy. *Diabetic Medicine*, 13, 259–265.

17. Okada R.D., Boucher C.A., Strauss H.W., Pohost G.M. (1980). Exercise radionuclide imaging approaches to coronary artery disease. *American Journal of Cardiology*, 16, 1188–1204.

18. Leppo J., Boucher C.A., Okada R.D., Newell J.B., Strauss H.W., Pohost G.M. (1982). Serial thallium 201 myocardial imaging after dipyridamole infusion; diagnostic utility in detecting coronary stenoses and relationship to regional wall motion. *Circulation*, 66, 649–657.

19. Josephson M.A., Brown B.G., Hecht H.S., Hopkins J., Pierce C.D., Petersen R.B. (1982). Noninvasive detection and localization of coronary stenoses in patients: comparison of resting dipyridamole and exercise thallium-201 myocardial perfusion imaging. *American Heart Journal*, 103, 1008–1018.

20. Eagle K.A., Singer D.E., Brewster D.C., Darling R.C., Mulley A.G., Boucher C.A. (1987). Dipyridamole-thallium scanning in patients undergoing vascular surgery: optimizing preoperative evaluation of cardiac risk. *Journal of the American Medical Association*, 257, 2185–2189.

21. Holley J.L., Fenton R.A., Arthur R.S. (1991). Thallium stress testing does not predict cardiovascular risk in diabetic patients with end-stage renal disease undergoing cadaveric renal transplantation. *American Journal of Medicine*, 90, 563–570.

22. Derfler K., Kletter K., Balcke., Heinze G., Dudczak R. (1991). Predictive value of thallium-201-dipyridamole myocardial stress scintigraphy in chronic hemodialysis patients and transplant recipients. *Clinical Nephrology*, 36, 192–202.

23. Camp A.D., Garvin P.J. Hoff J., Marsh J., Byers S.L., Chaitman B.R. (1990). Prognostic value of intravenous dipyridamole thallium imaging in patients with diabetes mellitus considered for renal transplantation. *American Journal of Cardiology*, 65, 1459–1463.

24. Brown K.A., Rimmer J., Haisch C. (1989). Noninvasive cardiac risk stratification of diabetic and nondiabetic uremic renal allograft candidates using dipyridamole-thallium-201 imaging and radionuclide ventriculography. *American Journal of Cardiology*, 64, 1017–1021.

25. Le A., Wilson R., Douek K., Pulliam L., Tozman D., Norman D., *et al.* (1994). Prospective risk stratification in renal transplant candidates for cardiac death. *American Journal of Kidney Diseases*, 24, 65–71.

26. Boudreau R.J., Strony J.T., duCret R.P., Kuni C.C., Wang Y., Wilson R.F., *et al.* (1990). Perfusion thallium imaging of type I diabetes patients with end stage renal disease: comparison of oral and intravenous dipyridamole administration. *Radiology*, 175, 103–105.

27. Marwick T.H., Steinmuller D.R., Underwood D.A., Hobbs R.E., Go R.T., Swift C., *et al.* (1990). Ineffectiveness of dipyridamole spect thallium imaging as a screening technique for coronary artery disease in patients with end-stage renal failure. *Transplantation*, 49, 100–103.

28. Yusuf S., Zucker D., Peduzzi P., Fisher L.D., Takaro T., Kennedy J.W., *et al.* (1994). Effect of coronary artery bypass graft surgery on survival: overview of 10-year results from randomised trials by the Coronary Artery Bypass Graft Surgery Trialist Collaboration. *Lancet*, 344, 563–570.

29. Beleslin B.D., Ostojik M., Stepanovic J., Djordjevic-Dikic A., Stojkovic S., Nedeljkovic M., *et al.* (1994). Stress echocardiography in detection of myocardial ischemia. *Circulation*, 90, 1168–1176.

30. Marwick T.H., D'Hondt A.-M., Baudhuin T., Willemart B., Wijns W., Detry J.M., *et al.* (1993). Optimal use of dobutamine stress for the detection and evaluation of coronary artery disease: combination with echocardiography, or scintigraphy, or both? *Journal of American College of Cardiology*, 22, 159–167.

31. Previtali M., Lanzarini L., Fetiveau R., Poli A., Ferrario M., Falcone C. (1993). Comparison of dobutamine stress echocardiography, dipyridamole stress echocardiography and exercise stress testing for diagnosis of coronary artery disease. *American Journal of Cardiology*, 72, 865–870.

32. Schroder K., Wieckhorst A., Voller H. (1997). Comparison of the prognostic value of dipyridamole and dobutamine stress echocardiography in patients with known or suspected coronary artery disease. *American Journal of Cardiology*, 79, 1516–1518.

33. Reis G., Marcovitz P.A., Leichtman A.B., Merion R.M., Fay W.P., Werns S.W., *et al.* (1995). Usefulness of dobutamine stress echocardiography in detecting coronary artery disease in end-stage renal disease. *American Journal of Cardiology*, 75, 707–710.

34. Valderrabano F., Jones E.H.P., Mallick N.P. (1995). Report on the management of renal failure in Europe XXIV. *Nephrology, Dialysis, Transplantation*, 10(Suppl. 5).

35. Pfeffer M.A., Braunwald E., Moye L.E., Basta L., Brown E.J., Cuddy T.E., *et al.* (1992). Effect of captopril on morbidity and mortality in patients with left ventricular dysfunction after myocardial infarction. Results of the survival and ventricular enlargement trial. The SAVE Investigators. *New England Journal of Medicine*, 327, 669–677.

36. NKF–DOQI clinical practice guidelines for the treatment of anemia of chronic renal failure (1997). *American Journal of Kidney Diseases*, 30(Suppl. 3), S192–S240.

37. Besarab A., Bolton W.K., Browne J.K., Egrie J.C., Nissenson A.R., Okamoto D.M., *et al.* (1998). The effects of normal as compared with low hematocrit values in patients with cardiac disease who are receiving hemodialysis and epoetin. *New England Journal of Medicine*, 339, 584–590.

38. Hoen B., Kessler M., Hestin D., Mayeux D. (1995). Risk factors for bacterial infections in chronic haemodialysis adult patients: a multicentre prospective survey. *Nephrology, Dialysis, Transplantation*, 10, 377–381.

39. Salonen J.T., Nyyssonen K., Korpela H., Tuomilehto J., Seppanen R., Salonen R. (1992). High stored iron levels are associated with excess risk of myocardial infarction in eastern Finnish men. *Circulation*, 86, 803–811.

40. Sempos C.T., Looker A.C., Gillum R.F., Makuc D.M. (1994). Body iron stores and the risk of coronary heart disease. *New England Journal of Medicine*, 330, 1119–1124.

41. Antiplatelet Trialists' Collaboration (1994). Collaborative overview of randomised trials of antiplatelet therapy. I: Prevention of death, myocardial infarction, and stroke by prolonged antiplatelet therapy in various categories of patients. *British Medical Journal*, 308, 81–106.

42. Kooistra M.P., van Es A., Marx J.J., Hertsig M. L., Struyrenberg A., (1994). Low-dose aspirin does not prevent thrombovascular accidents in low-risk haemodialysis patients during treatment with recombinant human erythropoietin. *Nephrology, Dialysis, Transplantation*, 9, 1115–1120.

43. Hebert M.J., Falardeau M., Picherte V., Houde M., Nolin L., Cardinal J., *et al.* (1995). Continuous ambulatory peritoneal dialysis for patients with severe left ventricular systolic dysfunction and end-stage renal disease. *American Journal of Kidney Diseases*, 25, 761–768.

44. Dolan M.J., Whipp B.J., Davidson W.D., Weitzman R.E., Wasserman K. (1981). Hypopnea associated with acetate hemodialysis: carbon dioxide-flow-dependent ventilation. *New England Journal of Medicine*, 305, 72–75.

45. Velez R.L., Woodard T.D., Henrich W.L. (1984). Acetate and bicarbonate hemodialysis in patients with and without autonomic dysfunction. *Kidney International*, 26, 59–65.

46. Cardoso M., Vinay P., Vinet B., Leveillee M., Prud'homme M., Tejedor A., *et al.* (1988). Hypoxemia during hemodialysis: a critical review of the facts. *American Journal of Kidney Diseases*, 11, 281–297.

47. Alderman E.L., Bourassa M.G., Cohen L.S., Davis K.B., Kaiser G.G., Killip T., *et al.* (1990). Ten-year follow-up of survival and myocardial infarction in the randomized Coronary Artery Surgery Study. *Circulation*, 82, 1629–1646.

48. Varnauskas E. (1988). Twelve-year follow-up of survival in the randomized European Coronary Surgery Study. *New England Journal of Medicine*, 319, 332–337.

49. Veterans Administration Coronary Artery Bypass Surgery Cooperative Study Group (1984). Eleven-year survival in the Veterans Administration randomized trial of coronary bypass surgery for stable angina. *New England Journal of Medicine*, 311, 1333–1339.

50. Loop F.D., Lytle B.W., Cosgrove D.M., Stewart R.W., Goormastic M., Wiliams G.W., *et al.* (1986). Influence of the internal-mammary-artery graft on 10-year survival and other cardiac events. *New England Journal of Medicine*, 314, 1–6.

51. Parisi A., Folland E.D., Hartigan P.A. (1992). A comparison of angioplasty with medical therapy in the treatment of single-vessel coronary artery disease. *New England Journal of Medicine*, 326, 10–16.

52. Pocock S.J., Henderson R.A., Rickards A.F., Hampton J.R., King S.B. III, Hamm C.W., *et al.* (1995). Meta-analysis of randomised trials comparing coronary angioplasty with bypass surgery. *Lancet*, 346, 1184–1189.

53. Bypass Angioplasty Revascularization Investigation (BARI) investigators (1996). Comparison of coronary bypass surgery with angioplasty in patients with multivessel disease. *New England Journal of Medicine*, 335, 217–252.

54. Faxon D.P., Kip K.E., Courrier J.W., Yeh W., Detre K. (1995). Diabetics have a significantly poorer eight-year outcome after angioplasty. *Circulation*, 92(Suppl. I), 76.

55. Serruys P.W., de Jaegere P., Kiemeneij F., Macaya C., Rutsch W., Heyndrickx G., *et al.* (1994). A comparison of balloon expandable stent implantation with balloon angioplasty in patients with coronary artery disease. *New England Journal of Medicine*, 331, 489–495.

56. Fischman D.L., Leon M.B., Baim D.S., Schatz R.A., Savage M.P., Penn I., *et al.* (1994). A randomized comparison of coronary-stent placement and balloon angioplasty in the treatment of coronary artery disease. Stent Restenosis Study Investigators. *New England Journal of Medicine*, 331, 496–501.

57. Versaci F., Gaspardone A., Tomai F., Crea F., Chiarello L., Gioffre P.A. (1997). A comparison of coronary artery stenting with angioplasty for isolated stenosis of the proximal left anterior descending coronary artery. *New England Journal of Medicine*, 336, 817–822.

58. Schomig A., Neumann F.J., Kastrati A., Schuhlen H., Blasini R., Hadamitzky M., *et al.* (1996). A randomized comparison of antiplatelet and anticoagulant therapy after the placement of coronary artery stents. *New England Journal of Medicine*, 334, 1084–1089.

59. The EPILOG Investigators (1997). Platelet glycoprotein IIb/IIIa receptor blockade and low-dose heparin during percutaneous coronary revascularization. *New England Journal of Medicine*, 336, 1689–1696.

60. Opsahl J.A., Husebye D.G., Helseth H.K., Collins A.J. (1988). Coronary artery bypass surgery in patients on maintenance dialysis: long-term survival. *American Journal of Kidney Diseases*, 12, 271–274.

61. Batiuk T.D., Kurtz S.B., Oh J.K., Orszulak T.A. (1991). Coronary artery bypass operation in dialysis patients. *Mayo Clinic Proceedings*, 66, 45–53.

62. Sauve C., Thaler F., Dubois C., Vinatier I., Aubert P., Loirat Ph. (1996). Results of cardiac surgery in chronic hemodialysis patients. *Nephrology, Dialysis, Transplantation*, 11, A135.

63. Hellerstedt W.L., Johnson W.J., Ascher N., Kjellstrand C.M., Knutson R., Sjapiro F.L., *et al.* (1984) Survival rates of 2728 patients with end-stage renal disease. *Mayo Clinic Proceedings*, 59, 776–783.

64. Reusser L.M., Osborn L.A., White H.J., Sexson R., Crawford M.H. (1994). Increased morbidity after coronary angioplasty in patients on chronic hemodialysis. *American Journal of Cardiology*, 73, 965–967.

65. Ahmed W.H., Shubrooks S.J., Gibson C.M., Baim D.S., Bittl J.A. (1994). Complications and long-term outcome after percutaneous coronary angioplasty in chronic hemodialysis patients. *American Heart Journal*, 128, 252–255.

66. Kahn J.K., Rutherford B.D., McConahay D.R., Johnson W.L., Giorgi L.V., Hartzler G.O. (1990). Short- and long-term outcome of percutaneous transluminal coronary angioplasty in chronic dialysis patients. *American Heart Journal*, 119, 484–489.

67. De Meyer M., Wyns W., Dion R., Khoury G., Pirson Y., van Ypersele de Strihou C. (1991). Myocardial revascularization in patients on renal replacement therapy. *Clinical Nephrology*, 36, 147–151.

68. Rinehart A.L., Herzog C.A., Collins A.J., Flack J.M., Ma J.Z., Opsahl J.A. (1995). A comparison of coronary angioplasty and coronary artery bypass grafting outcomes in chronic dialysis patients. *American Journal of Kidney Diseases*, 25, 281–290.

69. Francis G.S., Sharma B., Collins A.J., Helseth H.K., Comty C.M. (1980). Coronary artery surgery in patients with end-stage renal disease. *Annals of Internal Medicine*, 92, 499–503.

70. Monson B.K., Wickstrom P.H., Hagilin J.J., Francis G., Comty C.M., Helseth H.K. (1980). Cardiac operation and end-stage renal disease. *Annals of Thoracic Surgery*, 30, 267–272.

71. Laws K.H., Merrill W.H., Hammon J.W., Prager R.L., Bender H.W. (1986). Cardiac surgery in patients with chronic renal disease. *Annals of Thoracic Surgery*, 42, 152–157.

72. Marshall W.G., Rossi N.P., Meng R.L., Wedige-Stecher T. (1986). Coronary artery bypass grafting in dialysis patients. *Annals of Thoracic Surgery*, 42, S12–S15.

73. Albert F.W., Seyfert U.T., Grossman R., Schmidt U., Glunz H.G., Muller V., *et al.* (1987). Role of coronary angiography and heart surgery in care of kidney transplant recipients. *Transplantation Proceedings*, 19, 3689–3690.

74. Peper W.A., Taylor P.C., Paganini E.P., Svensson L.G., Ghattas M.A., Loop F.D. (1988). Mortality and results after cardiac surgery in patients with end-stage renal disease. *Cleveland Clinic Journal of Medicine*, 55, 63–67.

75. Rostand S.G., Kirk K., Rutsky E.A., Pacifico A.D. (1988). Results of coronary artery bypass grafting in end-stage renal disease. *American Journal of Kidney Diseases*, 12, 266–270.

76. Blakeman B.M., Pifarre R., Sullivan H.J., Montaya A., Bakhos M. (1989). Cardiac surgery for chronic renal dialysis patients. *Chest*, 95, 509–511.

77. Deutsch E., Bernstein R.C., Addonizio P., Kussmaul W.G. (1989). Coronary artery bypass surgery in patients on hemodialysis: a case-control study. *Annals of Internal Medicine*, 110, 369–372.

78. Ko W., Kreiger K.H., Isom O.W. (1993). Cardiopulmonary bypass procedures in dialysis patients. *Annals of Thoracic Surgery*, 55, 672–676

15

Hemodynamic instability, arrhythmias,
and dialysis reactions

K.M.L. Leunissen, J.P. Kooman, and F.M. van der Sande

Intermittent hemodialysis induces rapid changes in the fluid and solute status of the patient. This may lead to clinical symptoms which can vary from slight discomfort to life-threatening complications. The most frequently occurring symptom is hypotension. Other, less common complications are chest pain, cardiac arrhythmias, and anaphylactoid reactions. Although these complications are sometimes unavoidable, they can often be avoided with careful clinical judgment and modification of the dialysis regimen. This chapter will discuss the pathophysiology, treatment, and prevention of acute complications during intermittent dialysis.

Hemodialysis hypotension

Hypotension during dialysis may induce minor but troublesome side-effects to the patient, such as nausea, vomiting, and dizziness. It may also lead to more severe complications, such as cardiac or cerebral ischemia. Hypotension can also reduce the efficacy of the treatment, both because dialysis sometimes has to be (temporarily) terminated and because of reduced urea removal from the tissues due to vasoconstriction ('internal dialyzer'). Although many dialysis patients never suffer from hypotensive episodes, hemodialysis hypotension is especially frequent in the elderly and in those patients with a compromised cardiovascular system. Especially in the latter groups, hypotension may have serious consequences, such as myocardial and cerebral ischemia.

The pathogenesis of hemodialysis hypotension is multifactorial. Under normal circumstances, three major factors are of importance in the maintenance of hemodynamic stability during hypovolemia:

1. Refill of blood volume from the interstitium (blood volume preservation);

2. Constriction of the resistance vessels (small arteries and arterioles), leading to an increase in systemic vascular resistance; and

3. Maintenance of cardiac output, which occurs through an increase in myocardial contractility, heart rate, and constriction of the capacitance vessels (venules and veins), leading to centralization of blood volume. In this respect, not only an intact cardiovascular reflex but also an intact cardiovascular structure is of prime importance.[1]

In addition to a decline in blood volume, the two latter factors may also be impaired in dialysis patients. This explains why in healthy subjects, a blood volume decrease of 25% is generally well tolerated,[2] whereas in dialysis patients, hypotension often occurs with a much

Table 15.1 Factors affecting blood volume preservation during hemodialysis

Ultrafiltration rate
Fluid status
Dialysate sodium
Dialysate buffer
Treatment modality: hemodialysis vs. hemofiltration?
Dialysate temperature?
Food intake?
Venous compliance

lesser reduction in blood volume.[3] The importance of each of these factors may differ from patient to patient and from treatment to treatment.

Intravascular volume preservation

During ultrafiltration, fluid is removed from the intravascular space by convection owing to differences in hydrostatic pressure between the blood and dialysate compartments. Ultrafiltration can be performed with or without concomitant hemodialysis treatment ('isolated ultrafiltration').

In accordance with the Starling formula, the decrease in intravascular pressure and the increase in intravascular colloid osmotic pressure will induce a fluid shift from the interstitial to the intravascular space, which partly compensates for the fluid removed through the dialyzer. However, in most cases, the refill from the interstitial volume will not be complete and blood volume will decrease.[4,5] Intravascular hypovolemia may, therefore, even occur when the interstitial compartment is fluid-overloaded.

Several mechanisms, mainly related to the dialysis treatment but also patient-associated factors, will influence blood volume preservation and therefore influence hemodynamic stability during dialysis (Table 15.1).

Ultrafiltration rate

A main determinant of blood volume preservation is the ultrafiltration rate. Despite a rapid decrease in vascular hydrostatic pressure, the fluid that is removed from the intravascular compartment cannot be compensated completely by refill from the interstitium at high ultrafiltration rates.[3,6–8] The incidence of hypotension is significantly related to the ultrafiltration rate.[6] Patients with a compromised cardiovascular system appear to be particularly sensitive to the adverse hemodynamic effects of aggressive ultrafiltration.[7]

Fluid status of the patient

The fluid status of the patient has a major influence on changes in blood volume during dialysis, which can be explained by the hydration state of the interstitial tissue. When the patient is underhydrated, refill of blood volume is hampered because the interstitium is also fluid depleted and interstitial hydrostatic pressure is low. By contrast, interstitial pressure is high in hypervolemic patients, which will induce a volume shift into the intravascular space when fluid is removed during dialysis.[9–12]

Dialysate sodium

During dialysis, sodium that has accumulated during the interdialytic period needs to be removed. Usually a small gradient between plasma and dialysate sodium is present. In the earlier days of dialysis, lower sodium concentrations of the dialysate were frequently used. However, this approach was associated with an increased incidence of hypotensive periods compared with the use of higher sodium concentrations in the dialysate, which appeared to be related to impaired blood volume preservation.[12,13] One view attributes this phenomenon to a disequilibrium between the intracellular and extracellular spaces. During dialysis, urea diffuses into the dialysate. Urea equilibrates rapidly between the intravascular and interstitial compartments, whereas ion transport across the cellular membrane is delayed. Especially with a low dialysate sodium concentration, the extracellular compartment becomes hypotonic relative to the intracellular space, which will promote the movement of fluid into the cell.[13] A sodium shift from the dialysate into the patient would prevent the rapid fall in extracellular osmolality and, therefore, improve blood volume preservation.

Another viewpoint supports the hypothesis that the effect of dialysate sodium to the induction of an osmotic gradient between the intravascular and the interstitial compartments. During dialysis with a variable dialysate concentration, the intracellular volume (assessed by bioimpedance spectroscopy) remained stable, whereas changes in extracellular volume were largely confined to the intravascular space. This effect might be caused by the relatively slow sodium transport across the capillary wall.[14] Therefore, the effect of higher dialysate sodium concentrations on blood volume preservation[14,15] can also be explained by a fluid shift from the interstitial to the intravascular space due to an osmotic gradient across the capillary wall.[14]

Buffer substrate

The choice of dialysate buffer also influences blood volume preservation. Acetate induces arteriolar vasodilation, which increases precapillary hydrostatic pressure and provokes a shift from the intravascular to the interstitial space. Bicarbonate has less vasodilating properties and, therefore, exerts a more favorable effect on blood volume preservation.[12,16] Moreover, in patients with compromised cardiac function, acetate may further impair refill of blood volume because of increased pressure in the postcapillary venules secondary to left ventricular dysfunction.[17]

Treatment modality

Few authors have studied differences in blood volume preservation with various dialysis techniques. No differences in blood volume preservation were observed between isolated ultrafiltration and ultrafiltration combined with bicarbonate hemodialysis.[4,12]

By contrast, with hemodialysis, intracellular volume increased during hemodiafiltration, which can be explained by more effective removal of solutes leading to reduced osmolality of the extracellular space. However, no difference in plasma volume preservation was observed between these two techniques.[18] A recent study showed no differences in plasma refilling between standard hemodialysis and high efficiency hemodiafiltration.[19]

On the other hand, the decrease in blood volume was less pronounced during hemofiltration compared with hemodialysis at an equivalent ultrafiltration rate, which can be explained by decreased removal of low-molecular-weight substrates.[20] However, other investigators did not observe a difference in blood volume preservation between bicarbonate dialysis and hemofiltration.[21]

Temperature of the dialysate

Schneditz and colleagues observed a larger decline in relative blood volume with the use of cool versus normal temperature dialysate, despite better blood pressure control during cool dialysis.[22] Although this finding was not confirmed in other studies,[23] the negative effect of cool dialysis on blood volume preservation could be explained by a reduction in capillary surface area owing to peripheral vasoconstriction.[23]

Food intake

One study showed a rapid decline in blood volume during food intake, measured by continuous hematocrit monitoring. This effect can probably be explained by redistribution of blood from the large blood vessels (from which the hematocrit is measured) to peripheral blood vessels, in which the hematocrit is lower.[24]

Venous compliance

In patients with a reduced compliance (volume–pressure ratio) of the venous system, refill of blood volume from the interstitium is hampered because of a disturbance in the capillary Starling equilibrium. Venous compliance is especially reduced in dialysis patients with pre-existing hypertension, which appears to be due to structural abnormalities of the venous wall.[25,26]

The effect of venous compliance on blood volume preservation can be explained by the fact that in patients with a reduced venous compliance (i.e. increased stiffness of the venous wall), the pressure in the postcapillary venules is higher for a given level of plasma volume, which reduces the fluid shift from the interstitial to the intravascular compartment.[7] In patients with essential hypertension, the relation between blood volume and interstitial volume was found to be decreased in patients with essential hypertension with reduced venous compliance.[27] In agreement with this finding, during isolated ultrafiltration a steeper decline in blood volume was observed in patients with reduced venous compliance compared to patients with normal venous compliance.[28] This phenomenon is likely to be of greatest importance during the first part of a dialysis session because refill from the interstitium is initially dependent on the Starling equilibrium parameters before dialysis.[5] After 60–120 minutes the fall in venous pressure and the rise in colloid osmotic pressure result in the establishment of a new equilibrium.[5]

Systemic vascular resistance

During hypovolemia, constriction of the precapillary vessels, leading to an increase in systemic vascular resistance, is of primary importance for the maintenance of hemodynamic stability. This response appears to be disturbed during hemodialysis. In a minority of patients, autonomic neuropathy will certainly contribute to this phenomenon. However, the major cause of the impaired response appears to be a consequence of the treatment itself.

Autonomic neuropathy

Diabetes mellitus, which has a high prevalence amongst in hemodialysis patients, may lead to reduced arteriolar constriction because of autonomic neuropathy affecting the efferent sympathetic pathways.[28] However, the efferent sympathetic pathways appear generally to be intact in non-diabetic dialysis patients, as the vascular response is normal in response to a sympathetic stimulus like the cold pressor test. Moreover, the vasoconstrictor responses to hypovolemia are also preserved during isolated ultrafiltration and hemofiltration.[25,29] In addition, a reduced end-organ sensitivity for catecholamines has been observed in dialysis patients,[30] although this phenomenon may well be due to receptor downregulation in response to the general state of sympathetic overactivity that exists in the uremic state.[31]

Thus, as will be discussed later, the autonomic defect will primarily affect the heart rate response during hypovolemia. In non-diabetic dialysis patients, the hemodialysis treatment itself appears to be primarily responsible for the impaired vascular response.

Hemodialysis treatment

In contrast to isolated ultrafiltration and hemofiltration, hemodialysis thus appears to impair vasoreactivity during hypovolemia. In addition, the increase in plasma levels of vasoactive peptides, like catecholamines, vasopressin, and renin, was found to be less pronounced during hemodialysis compared with the other treatment modalities.[32–35] Impaired vascular reactivity appears to be the major determinant that explains the improved blood pressure response during the two latter treatment modalities compared with hemodialysis.[32] Acetate, which is now less frequently used, has a profound direct vasodilating effect,[32,33,36] possibly due to the effect of acetate itself or the formation of adenosine.[37] However, the constriction of the capacitance and resistance vessels is also reduced during bicarbonate dialysis. Factors such as changes in osmolality and ionized calcium do not appear to be responsible for this phenomenon.[38,39] It has been suggested that the excessive synthesis of cytokines, such as interleukin-1 (IL-1) and tumor necrosis factor-α (TNF-α) during dialysis, leads to an increased production of inducible nitric oxide synthase in smooth muscle, which attenuates the vasoconstriction response during hemodialysis.[40] Cytokine production is especially stimulated by the use of bioincompatible membranes in combination with contaminated dialysate.[41] Thus, nitric oxide was found to be increased in hemodialysis patients with symptomatic hypotension compared with patients without hemodynamic instability.[42] However, recent studies have failed to show any difference in hemodynamic stability between dialysis with bioincompatible versus biocompatible membranes.[43–45] Moreover, vascular reactivity was not improved by the use of ultrapure dialysate[46] or biocompatible membranes.[47] In addition, the time required for nitric oxide production is in disagreement with the fact that differences in vascular reactivity between isolated ultrafiltration and hemodialysis are present as early as 15–30 minutes into the dialysis run.[29–32] An increased concentration of the vasodilator peptide adenosine was found after episodes with severe symptomatic hypotension.[48] However, it is not known whether the increase in adenosine is of primary pathogenic importance or a consequence of increased release from ischemic tissue.

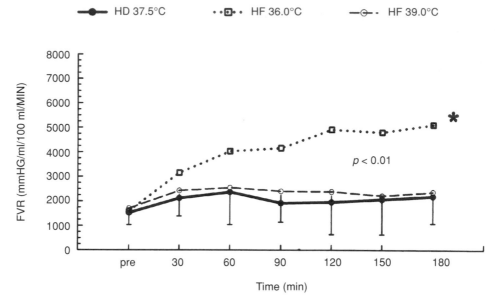

Fig. 15.1 Forearm vascular resistance (FVR) during hemodialysis (HD 37.5°C), cold hemofiltration (HF 36.0°C), and warm hemofiltration (HF 39.0°C). Reproduced from reference 21, with permission.

It is likely that the energy balance between the patient and the extracorporeal circuit plays an important role in the pathogenesis of the impaired vascular response during dialysis, as the hemodynamic reaction appears to differ between dialysis with standard (37–38°C) and cool (35–36°C) temperature of the dialysate. Both the blood pressure response and vascular reactivity are improved with the use of cool dialysate, whereas the blood returning from the extracorporeal circuit to the patient is also much cooler during isolated ultrafiltration and hemofiltration compared with 'standard' dialysis.[21,23,49,50] Interestingly, the differences in vascular reactivity between hemodialysis on one hand, and hemofiltration and isolated ultrafiltration, on the other hand, disappear when both treatment modalities are matched for blood temperature in the venous blood lines[23] (Fig. 15.1).

Dialysis treatment can affect body temperature control of the patient, which does not seem to be primarily related to an influx of heat from the extracorporeal circuit to the patient. In contrast, we observed an increase in blood temperature during hemodialysis with a bath temperature of 37.5°C despite net energy transfer from the patient to the extracorporeal circuit.[50] The mechanisms behind the thermal effects of dialysis have not yet been clarified. Nevertheless, the increase in body temperature during dialysis is likely to have a very important effect on the vascular response during dialysis, as at least part of the vasodilatation during dialysis can be explained by dilation of the (thermoregulatory) cutaneous blood vessels to get rid of the excess heat, counteracting the normal vascular response to hypovolemia. The beneficial hemodynamic effects of dialysate with lower bath temperatures (35–36°C) ('cool dialysis') could be due to removal of this excess heat. Another explanation for the improved vascular response during cool dialysis and the convective techniques is a constriction of the thermoregulatory blood vessels to maintain a constant blood temperature. Cool dialysis is particularly efficient in patients with a low pre-dialysis core temperature, which might be because in these patients, the rise in core temperature during dialysis is higher than in patients with normal pre-dialytic core temperature.[50]

Cardiac output

In addition to an increase in systemic vascular resistance, compensatory mechanisms will attempt to maintain cardiac output during hypovolemia to prevent hypotension. Major determinants of cardiac output are heart rate, myocardial contractility, and venous return, in combination with the compliance characteristics of the heart.

Physiological response of the heart and capacitance vessels to hypovolemia

Heart rate

In healthy subjects, heart rate will increase during hypovolemia in an attempt to compensate for the reduction in preload. This increase is mediated by an increased sympathetic tone due to a reduction in inhibitory impulses from the volume receptors in the atria and pulmonary veins and the high pressure receptors in the aorta and carotid sinus. There is some discussion regarding the importance of the heart rate response in the hemodynamic reaction to hypovolemia, as both in animal and in human experiments, blockade of the cardiac reflexes did not have a major effect on the blood pressure response during hemorrhage and lower body negative pressure.[51–53]

Myocardial contractility

An increase in sympathetic activity during hypovolemia will also stimulate myocardial contractility, which leads to a more efficient emptying of the heart. For the increase in myocardial contractility, adequate systolic function of the heart is a prerequisite.

Nevertheless, the importance of an increased myocardial contractility for blood pressure control during hypovolemia remains somewhat obscure; for example, beta-adrenergic blockade had only a minor effect on the blood pressure response to hypovolemia.[52,54]

Venous return

Of the total blood volume, 60–80% is located within the capacitance vessels. Therefore, the structure and function of the venous system have a major effect on the maintenance of cardiac output during hypovolemia. The venous system can be regarded both as a blood reservoir and as a conduction system for the return of blood from the tissues to the heart (Fig. 15.2). Regarding its function as a blood reservoir, it is of importance to note that under basal circumstances, a large amount of blood is hemodynamically inactive ('unstressed'). During hypovolemia, passive and active venoconstriction will result in centralization of blood volume. As the venous wall is very flexible, a reduction in blood volume will result in collapse of the venous wall, leading to passive venoconstriction (de Jager–Kroch phenomenon). Active venoconstriction occurs by contraction of smooth muscle in the venous wall.[51,55]

Regarding the function of the venous compartments as a conduction system for the hemodynamically active ('stressed') blood volume, the concept of venous compliance is of importance. Venous compliance is defined as the volume–pressure relationship of the venous system. It is determined mainly by the structure of the venous wall. A reduction in venous compliance

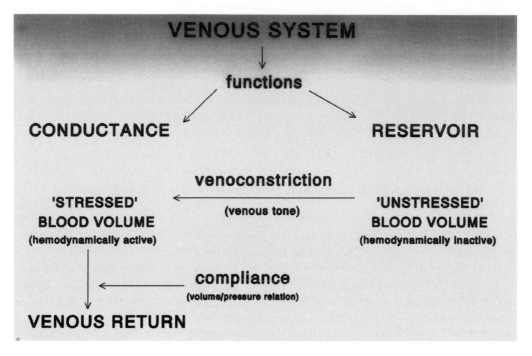

Fig. 15.2   The role of the venous system in the maintenance of hemodynamic stability during hypovolemia.

increases the sensitivity of the system to changes in blood volume. Thus an increase in blood volume results in a greater increase in central venous pressure and a decrease in blood volume will lead to a more pronounced decline in central venous pressure.[29,54,56]

Diastolic function of the heart

In addition to the systolic function of the heart, its diastolic function is of great importance in the hemodynamic response to hypovolemia. Diastolic dysfunction can be defined as an impaired capacity of the ventricle to accept blood without a disproportionate change in ventricular pressure, i.e. the compliance (volume–pressure ratio) of the ventricle is reduced.

Because of the increased sensitivity to changes in volume, a small increase in ventricular volume leads to a steep increase in ventricular pressure, and a small decrease in ventricular volume induces a steep decline in left ventricular pressure.[57–59] When the compliance (volume–pressure ratio) of the heart is reduced, the sensitivity of the heart to changes in filling volume increases. Therefore, patients with reduced left ventricular compliance have a very small margin between clinical over- and underhydration and are prone to both symptomatic hypotension and congestive heart failure.[57,58] The combination of reduced venous and ventricular compliance will be particularly disadvantageous in this aspect. A reduction in ventricular compliance also increases the importance of atrial contraction for cardiac filling. Therefore, patients with diastolic dysfunction are especially sensitive for supraventricular arrhythmias, such as atrial fibrillation.[57] Reduction of the compliance of the left ventricle (diastolic dysfunction) may be due to structural abnormalities of the cardiac wall, e.g. due to left ventricular hypertrophy, or to functional abnormalities resulting in impaired cardiac relaxation, such as coronary ischemia.

Response of the heart and capacitance vessels during hypovolemia during dialysis

Heart rate

Autonomic neuropathy Many hemodialysis patients have signs of autonomic neuropathy, characterized by dysfunction of the baroreceptor reflex arc. The autonomic defect is located primarily in the afferent part of the baroreceptor reflex arc and in the efferent parasympathetic response, which may impair the heart rate response during hypovolemia.[59,60]

Studies of the impact of autonomic neuropathy on hemodialysis hypotension have shown conflicting results. Although in some studies a relationship was observed between disturbances in the baroreceptor reflex arc and hemodialysis hypotension,[61–63] other authors did not find such a relationship.[64,65] In addition to pre-existing autonomic neuropathy, the hemodialysis treatment itself may interfere with the normal heart rate response. Zuchelli and colleagues observed acute dysfunction of the baroreceptors (assessed by the Valsalva maneuver) induced by the dialysis treatment itself,[66] although this finding was not confirmed by others.[65] In contrast, improvement in baroreceptor function was observed after hemofiltration.[66,67]

Acute sympathetic dysfunction Some episodes of acute hypotension during dialysis appear to be related to an acute decrease in sympathetic activity, which is preceded by a large burst in sympathetic activity.[68] This reduction in sympathetic activity leads to an acute decrease in peripheral vascular resistance and a reduction in heart rate. The acute reduction in sympathetic activity is probably due to the Bezold–Jarisch reflex, which is evoked by stimulation of left ventricular baroreceptors in response to severe left ventricular underfilling.

However, this reflex is probably only elicited during severe hypovolemia, as many episodes of symptomatic hypotension are accompanied by an increased or unchanged heart rate.[69,70] This reflex is also probably responsible for the acute collapse sometimes seen in dialysis patients during fluid removal.

Myocardial contractility

Influence of dialysis on cardiac function Myocardial contractility does not usually decrease during hemodialysis and may even increase. This is different from isolated ultrafiltration, during which cardiac output decreases according to the Frank–Starling mechanism, i.e. stroke volume decreases concomitantly with the decrease in preload.[71]

The increase in myocardial contractility has been attributed to fluid removal, an increase in ionized calcium, the removal of cardiodepressor uremic toxins, or a reduction in afterload (myocardial wall tension during systolic ejection) due to dilation of the resistance vessels.[72,73] Whereas the use of acetate does not appear to have a major impact on cardiac contractility in patients with normal cardiac function, it may have cardiodepressor effects in patients with systolic dysfunction of the heart.[17,74]

As ionized calcium has a direct effect on the contractility of the cardiac smooth muscle cells,[72,75,76] the use of lower calcium concentrations in the dialysate (1.25 mmol/l) may influence cardiac contractility. Indeed, in patients with reduced systolic function, cardiac contractility decreases during low-calcium dialysis but remains stable during high-calcium dialysis.[77]

Cardiac contractility is also increased with the use of cold dialysis, which contributes to improved hemodynamic stability.[78]

Systolic dysfunction   Reduced myocardial contractility, leading to systolic dysfunction of the heart, is present in a significant minority of dialysis patients. In patients with systolic dysfunction, dilated cardiomyopathy is often present.

Defined as a fractional decrease of less than 25% on echocardiography, systolic dysfunction is found in approximately 15% of dialysis patients. Systolic dysfunction has an adverse prognosis in dialysis patients[79,80] and predisposes the patient to symptomatic hypotension, because the heart cannot respond well to changes in filling pressure and it requires higher filling pressures to maintain an adequate cardiac output.

Risk factors for dilated cardiomyopathy in dialysis patients include chronic volume overload, hypertension, anemia, ischemic heart disease, arteriovenous fistula, carnitine deficiency, and older age. Systolic dysfunction is primarily associated with ischemic heart disease, anemia, and older age.[79,80]

Acute cardiac problems, such as coronary ischemia and cardiac arrhythmias, can also cause reduced cardiac contractility.

Venous return

Impaired venoconstriction   During hypovolemia, passive and active venoconstriction contribute to the maintenance of adequate cardiac filling pressures (preload) by centralization of blood volume. By analogy with its effect on the resistance vessels, hemodialysis can also impair the vasomotor responses of the capacitance vessels. This effect is present during both acetate and bicarbonate dialysis.[29,36,81] However, the effect of acetate dialysis is probably more pronounced, as preload was found to decrease more during acetate compared to bicarbonate dialysis despite equivalent ultrafiltration, suggesting a more pronounced reduction in venous return during hemodialysis.[82]

By contrast, significant venoconstriction occurs during isolated ultrafiltration and hemofiltration. By analogy to the resistance vessels, at least part of this effect is related to the energy balance during dialysis as venoconstriction is almost comparable between cool dialysis and isolated ultrafiltration.[23] Moreover, the clear difference in reactivity of the forearm veins between hemodialysis and hemofiltration disappears when both treatments are matched for extracorporeal blood temperature in the venous blood line.[21]

Reduced venous compliance   Independent of the effect on blood volume preservation, the fall in central venous pressure is greater in patients with reduced venous compliance.[28] As mentioned previously, venous compliance is especially reduced in dialysis patients with pre-existing hypertension. This is probably related to structural abnormalities of the venous wall as venous compliance does not change after administration of sympatholytic agents or non-endothelium-dependent vasodilating agents.[25] Moreover, structural abnormalities have been observed in veins of hypertensive uremic patients in contrast to normotensive subjects.[26] The larger decrease in central venous pressure in patients with reduced venous compliance is due to an increased sensitivity of the venous system to changes in volume status, owing to the steeper volume–pressure relationship.[29,55] This is in accordance with the more pronounced increase and decrease in central venous pressure, respectively, during volume loading and unloading in non-uremic hypertensive patients with reduced venous compliance.[56]

Diastolic dysfunction

Diastolic dysfunction of the left ventricle is frequent in dialysis patients, primarily because of the high prevalence of left ventricular hypertrophy. Abnormalities in cardiac ultrastructure and the frequent occurrence of cardiac ischemia also undoubtedly contribute to the high incidence of diastolic dysfunction in this patient group.[59,80,83] In clinical studies, it has been shown that dialysis patients with reduced left ventricular compliance are particularly sensitive to hemodialysis hypotension.[57,80] The relation between diastolic dysfunction and hemodialysis hypotension has been discussed in more detail in Chapters 2 and 7.

Summary

Symptomatic hypotension is a frequently occurring phenomenon in the dialysis population. Especially in elderly patients, who often suffer from cardiovascular disease, the incidence of symptomatic hypotension may be high, which can sometimes result in serious morbidity. Symptomatic hypotension may occur as a result of a fall in blood volume and reduced vasoreactivity during dialysis in combination with structural abnormalities of the cardiovascular system. The fall in blood volume is determined by multiple factors such as the hydration state of the patient, the ultrafiltration rate, the dialysate sodium concentration, and the dialysate buffer. Structural abnormalities of the venous system resulting in reduced venous compliance have also been found to impair blood volume preservation during dialysis (Fig. 15.3).

Constriction of the resistance and capacitance vessels is impaired during hemodialysis. This might be related to the treatment itself, as in non-diabetic dialysis patients vascular reactivity is normal during an efferent sympathetic stimulus and during isolated ultrafiltration and hemofiltration. The differences in vascular response between the latter treatment modalities and hemodialysis are at least partly related to differences in extracorporeal blood temperature. The reduced constriction of the resistance vessels results in an inadequate

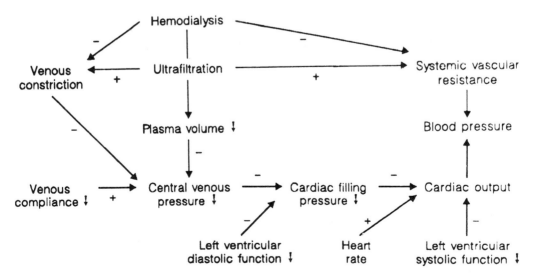

Fig. 15.3 Pathophysiological factors contributing to hemodialysis hypotension.

increase in systemic vascular resistance during hypovolemia, whereas the reduced constriction of the capacitance vessels may lead to a further reduction in venous return.

Regarding the cardiac response during hypovolemia, hemodialysis does not have a negative inotropic effect, except for the cardiodepressor effect of acetate in patients with severe cardiac dysfunction. In contrast, myocardial contractility may even increase due to an increase in heart rate, a reduction in afterload, and the influx of ionized calcium. The role of autonomic neuropathy in the pathogenesis of hemodialysis hypotension is uncertain, but possibly not very great. However, in the case of severe hypovolemia, cardiovascular collapse may ensue by an acute reduction in sympathetic activity (Bezold–Jarisch reflex).

Structural abnormalities of the cardiovascular system can further impair the blood pressure response during hemodialysis. A reduction in compliance (volume–pressure ratio), probably related to structural abnormalities of the venous wall, leads to a more rapid decrease in central venous pressure during fluid removal.

In addition to systolic dysfunction of the heart, diastolic dysfunction also appears to be of importance. Diastolic dysfunction (reduced ventricular compliance) increases the sensitivity of the heart to changes in filling volume and augments the risk of both over- and under-hydration. Diastolic dysfunction in dialysis patients occurs mainly as a result of concentric left ventricular hypertrophy, but may also be present in patients with a normal ventricular mass.

The relative importance of each of these factors may differ in the individual patient. Most often, a combination of these mechanisms will be responsible for hemodynamic instability during dialysis.

Treatment and prevention of hemodialysis hypotension

Acute treatment

During symptomatic hypotension, ultrafiltration is discontinued and the patient is placed in the Trendelenburg position. If blood pressure does not rise, isotonic or hypertonic saline, mannitol, or a colloid solution can be administered. Few reports have compared the efficacy of these maneuvers during hemodialysis hypotension. Gong and colleagues assessed the effect of 30 ml 7.5% hypertonic saline (80 mOsm), 10 ml 23% saturated hypertonic saline (80 mOsm), and 7.5% saline with 6% dextran 70 (100 mOsm). The increase in blood pressure was greater with the two latter solutions compared with 7.5% hypertonic saline, whereas the effect of the dextran solution was most prolonged.[84] Because a disequilibrium may exist during hemodialysis between an underfilled intravascular compartment and a still overhydrated interstitium, the use of hyperoncotic solutions, such as 20% albumin, dextran, and hydroxyethyl starch (HES), may induce a fluid shift from the interstitium to the intravascular compartment because of an increase in plasma colloid osmotic pressure. Indeed, we observed a more profound and longer lasting effect on plasma volume after HES and hyperoncotic albumin than with saline.[85] Nevertheless, there is some concern regarding the elimination of dextran and HES in patients with end-stage renal failure,[86] although Steinhoff and colleagues found only a very small amount of HES in the circulation of dialysis patients 48 hours after administration.[87] Accumulation in the reticuloendothelial system should also be taken into account. Moreover, the risk of anaphylactoid reactions, although small, is present with the use of human and synthetic colloids. Mannitol may also accumulate in patients with end-stage renal failure,[88] and large infusions of saline may lead to thirst and increased interdialytic weight gain. However, with the use of small amounts of hypertonic saline, no increase in interdialytic weight gain was observed in one study.[89]

Prevention of hemodialysis hypotension

To prevent symptomatic hypotension, a stepped approach is suggested. This approach is, of course, influenced by personal experience and is by no means meant to exclude other strategies (Table 15.2).

First steps

1. Estimation of dry weight   Adequate assessment of the fluid state prevents overhydration and hypovolemia. Hypovolemia occurs because of excessive removal of blood volume and reduced refill of blood volume from the interstitium, as discussed previously. Overhydration may lead to hypertension, left ventricular dilation, and occasionally pulmonary edema, whereas underhydration may provoke severe dialysis hypertension. Dry weight has been defined as the weight below which the patient is free of edema and is normotensive without symptomatic complaints during dialysis.[90] However, this strategy may fail to assess the optimal fluid status of the patient, as clinical symptoms may be a late symptom of underhydration. Therefore, more objective methods are needed. Physical examination, although of great importance, will often fail to detect subtle variations in fluid status. Radiography of the chest will only show severe overhydration. Biochemical markers, such as ANP and cGMP, which are released in response to left atrial stretch,[91,92] are difficult to apply in an acute clinical setting and their reliability in the assessment of underhydration is questionable.[90]

Table 15.2   Prevention of symptomatic hypotension

	BV preservation	Vasoconstriction	Cardiac response
First steps			
Optimal assessment of dry weight	+	0	0
Individualize ultrafiltration rate	+	0	0
Individualize dialysate sodium	+	0	0
Avoid acetate	+	+	+[a]
Avoid food intake	+?	+	0
Avoid vasoactive medication before dialysis	0	+	0
Prevent excessive interdialytic weight gain	+	0	0
Second steps			
Isolated ultrafiltration	0	+	0
Cool dialysis	0	+	+
Increase dialysate calcium	0	0	+
Blood volume monitoring	+	0	0
Other options			
Sodium profiling	+?	0	0
Hemofiltration	+?	+	0
Pharmacological treatment	0	+	0
CAPD			

BV, blood volume; CAPD, continuous ambulatory peritoneal dialysis.
[a]In patients with disturbed left ventricular function.

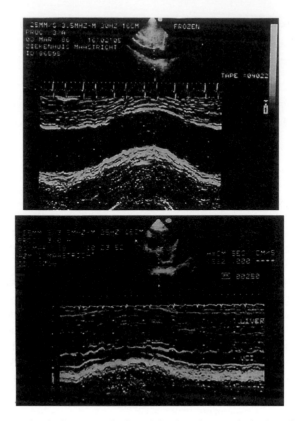

Fig. 15.4   The inferior caval vein in an overhydrated (top) and an underhydrated (bottom) patient.

Bioimpedance spectroscopy (BIS) is reproducible and rapid and generally correlates well with isotope dilution techniques.[93,94] However, a problem with the use of BIS in the assessment of dry weight is the absence of reference data for the dialysis population and the fact that in individual patients the difference between BIS and isotope dilution techniques may be clinically significant.[93,95] Some authors did not find BIS to be reliable in the assessment of acute changes in fluid state during dialysis.[96,97] Regional impedance ('conductivity') measurements, by contrast, were found to be fairly sensitive in the detection of fluid state during dialysis.[90,98] Echography of the inferior vena cava diameter (IVCD) correlates well with blood volume and right atrial pressure in dialysis patients and was found to be of clinical value in the assessment of dry weight in these patients (Fig. 15.4). Ideally, IVCD should be measured 1–2 hours after dialysis because of ongoing refill from the interstitium.[8] As IVCD is a derivative of right atrial pressure, one should be careful with its interpretation as a marker of dry weight in patients with severe left ventricular and/or valvular dysfunction.[99]

2. Individualization of ultrafiltration rate   The avoidance of high ultrafiltration rates will stimulate blood volume preservation because of increased refill from the interstitium. Whereas some patients tolerate high ultrafiltration rates well, others, mainly the elderly with cardiovascular disease, do not.[7] Problems can be avoided by using an empirically determined maximal ultrafiltration rate for each patient (which may differ for isolated ultrafiltration and ultrafiltration combined with hemodialysis). To obtain this goal, the duration of treatment might have to be extended. In one study, a better hemodynamic stability was observed with the use of an increased dialysis time.[100]

3. Dialysate sodium Low sodium dialysis (130–134 mmol/l) impairs blood volume preservation.[12–15] However, sodium gain during dialysis should be avoided as this might lead to interdialytic overhydration, thirst, and hypertension. A sodium concentration of 138–140 mmol/l will in most patients lead to a slightly negative sodium balance.[101] In patients with low pre-dialytic sodium levels, individualization of the dialysate sodium to the plasma sodium concentration may be advocated to prevent net sodium influx without the detrimental effects of low-sodium dialysis.

4. Avoidance of acetate as dialysate buffer Because of the untoward effects of acetate dialysis on blood volume preservation,[12,16] vascular reactivity,[32] and, in patients with severe left ventricular dysfunction, on cardiac function,[32] bicarbonate should be used as dialysate buffer.

5. Avoidance of food intake during dialysis Avoidance of food intake is advocated in dialysis patients with frequent symptomatic hypotensive periods. It has been observed that ingestion of a meal during dialysis leads to a more pronounced decrease in mean arterial pressure[102,103] and a reduction in large-vessel blood volume.[24] The pathophysiological mechanisms may involve a selective enhancement of splanchnical vasodilation or increased general vasodilation, possibly mediated partly by increased plasma insulin concentrations.[103–105] In contrast to studies in non-uremic patients, caffeine had no effect on postprandial hemodynamics during dialysis.[102]

6. Avoidance of vasoactive medication before dialysis Vasoactive medication taken before dialysis may further impair the vascular response during dialysis. Especially in patients prone to hemodialysis hypotension, one should pay attention to the timing of intake.

7. Prevention of excessive weight gain Because a large amount of fluid has to be removed in a relatively short period of time, excessive interdialytic weight gain greatly increases the risk of hypotensive episodes. Dietary counseling and restriction of sodium and water intake may be of help.

Second steps

If these simple maneuvers fail to control hemodialysis hypotension, several approaches can be taken to improve hemodynamic stability during dialysis.

1. Isolated ultrafiltration Fluid removal during isolated ultrafiltration has the hemodynamic advantage of enhancing constriction of the resistance and capacitance vessels compared to hemodialysis.[29,32] However, in contrast to hemodialysis, stroke volume decreases with a reduction in preload according to the Frank–Starling mechanism.[71] Clinical studies have shown the superior blood pressure response during isolated ultrafiltration compared to hemodialysis in patients with normal and abnormal ventricular function.[7,32] We use isolated ultrafiltration, especially in cases of excessive interdialytic weight gain, when the amount of fluid which has to be removed during hemodialysis exceeds the individualized maximal ultrafiltration rate.

2. Cool dialysis   Hemodynamic stability can also be improved by the use of cool dialysate (35–36°C) as a consequence of increased cardiac contractility and vasoconstriction compared to standard dialysis.[23,49,78,106,107] Despite the lowering of the venous blood temperature, blood temperature did not decrease below 35°C during cool dialysis with a dialysate temperature of 35.5°C.[50] Except for occasional chills, few side-effects have been described. In addition, we did not observe rebound hypotension after the use of cool dialysate (K.M.L. Leunissen et al., unpublished results).

One study found the efficacy of cool dialysis to be related to the individual core temperature of the patient.[108] Thus, individualization of dialysate temperature might be an option in the future.

3. Dialysate calcium   Calcium ions have an important role in the contractility of cardiac and vascular smooth muscle cells and in the release of catecholamines from adrenergic nerves.[109] A dialysate calcium concentration in the range of 1.5–1.75 mmol/l results in an increase in plasma ionized calcium of ±0.20 mmol/l, whereas plasma ionized calcium remains more or less unchanged with a dialysate calcium concentration of 1.25 mmol/l.[110] The latter concentration has become popular as a tool to prevent hypercalcemia in the treatment of secondary hyperparathyroidism. The change in ionized calcium during dialysis probably exerts an important inotropic effect. Several studies reported a difference in the blood pressure response between dialysis with low and normal dialysate calcium concentrations. This effect was not due to an effect on vascular reactivity but was primarily related to an increase in left ventricular contractility.[39,72,75–77] The hemodynamic effects of dialysate calcium appear to be especially important in patients with impaired left ventricular systolic function in whom blood pressure was found to decrease with the use of low dialysate calcium but remained stable with the use of higher dialysate calcium concentrations.[77] Although no severe adverse effects have been reported with the use of high calcium dialysate, one should keep in mind that an excessive rise in serum calcium may exert arrhythmogenic effects.

4. Membranes?   The use of biocompatible dialysis membranes probably has no effect on the prevention of hemodialysis hypotension. Although an earlier report suggested an improvement in hemodynamic stability with the use of cellulose acetate compared with cuprophane membranes,[111] recent larger trials have failed to show a difference in the incidence of hemodialysis hypotension between dialysis with biocompatible and bioincompatible membranes.[43–45]

5. Blood volume monitoring   Recent developments have made it possible to monitor relative changes in blood volume continuously during dialysis. The basis of these techniques is the continuous monitoring of hematocrit, total protein, or hemoglobin from lysed erythrocytes from which the fall in blood volume can be estimated.[22,112,113] In some newer dialysis machines, options for continuous blood volume monitoring have become standard.

With continuous blood volume monitoring, it may be possible to detect a fall in plasma volume before this leads to symptomatic hypotension. If a steep fall in plasma volume occurs, one might prevent a further decline, e.g. by slowing the ultrafiltration rate.[3,6] It has been suggested that hypotensive periods occur at a patient-specific hematocrit.[114] However, differences in ultrafiltration rate, changes in hydration state, and changes in erythrocyte volume between various dialysis treatments by the use of erythropoietin may lead to errors when applying this method too rigidly.

Despite these limitations, the use of blood volume monitoring may enable the clinician to individualize ultrafiltration and may prevent hemodialysis hypotension in individual patients. However, the use of blood volume monitoring in all dialysis patients is still rather expensive. In the future, it may become possible to integrate blood volume monitoring within a 'closed-loop' system, which automatically adjusts ultrafiltration rate or the sodium concentration of the dialysate according to the blood volume profile of the patient.[115]

Other options

If hemodialysis hypotension persists, some authors advocate more experimental approaches, such as sodium profiling. The use of vasoactive medication during dialysis has been suggested as a means to improve blood pressure stability during dialysis. However, especially with the use of vasoactive medication, clinical experience is still limited. In very hypotensive-prone patients, it is probably better to switch to other treatment modalities, such as hemofiltration or continuous ambulatory peritoneal dialysis, as will be discussed later.

1. Sodium profiling Sodium profiling with a variable sodium concentration in the dialysate has been proposed as a tool to decrease morbidity without a concomitant increase in sodium load. Profiles with an increased sodium concentration throughout the dialysate reduce cramps in the last part of dialysis. However, they may aggravate the fall in osmolality and therefore increase the incidence of symptomatic hypotension at the start of dialysis.[116,117] Decreasing sodium profiles reduces the fall in osmolality during the first part of dialysis and may therefore reduce the incidence of symptomatic hypotension at the start of dialysis, especially when used in combination with a decreasing ultrafiltration profile.[116] Sodium modeling allows one to obtain a greater individualization of dialysis therapy profiling and has been found to have a beneficial effect on dialysis blood pressure.[116-119] Nevertheless, not all authors found a beneficial effect on hemodynamic stability and there is also a risk of sodium retention with the use of some profiles.[117,120,121] Moreover, owing to the relative complexity of the method and technical limitations of various dialysis machines, the routine use of sodium profiling is still limited and the optimal sodium profile has not yet been elucidated. We think that an algorithm for sodium profiling should be based on the individual blood volume response of the patient as assessed by continuous blood volume monitoring and also on the estimation of individual Na overload between sessions, in addition to that of water overload.

2. Pharmacological maneuvers In several studies in dialysis patients with frequent hemodialysis hypotension, blood pressure stability was improved with the administration of vasoactive substances. Sympathomimetic agents, such as the norepinephrine precursor L-threo-3,4-dihydroxyphenylserine (L-DOPS),[122] amezinium methylsulfate,[123] and midodrine,[124] and other vasoactive agents, such as lysine vasopressin,[125] have been used successfully. However, the first of these agents, in particular, is associated with significant side-effects.

The serotonin reuptake inhibitor sertraline has recently been shown to reduce the frequency of hemodialysis hypotension in some patients by attenuating paradoxical sympathetic withdrawal.[126] However, to date, the clinical experience with the use of antihypotensive agents is still limited in dialysis patients.

In some patients, all the maneuvers discussed previously will fail. In these patients, changing to another technique may be the only option.

3. Hemofiltration Cardiovascular stability is better maintained during hemofiltration compared with hemodialysis. Although differences in blood volume preservation[20] and baroreceptor functioning[66,67] may play a role, the most important determinant of improved blood pressure stability during hemofiltration appears to be enhanced vascular reactivity compared to hemodialysis.[21,34,127,128] The possible pathogenetic mechanisms behind the different vascular responses of hemodialysis and hemofiltration have been addressed previously. At least part of this difference is related to differences in extracorporeal blood temperature. It has been suggested that increased convective clearance of vasodilator peptides, like calcitonin-gene-related peptide, could also contribute to the improved vascular response during hemofiltration, although direct evidence for this hypothesis is not yet available.

Cardiac contractility does not differ to a great extent between hemodialysis and hemofiltration, and cardiac output may even be greater during hemodialysis due to the reduction in afterload and the increase in heart rate.[127]

Surprisingly few hemodynamic studies have been performed during hemodiafiltration. In a study in patients with acute renal failure, vascular reactivity was reduced compared with hemofiltration but increased compared with hemodialysis.[129] An improvement in blood pressure stability was noted with hemodiafiltration and acetate-free biofiltration compared to hemodialysis in elderly dialysis patients,[130] although in another study, no difference in hemodynamic stability between hemodialysis and hemodiafiltration was observed.[19]

4. Continuous ambulatory peritoneal dialysis (CAPD) CAPD leads to a more gradual removal of fluid compared with hemodialysis. Although hypotension may be observed during acute peritoneal dialysis with frequent exchanges of a high-glucose dialysate, it does not usually occur during chronic peritoneal dialysis. Therefore, CAPD can be a good option in patients with frequent symptomatic hypotension.

Coronary ischemia

Myocardial ischemia occurs frequently in dialysis patients, as discussed in Chapter 3. During hemodialysis, hypotension or arrhythmias can exacerbate myocardial ischemia. In addition, overhydration or severe hypertension may decrease myocardial perfusion and increase oxygen consumption because of increased ventricular wall stress.[131] Myocardial ischemia by itself may lead to hemodialysis hypotension, both by an acute reduction in cardiac contractility, leading to systolic dysfunction and by the induction of acute diastolic dysfunction of the heart due to reduced ventricular relaxation.[58,83]

Treatment and prevention

When angina pectoris occurs during hemodialysis and blood pressure is low, hypovolemia is probably implicated. In this case, ultrafiltration should be stopped and hypovolemia corrected. Electrocardiography should also be performed to assess the presence of arrhythmias. In case blood pressure is not too low, sublingual nitroglycerine may be given cautiously. One should, however, be extremely careful with the administration of nitroglycerine in hypovolemic patients as this may further aggravate hypotension due to venodilatation and may lead to circulatory collapse. In the case of ongoing anginal complaints, dialysis should be terminated and expert cardiological help sought.

On the other hand, in case of overhydration, ultrafiltration of excess fluid is appropriate and should be performed under cardiac monitoring in an intensive care setting. The difference between coronary ischemia due to under- or overhydration will usually be evident from clinical findings.

In hemodialysis patients with coronary artery disease, prevention of symptomatic hypotension is of utmost importance. Careful estimation of dry weight, correction of anemia, and avoidance of excessive ultrafiltration rates, e.g. by increasing dialysis time, are recommended. Acetate should not be used. In some patients transfer to CAPD or hemofiltration may be the only options. Overhydration may be prevented with a careful estimation of dry weight and dietary counseling with special attention to the sodium and water intake.

Arrhythmias

In studies using Holter electrocardiography, a high incidence of arrhythmias, including multiform ventricular premature depolarizations, extrasystoles, couplets, and longer runs of ventricular premature depolarizations, was observed in more than 50% of dialysis patients.[132,133] Most of these arrhythmias are asymptomatic and of unknown clinical significance.[134] However, more severe symptomatic atrial and ventricular tachycardias may also occur. The most commonly encountered symptomatic arrhythmia is atrial fibrillation. Atrial fibrillation is particularly troublesome in patients with diastolic dysfunction of the heart, as in these patients ventricular filling is primarily dependent on the atrial contraction. Therefore, the combination of hypovolemia, atrial fibrillation, and reduced left ventricular compliance may lead to severe hypotension.[58]

Although not all authors agree on this subject,[132,135] dialysis appears to increase the risk of arrhythmias.[132,134–138] Rapid changes in serum potassium have received attention as a contributing factor,[139] but also changes in acid–base status,[140] serum calcium,[141] and a rapid decrease in circulating blood volume[137] have been implicated. Patients with cardiovascular abnormalities, such as left ventricular hypertrophy[132,136] and coronary artery disease,[135,142] appear to be at particular risk for dialysis-associated arrhythmias.

Hypokalemia increases the vulnerability of the heart for arrhythmias because of an increased ratio between intracellular and extracellular potassium, resulting in a negative membrane potential. Hemodialysis leads to rapid changes in serum potassium levels, especially when a low potassium bath is used. The concomitant use of digoxin increases the sensitivity of the heart to rapid changes in serum potassium and may augment the risk for arrhythmias in dialysis patients.[142,143]

The use of acetate has also been implicated in the pathogenesis of arrhythmias during dialysis. One study in dialysis patients with frequent and dangerous ventricular arrhythmias showed a clear reduction in these episodes with the use of bicarbonate versus acetate as the dialysate buffer,[140] although this was not confirmed in another study.[135]

Dialysis calcium concentrations have also been implicated in the pathogenesis of arrhythmias. A higher incidence of non-symptomatic arrhythmias was observed in the group treated with higher calcium dialysate (1.75 mmol/l) versus the group treated with 1.25 mmol/l calcium dialysate. This phenomenon was explained by an increase in re-entry or triggered activity by an increased extra- or intracellular calcium concentration.[141] However, we did not observe an increase in symptomatic arrhythmias with the use of a dialysate calcium concentration of 1.75 mmol/l in patients with myocardial dysfunction.[77]

Prevention

The acute treatment of arrhythmias does not differ from that for non-uremic patients. For a detailed discussion on this issue, the reader is referred to standard textbooks. It is very important to correct abnormalities in the volume status of the patient. When pharmacological treatment or prevention is needed, one should keep in mind that in dialysis patients, a dose-adjustment is needed for various anti-arrhythmic drugs, such as sotalol, digoxin, disopyramide, flecainamide, and procainamide.

Regarding the prevention of dialysis-associated arrhythmias, special care should be taken with the composition of the dialysate. An excessive lowering of serum potassium should be avoided. Factors which influence potassium homeostasis during dialysis include the acid–base status of the patient and the glucose concentration in the dialysate. Especially in acidemic patients, influx of bicarbonate may promote a shift of potassium from the extracellular to the intracellular space, which may lead to a more rapid decline in serum potassium.[144] The use of glucose-free dialysate may increase potassium removal because of an outward shift of potassium from the cell due to lower insulin levels.[145]

During standard hemodialysis, approximately 50–80 mmol of potassium is removed.[146] In patients with pre-dialysis serum potassium below 4.5 mmol/l, we give potassium supplementation with a perfusor attached to the venous blood line using the following scheme (using a dialysate potassium concentration of 2.0 mmol/l).

K^+ 4.0–4.5 mmol/l:	5 mmol/h
K^+ 3.5–4.0 mmol/l:	10 mmol/h
K^+ 3.0–3.5 mmol/l:	15 mmol/h
K^+ below 3.0 mmol/l:	20 mmol/h or more

However, an increase in the potassium concentration of the dialysate of 3.0 or 4.0 mmol/l can also be used as well.

In addition, special care should be given to the prevention of over- and underhydration.[143] Digoxin should be used only for strict indications.

It has been suggested that hemofiltration reduces the risk for arrhythmias. In an uncontrolled study, a reduced incidence in complex ventricular extrasystoles was observed in patients treated with hemofiltration compared to hemodialysis.[147] Another study, however, did not confirm these findings.[135]

Dialysis reactions

Anaphylactoid reactions during dialysis may occur as a result of contact between blood and different components of the extracorporeal circuit, such as the tubing system, the dialysis membrane, and remnants of the sterilization procedure, or as a result of medication administered during the dialysis treatment. Two main types of dialysis reactions can be distinguished: Type A (I), or anaphylactoid reactions, and type B (II) reactions. As will be discussed later, the latter type is probably not related to an allergic phenomenon.

Type A reactions

Type A reactions are anaphylactoid in nature and occur mainly during the first 5–10 (maximal 20) minutes of hemodialysis. These reactions are characterized by dyspnea, angioedema, urticaria, nausea, and diarrhea, and may even result in cardiorespiratory arrest and death. Most type A reactions are Ig-E mediated. Hypersensitivity reactions to ethylene dioxide or to disinfectants employed for reuse procedures are primarily responsible.[148,149] In recent years, the incidence of these reactions has diminished, probably as a result of the less frequent use of ethylene oxide sterilized membranes.[150] Although dialysis reactions have been reported with the use of various dialysis membranes, in recent years hypersensitivity reactions to polyacrylonitrile (PAN) membranes have received much attention. Hypersensitivity reactions to PAN membranes appear to be primarily mediated through the release of bradykinin via activation of factor XII (Hageman factor). This reaction may be enhanced by the use of angiotensin-converting enzyme (ACE) inhibitors, which inhibit the breakdown of bradykinin.[148,149,151] Hypotensive reactions with PAN membranes occur in a rather hetero-geneous way, which has been attributed to the fact that contact phase inhibition by PAN membranes is a pH-dependent mechanism and might, therefore, depend on the acid–base status of the patient.[152]

Administration of medication during dialysis may also lead to allergic reactions. Thus, the intravenous infusion of iron dextran in iron-deficient dialysis patients sometimes leads to severe anaphylaxis.[153] Such reactions can also occur after administration of synthetic or human colloid solutions.

Type B reactions

Type B reactions occur later during the dialysis session (after 20–40 minutes) and are mainly characterized by chest or back pain. These reactions are usually milder and can be distinguished easily from type A reactions, although the distinction may be difficult in the case of severe chest pain and dyspnea. The incidence of type B reactions also appears to be diminishing. The pathogenesis of type B reactions is not entirely clear. It has been related to complement release, as these reactions were primarily observed after 'first-use' of unsubstituted cellulose membranes and abated with reuse.[154] However, in one large randomized study, no difference in dialysis reactions was observed between biocompatible and bioincompatible membranes.[43]

Treatment and prevention

When type A reactions occur during hemodialysis, dialysis must be terminated immediately and the blood should not be returned to the patients. Other catastrophes, such as air embolism and massive hemolysis, have to be excluded. Antihistamines (H_1 and H_2 inhibitors) should be given (clemastine 2 mg i.v. and ranitidine 50 mg i.v.). Steroids may prevent a delayed reaction. In severe cases, epinephrine (1 ml 1:1000 s.c. or 1 ml 1:10.000 i.v. should be administered). Plasma expanders may be needed to maintain hemodynamic stability. In the case of cardiopulmonary arrest, standard resuscitation approaches should be followed.

When a type A reaction has occurred, preventive measures should be taken, including the rinsing of the dialyzer immediately before use, refraining from the use of ethylene oxide-sterilized membranes, and, if PAN membranes were implicated, changing to another mem-brane and stopping ACE inhibitor therapy. Intravenous injection of iron dextran should only be used with caution. Iron saccharate or iron gluconate are reasonable alternatives which may lead to less frequent allergic reactions.[148,149]

As type B reactions are usually much milder, dialysis does not always have to be termi-nated. In the case of chest pain, coronary ischemia should be excluded. Administration of oxygen has been advocated by some authors. However, in the case of severe reactions, dialy-sis has to be discontinued here as well.[148,149]

References

1. Leunissen KM, Kooman JP, van Kuijk W, Luik AJ, van der Sande F, *et al.* (1996). Preventing haemodynamic instability in patients at risk for intra-dialytic hypotension. *Nephrology Dialysis Transplantation* 11:11–15.
2. Hinds CJ, Watson D (1996). *Intensive Care*, p. 72. WB Saunders.

3. Mann H, Ernst E, Gladziwa U, Schallenberg U, Stiller S (1989). Changes in blood volume during dialysis are dependent upon the rate and amount of ultrafiltrate. *Transactions of the American Society of Artificial Organs* 35:250–252.

4. Rodriguez M, Pederson JA, Llach F (1985). Effect of dialysis and ultrafiltration on osmolality, colloid osmotic pressure, and vascular refilling rate. *Kidney International* 28:808–813.

5. Fauchald P (1989). Effect of ultrafiltration on body fluid volumes and transcapillary colloid osmotic gradient in hemodialysis patients. *Contributions to Nephrology* 74:170–175.

6. Ronco C, Fabris A, Chiaramonte S, De Dominicis E, Feriani M, Brendolan A, *et al.* (1988). Comparison of four different short dialysis techniques. *International Journal of Artificial Organs* 11:169–174.

7. van der Sande FM, Kooman JP, Mulder AW, van Kuijk WH, Leunissen KL (1998). Effects of different ultrafiltration rates on hemodynamic parameters in cardiac compromised patients and patients with a normal cardiac function. *Clinical Nephrology* 50:301–308.

8. Katzarski KS, Nisell J, Randmaa I, Danielsson A, Freyschuss U, Bergström J (1997). A critical evaluation of ultrasound measurement of inferior vena cava diameter in assessing dry weight in normotensive and hypertensive dialysis patients. *American Journal of Kidney Diseases* 30:459–465.

9. Koomans HA, Geers AB, Dorhout Mees EJ (1984). Plasma volume recovery after ultrafiltration in patients with chronic renal failure. *Kidney International* 26:848–854.

10. Lopot F, Kotyk P, Blaha J, Forejt J (1996). Use of continuous blood volume monitoring for detecting inadequately high dry weight. *International Journal of Artificial Organs* 19:411–414.

11. Bogaard H, de Vries JP, de Vries PM (1994). Assessment of refill and hypovolemia by continuous surveillance of blood volume and extracellular blood volume. *Nephrology Dialysis Transplantation* 9:1283–1287.

12. Leunissen KM, Noordzij TC, van Hooff JP (1990). Pathophysiologic aspects of plasma volume preservation during dialysis and ultrafiltration. *Contributions to Nephrology* 78:201–211.

13. Fleming SJ, Wilkinson JS, Greenwood RN, Aldridge C, Baker LR, Cattel WR (1984). Effect of dialysate composition on intercompartmental fluid shift. *Kidney International* 26:848–854.

14. van Stone JC, Bauer J, Carey J (1980). The effect of dialysate sodium on body fluid distribution during dialysis. *Transactions of the American Society of Artificial Internal Organs* 26:383–386.

15. Kouw PM, Olthof CG, Gruteke P (1991). Influence of high and low sodium dialysis on blood volume preservation. *Nephrology Dialysis Transplantation* 1991 6:876–880.

16. Hsu CH, Swartz RD, Somermeyer MG (1984). Bicarbonate hemodialysis: influence on plasma refilling and hemodynamic stability. *Nephron* 38:202–208.

17. Leunissen KM, Cheriex EC, Janssen JH, Teule GJ, Mooy JM, Ramentol M, *et al.* (1987). Influence of left ventricular function on changes in plasma volume during acetate and bicarbonate dialysis. *Nephrology Dialysis Transplantation* 2:99–103.

18. Kouw PM, van Es A, Olthof CG, Oe PL, de Vries PM, Donker AJ (1992). High efficiency dialysis strategies: effects on fluid balance by means of conductivity measurements. In: Kouw PM. *Determinants of intra- and extracellular fluid volume by means of non-invasive conductivity measurements. In vivo* validation and clinical application. Free University of Amsterdam Press.

19. Takenaka T, Tsuchiya Y, Suzuki H (1997). High-performance hemodiafiltration and blood pressure stability. *Nephron* 73:30–35.

20. de Vries PM, Olthof CG, Solf A, Schuenemann B, Oe PL, Quellhorst E, *et al.* (1991). Fluid balance between haemodialysis and haemofiltration: the effect of dialysate sodium and a variable ultrafiltration rate. *Nephrology Dialysis Transplantation* 6:257–263

21. van Kuijk WH, Hillion D, Savoiu C, Leunissen KM (1997). Critical role of the extracorporeal blood temperature in the hemodynamic response during hemofiltration. *Journal of the American Society of Nephrology* 1997 8:949–955.

22. Schneditz D, Martin K, Kramer M, Kenner T, Skrabal F (1997). Effect of controlled extracorporeal blood cooling on ultrafiltration-induced blood volume changes during hemodialysis. *Journal of the American Society of Nephrology* 8:956–964.

23. van Kuijk WH, Luik AJ, de Leeuw PW, van Hooff JP, Nieman FH, Habets HM, *et al.* (1995). Vascular reactivity during hemodialysis and isolated ultrafiltration: thermal influences. *Nephrology Dialysis Transplantation* 16:1852–1858.

24. Shibagaki Y, Takaichi K (1998). Significant reduction of the large-vessel blood volume by food intake during hemodialysis. *Clinical Nephrology* 49:49–54.

25. Kooman JP, Wijnen JA, Draaijer P, van Bortel L, Gladziwa U, Struyker Boudier HA, *et al.* (1992). Compliance and reactivity of the peripheral venous system in patients treated with chronic intermittent hemodialysis. *Kidney International* 41:1041–1048.

26. Kooman JP, Daemen MJ, Wijnen R, Verluyten-Goessens MJ, van Hooff JP, Leunissen KM (1995). Morphological changes of the venous system in uremic patients. *Nephron* 69:454–458.

27. London GM, Safar ME, Levenson JA, Simon AC, Temmar MA (1981). Renal filtration fraction, effective vascular compliance, and partition of fluid volumes in sustained essential hypertension. *Kidney International* 20:97–103.

28. Henrich WL (1982). Autonomous insufficiency. *Archives of Internal Medicine* 142:339–344.

29. Kooman JP, Gladziwa U, Böcker G, van Bortel LM, van Hooff JP, Leunissen KM (1992). Role of the venous system in hemodynamics during ultrafiltration and bicarbonate dialysis. *Kidney International* 42:718–726.

30. McGrath BP, Ledingham JG, Benedict CR (1978). Catecholamines in peripheral venous plasma in patients on chronic hemodialysis. *Clinical Science in Molecular Medicine* 55:89–96.

31. Converse RL, Jacobson TN, Jost CM, Toto RD, Joot CM, Cosentino F, *et al.* (1992). Sympathetic overactivity in patients with chronic renal failure. *New England Journal of Medicine* 327:1912–1918.

32. Baldamus CA, Ernst W, Frei UW, Koch KM (1982). Sympathetic and hemodynamic response to volume removal during different forms of renal replacement therapy. *Nephron* 31:324–332.

33. Hegbrant J, Thysell H, Martensson L, Ekman R, Boberg U (1993). Changes in plasma levels of vasoactive peptides during sequential bicarbonate dialysate. *Nephron* 63:309–313.

34. Bergström J (1988). Catecholamines and control of blood pressure during hemodialysis and hemofiltration. *Kidney International* 34:S110–S114.

35. Odar-Cederlof I, Theodorsson E, Eriksson CG, Hamberger B, Tidgren B, Kjellstrand CM (1993). Vasoactive agents and blood pressure regulation in sequential ultrafiltration and hemodialysis. *International Journal of Artificial Organs* 16:662–669.

36. Nakamura Y, Ikeda T, Takata S, Yokoi H, Hirono M, Abe T, *et al.* (1991). The role of peripheral capacitance and resistance vessels in hypotension following hemodialysis. *American Heart Journal* 121:1170–1177.

37. Carmichael FJ, Salvidia V, Varghese GA, Israel Y, Orrego H (1988). Ethanol-induced increase in portal blood flow: role of acetate and A1- and A2-adenosine receptors. *American Journal of Physiology* 255:G417–G423.

38. van Kuijk WH, Wirtz JJ, Grave W, de Heer F, Menheere PP, van Hooff JP, *et al.* (1996). Vascular reactivity during combined ultrafiltration–haemodialysis. Influence of dialysate sodium. *Nephrology Dialysis Transplantation* 11:323–328.

39. van Kuijk WH, Mulder WA, Hanff GA, Leunissen KML (1997). The effect of changes in plasma ionized calcium on blood pressure and vascular reactivity during ultrafiltration and hemodialysis. *Clinical Nephrology* 47:190–196.

40. Henderson LW, Koch KM, Dinarello CA, Shaldon S (1983). Hemodialysis hypotension: the interleukin-1 hypothesis. *Blood Purification* 1:3–8.

41. Dinarello CA (1992). Interleukin-1 and tumor necrosis factor and their naturally occurring antagonists during hemodialysis. *Kidney International* 42(Suppl 38):S68–S72.

42. Yokokawa K, Mankus R, Saklayen MG, Kohno M, Yasunari K, Minami M, *et al.* (1995). Increased nitric oxide production in patients with hypotension during hemodialysis. *Annals of Internal Medicine* 123:35–37.

43. Bergamo Collaborative Dialysis Study Group (1991). Acute intradialytic well-being results of a clinical trial comparing polysulfone with cuprophane. *Kidney International* 40:714–719.
44. Collins DM, Lambert MB, Tannenbaum JS, Oliverio M, Schwab SJ (1993). Tolerance of hemodialysis: a randomized prospective trial of high-flux versus conventional high-efficiency hemodialysis. *Journal of the American Society of Nephrology* 4:148–154.
45. Skroeder NR, Jacobson SH, Lins LE, Kjellstrand CM (1994). Acute symptoms during and between hemodialysis: the relative role of speed, duration, and biocompatibility of dialysis. *Artificial Organs* 18:880–887.
46. van Kuijk WA, Buurman WA, Gerlag PG, Leunissen KM (1996). Vascular reactivity during combined ultrafiltration–hemodialysis: influence of dialysate derived contaminants. *Journal of the American Society of Nephrology* 7:2664–2669.
47. Aakhus S, Bjoernstad K, Jorstad S (1995). Systemic cardiovascular response in hemodialysis without and with ultrafiltration with membranes of high and low biocompatibility. *Blood Purification* 13:229–240.
48. Shinzato T, Milwa M, Nakai S, Morita H, Odani H, Inove I, *et al.* (1994). Role of adenosine in dialysis-induced hypotension. *Journal of the American Society of Nephrology* 4:1987–1994.
49. Coli U, Landini S, Lucatello S, Fracasso A, Morachiello P, Righetto F, *et al.* (1983). Cold as cardiovascular stabilizing function in hemodialysis: hemodynamic evaluation. *Transactions of the American Society of Artificial Internal Organs* 29:71–75.
50. van der Sande FM, Kooman JP, Burema JH, Hameleers P, Kerkhofs AM, Barendregt JM, *et al.* The effect of dialysate temperature on energy balance during hemodialysis. *American Journal of Kidney Diseases* 33:1115–1121.
51. Daugirdas JT (1991). Dialysis hypotension a hemodynamic analysis. *Kidney International* 39:233–246.
52. Ushioda E, Nuwayhid B, Kleinman G, Tabsh K, Brinkman CR III, Assali NS (1983). The contribution of the beta-adrenergic system to the cardiovascular response to hypovolemia. *American Journal of Obstetrics and Gynaecology* 147:423–429.
53. Sander-Jensen K, Mehlsen J, Stadeager C, Christensen NJ, Fahrenkrug J, Schwartz TW, *et al.* (1988). Increase in vagal activity during hypotensive lower body negative pressure in humans. *American Journal of Physiology* 255:R149–R156.
54. Hintze TH, Vatner SF. (1982) Cardiac dynamics during haemorrhage: relative unimportance of adrenergic inotropic responses. *Circulation Research* 50:705–713.
55. Greenway CV, Wayne Lautt W (1986). Blood volume, the venous system, preload, and cardiac output. *Canadian Journal of Physiology and Pharmacology* 64:383–387.
56. Safar ME, London GM, Levenson JA, Simon AC, Chau NP (1979). Rapid dextran infusion in essential hypertension. *Hypertension* 1:615–623.
57. Cohen-Solal A (1998). Left ventricular diastolic dysfunction: pathophysiology, diagnosis and treatment. *Nephrology Dialysis Transplantation* 13(Suppl 4):3–5.
58. Ritz E, Rambausek M, Mall G, Ruffman K, Mandelbaum A (1990). Cardiac changes to uremia and their possible relation to cardiovascular instability on dialysis. *Contributions to Nephrology* 78:221–229.
59. Bondia A, Tabernero JM, Macias JF, Martin-Luengo C (1988). Autonomic nervous system in hemodialysis. *Nephrology Dialysis Transplantation* 2:174–180.
60. Nakashima Y, Fouad FM, Nakamoto S, Textor SC, Bravo EL, Tarazi RC (1987). Localisation of autonomic nervous system dysfunction in dialysis patients. *American Journal of Nephrology* 7:375–381.
61. Heber ME, Lahiri A, Thompson D, Raftery EB (1989). Baroreceptor, not left ventricular, dysfunction is the cause of hemodialysis hypotension. *Clinical Nephrology* 32:79–86.
62. Lin YF, Wang JY, Shum AY, Jiang HK, Lai WY, Lu KC, *et al.* (1993). Role of plasma catecholamines, autonomic, and left ventricular function in normotensive and hypotension

prone dialysis patients. *Transactions of the American Society of Artificial Internal Organs* 39:946–953.

63. Stojceva-Taneva O, Masin G, Polenakovic M, Stojcev S, Stojkovski L (1991). Autonomic nervous system dysfunction and volume nonresponsive hypotension in hemodialysis patients. *American Journal of Nephrology* 11:123–126.

64. Nies AS, Robertson D, Stone WJ (1979). Hemodialysis hypotension is not the result of uremic peripheral autonomous neuropathy. *Journal of Laboratory and Clinical Medicine* 94:395–402.

65. Ligtenberg G, Blankestijn PJ, Boomsma F, Koomans HA (1996). No change in automatic function tests during uncomplicated haemodialysis. *Nephrology Dialysis Transplantation* 11:651–656.

66. Zuchelli P, Santoro A, Sturani A, Degli Esposti E, Chiarini C, *et al.* (1984). Effects of hemodialysis and hemofiltration on the autonomic control of circulation. *Transactions of the American Society of Artificial Internal Organs* 30:163–167.

67. Baldamus CA, Mantz P, Kachel HG, Koch KM, Schoeppe W (1984). Baroreflex in patients undergoing hemodialysis and hemofiltration. *Contributions to Nephrology* 41:409–414.

68. Converse RL, Jacobsen TN, Jost CM, Toto RD, Grayburn PA, Obregon TM, *et al.* (1992). Paradoxical withdrawal of reflex vasoconstriction as a cause of haemodialysis-induced hypotension. *Journal of Clinical Investigation* 90:1657–1665.

69. Santoro A, Mancini E, Spongano M, Rossi M, Paolini F, Zucchelli P (1990). A haemodynamic study of hypotension during haemodialysis using electrical bioimpedance cardiography. *Nephrology Dialysis Transplantation* 5(Suppl 1):147–153.

70. Zoccali C, Tripepi G, Mallamaci F, Pannucciov (1997). The heart rate response to dialysis hypotension in haemodialysis patients. *Nephrology Dialysis Transplantation* 12:519–523.

71. Nixon JV, Mitchell JH, McPhaul JJ Jr, Henrich WL (1983). Effect of hemodialysis on left ventricular function. Dissociation of changes in filling volume and in contractile state. *Journal of Clinical Investigation* 71:377–384.

72. Henrich WL, Hunt JM, Nixon JV (1984). Increased ionized calcium and left ventricular contractility during hemodialysis. *New England Journal of Medicine* 310:19–23.

73. Drüeke T, Le Pailleur C (1986). Cardiomyopathy in patients on maintenance haemodialysis. *Contributions to Nephrology* 52:27–33.

74. Leunissen KM, Hoorntje SJ, Fiers HA (1986). Acetate versus bicarbonate dialysis in critically ill patients. *Nephron* 42:146–151.

75. Lang RM, Fellner SK, Neumann A, Bushinsky DA, Borow KM (1988). Left ventricular contractility varies directly with blood ionized calcium. *Annals of Internal Medicine* 108:524–529.

76. Leunissen KM, van den Berg BW, van Hooff JP (1989). Ionized calcium plays a pivotal role in controlling blood pressure during hemodialysis. *Blood Purification* 7:233–239.

77. van der Sande FM, Cheriex ET, van Kuijk WH, Leunissen KM (1998). The effect of low calcium (1.25 mmol/l) and high calcium dialysate (1.75 mmol/l) on haemodynamics during ultrafiltration and dialysis in cardiac compromised patients. *American Journal of Kidney Diseases* 32:125–131.

78. Levy FL, Grayburn PA, Foulks CJ, Brickner ME, Henrich WL (1992). Improved left ventricular contractility with cool temperature hemodialysis. *Kidney International* 41:961–965.

79. Parfrey PS, Harnett Foley RN, Parfrey PS, Harnett JD (1992). Left ventricular hypertrophy in dialysis patients. *Seminars in dialysis* 5:34–41.

80. Kooman JP, Leunissen KM (1993). Cardiovascular aspects in renal disease. Current Opinion in *Nephrology and Hypertension* 2:791–797.

81. Bradley JR, Evans DB, Gore SM, Cowley AJ (1988). Is dialysis hypotension caused by an - abnormality of venous tone? *British Medical Journal* 296:1634–1637.

82. Jahn H, Schohn D, Schmitt R (1983). Hemodynamic modifications induced by fluid removal and treatment modalities in chronic hemodialysis patients. *Blood Purification* 1:80–89.

83. Wizemann V, Blank S, Kramer W (1994). Diastolic dysfunction of the left ventricle in dialysis patients. *Contributions to Nephrology* 106:106–109.
84. Gong R, Lindberg J, Abrams J, Whitaker WR, Wade CE, Gouge S (1993). Comparison of hypertonic saline solutions and dextran in dialysis-induced hypotension. *Journal of the American Society of Nephrology* 3:1808–1812.
85. van der Sande FM, Kooman JP, Barendregt JN, Nieman FH, Leunissen KM (1999). Effect of iv fluids on plasma volume preservation. *Journal of the American Society of Nephrology* 55:2598–2608.
86. Köhler H (1997). Einfluss der nierenfunktion auf die elimination und wirkung von kolloidalen plasma ersatzmitteln (influence of renal function on elimination and action of colloid fluids). *Fortschritt in Medizin* 40:S1809–S1813.
87. Steinhoff J, Mansky T, Reitz M, Schulz E, Sack K (1988). Pharmakokinetic von hydroxyäthyl-stärke bei patienten unter hämodialyse und hämofiltration (pharmacokinetics of hydroxy-ethylstarch in patients treated with hemodialysis and hemofiltration). *Nieren und Hochdrückkrankheiten* 17:S411–S414.
88. Better OS, Rubinstein I, Winaver JM, Knochel JP (1997). Mannitol therapy revisited. *Kidney International* 51:886–894.
89. Canzanello VJ, Hylander-Rossner B, Sands RE, Morgan TM, Jordan J, Burkart JM (1991). Comparison of 50% dextrose water, 25% mannitol, and 23.5% saline for the treatment of hemodialysis-associated muscle cramps. *Transactions of the American Society of Artificial Internal Organs* 37:649–652.
90. Lauster F, Gerzer R, Weil J, Fulle HJ, Schiffl H (1990). Assessment of dry body weight in hemodialysis patients by the biochemical marker cGMP. *Nephrology Dialysis Transplantation* 5:356–361.
91. Kouw PM, Kooman JP, Cheriex EC, Olthof CG, de Vries PM, Leunissen KM (1993). Assessment of postdialysis dry weight: a comparison of techniques. *Journal of the American Society of Nephrology* 4:98–104.
92. Leunissen KM, Menheere PP, Cheriex EC, van den Berg BW, Noordzij TC, van Hooff JP (1989). Plasma alpha-human atrial natriuretic peptide and volume status in chronic haemodialysis patients. *Nephrology Dialysis Transplantation* 4:382–386.
93. Kong CH, Thompson CM, Lewis CA, Hill PD, Thompson FD (1993). Determination of total body water in uraemic patients by bioelectrical impedance. *Nephrology Dialysis Transplantation* 8:716–719.
94. Segal KR, Burastero S, Chun A, Coronel P, Pierson RN, Wang J (1991). Estimation of extracellular and total body water by multiple-frequency bioelectrical-impedance measurement. *American Journal of Clinical Nutrition* 54:26–29.
95. Chertow GM, Lowrie EG, Wilmore DW, Gonzalez J, Lew NL, Ling J, *et al.* (1995). Nutritional assessment with bioelectrical impedance analysis in maintenance hemodialysis. *Journal of the American Society of Nephrology* 6:75–81.
96. Formica C, Atkinson MG, Nyulasi I, McKay J, Heale W, Seeman E (1993). Body composition following hemodialysis: studies using dual-energy x-ray absorptiometry and bioelectrical impedance analysis. *Osteoporosis International* 3:192–197.
97. Mandolfo S, Farina M, Imbasciati E (1995). Bioelectrical impedance and hemodialysis. *International Journal of Artificial Organs* 18:700–704.
98. Kouw PM, Kooman JP, Cheriex EC, Olthof CG, de Vries PM, Leunissen KM (1993). Assessment of postdialysis dry weight: a comparison of techniques. *Journal of the American Society of Nephrology* 4:98–104.
99. Mandelbaum A, Ritz E (1996). Vena cava diameter measurement for estimation of dry weight in haemodialysis patients. *Nephrology Dialysis Transplantation* 11(Suppl 2):24–27.
100. Brunet P, Saingra Y, Leonetti F, Vacher-Coponat H, Ramananarivo P, Berland Y (1996). Tolerance of haemodialysis: a randomized cross-over trial of 5-h versus 4-h treatment time. *Nephrology Dialysis Transplantation* 11(Suppl 8):46–51.

101. Locatelli F, Ponti R, Pedrini L, di Filippo S (1989). Sodium and dialysis: a deeper insight. *International Journal of Artificial Organs* 12:71–74.

102. Sherman RA, Torres F, Cody RP (1988). Postprandial blood pressure changes during hemodialysis. *American Journal of Kidney Diseases* 12:37–39.

103. Barakat MM, Nawab ZM, Yu AW, Lau AH, Ing TS, Daugirdas JT (1993). Hemodynamic effects of intradialytic food ingestion and the effects of caffeine. *Journal of the American Society of Nephrology* 3:1813–1818.

104. Brandt JL, Castleman L, Ruskin HD, Greenwald J, Kelly JJ (1955). The effect of oral protein and glucose feeding on splanchnic blood flow and oxygen utilization in normal and cirrhotic subjects. *Journal of Clinical Investigation* 34:1017–1025.

105. Kahn AM, Husid A, Song T (1997). Relationship between insulin and hemodialysis-associated hypotension. *Current Opinion in Nephrology and Hypertension* 6:1–5.

106. Jost CM, Agrawal R, Khair-el-Din T, Grayburn PA, Victor RG, Henrich WL (1993). Effects of cooler temperature dialysate on hemodynamic stability in 'problem' dialysis patients. *Kidney International* 44:606–612.

107. Mahida BH, Dumler F, Zasuwa G, Fleig G, Levin NW (1983). Effect of cooled dialysate on serum catecholamines and blood pressure stability. *Transactions of the American Society of Artificial Internal Organs* 24:383–389.

108. Fine A, Penner B (1996). The protective effect of cool dialysate is dependent on patients' predialysis temperature. *American Journal of Kidney Diseases* 28:262–265.

109. Rubin RP (1970). Neurotransmitter substances and hormones. *Pharmacological Reviews* 22:389–428.

110. Argiles A, Kerr PG, Canaud B, Flavier JL, Mion C (1993). Calcium kinetics and the long-term effects of lowering dialysate calcium concentration. *Kidney International* 43:630–640.

111. Branger B, Deschodt G, Oules R, Balducchi JP, Granolleras C, Alsadabani B, *et al.* (1988). Biocompatible membranes and hemodynamic tolerance to hemodialysis. *Kidney International* 33(Suppl 24):S196–S197.

112. Steuer R, Leypoldt JK, Cheung A, Senekjian H, Connis J (1996). Reducing symptoms during dialysis by continuously monitoring the hematocrit. *American Journal of Kidney Diseases* 27:525–532.

113. Schallenberg U, Stiller S, Mann H (1987). A new method of continuous hemoglobinometric measurements of blood volume during dialysis. *Life Support Systems* 5:293–305.

114. Steuer R, Leypoldt JK, Cheung A, Harris D, Conis J (1983). Hematocrit as an indicator of blood volume and a predictor of intradialytic morbid events. *Transactions of the American Society of Artificial Internal Organs* 24:383–389.

115. Ishihara T, Igarashi I, Kitano T, Shinzato T, Maeda K (1993). Continuous hematocrit monitoring method in an extracorporeal circulation system and its application for automatic control of blood volume during artificial kidney treatment. *Artificial Organs* 17:708–716.

116. Churchill DN (1996). Sodium and water profiling in chronic uremia. *Nephrology Dialysis Transplantation* 11(Suppl 8):38–41.

117. Raja RM (1996). Sodium profiling in elderly haemodialysis patients. *Nephrology Dialysis Transplantation* 11(Suppl 8):42–45

118. Acchiardo SR, Hayden AJ (1991). Is Na modeling necessary in high flux dialysis. *Transactions of the American Society of Artificial Internal Organs* 37:M135–M137.

119. Sadowski RH, Allred EN, Jabs K (1993). Sodium modeling ameliorates intradialytic and interdialytic symptoms in young hemodialysis patients. *Journal of the American Society of Nephrology* 4:1192–1198.

120. Flanigan MJ, Khairullah QT, Lim VS (1997). Dialysate sodium delivery can alter chronic blood pressure management. *American Journal of Kidney Diseases* 29:383–389.

121. Daugirdas JT, Al-Kudsi RR, Ing TS, Norusis MJ (1985). A double-blind evaluation of sodium gradient hemodialysis. *American Journal of Nephrology* 5:163–168.

122. Iida N, Tsubakihara Y, Shirai D, Imada A, Suzuki M (1994). Treatment of dialysis induced hypotension with L-threo-3,4-dihydroxyphenylserine. *Nephrology Dialysis Transplantation* 6:1130–1135.

123. Kanamura M, Nagashima S, Nakashima M (1988). Clinical effect of amezinium methylsulfate (LU-1631) on hypotensive agents undergoing intermittent hemodialysis therapy. *Journal of Clinical and Therapeutical Medicine* 4:1311–1319.

124. Flynn JJ III, Mitchell MC, Caruso FS, McElligott MA (1996). Midodrine treatment for patients with hemodialysis hypotension. *Clinical Nephrology* 45:261–267.

125. Lindberg JS, Copley JB, Melton K, Wade CE, Abrams J, Goode D (1990). Lysine vasopressin in the treatment of refractory hemodialysis-induced hypotension. *American Journal of Nephrology* 10:269–275.

126. Dheenan S, Venkatesan J, Grubb BP, Henrich WL (1998). Effect of sertraline hydrochloride on dialysis hypotension. *American Journal of Kidney Diseases* 31:624–630.

127. Fox SD, Henderson LW (1993). Cardiovascular response during hemodialysis and hemofiltration: thermal, membrane and catecholamine influences. *Blood Purification* 11:224–226.

128. Hampl H, Paeprer H, Unger V, Fischer C, Resa I, Kessel M (1980). Hemodynamic changes during hemodialysis, sequential ultrafiltration, and hemofiltration. *Kidney International* 18:S83–S88.

129. Wizemann V, Kramer W, Knopp G, Sychla M, Schmidt H, Rawer P, *et al.* (1981). Cardiovascular function during hemodialysis, hemofiltration, hemodiafiltration. In: Schütterle G, Wizemann V, Seyfart G, editors. *Hemodiafiltration*, pp. 89–104. Proceedings 1. Symposium Giessen. Hygieneplan, Oberursel.

130. Movilli E, Camerini C, Zein H, D'Avolio G, Sandrini M, Strada A, *et al.* (1996). A prospective comparison of bicarbonate dialysis, hemodiafiltration, and acetate-free biofiltration in the elderly. *American Journal of Kidney Diseases* 27:541–547.

131. Wizemann V (1996). Coronary artery disease in dialysis patients. *Nephron* 74:642–651.

132. De Lima JJ, Lopes HF, Grupi CJ, Abensur H, Giorgi P, Krieger EM, *et al.* (1995). Blood pressure influences the occurrence of complex ventricular arrhythmias in hemodialysis patients. *Hypertension* 26:1200–1203.

133. Shapira OM, Bar-Khayim Y (1992). ECG changes and cardiac arrhythmias in chronic renal failure patients on hemodialysis. *Journal of Electrocardiology* 53:273–279.

134. Sforzini S, Latini R, Mingardi G, Vincenti A, Redaelli B (1992). Ventricular arrhythmias and four-year mortality in haemodialysis patients. *Lancet* 339:212–213.

135. Wizemann V, Kramer W, Funke T, Schütterle G (1985). Dialysis-induced cardiac arrhythmias: fact or fiction? *Nephron* 39:356–360.

136. Saragoca MA, Canziani E, Cassiolato JL, Gil MA, Andrade JL, Draibe SA, *et al.* (1991). Left ventricular hypertrophy as a risk factor for arrhythmias in hemodialysis patients. *Journal of Cardiovascular Pharmacology* 17(Suppl 2):S136–S138.

137. Abe S, Yoshizawa M, Nakanishi N, Yazawa T, Yokota K, Honda M, *et al.* (1996). Electrocardiographic abnormalities in patients receiving hemodialysis. *American Heart Journal* 131:1137–1144.

138. Morrison G, Michelson EL, Brown S, Morganroth J (1980). Mechanism and prevention of cardiac arrhythmias in chronic hemodialysis patients. *Kidney International* 17:811–819.

139. Ramirez G, Brueggemeyer CD, Newton JL (1984). Cardiac arrhythmias on hemodialysis on chronic renal failure patients. *Nephron* 36:212–218.

140. Fantuzzi S, Caico C, Amatruda O, Cervini P, Abu-Turky H, Baratelli L, *et al.* (1991). Hemodialysis-associated cardiac arrhythmias: a lower risk with bicarbonate? *Nephron* 58:196–200.

141. Nishimura M, Nakanishi T, Yasui A, Tsuji Y, Kunishige H, Hirabayashi M, *et al.* (1992). Serum calcium increases the risk of arrhythmias during acetate hemodialysis. *American Journal of Kidney Diseases* 19:149–155.

142. Blumberg A, Häusermann M, Strub B, Jenzer HR (1983). Cardiac arrhythmias in patients on maintenance hemodialysis. *Nephron* 33:91–95.
143. Kimura KI, Tabei K, Asano Y, Hosoda S (1989). Cardiac arrhythmias in hemodialysis patients. *Nephron* 53:201–207.
144. Wiegand CF, Davin TD, Raij L, Kjellstrand CM (1981). Severe hypokalemia induced by hemodialysis. *Archives of Internal Medicine* 141:167–170.
145. Ward RA, Wathen RL, Williams TE, Harding GB (1987). Hemodialysate composition and intradialytic metabolic, acid–base and potassium changes. *Kidney International* 32:129–135.
146. Ketchersid TL, van Stone JC (1991). Dialysate potassium. *Seminars in Dialysis* 4:46–51.
147. Quellhorst E, Schuenemann B, Mietzsch G (1987). Long-term hemofiltration in 'poor-risk' patients. *Transactions of the American Society of Artificial Internal Organs* 33:758–764.
148. Jaber BJ, Pereira BJG (1997). Dialysis reactions. *Seminars in Dialysis* 10:158–165.
149. Salem M, Ivanovich PT, Ing TS, Daugirdas JT (1994). Adverse effect of dialyzers manifesting during the dialysis session. *Nephrology Dialysis Transplantation* (Suppl 2):127–137.
150. de Filippi C, Piazza V, Efficace E, Galli F, Pisati P, Aprile C, *et al.* (1998). Dialysis hypersensitivity: a fading problem? *Blood Purification* 16:66–71.
151. Verresen L, Waer M, Vanrenterghem Y, Michielsen P (1990). Angiotensin converting enzyme inhibitors and anaphylactoid reactions to high flux membrane dialysis. *Lancet* 336:1360–1362.
152. Renaux JL, Thomas M, Crost T, Loughraieb N, Vantard G (1999). Activation of the kallikrein-kinin system in hemodialysis: role of membrane electronegativity, blood dilution, and pH. *Kidney International* 55:1097–1103.
153. Novey HS, Pahl M, Haydik I, Vaziri ND (1994). Immunologic studies of anaphylaxis to iron dextran in patients on renal dialysis. *Annals of Allergy* 72:224–228.
154. Daugirdas JT, Ing TS (1988). First use reactions during hemodialysis: a definition of subtypes. *Kidney International* 24:S37–S43.

16

Dialysis therapy in the cardiothoracic intensive care unit

Eduardo K. Lacson and William F. Owen

Introduction

In the United States in 1996[1] there were over 300 000 patients with end-stage renal failure (ESRF), who, by definition, required a life-long course of dialysis. Cardiovascular causes (cardiac arrest, acute myocardial infarction, and other cardiac events) accounted for half the reported deaths in this population.[1] This is unsurprising as cardiac disorders are present in a large fraction of patients when they begin dialysis. In one study, the investigators noted that 42% of patients had a previous myocardial infarction (MI) or coronary revascularization (also known as coronary artery bypass surgery, CABG) and up to 40% had a previous episode of congestive heart failure (CHF).[2] In addition, the prevalence of left ventricular hypertrophy (LVH) in this patient population was approximately 75%.[3–5] Furthermore, the development of incident ischemic heart disease in a prospective cohort was 3% per year,[6] while new-onset CHF occurred at approximately 7% per year.[7] Thus, coronary artery disease is a substantial problem in the ESRF population.

The exact number of procedures, outcomes, or costs related to cardiothoracic surgery is not well documented in the literature. However, in 1996, out of 344 383 hospital admissions, 1652 were directly related to CABG as the primary diagnosis-related group (DRG) designation.[1] This may be an underestimation, especially with the high incidence of cardiovascular disease in the pre-ESRF population. Such under-reporting may arise because of several factors. First, the high mortality rate for patients with ESRF (~20% annually[1]) may preclude intervention in many cases. Second, the ESRF population is older with a greater prevalence of diabetes mellitus; this case-mix may portend an increased mortality.[1,8,9] Thus, the percentage of available candidates for major cardiac surgical intervention may be limited. Third, recent evidence describes a relatively poor survival after anterior MI for ESRF patients compared with the general population.[10] Such inevitably poor outcomes may limit the aggressive approach to surgery in this population. In summary, these factors may all contribute to the less-than-expected use of surgical interventions for cardiovascular disease in the ESRF population.

In addition to patients with ESRF, patients with chronic renal failure (CRF), especially those with borderline renal function, are also at increased risk of cardiovascular disease.[11] A significant association is present between declining renal function and the prevalence of LVH,[12,13] which may be a predictor of significant cardiac morbidity.[2] A cohort study of CRF patients revealed a 38% incidence of LVH.[13] It is likely that a portion of these patients is at risk for future cardiac events and surgical interventions.

In addition to the prevalence of substantial cardiac disease in patients with renal insufficiency, there is the occurrence of *de novo* renal failure associated with cardiac procedures. The incidence of acute renal failure (ARF) that requires hemodialysis as a complication of CABG is reported as 0.6–3.7%.[14–16] For thoraco-abdominal aneurysm resection and repair, the incidence increases to 8–15%.[17,18] It is noteworthy that a major risk factor for ARF is pre-existing CRF.[14–18]

Therefore, it is not uncommon for the multidisciplinary staff of the cardiothoracic intensive care unit (CT-ICU) to face the issue of dialytic management of the postoperative patient. The current practice standard is for patients to undergo dialysis for either ESRF, in which the azotemia is the consequence of pre-existing irreversible, structural renal insufficiency, or for ARF, which describes a wide variety of disorders associated with the acute retention of nitrogenous products of metabolism. Because ARF is potentially reversible, an aggressive pursuit should be undertaken to identify and correct the cause. Within the ICU setting, most cases of renal failure that require dialytic support are acute in nature. Except where specifically denoted, all subsequent discussions are applicable to patients with ESRF or ARF, with or without pre-existing CRF.

Despite vastly improved medical, surgical, and nursing care within the ICU, the use of mechanical ventilators, inotropes, intracardiac pressure monitoring, total parenteral nutrition, an expanded choice of antimicrobial agents, and the ready availability of multiple dialysis techniques, mortality from ARF greatly exceeds that of CRF. Whereas the annual mortality from incident ESRF has declined from 36% to approximately 25% over the last 10 years,[1] the mortality for ARF has remained relatively unchanged. Since the 1950s, the mortality has ranged from 36 to 88%.[19–23] Specifically focusing on postoperative cardiothoracic procedures, several case series of ESRF patients reveal a perioperative mortality rate of 8%–42%. The most powerful adverse prognostic factor was a diagnosis of New York Heart Association's Class IV heart failure.[24–27] For patients with ARF, with or without a background history of CRF, the mortality rate was 44–70%,[14–16,28] which is not substantially different from the previously reported mortality rates for ARF in the general population.[19–23] Specific factors associated with poor prognosis include postoperative low cardiac output,[29] use of intermittent positive pressure ventilation,[30] sepsis,[23,29] and multiorgan system failure post-CABG.[28,31] Despite their comorbidity, a vast majority of patients with ARF do not require dialytic support. In a series of over 2000 consecutive patients undergoing CABG from 1987 to 1990, only 297 (15.1%) developed ARF (defined as 50% increase in serum creatinine) with 25 (1.2%) requiring dialysis. However, mortality was 44% in this subset with advanced renal failure.[15] In another series of 775 patients, 111 (15.1%) developed ARF (defined as creatinine up to 2.5 mg/dl), and 27 (3.7%) needing renal replacement therapy.[16]

Because of the potential for recovery, all patients with ARF should be considered for renal replacement therapy.[32] The exceptions are patients with aggressive terminal neoplastic disease who are no longer candidates for chemotherapy with a significantly abbreviated expected lifespan, patients in a persistent vegetative state, and those with such severe medical complications that dialysis cannot be technically performed. Dialysis fulfills two biophysical goals: (1) solute removal, as is the case for potassium and urea, or the addition of solute, as is the case for bicarbonate and calcium ('clearance'); and (2) the elimination of volume from the patient ('ultrafiltration'). These two processes can be performed simultaneously or at different times. The dialysis procedures used are hemodialysis, hemofiltration, a combination of these, and peritoneal dialysis (Table 16.1).

Table 16.1 Dialytic modalities

Technique	Dialyzer	Blood flow (ml/min)	Physical principle
Intermittent			
Conventional hemodialysis	Hemodialyzer	200–500 (with blood pump)	Diffusive solute clearance and UF concurrently
Ultrafiltration (UF)	Hemodialyzer	200–500 (with blood pump)	UF alone
Sequential UF–clearance	Hemodialyzer	200–500 (with blood pump)	UF followed by diffusive clearance
Continuous			
Slow continuous ultrafiltration (SCUF)	Hemofilter	50–100	UF alone
Continuous arteriovenous hemofiltration (CAVH)	Hemofilter	50–200	UF with solute clearance by convective transport
Continuous venovenous hemofiltration (CVVH)	Hemodialyzer	50–200 (with blood pump)	UF with solute clearance by convective transport
Continuous arteriovenous hemodialysis (CAVHD)	Hemodialyzer	50–200	Diffusive solute clearance and UF concurrently
Continuous venovenous hemodialysis (CVVHD)	Hemodialyzer	50–200 (with blood pump)	Diffusive solute clearance and UF concurrently
Continuous arteriovenous hemodiafiltration (CAVHDF)	Hemodialyzer	50–200	Simultaneous diffusive and convective clearance with dialysate and replacement solution
Continuous venovenous hemodiafiltration (CVVHDF)	Hemodialyzer	50–200 (with blood pump)	Simultaneous diffusive and convective clearance with dialysate and replacement solution
Peritoneal			
Continuous ambulatory/cycling (CAPD/CCPD)	None	N/A	Exchanges performed continuously at varying intervals
Intermittent (IPD)	None	N/A	Exchanges performed for 10–12 hours every 2–3 days

Hemodialysis

Hemodialysis is a diffusion-driven and size-discriminatory process for the efficient clearance of relatively small solutes such as electrolytes and urea (<300 Da). The clearance of larger solutes is typically far less effective. During hemodialysis, ultrafiltration is driven by the generation of negative hydraulic pressure on the dialysate side of the dialyzer. The major components of the hemodialytic process are: (1) the artificial kidney or dialyzer; (2) the delivery system, which comprises the mechanical devices that pump the patient's blood and the dialysate through the dialyzer; and (3) the dialysate, which is the fluid having a defined chemical composition used for solute clearance. The hemodialyzer is configured as a cylinder that is filled with thousands of parallel hollow fibers traversing the length of the cylinder. The hollow fibers are composed of a semipermeable membrane material. The patient's blood is pumped into the dialyzer, thus through the fibers, by a peristaltic pump. In parallel, dialysate solution is pumped around the fibers. During the performance of 'conventional' intermittent hemodialysis (HD), the patient's blood and dialysate are pumped continuously through the dialyzer in opposite (countercurrent) directions at flow rates of approximately 300 and 500 ml/min, respectively. The dialysate passes through the dialyzer only once (single pass system) and is discarded after interaction with the blood across the dialyzer's semipermeable membrane. The efficiency of hemodialysis can be augmented by the use of dialyzers that are more porous to water and solutes. These kidneys with enhanced performance characteristics are described as high-efficiency or high-flux dialyzers, depending on their ultrafiltration capacity.[33] High-efficiency hemodialysis uses a high-porosity dialyzer that has an ultrafiltration coefficient greater than 10 and less than 20 ml/mmHg/hour. High-flux hemodialysis uses an even more porous dialyzer with an ultrafiltration coefficient greater than 20 ml/mmHg/hour. Typically, these enhanced performance dialyzers have relatively greater clearances of solutes of large molecular weight (>300 Da).

Variables of the hemodialysis procedure that may be manipulated by the dialysis care team are the type of dialyzer (determines the solute clearance and ultrafiltration capacity), the dialysate composition (influences solute clearance and loading), the blood and dialysate flow (influences solute clearance), the hydraulic pressure that drives ultrafiltration, and the duration of dialysis. Although not directly related to the biophysical specifics of the dialysis procedure, the time spent on dialysis has a large impact on the amount or 'dose' of dialysis.

The provision of hemodialysis should be quantitated, so that patients can derive the maximal benefit from the intervention. Numerous patient outcome studies have demonstrated a strong statistical relationship between the measured dose of hemodialysis and ESRF patient survival.[34-38] Therefore, the delivered dose of hemodialysis should be measured routinely,[39] understanding the caveat that this has only been demonstrated (in patients with ARF) in one study.[40] The current, most complete measurement of the dose of hemodialysis is the volume-adjusted fractional clearance of urea, Kt/V, in which K is the dialyzer urea clearance, t the time on dialysis, and V the volume of distribution of urea.[41] Alternatively, the dose of hemodialysis can be expressed as the fractional reduction in urea during a single hemodialysis treatment, the urea reduction ratio (URR), which is defined mathematically as:[42]

$$[1 - (\text{postdialysis} \div \text{predialysis BUN concentrations})] \times 100$$

where BUN is blood urea nitrogen. There is inadequate information to recommend a minimum or optimal dose of dialysis for patients with ARF. Recent evidence only suggests that a higher dose of dialysis may be beneficial to survival, but the design of the observational study did not support the development of a benchmark dialysis dose.[40] In view of the absence of evidence that patient with ARF require different dialysis doses than patients with ESRF, current recommendations derived from outcomes in maintenance dialysis patients have been adopted, i.e. URR $\geq$ 65% or $Kt/V \geq 1.2$.[39]

Hemofiltration and hemodiafiltration

Compared with the diffusion-driven solute clearance of hemodialysis, hemofiltration depends on convective transport. Specifically, the patient's blood is conveyed through an extremely high-porosity dialyzer (hemofilter). The result is the formation of a protein-free hemofiltrate that resembles plasma water in composition. The driving force for perfusion of the hemofilter is typically the patient's mean arterial pressure, whereas the hydrostatic pressure in the hemofiltrate compartment provides the driving force for the formation of the filtrate. For effective hemofiltration, the mean arterial pressure should be maintained above 70 mmHg. Blood is usually conveyed into the hemofilter from an arterial cannula and is returned into a large-caliber vein. If the hemofiltrate is formed and is not replaced by a replacement solution, the process is described as *slow continuous ultrafiltration* (SCUF). Little solute clearance occurs during SCUF. An alternative technique that enhances solute clearance is to replace the lost volume continually with a solution that lacks the solute being removed. If an arteriovenous blood path is used, the process is called *continuous arteriovenous hemofiltration* (CAVH). If a venovenous path is used (blood flow driven by a blood pump), the procedure is described as *continuous venovenous hemofiltration* (CVVH). Optimal solute clearance is achieved by combining diffusive clearance and convective transport. This is accomplished by circulating a dialysate through the hemofilter with or without high ultrafiltration rates (*continuous arteriovenous hemodiafiltration* (CAVHDF) and *continuous arteriovenous hemodialysis* (CAVHD), respectively). Alternatively, these procedures may be performed using venovenous access with a blood pump to generate adequate flow rates (CVVHDF and CVVHD, respectively). Hemodiafiltration combines both high ultrafiltration rate (requiring replacement fluid) and dialysate flow for clearance. Collectively, these modalities are termed continuous renal replacement therapy (CRRT).[43] Among CRRT modalities, venovenous blood paths have become the prevalent treatment modality. This is because of the greater ease and the lesser risk associated with establishing venous angioaccess in comparison to arterial access. However, hemodialysis, not CRRT, remains the prevalent treatment modality in ICUs. The reasons for the limited penetration of CRRT are complex, but are a consequence of the need for capital investment in new delivery systems for CRRT, increased need for uniquely trained ICU nursing personnel, increased costs of CRRT, and absence of evidence demonstrating unique benefit of CRRT over conventional hemodialysis.

Peritoneal dialysis

Peritoneal dialysis (PD) relies on the diffuse clearance of solutes across the peritoneal membrane, whereas ultrafiltration during peritoneal dialysis depends on the instillation of a hyperosmolal solution.[44] Typically, maintenance peritoneal dialysis is performed daily, either by the performance of manual instillation and drainage of the dialysate during waking hours (*continuous ambulatory peritoneal dialysis*, CAPD) or while sleeping using an automated dialysate cycling device (*continuous cycling peritoneal dialysis*, CCPD).[45] The dialysate volume is usually 2–3 liters per instillation, and it dwells in the peritoneal cavity for variable intervals depending on the clearance and ultrafiltration goals (described as an 'exchange'). In the setting of acute dialysis, peritoneal dialysis can be managed as an intermittent therapy or be extended continuously. Intermittent therapy denotes use of usually 60–80 liters of dialysate over 48–72 hours, discontinued, and then repeated. The alternative approach is to perform PD in a continuous fashion, manually as in CAPD, or using an automated cycler device which will regulate the volume of dialysate and interval between drainage. Access for acute PD may be through a stiff catheter, but this catheter must be changed/removed after 72 hours, as the risk of peritonitis increases significantly, thereafter. A soft Dacron cuffed catheter is preferred if extended periods of PD are expected. A major disadvantage of PD is its relative inefficiency for solute clearance, which may be problematic for patients in the intensive care unit who are often hypercatabolic and require high solute clearance for azotemia control. The advantages of PD are that it obviates the use of anticoagulation. Also, an inherently biocompatible biological membrane (the peritoneum) is used for dialysis, so the likelihood of adverse interactions between blood and dialysis materials is minimized. Finally, the demand for nursing time is less if automated peritoneal dialysis cycling is used. Careful attention has to be paid to the patient's nutrition as substantial losses of protein and amino acid may occur in the dialysate.[46] Very few programs in the US resort to acute PD regimens with the advent of other CRRTs. However, patients who were on PD preoperatively may be kept on PD as long as they do not have any suspicion of having any intraoperative bowel or peritoneal complication and the technique is able to meet the patient's need for solute clearance.

Indications and goals for dialysis in renal failure

In patients with ARF, the goal of dialytic therapy is to support the patient while awaiting the recovery of adequate renal function; in chronic renal failure, the objective is for dialysis to substitute indefinitely for absent renal function. Because there has been inadequate time for the establishment of compensatory or adaptive alterations, it is mandatory that dialysis be speedily initiated in patients with ARF. Premorbid conditions that can be corrected by dialysis are absolute indications for its initiation. These absolute indications for the initiation of dialysis are uremic serositis, uremic encephalopathy, hyperkalemia that is inadequately corrected with conservative therapy, hypervolemia that is inadequately corrected with optimal doses of diuretics, and acidosis that is not adequately corrected with alkali. In addition, there are selected conditions that typically are not life-threatening and that can be managed by more conservative means. These conditions are relative indications for the initiation of dialysis. Examples include azotemia in the absence of uremia, hypercalcemia, hyperuricemia, hypermagnesemia, and uremic bleeding.

Absolute indications

Uremic encephalopathy and serositis
Historically, aside from hyperkalemia, uremic encephalopathy was the principal absolute indication for the initiation of dialysis.[47] Tremor, asterixis, diminished cognitive function, neuromuscular irritability, seizures, somnolence, and coma are all reversible manifestations of uremia that merit the provision of dialysis.[48] Of the complications of uremia, none is cor-

rected as dramatically with dialysis as those of the central nervous system (CNS). This complication of renal failure improves rapidly with the institution of an adequate dialysis regimen. If the neurological abnormalities are not abated after several dialysis sessions, other etiologies should be sought.

Reversible cardiopulmonary complications of uremia, such as uremic pericarditis and uremic lung, respond to the initiation of an adequate dialysis regimen, but clinical resolution is more protracted than for the CNS manifestations of uremia.[49,50] Uremic pericarditis is characterized by the presence of sterile inflammation of both layers of the pericardium. It is accompanied by pericardial neovascularization and the development of a serofibrinous exudative effusion. As a consequence of the injudicious use of systemic anticoagulation during dialysis for uremic pericarditis, intrapericardial hemorrhage and cardiac tamponade may occur. Similarly, in untreated patients, spontaneous hemorrhage and cardiac tamponade may arise.[51] In addition, uremic pericarditis may be associated with systolic dysfunction of the left ventricle as well as serosal inflammation with pleural hemorrhage. This is not commonly encountered in patients for CABG since they are usually screened and managed preoperatively. Uremic lung is a poorly understood late pulmonary complication of uremia that refers to a roentgenographic pattern of atypical pulmonary edema that is not necessarily associated with elevated pulmonary capillary wedge pressures.[50] It is treated by the initiation of dialysis.

There is a poor correlation between the BUN concentration and the development of uremic signs and symptoms.[52] The BUN concentration is determined by the degree of renal insufficiency, dietary protein intake, hepatocellular function, and protein catabolic rate. Thus, it is unsurprising that uremic manifestations can occur with a BUN concentration ≤ 100 mg/dl. In addition to its absolute value, the temporal rate of increase of the BUN seems to influence the development of uremia. Patients with a sudden and rapid decline in renal function, such as those with ARF, typically manifest uremic symptoms at lesser degrees of azotemia than do patients with more gradual declines in renal function, such as those with chronic progressive renal failure. This is especially true for uremic encephalopathy. Finally, selected patient populations, such as children, the elderly, and individuals with diabetes mellitus, manifest uremic symptoms sooner. These clinical observations, and the absence of studies that rigorously link patient outcome to a range of BUN concentrations, indicate that there are no benchmark values to initiate dialysis for ARF or target value to maintain the BUN concentration with dialysis. The goal is to provide adequate clearance of endogenous nitrogenous waste in the setting of adequate nutritional therapy.[53,54]

Hyperkalemia

During the course of progressive renal insufficiency, the capacity to excrete potassium is compromised, and the adaptive cellular uptake declines.[55] Although hyperkalemia is a frequent complication in the course of renal failure,[56] its severity and the degree of renal insufficiency at which it is first manifested are influenced by the cause of the renal failure, exogenous and endogenous potassium load, comorbid conditions, and medications administered, such as angiotensin-converting enzyme inhibitors and non-selective beta blockers. For example, ARF that complicates hemolysis, tumor lysis syndrome, crush injuries, rhabdomyolysis, hyperthermia, burns, hemolytic uremic syndrome/thrombotic thrombocytopenic purpura, sepsis with high fever, and disseminated intravascular coagulopathy may be associated with severe and rapidly developing hyperkalemia due to hypercatabolism and cytolysis. Upper gastrointestinal bleeding, a frequent occurrence in ICU patients with ARF, predisposes to the development of hyperkalemia. The contributions of blood transfusion to the development of hyperkalemia in patients with renal insufficiency is uncertain. During prolonged *ex vivo* storage, erythrocytes spontaneously release intracellular potassium, and their half-life *in vivo* is abbreviated.[57] The transfusion of senescent erythrocytes and their relatively hyperkalemic preservative may account for the increase in serum potassium, although the reported increment was quite modest.[58]

The need for emergent treatment is based on the degree of hyperkalemia, rate of rise, symptoms, and presence of ECG changes. It should be noted that patients with CRF develop adaptive mechanisms to excrete potassium[59] and are able to acclimatize to this deranged environment. In contrast, hyperkalemia in the setting of ARF is poorly tolerated in most instances. In the absence of indications for urgent treatment, such as electrocardiographic (ECG) signs of cardiac toxicity, conservative measures are adequate. These include limiting daily intake of potassium (oral or parenteral), discontinuing provocative medications, and augmenting potassium excretion through urine output or the gastrointestinal tract (if oliguric). Cation exchange resins are the mainstay of conservative therapy. However, if hyperkalemia is severe enough to produce symptoms and/or ECG changes, therapy is of great urgency. Non-dialytic measures to lower potassium rapidly and strategies to minimize cardiotoxicity must be implemented. This can be accomplished by administration of calcium salts,[60] insulin and β_2 agonists (administered intravenously or in nebulized form).[55,61] Despite the prior convention of administering sodium bicarbonate, recent data demonstrate that it is of little benefit.[62] The rapidity of onset and, most importantly, their limited duration of action should be considered in deciding the appropriateness for their use. However, the combination of therapies can allow adequate time for concurrent measures to be instituted to eliminate potassium from the body. This can be achieved by exchange resins and/or dialysis.

Although, intuitively, hemodialysis seems to be the quickest way to remove potassium, its efficiency is not much more than an optimal response to a cation exchange resin. An operational reality is that for many dialysis units, it may take ≥1 hour to set up and initiate hemodialysis. Conservative measures can and should be started in the interim.

Hypervolemia

The obligatory volume of fluids, medications, and food administered to care for the patient can often exceed the excretory capacity of even patients with non-oliguric ARF. In the absence of intravascular volume monitoring, parenteral fluid challenges are typically administered to patients with ARF to correct putative hypovolemia. In such cases, the therapeutic result is often the development of mild hypervolemia. An excessive sodium load administered as the sodium salt of medications (such as sodium penicillins), hyperalimentation, alkali loads (such as sodium citrate or bicarbonate), and cation exchange resins (such as sodium polystyrene sulfonate) are often unappreciated contributors to the development of hypervolemia. Another scenario for the development of hypervolemia is a critically ill patient whose nutritional needs have not been met during hospitalization. Many catabolic patients with renal failure can lose up to 0.5–1.0 kg of lean mass daily. The inappropriate matching of sensible and insensible losses in these patients results in the maintenance of a stable weight at the expense of expansion of the patient's total body water. Lastly, postoperative intensive care patients are also subject to fluid resuscitation to maintain blood pressure and replace fluid losses in surgery. In a study of 150 patients in an ICU who underwent elective thoracic surgery or abdominal surgeries, weight gains of 2.6 ± 2.8% and 7.5 ± 5.7%, respectively, were observed.[63]

The principal intervention for hypervolemia is the diuretics.[64] Even patients with advanced renal insufficiency (glomerular filtration rate <15 ml/min) may respond to optimal doses of diuretics that affect the loop of Henle and cortical diluting segments of the nephron. Because these agents are highly protein-bound, depend on tubular secretion for the intraluminal effect,[65] and operate on the basis of the achievement of a threshold dose,[66] an inadequate response should prompt the following responses: (1) double the dose up to a maximal dose of 200 mg of furosemide or 10 mg of bumetanide intravenously, (2) administer the diuretic as a continuous infusion that maintains the tubular concentration in excess of the threshold,[67] (3) administer the diuretic mixed with albumin to diminish its volume of distribution,[68] and/or (4) include a thiazide diuretic to diminish sodium reabsorption at an additional nephron segment.[69] Because of the increased risk of irreversible ototoxicity, ethacrynic acid should be a last choice.

Even in the absence of a diuretic effect, the vasodilatory response to parenteral furosemide can be of therapeutic benefit in cases of emergent hypervolemia;[70] they will reduce the pulmonary capillary wedge pressure even in oligoanuric patients. Therefore, furosemide can be used as an adjunct to acutely treat hypervolemia in dialysis patients. Osmotic cathartics such as sorbitol can be used to induce significant gastrointestinal losses of fluid. In additional, nitrates and parenteral narcotics that reduce afterload can be used to temporize the patient until more definitive therapy is instituted. Diuretics may also increase the urine output of an oliguric patient with ARF so that they become non-oliguric.[71] However, outcome studies demonstrate no change in the patients' survival,[72] but the management of other volume-dependent issues becomes more facile, such as nutrition supplementation. Diuretic administration with dialysis is employed on occasion to supplement fluid removal in non-oliguric patients who require solute clearance. Arguably, this strategy may limit the need for ultrafiltration during dialysis, which may be a provocateur for intradialytic hypotension. In turn, recurrent hypotension with intermittent hemodialysis therapy may cause further ischemic renal damage and potentially delay recovery of renal function.[65,73]

However, the absence of an adequate diuretic response is an absolute indication for dialysis, e.g. diuresis that is inadequate to meet the volume expansion resulting from obligatory fluids. Fluid removal can be accomplished by hemodialysis, hemofiltration, or peritoneal dialysis (ultrafiltration). Ultrafiltration rates of more than 3 liters per hour can be achieved during hemodialysis, 1–3 liters per hour during hemofiltration, and usually less than 1 liter per hour during peritoneal dialysis. Each dialysis technique has its advantages and disadvantages which will be discussed later in the chapter.

Acidosis

As renal function declines, endogenously generated organic acids and exogenously ingested acids are retained. In parallel, the capacity to generate and reclaim bicarbonate becomes increasingly compromised.[74] Typically, endogenous acid generation occurs at a rate of 1 meq/kg/day, resulting in a typical decline in serum bicarbonate concentration to a steady-state plasma concentration of 12 meq/L.[75] Therefore, in patients with renal failure, metabolic acidosis is the typical acid–base disturbance. The severity of the acidosis in ICU patients with ARF will be influenced by comorbid occurrences that may further contribute to the acidemia, such as lactic acidosis secondary to sepsis or poor cardiac output, hypercapnia secondary to ventilatory failure, ketoacidosis secondary to uncontrolled diabetes mellitus, and bicarbonate dilution secondary to volume expansion without alkali.

Metabolic acidosis in renal insufficiency is usually well tolerated until the systemic pH falls to 7.25 or less and/or the serum bicarbonate concentration is ≤15 meq/L. However, such tolerance is highly dependent on the compensatory hyperventilation. In ESRF patients, the steady-state serum bicarbonate concentration is influenced by the dialytic modality, type of alkali in the dialysate, frequency of dialysis, and the interdialytic weight gain.[74] For those treated with conventional bicarbonate-buffered dialysis, the steady-state serum bicarbonate concentration is 21 meq/L. It is noteworthy that lactate is the buffer used in most dialysates for PD, and so can be problematic for patients with liver disease and those already generating large lactate loads. However, in healthy PD patients, the steady-state serum bicarbonate concentration is approximately 26 meq/L.

Severe acidosis can result in changes in mental state leading to coma, and can provoke hypotension by depressing myocardial contractility and causing vasodilatation. The correction of acidosis is thus a major concern, especially in the ICU. Less severe acidosis may be corrected by administration of exogenous oral alkali therapy, whereas the inability to ingest oral medications mandates the use of parenteral supplements. Sodium bicarbonate is the preferred intervention. Sodium citrate, a metabolized alkali equivalent, is an alternative oral option and may be more palatable. However, sodium citrate can markedly increase passive aluminum absorption, leading to toxic levels, if ingested with aluminum-containing antacids (the latter is frequently used as a phosphate binder in renal failure).[76,77] The use of alkali agents should be judicious in patients with renal failure. Because bicarbonate and citrate are administered as sodium salts, volume expansion will occur if the sodium load is not excreted. If large doses of alkali are required to control acidosis in renal failure, dialysis is indicated. This will permit alkali loading with control of volume expansion.

Too rapid a correction of severe metabolic acidosis (plasma bicarbonate <10 meq/L) may be deleterious. Because bicarbonate cannot be conducted rapidly into the cerebrospinal fluid (CSF), paradoxical acidification of the CSF may occur. Also, if compensatory respiratory alkalosis has been manifest, the return to a normal ventilatory pattern can be delayed with excessively rapid correction. Alkalemia from relative excessive alkaline may also have grave consequences.[78] An initial partial correction of hypobicarbonatemia to 15–20 meq/L is appropriate. The final goal is to keep serum levels at 22–24 meq/L to prevent protein degradation.[79]

Relative indications

Non-life-threatening indications for dialysis can typically be managed by more conservative interventions. The physician must avoid the temptation to intervene in the course of ARF to dialyze to a set BUN concentration without proper consideration of the overall condition of the patient, the expected course of the type of renal failure suffered, fluid and nutritional requirements, and the presence of comorbid conditions. Although dialytic therapy is an essential tool in the management of ARF, its use or abuse may have detrimental effects. For example, it has been observed that in many patients with advanced renal failure, the institution of hemodialysis results in progressive deterioration in glomerular filtration rate (GFR) over several months.[80] Peritoneal dialysis does not provoke a similar relentless decline in residual renal function.[81] As will be discussed later, this may be a consequence of combined dialysis-induced hypotension with abnormal vascular compensation, and complement-mediated immunological injury resulting from bioincompatible dialyzer membrane materials.[82,83] Preserving residual renal function is of significant benefit in managing patients with advanced renal insufficiency.[84] Even modest preservation of GFR may ease fluid management in these patients. In terms of solute clearance, a residual GFR of approximately 15 ml/min is equivalent to 5 hours of hemodialysis with a dialyzer having a urea clearance of 160 ml/min. In addition, endogenous renal clearance of mid-molecular-weight molecules greatly surpasses that from hemodialysis.

All of the absolute indications defined in the previous section may provoke consideration of dialysis when present to a lesser extent. For example, a hypercatabolic trauma patient with ARF manifest by a rapidly increasing serum potassium concentration, declining serum bicarbonate concentration, falling urine output, and a mildly diminished sensorium does not fulfill any of the absolute criteria for the initiation of dialysis. In such a case, the need for dialysis is inevitable, and the patient's care is not improved by withholding dialysis until one of the life-threatening complications of renal failure has developed. Certainly, other clinical conditions such as hypercalcemia, hyperuricemia, hypermagnesemia, or uremic bleeding combined with other indications may prompt intervention with dialysis therapy.

Although not commonly seen in the CT-ICU, hypercalcemia and hyperuricemia associated with ARF may be encountered in patients with malignancies and tumor lysis syndrome, respectively.[85,86] Hypermagnesemia in renal failure is usually the result of the injudicious use of magnesium-containing cathartics or antacids.[87] These metabolic disorders are readily corrected by deletion of the excessive electrolyte from the dialysate. For example, hypercalcemia that is unresponsive to conventional conservative interventions may be corrected by hemodialysis with a reduced calcium dialysate (<2.5 meq/L).

Gastrointestinal and dermatological bleeding are common manifestations of platelet dysfunction in renal insufficiency. The hemostatic defect of renal insufficiency that best illustrates the impairment of platelet aggregation and adherence is the typical threefold prolongation of the bleeding time.[88] Some of the determinants of the platelet dysfunction of renal insufficiency include: (1) anemia that alters the flow pattern within the vasculature, thereby diminishing the physical interaction between the platelets and the endothelium; (2) decreased binding of von Willebrand factor to the platelet receptor; and (3) increased endothelial generation of nitric oxide.[89-91] Although either peritoneal or hemodialysis may correct the platelet defect,[92,93] more conservative therapies are available. Platelet dysfunction can be rapidly corrected by: (1) erythrocyte transfusion to a hematocrit level above 35%,[89] (2) infusion of 10 units of cryoprecipitate, which is rich in von Willebrand factor, every 12–24 hours,[94] or (3) intravenous (0.3 mcg/kg) or subcutaneous (0.3 mcg/kg) administration of deamino-8-D-arginine vasopressin (DDAVP), which induces the endothelial release of factor VIII—von Willebrand multimers.[95] Although not uniformly effective, and of diminishing benefit after repeated administration, DDAVP is the safest and most rapid way to correct the platelet defect of renal insufficiency. However, the use of cryoprecipitate is preferred when contemplating major surgical procedures. Interventions that produce a more protracted response that have a delayed onset of action are the administration of erythropoietin to increase red cell production,[96] intravenous conjugated estrogens (0.6 mg/kg for 5 days),[97] oral Premarin (50 mg/day for 7 days),[98] or low-dose transdermal estrogen (50–100 μg patch every 3.5 days).[99] The platelet defect is not always fully corrected with dialysis therapy.[93]

Other 'non-renal' indications for dialysis therapy have been advocated.[100,101] A relatively common indication is drug overdosage with water-soluble drugs such as lithium, procainamide, and aminoglycosides.[102,103] Hypothermia induced by continuous arteriovenous hemofiltration has been suggested as a treatment for adult inflammatory distress syndrome

(ARDS).[104] Another uncontrolled study found a trend for better survival in patients with ARDS treated by CAVH in comparison to supportive therapy.[105] CAVHD has also been suggested for prophylactic extracorporeal removal of myoglobin in crush injuries,[106] but this has not been validated.[107] CRRT has been suggested as a principal treatment for patients with severe hyperthermia resistant to conventional warming technique.[100] Isolated ultrafiltration has been advocated for intractable CHF, regardless of the degree of renal function.[100] This intervention is supported by data which demonstrate a more sustained improvement in functional status with fluid removal by extracorporeal ultrafiltration in comparison to diuretics alone.[108] It is important to realize that other than toxicological indications, there is currently no evidence-based consensus on the utility of dialysis interventions for indications other than renal replacement therapy.

Continuous versus intermittent dialytic therapy

The subsequent discussion will be restricted to intermittent hemodialysis and CRRT and will exclude PD, which is used infrequently in the ICU. Advocates of CRRT have expounded several potential advantages of CRRT over intermittent hemodialysis (Table 16.2). One of the putative advantages is hemodynamic stability during ultrafiltration. Fluid removal can be achieved by CRRT or hemodialysis. Hypotension can occur if too much fluid is removed or if fluid is removed too quickly. Because of its intermittent nature, significant volume expansion can occur between hemodialysis treatments, especially if the patient is receiving parenteral nutrition and hemodialysis is performed every other day. In contrast, CRRT allows for relatively precise hourly adjustments of the ultrafiltration rate that permits the total removal of 8–24 L/day. Because ultrafiltration with CRRT is gradual, hemodynamic stability with ultrafiltration may be more readily maintained.[109] Therefore, a principal advantage of CRRT is that it permits the allocation of nutrition, obligate medications, and blood products without the limitation of volume overload.[110] The only randomized cross-over trial to evaluate this chain of logic was performed in 27 patients with septic and/or postoperative renal failure. No difference was observed with CRRT in comparison to HD.[111] A decline in mean arterial pressure of >10 mmHg occurred in 25% and 26% of patients, respectively. A trend for less use of adrenergic drugs was noted for the former but did not reach statistical significance.

Arguably, the continuous, dynamic nature of CRRT may allow for better correction of azotemia and acidemia than hemodialysis.[112] Four hours of daily HD is calculated to be equivalent to 1 week of CVVH. In a comparison of CVVH and hemodialysis in patients with ARF, CRRT provided better control of azotemia for equal amounts of therapy.[113] In addition to the augmented clearance provided by the continuous nature of CRRT is the potential to minimize the risk of cerebral edema. The relative impediment of urea movement from the CNS into plasma water and alkalinization of CSF result in paradoxical cerebral hyperosmolality and acidification with rapid dialysis. Arguably, patients at high risk for cerebral edema, such as those with hepatorenal syndrome, may benefit from a more deliberate form of solute clearance such as that provided by CRRT. Validation of this chain of logic was demonstrated in 30 randomized patients with acute renal and fulminant hepatic failure. Increased intracranial pressure occurred with the use of intermittent hemofiltration compared to CAVHF or CAVHD.[114]

Sepsis syndrome and multiorgan dysfunction syndrome (MODS) predict poor outcome in acute renal failure.[115] The inflammatory milieu that results from adaptive immunity may be

Table 16.2 Comparison of continuous renal replacement therapy (CRRT) with intermittent hemodialysis techniques (HD)

Criteria	CRRT	HD	Comments
Solute removal	Continuous removal	Rapid removal	
Hemodynamic stability	Indicated for low BP (<90 mmHg)	Improved stability with sequential UF, cool dialysate, and sodium modeling	Pharmacological agents may improve stability in HD (e.g midodrine)
Fluid balance	Slow, large volume removal	Limited but rapid removal of fluid	Related to hemodynamic status
Nutritional support	Ideal for TPN, especially with large obligate volume load	Usually adequate but may be limited by need for fluid removal	Link between TPN vs. enteral nutrition and improved survival not validated
Metabolic control	Some studies show excellent control	Excellent to good control, depending on solute load	Unclear relationship to mortality
Removal of toxins or electrolytes	Continuous removal including some intracellular ions	Rapid removal	Especially for life-threatening states
Anticoagulation	Usually necessary	May be done with minimal or none	Principal cause of complications with CRRT
Nursing support	Intensive	HD nurse needed	Facility-specific
Patient mobility	Limited mobility; disassembly needed	Flexible schedule around procedures	
Cost	Higher	Lower	CRRT costs lower with patient volume
Survival	May be as good as HD	May be limited by uncertainty of requirement	Affected by other organ failure

deleterious to patients' outcomes.[116] Because of their improved absorption of inflammatory mediators to the dialysis membrane and/or their clearance into the dialysate in CRRT in comparison to conventional dialysis, it has been suggested that a continuous treatment modality may improve patients' outcomes in sepsis and MODS with renal failure. Several human studies have demonstrated that hemofiltration removes inflammatory mediators such as tumor necrosis factor alpha (TNF-α), interleukin (IL)-1β, IL-6, platelet activating factor, and activated complement fragments from circulation.[117,118] The specific mechanism of removal is through convective clearance and/or their direct adsorption to the hemofilter membrane. However, counter to this argument is the observation that serum levels of these immunological provocateurs are not substantially altered by CRRT.[117,119] Furthermore, CRRT may also eliminate beneficial humoral mediators. A recent study demonstrated removal of both IL-1 receptor antagonist and IL-10, modulators of the pro-inflammatory effects of IL-1 and TNF-α, respectively.[120]

Despite these theoretical advantages, CRRT has not been demonstrated to be of added benefit over conventional dialysis in terms of patient outcomes. Based on an analysis of data from 15 studies performed between 1986 and 1993, CRRT was not observed to improve the outcome of patients in comparison to the intermittent hemodialysis.[121] Furthermore, in a randomized, cross-over, intervention trial comparing the hemodynamic response to intermittent hemodialysis versus CAVH in ICU patients with ARF, no difference in mean arterial pressure, use of adrenergic drugs, and change in body weight occurred across the two methods.[111] A prospective trial to determine prognostic factors of hospital mortality did not find the manner of renal replacement therapy a significant factor.[122] Recently, another multi-center, randomized, controlled trial of 166 patients with ARF found that intermittent hemodialysis resulted in lower mortality (41.5%) in comparison with CRRT (59.5%).[123] It is noteworthy that despite randomization, patients allocated to CRRT had higher severity of illness scores. However, after statistical adjustment for this difference, no survival advantage was noted for CRRT treatment. The failure to demonstrate a clear favorable effect of CRRT on patient mortality may be a consequence of a patient selection bias such that patients who are more ill are referred for CRRT.

There are operational drawbacks in the use of CRRT that have limited its penetration into clinical practice in the ICU.[124] These include the customary need for anticoagulation (unless the patient has a pre-existing coagulopathy), increased frequency of access-related problems due to their continuous use, need for intensive nursing support and specialized training, need for patient immobility, slower onset of electrolyte correction, and the cost. CRRT is estimated to be 2.5 times more expensive than conventional hemodialysis. Absolute cost differences range by technique and locale.[118,123,125,126] Several programs have tried to decrease operating costs by employing an economy of scale.[127]

Experience with using CRRT in the CT-ICU is increasing. Ultrafiltration may be performed intra-operatively while the patient is on cardiopulmonary bypass,[128] postoperatively,[129] or both[130] to restore fluid balance in patients with ARF or ESRF. Although ARF increases the mortality in patients post-CABG by as much as eightfold,[131] the 63.7% mortality rate is no different from any other causes of ARF.[19–23] In such cases, CRRT has been used with technical success, but with no impact on patient mortality.[132–134] For patients with end-stage cardiomyopathies, the hemofilter may be placed in series with the ventricular assist device(s).[135] Closer scrutiny of expensive treatment interventions, such as CRRT, can be expected to increasingly demand evidence of their outcome benefit.[136]

Matching the treatment modality with the patient

There is currently no consensus regarding the definitive dialysis modality for a particular clinical situation. Before the advent of CRRT, most cases of ARF were treated with HD. The small number of cases that were intolerant of modified hemodialysis prescriptions were treated with PD or were considered not amenable to renal replacement therapy.[137] Now that CRRT has greater penetration in ICU settings, patients who are increasingly ill and whose outcome is defined by non-renal related morbidity are the recipients of renal replacement therapy. As such, the following are guidelines that reflect the experiences and bias of the authors in the context of currently available data.

Acute peritoneal dialysis

The use of acute PD in the US is largely historical, especially in the CT-ICU.[138,139] Currently, the settings in which it may be employed include: (1) a stable CAPD patient who undergoes a surgical procedure or an illness which does not violate the integrity of the peritoneum. This is usually in the setting of adequate nutrition and preservation of residual renal function such that balanced solute and volume clearance occur; (2) a patient without the benefit of any sustainable vascular access, but who has an intact peritoneum, low demand for clearance, and a reasonable prognosis; (3) a patient with an intact peritoneum, low demand for clearance, and absent dialysis nursing or technical support for HD or CRRT; and (4) a patient with an intact peritoneum, increased intracranial pressure, who is at high risk of developing cerebral edema, but dialysis nursing or technical support for CRRT is absent.

Continuous renal replacement therapy

CRRT in one or more of its forms is indicated for: (1) patients who have large mandatory ultrafiltration needs and potential hemodynamic compromise; (2) hemodynamically unstable patients who are intolerant of HD, who meet the criteria for initiation of renal replacement therapy but do not have any contraindication for CRRT (e.g. lack of adequate vascular access); and (3) patients with increased intracranial pressure and high risk for cerebral edema. All other indications are not validated by substantial evidence.[100,101]

The first point requires special emphasis for the renal failure patient in the ICU, where the provision of nutrition through TPN is a common volume challenge. The importance of adequate nutrition to optimize the survival of patients with renal insufficiency has been definitively demonstrated.[54,140] Similarly, critically ill patients with ARF are at high risk of malnutrition because of reduced nutritional intake and hypercatabolic processes, such as sepsis, glucocorticoid therapy, surgical trauma, and especially multiple organ failure.[53,141] Dialysis itself may also adversely affect the patient's nutritional status. For example, amino acids and water-soluble vitamins are readily removed with all forms of dialysis, so should be repleted daily.[142,143] Peritoneal dialysis can result in substantial protein loss,[46] far more so than conventional hemodialysis or CRRT. On the other hand, hemodialysis with selected membrane materials may accelerate catabolism and compromise patients' outcomes.[144,145] Current recommendations for nutrition in patients with renal failure are for the enteral or parenteral administration of ≥35 kcal/kg/day including 1.2–1.4 gm of protein/kg.[53,146]

In past years, protein intake was severely restricted in patients with acute renal failure, in an effort to reduce uremic symptoms. However, early and aggressive institution of nutritional support has appropriately become an appropriate standard practice in many centers. As stated earlier, dialysis should be initiated relatively early for ARF to permit adequate nutritional support, especially in catabolic patients. Once begun, dialysis may need to be more intensive, so that resultant nitrogenous waste products can be sufficiently cleared and adequate volume removed. Dialysis should be prescribed and delivered at a level to control azotemia without compromising nutrition, even if treatments are prolonged (5–6 hours per treatment) and/or more frequent (4–6 treatments per week). CRRT may be an especially practical and effective modality for critically ill patients who require large volumes of hyperalimentation with their other obligate fluid intake.[100,101] It is noteworthy that neither oral nor parenteral nutrition has been shown to improve outcome in ARF, pre-ESRF, or ESRF patients.[146,147] Therefore, some critics of CRRT have questioned the use of high cost interventions of unproven benefit, such as TPN.[125] Their chain of logic goes that administering TPN over enteral nutrition artificially creates the need for CRRT, so further increasing healthcare costs without providing a definitive survival advantage.[121] Supporters of CRRT counter that the retrospective data show improved outcome for patients using CRRT and improvement in the designs of prospective trials will eventually resolve the issue.[148] We feel that CRRT remains a viable option to consider at the present time to provide adequate nutritional support, regardless of the route or volume of administration.[126]

Intermittent hemodialysis and ultrafiltration

We feel that intermittent HD therapy remains the primary option for patients meeting the criteria for initiation of dialysis enumerated earlier, except for the specific situations noted for CRRT and, much less commonly, acute PD. It is specifically indicated if rapid fluid, electrolyte, solute, or drug and poison removal is indicated in a patient who is likely to tolerate the procedure. In fact, recent techniques such as sequential ultrafiltration have made it possible to dialyze patients who were previously perceived as unable to tolerate the procedure. An advantage of HD over CRRT is the ability to provide the former without anticoagulation for patients with high risk of bleeding complications.[149] Lastly, patients who will need radiology or nuclear medicine tests as well as repeated debridement or surgery (not to mention conscious or recovering patients) will benefit from the added mobility and flexibility in scheduling afforded by HD therapy. In conclusion, our first option for patients requiring renal replacement therapy is HD, unless otherwise contraindicated. Regardless of the dialysis modality selected, it is critical that the full range of dialysis techniques be used as necessary. The selection of one form of therapy does not preclude change to another when the dynamics of the patient's clinical condition alter.

Components of the dialysis process

Hemodialysis and hemofiltration

Dialyzers and hemofilters

Most of the commercial dialyzers available for hemodialysis in the US are configured as large cylinders packed with hollow fibers through which the blood flows (hollow fiber dialyzer). The dialysate flows through the dialyzer and around these fibers, usually in a countercurrent direction. The membrane for these dialyzers is composed of a variety of modified biological or synthetic materials such as regenerated cellulose, cuprophane, hemophan, cellulose acetate, polysulfone (PS), polymethylmethacrylate (PMMA), and polyacrylonitrile (PAN).[150] The surface area available for solute transport and the filling volume of the blood and dialysate compartments vary significantly among different dialyzers and are a function of the membrane material. These materials vary in their characteristics for solute transport and ultrafiltration,[33] capacity to interact with cellular and soluble components of the blood ('biocompatibility'),[151] and cost and reuse capacity.[152] The choices of dialyzer for the management of either acute or chronic renal failure are usually dictated by these three variables in this exact rank order.

Membrane transport characteristics The impetus for the development of more efficient dialyzers stems from the desire to decrease time on hemodialysis by augmenting solute clearance per unit time. A secondary goal is to improve clearance of larger solutes that may be toxic, such as β_2-microglobulin. The relative inability of dialyzers to clear these larger solutes may contribute to the development of neuropathy and dialysis-associated amyloidosis.[153,154] A putative disadvantage of these efficient and relatively open-pore dialyzers is that they may more readily permit the transmembrane back-flux of bacterial-derived lipopolysaccharides from the dialysate into the dialyzer blood compartment (backfiltration).[155] The resultant patient exposure to the pyrogen results in a febrile illness without bacteremia, described as a pyrogen reaction, and may occur more often with high-flux dialyzers. The use of bicarbonate-buffered dialysates, which are permissive for the growth of gram-negative bacteria, and ultrafiltration controllers that limit the rate of ultrafiltration may also contribute to the occurrence of pyrogen reactions.[156,157]

The characteristic requirements of a dialyzer or hemofilter used in CRRT must be considered from a different perspective. Because the driving force for hemofiltration is the mean arterial pressure or a low speed venous pump, and clearance is disproportionately dependent on convection,[118] a low resistance, high Kuf hemofilter in required. Hemofilters are usually composed of PS, PMMA, or PAN because cuprophan does not have sufficient hydraulic permeability at a transmembrane pressure of 30–70 mmHg. In continuous hemodialysis techniques (CAVHD, CVVHD, CAVHDF, CVVHDF), solute transport is limited by the dialysate flow rate, unlike conventional intermittent hemodialysis. The blood flow rate is usually 100–150 ml/min, and dialysate flow rate is generally 16–30 ml/min. The rapidity of solute equilibration across the dialysis membrane, which is a function of the hemofilter, determines the type of hemofilter that can be used.[43]

Membrane biocompatibility The development of a wide array of dialyzers allows an easier selection to fulfill the dialytic solute and ultrafiltration needs of the patient. However, with the advent of these newer membranes, an added criterion for selection of membranes in the management of ARF and the ESRF population is its biocompatibility.[158] The interaction of both soluble and cellular components within the blood with the dialysis membrane may be important in the pathobiology of such varied issues as duration of recovery from acute ischemic renal failure,[77] adverse intradialytic symptoms and signs such as fever, hypotension and hypoxemia,[159,160] immunological dysfunction and infectious susceptibility,[161-165] maintenance of an anabolic state,[144,166] faster loss of residual renal function,[167] development of β_2-microglobulin amyloidosis,[168] and the severity of hyperlipidemia.[169]

A plethora of alterations of cellular functions and physiological responses have been described in association with hemodialysis using cellulosic-based membranes, including the intradialytic generation of complement-derived anaphylatoxins such as C3a and C5a via the alternate complement pathway *in vivo*,[170] induction of enhanced membrane expression of selected granulocyte adhesion molecules such as MAC-1 and LAM-1 *in vivo*,[171] inappropriate production of reactive oxygen species such as superoxide by granulocytes *in vivo*,[172] activation of the coagulation pathway *in vitro*,[173] formation of kallikrein and bradykinin,[174] enhanced monocyte elaboration of cytokines such as IL-1, IL-6, and TNF *in vitro* and perhaps *in vivo*,[162,175,176] altered IL-2 receptor expression *in vivo*,[177] altered monocyte phagocytosis *in vitro*,[164] and defective natural killer cell function.[178] Dialysis membranes with these properties are described as bioincompatible. By contrast, membranes without these proinflammatory effects are biocompatible. In addition, another aspect of biocompatibility is the ability of the membrane to adsorb activated proinflammatory substances. Highly adsorptive membranes can efficiently reduce factor D (an essential enzyme of the alternative pathway activation),[179] bradykinin, and pyrogenic cytokines such as IL-1 and TNF, all of which may adversely affect the outcome of patients.[180] Bioincompatible membrane dialyzers are typically composed of cellulose, whereas biocompatible membrane dialyzers are synthetic materials, such as PS, PMMA, polyamide, or PAN. Many of the adverse pathobiological consequences of hemodialysis that arise from membrane interactions are thought to be attenuated by using biocompatible membranes.[158] This has led to an increased selection of these membrane materials for dialyzers in maintenance hemodialysis.[181] Many of these issues are discussed in greater detail in two reviews.[282,183]

Based on *in vitro* models of ischemic ARF[184] and several *in vivo* interventional trials,[77,185] the use of biocompatible membranes has been espoused to enhance patient survival, expedite recovery from ARF, and diminish the need for dialytic support.[186] However, the beneficial effects of biocompatible membranes are far from being conclusively demonstrated, both in ARF and ESRF. Two groups of investigators observed no difference in patient survival or renal recovery using cellulosic or synthetic biocompatible membranes dialyzers.[187,188] In fairness to proponents of using biocompatible membranes, these studies were not designed specifically to look at this difference. Another study addressing patients' symptoms such as hypotensive episodes, angina, and bronchospasm during hemodialysis did not indicate any difference between membranes in a single session per matched patient pair.[189] Although catabolic effects have been demonstrated in experimental single hemodialysis sessions with bioincompatible membrane,[144] a long-term study found an increase in serum albumin in two groups of patients treated with both membrane types, with the difference being an earlier and more marked increase in albumin for the group treated with the biocompatible membrane.[166] However, there was a significant difference in the increase of patients' dry weight in this group compared with those treated with cellulosic membranes. In the same study, flux characteristics of the membranes were not found to have a significant effect on nutritional parameters.

Because of the non-conclusive evidence presented to date, it is not justifiable to recommend the routine exclusion of relatively 'non-biocompatible' (i.e. cellulosic and modified cellulosic such as cellulose triacetate) membrane dialyzers.[190,191] The major limitation of biocompatible membrane dialyzers is their cost. A synthetic biocompatible membrane dialyzer is at least twice the price of a cellulosic membrane dialyzer. However, the benefits of biocompatible membrane materials are not conclusive; the two well-controlled, prospective studies supporting their use demonstrated no detrimental effect when compared with cuprophan.[77,185] In summary, choosing a biocompatible membrane is paying more for uncertain but potentially improved patient outcomes.[181,191,92] In 1996, despite the inconclusive evidence, the fraction of cellulosic dialyzers used in the US dropped to 20%, compared with 70% in 1990.[181] Most dialysis programs now use biocompatible dialyzer membrane materials for ARF. On the other hand, because of the high ultrafiltration requirement for continuous dialytic therapy and the inability of cellulosic dialyzers to fulfill this requirement, CRRT is always performed with highly porous, biocompatible dialyzers.

Membrane reuse   Although the many dialyzer manufacturers label the device as intended for a single use, it is conventional practice to reuse dialyzers for a given patient. The practice involves sterilizing the dialyzer with formaldehyde, glutaraldehyde, periacetic acid, or heat and citric acid. The dialyzer is cleansed with bleach and thereafter undergoes limited functional testing.[193] The principal reason for dialyzer reuse is economical.[152] There is no conclusive evidence to substantiate the suggestion that either morbidity or mortality associated with single use or reuse is different. Because of operational constraints, many units do not reuse dialyzers for hospitalized patients. Readers interested in learning more about dialyzer reuse are referred to other sources.[39,152,193]

Dialysates for hemodialysis

The composition of the dialysate is a major component of the dialysis process that determines the outcome of the procedure on the blood chemistry. Although sodium and potassium are typically the only components of the dialysate that are altered in response to different clinical situations, the other constituents are equally critical. The dialysate is stored as a liquid or powdered concentrate that is diluted in a fixed ratio to yield the final solute concentration. Dialysate concentrates and water can be appropriately and safely proportioned by using on-line measurements of the conductivity of the dialysate prior to its entry into the hemodialyzer.

Glucose   Before hydraulic-driven ultrafiltration became available, the dialysate glucose concentration was maintained at above 1.8 g/dl to generate an osmotic gradient between the blood and the dialysate. Although this was effective for inducing ultrafiltration, some patients developed morbid symptoms and signs of hyperosmolality, especially at glucose concentrations greater than 2.2 g/dl.[194] Currently, dialysates are either glucose-free, normoglycemic (0.0–0.25% dextrose) or modestly hyperglycemic (>0.25% dextrose). Hemodialysis with a glucose-free dialysate results in a net glucose loss of approximately 30 g and stimulates ketogenesis and gluconeogenesis.[195] Such alterations in intermediary metabolism may be particularly deleterious in chronically or acutely ill hemodialysis patients who are malnourished or on a medication such as propranolol that is provocative for hypoglycemia.[197,197] These effects are ameliorated by the use of a normoglycemic dialysate. Additional metabolic consequences occurring from the use a glucose-free dialysate include an accelerated loss of free amino acids into the dialysate,[198] a decline in serum amino acids,[199] and enhanced potassium clearance because of relative hypoinsulinemia.[195] Therefore, the dialysate glucose concentration should be maintained close to normoglycemic concentrations, which in most units is prepared at 0.2 g/dl.

Sodium   Historically, the dialysate sodium concentration was maintained at hypo-osmolal levels (<135 meq/L) to prevent interdialytic hypertension, exaggerated thirst, and excessive weight gain. However, hyponatremic dialysates increase the likelihood of intradialytic hypotension, cramps, headaches, nausea, and vomiting, and are provocative for the dialysis dysequilibrium syndrome.[200–204] During hemodialysis, the volume ultrafiltered may exceed the extracellular volume. As solute is removed from the extracellular compartment, there is a relative increase in intracellular osmolality, which drives transcellular volume movement.[205] These hemodynamic alterations are absent in the setting of equal dialysate and serum sodium concentrations. Thus, there has been an appropriate increase in the dialysate sodium to 140–145 meq/L.

Unfortunately, an increase in the dialysate sodium can result in polydypsia and increased interdialytic weight gain.[202] However, the enhanced capacity to ultrafilter these patients offsets this problem. The pressor response to an increased dialysate sodium varies. In patients who are hypertensive because of hyperreninemia during ultrafiltration, a higher dialysate sodium may be associated with a reduction in blood pressure. However, most patients exhibit no increment in blood pressure with physiological dialysate sodium concentrations.[202] A minority of patients who typically are hypertensive at baseline have worsened pressor control with a higher sodium dialysate.[201–203]

The newer dialysate delivery systems permit active alteration of the dialysate sodium concentration during hemodialysis by the use of variable-dilution proportioning systems. The technique of 'sodium profiling' or 'sodium modeling' to fit a patient's hemodynamic needs has been espoused as a mean of accomplishing optimal blood pressure support without increased thirst at the completion of the treatment.[206–210] The alteration in the dialysate sodium can be executed in several patterns. It can be performed in a step fashion in which the dialysate sodium concentration is initially high (≥145 meq/L) and is promptly reduced (<135 meq/L) during the second half of the dialysis session. Alternatively, the sodium concentration can be reduced as a linear gradient from above 145 meq/L to approximately 135 meq/L.[206] Logarithmic declining sodium profiles can also be performed. Sodium profiling reduces the frequency of hypotension during ultrafiltration without decreasing the dialysis time committed to diffusive clearance, as is the case with sequential ultrafiltration–clearance. However, it is unclear whether this technique offers any advantage over a fixed dialysate sodium of 140–145 meq/L;[207,208] two recent studies suggested that it does.[209,210] The beneficial effect of sodium manipulation may be seen in some patients, although currently there are no criteria to select patients who will be responsive to this therapy. Therefore, for most hemodialysis patients, the dialysate sodium concentration should be maintained at 140–145 meq/L.

Potassium   Unlike urea, which usually behaves as a solute distributed in a single pool with a variable volume of distribution, only 1–2% of the total body store of 3000–3500 meq of potassium is present in the extracellular space.[211] The flux of potassium from the intracellular compartment to the extracellular space, and subsequently across the dialysis membrane to the dialysate compartment, is unequal. Therefore, the efficacy of potassium removal in hemodialysis is highly variable, difficult to predict, and influenced by dialysis-specific and patient-specific factors.[212] In a study that controlled for dialyzer-specific components of the dialysis procedure (blood and dialysate flow, dialyzer type and surface area, duration of dialysis, dialysate composition), potassium removal varied by approximately 70%. Even for the same patient, approximately 20% variability in potassium removal was noted using identical hemodialysis conditions.[213]

During hemodialysis, approximately 70% of the potassium removed is derived from the intracellular compartment.[195] As 50–80 meq of potassium are removed in a single dialysis session, and only 15–20 meq of potassium are present in the plasma, life-threatening hypokalemia would be the consequence of hemodialysis if this was not the case.[212] However, the volume of distribution of potassium is not constant. The greater the total body potassium, the lower is its volume of distribution.[214] The practical consequence of these observations is that the fractional decline in the plasma potassium during a single dialysis session will be greater if the pre-hemodialysis potassium is higher. Therefore, optimal potassium elimination by hemodialysis is accomplished by daily short hemodialysis treatments, instead of protracted sessions every other day. The transfer of potassium from the intracellular compartment to the extracellular compartment usually occurs more slowly than the transfer from the plasma across the dialysis membrane.[215,216] This discrepancy further complicates predicting the quantity of potassium removed during hemodialysis. A practical consequence of the discordant transfer rates is that the plasma potassium measured immediately after the completion of hemodialysis is approximately 30% less than the steady-state value measured after 5 hours. Therefore, hypokalemia diagnosed immediately after the completion of hemodialysis should not be treated with potassium supplements.

The transcellular distribution of potassium is influenced by several variables, including the relative degree of hyperinsulinemia (promotes potassium uptake into cells and lowers its intradialytic clearance),[56,195] catecholamine tone (β-agonists promote cellular uptake of potassium and α agonists stimulate the cellular egress of potassium—attenuate and increase the intradialytic clearance of potassium, respectively),[61,211] sodium–potassium ATPase activity (pharmacological inhibition diminishes potassium uptake into cells, which may enhance intradialytic clearance),[216] and systemic pH (alkalemia augments transcellular potassium uptake, which may diminish dialytic clearance of potassium).[211] Surprisingly, although the degree of systemic alkalization is greater and more rapid in onset with bicarbonate-buffered dialysates than with acetate-buffered dialysates, the choice of buffer does not appear to be critical in determining potassium removal during hemodialysis.[195,217] Paradoxically, it has been observed that as the gradient for potassium clearance from blood into the dialysate is increased by decreasing the dialysate potassium concentration, the uptake of bicarbonate from the dialysate declines.[218] This interaction between alkali and potassium in the dialysate is sizable; a 1 meq increase in the potassium gradient results in a decline in bicarbonate dialysance of 50 meq. This interaction should not be overlooked in planning the dialysate prescription for patients being dialyzed for severe acidosis.

As the selection of the dialysate potassium is empirical, most patients are dialyzed with a potassium concentration of 1–3 meq/L. However, it is also possible to vary the potassium concentration within a dialysis treatment, depending on the needs of the patient as determined by the nephrologist and the ICU care team. For patients who have excessive potassium loads from their diet, medications, hemolysis, trauma, or gastrointestinal bleeding, the dialysate potassium concentration should be 0–1 meq/L (although we rarely have patients maintained on a zero potassium bath for the entire duration of a treatment on a regular basis). For stable patients who do not have significant cardiac disease or who are not taking cardiac glycosides, a dialysate potassium concentration of 2–3 meq/L is appropriate.

In a patient with a history of cardiac disease, especially with arrhythmias and cardiac glycoside (i.e. digoxin) usage, the dialysate potassium should be increased to 3–4 meq/L.[219] Such patients are at the greatest risk for the development of dysrhythmias associated with the rapidity of the change in potassium flux during the first half of dialysis. Such high-risk patients are best managed by tolerating a greater degree of interdialytic hyperkalemia managed by the concomitant administration of kayexalate. Most of the cardiac morbidity (i.e. arrythmias) that arise from the dialysate potassium concentration occur during the first half of the dialysis sessions.[220] The rapidity of the fall in the plasma potassium concentration, rather than the absolute plasma concentration, determines the risk of cardiac arrhythmias.[215,219] For this reason, hyperkalemic patients should be managed by an incremental decline in the dialysate potassium concentration. If the patient has a significant deficit in total body potassium, post-dialysis hypokalemia can occur, even if the dialysate potassium concentration is greater than the serum potassium concentration.[221] This seemingly contradictory situation arises because of the potential for a delayed conductance of potassium from the dialysate into the patient, in comparison to its movement from the extracellular space into the intracellular compartment. Two recent studies using a modified (potassium modeling) Fersenius E machine recommend either an initial dialysate potassium concentration of 1.5 meq/L less than the serum predialysis potassium concentration, then modeled to approach 2.5 meq/L (less) by the end of the treatment,[220] or removing 15% of serum potassium per hour of dialysis.[222] The first study decreased hourly premature ventricular contractions (PVCs) and couplets by 60% in the first 2 hours of dialysis, while the second study decreased PVCs over the entire dialysis session and improved the Lown classification.

Bases   Initially, bicarbonate was used as the base in the dialysate. In the early 1960s, it was superseded by acetate, which is stable in aqueous solution at neutral pH in the presence of divalent cations. Acetate is metabolized in skeletal muscle and to a lesser extent in the liver to acetyl CoA, which is subsequently metabolized further via the Krebs cycle to carbon dioxide and water. In the latter process, one proton is consumed and one molecule of bicarbonate is liberated.[223] During conventional hemodialysis with large surface area dialyzers, acetate flux above 300 mmol per hour can occur, resulting in acetate accumulation as the amount translocated exceeds the capacity to metabolize the base. This complication occurs most often in women, elderly patients, and patients who are malnourished.[224] The resultant clinical consequences of acetate accumulation include variable degrees of nausea, vomiting, headache, fatigue, peripheral vasodilatation, decreased myocardial contractility, metabolic acidosis, and arterial hypoxemia.[225–228] Therefore, it is not surprising that vascular instability is much more problematic with predominant acetate-containing dialysates than bicarbonate-containing dialysates. The hemodynamic instability associated with acetate is worsened by a hyponatremic dialysate and is lessened with a normonatremic dialysate.[226,229,230]

Hemodialysis using a bicarbonate-buffered dialysate prevents these complications. The paradoxical anion gap metabolic acidosis associated with acetate dialysis occurs because the intradialytic loss of bicarbonate from blood into the dialysate exceeds the patient's capacity to generate alkali from metabolized acetate. A raised bicarbonate concentration in the dialysate attenuates the diffusive gradient from blood to dialysate. Similarly, dialysis-induced hypoxemia is attenuated by a bicarbonate dialysate. During hemodialysis with acetate, there is a large diffusive loss of carbon dioxide into the dialysate such that the minute ventilation falls by approximately 25%. Therefore, despite the loss of carbon dioxide across the dialytic circuit, there is little decline in the arterial carbon dioxide tension (normocapneic hypoventilation). During hemodialysis with acetate, hypoxemia is most prominent during the first 60 minutes of hemodialysis and may be associated with an approximately 35 mmHg decline in arterial oxygen tension.[161,231]

Because of the amelioration of many intradialytic symptoms with bicarbonate-containing dialysates and the increased use of high-efficiency and high-flux hemodialysis, acetate is used for hemodialysis in less than 20% of the dialysis facilities in the US.[1] Bicarbonate dialysis is now feasible because of the widespread availability of proportioning systems that permit mixing of the separate concentrates containing bicarbonate and divalent cations close to the final entry point of the dialysate into the dialyzer. Unlike the more acidic and hyperosmolal acetate-based dialysate, liquid bicarbonate concentrates and reconstituted bicarbonate dialysates support the growth of gram-negative bacteria such as *Pseudomonas*, *Acinetobacter*, *Flavobacterium*, and *Achromobacter*, filamentous fungi, and yeast.[156,157] Because of the propensity of the dialysate to support bacterial growth and the morbidity associated with the presence of such growth in the dialysate, strict guidelines exist for the acceptable limit of bacterial growth, the presence of lipopolysaccharide in the dialysate, and dialyzer reuse.[193,232] Some units have begun using polysulfone hollow-fiber filters along the path of the dialysate prior to reaching the dialyzer, intending to remove bacteria and endotoxins (ultrapure dialysate).[233]

A bicarbonate-based dialysate of 30–38 meq/L should be used. Bicarbonate concentrations above 38 meq/L may result in the development of a metabolic alkalosis with secondary hypoventilation, hypercapnia, and hypoxemia. If a bicarbonate dialysate is unavailable, acetate at an equivalent concentration is suitable, but large-surface-area dialyzers or dialyzers with high-efficiency or high-flux transport characteristics cannot be used.[104]

Calcium   Patients with renal failure are prone to develop hypocalcemia, hyperphosphatemia, hypovitaminosis D, and hyperparathyroidism. Therefore, historically, positive calcium balance has been useful as an adjunct during hemodialysis for controlling metabolic bone disease.[234–236] In patients with renal failure requiring dialysis, 61% of the calcium is not bound to plasma proteins and is in a diffusible equilibrium during hemodialysis.[237] Assuming free conductance of calcium across the dialysis membrane secondary to diffusive clearance and an additional contribution secondary to convective losses, a dialysate calcium concentration of roughly 3.5 meq/L (7.0 mg/dl) is necessary to prevent intradialytic calcium losses.[238] Because such elevated calcium dialysates induce hypercalcemia transiently, it temporarily reduces parathyroid hormone secretion,[239] and in the past had been the standard dialysate calcium concentration.

Over the last decade, increasing and appropriate concerns arose for the development of aluminum intoxication syndromes secondary to the protracted use of oral aluminum hydroxide as a phosphate binder. Short-term use of aluminum-containing antacids in ICUs were not uncommon but have recently been replaced with H_2-blockers and proton pump inhibitors. The three aluminum intoxication disorders, which arise because of the intestinal absorption and retention of ingested aluminum, are progressive osteomalacia, iron-resistant microcytic anemia, and progressive encephalopathy.[240–240] Instead of using aluminum salts alone, calcium carbonate or calcium acetate have been increasingly employed alone or with small quantities of aluminum hydroxide as oral phosphate binders.[243,244] However, because variable amounts of calcium are absorbed from the ingested calcium salt, persistent hypercalcemia is a frequent complication of a dialysate calcium of greater than 3.0 meq/L, especially if a vitamin D supplement is also used. To minimize the likelihood of hypercalcemia and potentially soft tissue calcification,[245] there is a trend towards lower dialysate calcium concentrations.[234] In most dialysis facilities, a dialysate calcium concentration of 2.5–3.0 meq/L is used. Despite these reduced dialysate calcium concentrations, some patients are still hypercalcemic between dialysis sessions. The combination of a reduced ingested dose of calcium salt and the inclusion of a small quantity of aluminum hydroxide can minimize the risk of hypercalcemia and treat hyperphosphatemia. Recently, a non-calcium, non-aluminum phosphate binding polymer was introduced for patients who remain hypercalcemic despite these measures, but at greater cost than conventional phosphate binders.[246] Newer drugs, including vitamin D analogs such as 22-oxacalcitriol,[247] 1α-hydroxyvitamin D_2,[248] and 19-nor-1-α-25-dihydroxyvitamin D_2,[249] are reported to cause less hypercalcemia in comparison to calcitriol. In addition, a new class of agents called calcimimetics (e.g. R-568)[250] also inhibit PTH secretion by activating a calcium-sensing receptor on the parathyroid glands. The efficacy of these compounds has not been evaluated extensively.

A reduction in the dialysate calcium may increase vascular instability during hemodialysis.[251,252] Dialysis-induced changes in the serum calcium concentration correlate with the intradialytic systolic and diastolic blood pressures. This interaction is secondary to alterations in left ventricular performance without an accompanying alteration in the peripheral vascular resistance.[253] Our current practice is to use 2.5 meq/L of calcium unless otherwise indicated.

Magnesium   Like potassium, the serum magnesium concentration is a poor determinant of total body magnesium stores. Only approximately 1% of the total body magnesium is present in the extracellular fluid, and only 60% of this amount (approximately 25 meq) is free and diffusible.[254] Because of scant extrarenal clearance, removal during hemodialysis is the primary route of elimination for magnesium in renal failure. The magnesium flux that occurs during a dialysis session is difficult to predict despite knowledge of the serum and dialysate magnesium concentrations. When using a low magnesium dialysate, the postdialytic decline in serum magnesium concentration is virtually resolved after 24 hours.[255]

Because the ideal serum magnesium concentration in patients with ESRF is debatable, the appropriate dialysate magnesium concentration is unresolved. Many centers use a 1.0 meq/L dialysate magnesium concentration, and mild interdialytic hypermagnesemia is often observed. Although elevated magnesium concentrations impair bone formation *in vitro* and *in vivo*, its clinical significance is unresolved.[254,256–258] A reduction of the dialysate magnesium concentration to less than 0.5 meq/L has been reported to improve osteomalacic bone pathology and symptoms.

Magnesium intake has recently been shown to decrease the frequency of arrhythmias in patients with normal kidney function.[259] Early studies indicated that the antiarrhythmic effect of magnesium may be mediated by a direct effect on calcium and potassium flux across the myocardial cell membranes.[260] One proposed mechanism is its inhibitory effect on lysophosphatidyl choline, a phospholipid released by ischemic myocardial cells causing accumulation of intracellular ionized calcium with subsequent coronary artery spasm.[261] Another is an inhibitory effect of the lack of magnesium on nitric oxide release from the coronary endothelium, thus leading to vasoconstriction and thrombosis early in the postoperative course of CABG.[262] The coronary spasms and/or thrombosis may lead, in turn, to an increased risk of cardiac arrhythmia. Hypomagnesemia is common in patients after cardiac surgery,[263] and a decreased incidence of arrythmias has been demonstrated in this population with magnesium supplementation.[262–266] There is no direct relationship between both total and ionized serum magnesium levels and the incidence of arrhythmia.[267,268]

Because magnesium is primarily excreted by the kidneys, it accumulates in most patients who have impaired renal function.[269,270] Therefore, patients who undergo dialysis treatments in the CT-ICU will usually have higher magnesium levels and do not require magnesium supplementation. A magnesium dialysate concentration of 1.0 meq/L is conventional for HD.

Chloride   Chloride is the major anion in the dialysate. Because its concentration is defined by the constraints of maintaining electrical neutrality in the dialysate, chloride concentration varies depending on the concentration of cations.

Dialysates for continuous hemodialysis and hemodiafiltration

An advantage of CAVHD, CVVHD, CAVHDF, and CVVHDF over conventional hemodialysis is the lack of need for complex blood and dialysate delivery systems. Typical dialysate flow rates for continuous hemodialysis or hemodiafiltration are 800–1000 ml/hour (versus 500–800 ml/min for conventional hemodialysis), and the dialysate is usually delivered into the dialyzer by a continuous infusion pump. Because it is impractical to mix and store conventional hemodialysis dialysate for continuous hemodialysis and hemodiafiltration, and the formation of a custom dialysate in the volumes required for these techniques is cumbersome and costly. Instead, conventional peritoneal dialysate is often used for CRRT. Despite the use of commercially prepared peritoneal dialysates that typically are less costly than custom preparations, the dialysate costs associated with CAVHD and CVVHD make these techniques more expensive than CAVH or CVVH. Although peritoneal dialysate presents the most conveniently available fluid for use, its glucose concentration is higher than optimally desired. A further drawback is that it uses lactate as the buffer, instead of bicarbonate. High concentrations of bicarbonate cannot be used in a dialysate containing divalent cations, as it will form an insoluble precipitate. Lastly, peritoneal dialysate is relatively hyponatremic (sodium concentration of 132 meq/L).

The need for a custom dialysate for hemofiltration arises most often in situations in which the calcium concentration requires modification[271] or the patient cannot tolerate a lactate-buffered dialysate.[272] Commercial dialysates for peritoneal dialysis are usually available in three calcium concentrations: 3.5, 3.0, and 2.5 meq/L. Such a limited selection compromises the treatment of hypercalcemic patients by these modalities. When such circumstances arise, the dialysate formula should be tailored to the individual using an appropriately reduced calcium concentration. The standard lactate-buffering of peritoneal dialysates may become problematic for patients with an impaired capacity to metabolize lactate, such as those with lactic acidosis secondary to impaired hepatic and renal function, and hypotensive patients with ongoing tissue ischemia and tissue lactate generation. Hyperlactatemia has been shown to occur in hemodiafiltration using lactate-buffered dialysate.[273] In these circumstances, a custom dialysate should be formulated with bicarbonate as the buffer. A recent report describes the successful experience with a custom bicarbonate dialysate containing 144 meq/L sodium, 37 meq/L bicarbonate, 3 or 4 meq/L potassium, 3 meq/L calcium, and 1.4 mg/dl magnesium. No solute precipitation was observed, and numerous bacteriological cultures were negatives.[274] Recently, custom-made dialysates have been used as replacement solutions and vice versa, depending on the individual patient's needs.

Replacement solutions for continuous hemofiltration

The principal mechanism for solute clearance in techniques employing hemofiltration is by convection. To achieve adequate solute clearance, the ultrafiltered volume must be large (12–24 L/day), which makes fluid replacement obligatory. Because the composition of the ultrafiltrate is similar to plasma water, the ideal replacement solution should approximate the normal plasma composition minus the solutes that need removal. Numerous replacement solutions have been used. Lactated Ringer's solution and peritoneal dialysate are two commonly used commercial replacement solutions. Although convenient, they do not offer the

Table 16.3　Commercial peritoneal dialysis (PD) solution and lactated Ringer's as replacement fluid for continuous renal replacement therapy (CRRT)

Solute	Dianeal PD–2	Lactated Ringer's
Sodium (meq/L)	132	130
Potassium (meq/L)	0	4.0
Chloride (meq/L)	96	109
Calcium (meq/L)	3.5	3.0
Magnesium (meq/L)	0.5	0
Lactate (meq/L)	40	28
Glucose (gm/dl)	1.5, 2.5, 4.25	0

same flexibility in composition as custom formulations. Both lactated Ringer's and peritoneal dialysate have lactate as buffer and may not be suitable in association with liver failure and lactic acidosis.[273] It should also be recognized that lactated Ringer's provides an obligate potassium load and peritoneal dialysate has a high glucose content. A specially formulated hemodiafiltration fluid is currently marketed. Although it contains lactate, it is normoglycemic and has a higher sodium concentration than peritoneal fluid or Ringer's solution. This preparation can also be used as a dialysate for CRRT (Table 16.3).

In situations where lactate buffer is less than ideal and a bicarbonate solution is preferred, it can be prepared on site, but must be used soon after preparation because of its inherent instability and the risk of bacterial growth. Custom replacement solutions can be made by the addition of various solutes to 5% dextrose water or saline. The 'single bag' approach is easiest, in which bicarbonate is mixed with calcium and magnesium. Because of the potential for solute precipitation, single bags have limited use. Alternately, bicarbonate can be prepared separately from the calcium- and magnesium-containing solution, and the two bags of replacement solutions can be infused sequentially or concurrently through different infusion ports.[272] Ideally, a balance needs to be reached when using dialysate with the replacement solution such that concentrations can be manipulated on both sides to achieve homeostasis for the critically ill patient.

Occasionally, patients can be rendered hypophosphatemic on CRRT because of continuous phosphate removal; they may need supplementation.[273] The effect of losses of selenium, copper, chromium, zinc, or other trace elements during CRRT is unknown.[275,276] In summary, since the replacement fluids can be prepared as needed, they can be customized to respond to the patient's requirements for concentrations of sodium, calcium, magnesium, potassium, and base (lactate, acetate, or bicarbonate).

Anticoagulation for intermittent hemodialysis

Despite the impaired capacity of platelets to aggregate and adhere in most patients with advanced renal failure, the interaction of plasma with the dialysis membrane results in activation of the clotting cascade, thrombosis in the extracorporeal circuit, and the resultant dysfunction of the dialyzer.[277] Dialyzer thrombogenicity is determined by its composition, surface charge, surface area, and configuration.[278] In addition, the propensity for intradialytic clotting is influenced by the blood flow through the dialyzer, the extent of blood recirculation in the extracorporeal circuit (previously dialyzed blood re-entering the dialyzer), the amount of ultrafiltration, and the length, diameter, and composition of the lines between the patient and the dialyzer. Patient-specific variables that influence thrombogenicity and determine the requirements for anticoagulants include the presence of congestive heart failure, malnutrition, neoplasia, blood transfusions, and comorbid coagulopathies such as disseminated intravascular coagulation, warfarin therapy, or hepatic synthetic dysfunction.[279]

Because of its low cost, ready availability, ease of administration, simplicity of monitoring, and relatively short biological half-life, the glycosaminoglycan heparin is the most widely used anticoagulant for dialysis. Historically, the time constraints of hemodialysis are such that the activated partial thromboplastin time (PTT) cannot be used to monitor the effectiveness of anticoagulation. Instead, an activated clotting time (ACT) is sometimes used. In this assay, whole blood is mixed with an activator of the extrinsic clotting cascade such as kaolin, diatomaceous earth, or ground glass, and the time necessary for the blood to first congeal is monitored. The normal range is 90–140 seconds.[279] The subsequent anticoagulation regimens described for HD are therefore based on ACT measurements. A new test to monitor PTT at the bedside (with a turnaround time of 3 minutes) has recently been described in Europe.[280]

The precise method of administration of heparin is influenced by the patient's comorbid illness and varies among dialysis providers. The simplest method of heparin administration is 'systemic' administration, in which 2000–5000 units of heparin are administered at the initiation of dialysis followed by a constant infusion of 500–1000 units/hour (total dose of 25 units per kilogram of dry weight per hour of dialysis). The target ACT is approximately 50% above baseline. Another method of systemic anticoagulation is to administer a bolus of heparin (100 units per kilogram of dry weight at the start) with repeated smaller boluses only when the ACT falls below target. Because the degree of anticoagulation during systemic anticoagulation is relatively intensive, it is appropriate only for stable patients who are at no risk for bleeding. Therefore, in the ICU, systemic anticoagulation is rarely used. Less intensive anticoagulation is achieved with 'fractional' heparinization, in which the target ACT is maintained at 15% ('tight fractional') or 25% ('fractional') greater than the baseline value. Five hundred to 3000 units of heparin are administered at the initiation of dialysis, followed by a continuous heparin infusion at an initial rate of 500–1000 units/hour.[278,279]

Alternatively, regional anticoagulation may be achieved with sodium citrate as the anticoagulant.[281] Citrate binds to calcium and forms a dialyzable salt, thereby depleting the extrinsic and intrinsic clotting cascades of the obligatory cofactor, calcium. A 4% solution of trisodium citrate is initially infused into the arterial line at 200 ml/hour, and the infusion rate is adjusted after 20 minutes to maintain the ACT of the machine at 25% over baseline. This process is reversed on the venous side distal to the filter by infusion of 10% calcium chloride at 30 ml/hour. Although very effective,[278,281] the principal disadvantages of this technique are the requirements for additional infusions and close monitoring of patient's calcium and acid–base status (as citrate is metabolized to generate bicarbonate, thus increasing the risk of alkalemia). The dialysate used in citrate regional anticoagulation must have lower sodium and bicarbonate concentrations and was calcium free in initial protocols.[278,282] However, successful regional anticoagulation has been achieved with a standard dialysates.[281,283]

If the dialysis personnel are not experienced with regional (citrate) anticoagulation, this technique can be associated with significant side-effects including alkalosis and hypocalcemia (paresthesias, cramps, hypotension, and/or tetany).[278,284] Therefore, in high-risk situations in which fractional and regional anticoagulation is not an option, dialysis may be performed without heparin.[149,285] In this technique, the hemodialyzer is first rinsed with 1 liter of

0.45% saline containing 3000–5000 units of heparin. Hemodialysis is immediately initiated using the greatest blood flow that can be tolerated, and the dialyzer is flushed every 15–30 min with 50 ml of saline. Although not conducive to large-volume ultrafiltration, compromised blood flow, or the intradialytic administration of blood products, heparin-free techniques have been largely successful and may be the safest choice for any ICU patient at risk of bleeding.

Other methods of anticoagulation have been tried but are not routinely used in the CT-ICU. These includes 'regional' heparinization (using protamine) which can be difficult because of complexity in balancing the infusions rates,[278] bleeding from rebound anticoagulation due to the dissociation of the heparin–protamine complex,[387] and direct complications of protamine (flushing, bradycardia, dyspnoea, and hypotension).[278] Protamine may also cause increased pulmonary pressures and hypotension in patients undergoing CABG.[286] Alternative anticoagulants include the use of low-molecular-weight heparin,[288] dermatan sulfate,[289] and recombinant hirudin.[290,291]

Anticoagulation must be individualized based on the patient's risk of hemorrhage. Clearly, the risk of thrombosis of the dialytic circuit is a secondary consideration. Guidelines for anticoagulation based on comorbid conditions are:

1   Patients who are bleeding, at significant risk of bleeding, have a baseline major thrombostatic defect, or are within 7 days of a major operative procedure or within 14 days of intracranial surgery should be dialyzed without heparin or by regional anticoagulation.

2   Patients who are within 72 hours of a needle or forceps biopsy of a visceral organ should be dialyzed without heparin or by regional anticoagulation.

3   Patients who are beyond the temporal limits established for items 1 and 2 can be dialyzed by fractional heparinization. If they have previously received fractional heparinization, they can now be considered for systemic anticoagulation.

4   Patients with pericarditis should be dialyzed without heparin or by regional anticoagulation.

5   Patients who have undergone minor surgical procedures within the previous 72 hours should be dialyzed under fractional anticoagulation.

6   Patients anticipated to receive a major surgical procedure within 8 hours of hemodialysis should be dialyzed without heparin or by regional anticoagulation. If they are within 8 hours of a minor procedure, fractional anticoagulation is appropriate.

It is our practice to use HD without heparin for patients who are suitable candidates and are within 7 days of their cardiac procedure while within the CT-ICU. Similarly, should there be any planned surgical procedure after the initial surgery, we continue dialysis without any heparin. For subsequent dialysis treatments after the initial period of highest risk for bleeding complications and the patients is stable, we use fractional heparinization.

Anticoagulation for CRRT

The need for anticoagulation in CRRT is a consequence of the lower blood flow rates (100–150 ml/min), the prolonged continuous exposure of blood to the dialyzer membrane, and aggressive ultrafiltration that results in hemoconcentration. In addition, reduced blood flow through long venous lines is very thrombogenic.[292] Thus, even by modifying the procedure to minimize thrombogenicity (using relatively short arterial and venous lines, changing to a parallel-plate configuration for the hemofilter, performing pre-dilutional hemofiltration), anticoagulation is usually required.[292] In CRRT, the required intensity of anticoagulation is similar to that associated with systemic heparinization for hemodialysis. After a systemic loading dose of heparin, an initial maintenance infusion of approximately 10 units/kg/hour is administered and titrated to maintain the PTT in the arterial line 50% greater than control (or the ACT at 180–220 seconds). Obviously, such concentrated heparinization compromises the use of this technique for patients at risk for bleeding.

Alternatives to the standard systemic heparinization described above have been proposed for patients with high risk of bleeding. These include citrate regional anticoagulation,[293] use of heparin with prostacyclin,[294] low-molecular-weight heparin,[295] and more novel agents[291,296] (mostly derived from experience with HD). Regional citrate anticoagulation can be performed using 40 meq/L of trisodium citrate (calcium free) in the replacement solution during hemofiltration with a separate infusion of calcium gluconate to maintain ionized calcium at 1.0 mmol/L.[293,297–300] Divalent cations like magnesium and calcium should be monitored at least every 6 hours. Usually, no ACT or PTT measurements are needed because they are unchanged. In a study in CVVH, no hemorrhagic episodes occurred for 17 patients with a mean filter lifespan of 29.5 ± 17.9 hours.[300] Citrate toxicity can result in alkalosis,[288] hypocalcemia,[278] hypernatremia,[296] and in patients with impaired ability to metabolize citrate to bicarbonate (such as with liver failure), lactic acidosis.[301] Low-molecular-weight heparin has been successfully employed in a CRRT. It has the theoretical advantage of over standard heparin of less bleeding while providing anticoagulation. A loading dose of 8 units/kg and 5 units/kg/hour for a maintenance infusion is suggested.[295]

CRRT can be performed without anticoagulation. However, unless the hemofilter is changed frequently its performance is compromised secondary to thrombosis. This technique involves rinsing the kidney and lines with heparinized saline in the method described for heparin-free hemodialysis, followed by frequent saline flushes (i.e. every 20–30 minutes as needed).[302] It is most successful in patients with thrombocytopenia (<60 000/μl).[296] It must be emphasized that the choice of anticoagulation in CRRT must primarily be governed by the condition of the patient. In patients with a high risk of bleeding, it may be better to abandon CRRT for heparin-free hemodialysis.

Thrombosis within the hemofilter is easy to recognize by the characteristic striped clotting of the usually white fibers within the hollow-fiber dialyzer. Unfortunately, the parallel-plate configuration is assembled in such a manner that the interior of the hemofilter cannot be visualized. In this circumstance, clotting of the hemofilter can be defined inferentially by the decline in the ultrafiltration rate and/or decrease in dialysate urea nitrogen to BUN ratio (less than 0.6 is significant).[292]

Hemodialysis angioaccess

An adequately functioning angioaccess is a prerequisite for any blood-based dialytic techniques. There are two categories of access-related issues in the intensive care setting: ESRF patients with established permanent access and patients with ARF requiring temporary angioaccess for hemodialysis or CRRT. The care and maintenance of these permanent or temporary accesses are of crucial importance for the support of patients needing dialysis treatments.

Relevant to care within the ICU, it should be appreciated that in patients with ESRF, acute thrombosis of either a native vein or graft fistula may occur from intravascular volume depletion secondary to overzealous ultrafiltration, systemic hypotension from a comorbid condition like sepsis, or excessive local pressure for hemostasis after removal of the hemodialysis needles. Judicious care must be given to ensure patency of these fistulas. This includes their exclusion from use for routine cannulation or phlebotomy, and prohibition of blood pressure measurements or application of constricting dressings on the fistula-side limb. An early sign of thrombotic graft failure is the observation of an increase in the pressure of the venous limb of the dialysis circuit (venous pressure).[303] Although hemodialysis may still be performed at this stage, the efficiency of the treatment will be compromised as turbulent non-laminar blood flow occurs together with regurgitation of venous side blood back to the arterial side (access recirculation). The occurrence of blood recirculation will decrease the efficiency of the prescribed dialysis treatment.[304]

The type of angioaccess needed for dialysis in the setting of ARF in the ICU is determined by the chosen modality of dialytic therapy. If hemodialysis is adopted, a venous catheter will suffice. Should CRRT be preferred, there is the option of using arteriovenous or venovenous methods. The latter takes precedence in most modern-day ICUs because it allows for direct regulation of blood flow and, consequently, higher blood flows can be achieved relatively independent of the mean arterial pressure.[305] Also, establishing arterial angioaccess with a large-bore double-lumen catheter may be problematic, especially in patients with pre-existing arterial vascular disease.

Acute angioaccess for hemodialysis or venovenous CRRT may be achieved with vascular catheters. Femoral vein catheters are available in a number of lengths and diameters. The 24-cm length is preferable, because it causes less blood recirculation.[306] Ideally, catheters should be removed within 7 days to minimize the risk of infection and thrombosis. The typical pathogenesis for catheter infections is from bacteria colonizing the skin adjacent to the catheter entry site that migrate down the catheter sheath.[307] Femoral venous access is preferable in patients with coagulopathy. If arterial puncture inadvertently occurs, the site is easily compressible. In contrast, puncture of the subclavian or carotid artery (located beside the internal jugular vein) may result in hemothorax or stroke, respectively, among other complications. In critically ill patients on mechanical ventilation and at increased risk for pneumothorax, femoral catheterization should be considered when acute hemodialysis is required.

Alternative sites for catheter-based angioaccess are the subclavian or internal jugular veins. In comparison with the femoral vein, these sites have the advantages of fewer local infections, longer local positioning, and enhanced patient mobility.[308] In comparison with femoral vein catheters, the subclavian vein offers the advantages of increased patient comfort and mobility, and a lower risk of local infection. For the patient with acute renal failure, the subclavian vein is a useful angioaccess site, particularly if the patient is too unstable to undergo surgical placement of a tunneled internal jugular vein dialysis catheter. Unfortunately, subclavian vein stenosis is a frequent complication of long-term subclavian vein cannulation, and may seriously impair venous drainage of any permanent ipsilateral hemodialysis access which might be used if renal function does not recover.[309] This scenario is not uncommon in patients with atherosclerotic cardiovascular disease and chronic renal failure who eventually requires chronic dialysis after cardiothoracic surgery such as CABG.

The placement of temporary or semi-permanent hemodialysis catheters in the internal jugular vein has emerged in recent years as the optimal angioaccess for patients with ESRF, especially with catheters surrounded by a Dacron cuff.[310–312] Although a tunneled technique performed within a sterile environment with fluoroscopy is more often used for long-term, internal jugular vein catheter placement, direct percutaneous internal jugular venous cannulation is used most often in the acute setting. The right internal jugular vein is preferred,[313] as its passage into the superior vena cava is more direct and reliably performed.

Because a large dialysis catheter may be easily displaced, long-term internal jugular catheters should be surgically placed and tunneled beneath the skin under fluoroscopic guidance. A tunneled catheter in the internal jugular vein offers several distinct advantages over a percutaneous temporary dialysis catheter, even for patients with ARF in the ICU. Tunneled internal jugular vein catheters, such as the modified Hickman–Broviac or Tesio catheters, are more comfortable, do not require immobility (especially in the supine position), and have a Dacron cuff, which may reduce the risk of infection.[309–312] Although suboptimal to an endogenous fistula or a prosthetic graft permanent angioaccess, tunneled internal jugular vein catheters have been used in some patients for months to years. Therefore, they offer a reasonable compromise angioaccess for patients with ARF whose renal recovery seems protracted or even unlikely. Fortunately, the internal jugular veins are less prone to stenosis than the subclavian veins, even after long-term cannulation,[314] so that compromised permanent angioaccess is less of a concern. Unfortunately, the internal jugular vein site may be more prone to direct bacterial contamination in patients with a tracheostomy. Therefore, they should be avoided in this patient subset.

Hemofiltration angioaccess

The venous access for CVVH or CVVHD is exactly as described above. The principal advantage of an arteriovenous access for CRRT is that it allows the use of a very simple extracorporeal circuit without a blood pump or an air embolus monitor. There are only two forms of arteriovenous access: wide-bore single-lumen femoral artery and vein catheters[315] and, much less commonly, the Scribner shunt (an external plastic arteriovenous fistula).[316] Scribner shunts should not be placed in patients with peripheral vascular disease who may develop digital ischemia.

Vascular access is usually achieved by percutaneous cannulation of the common femoral artery and vein. Alternative sites, including the axillary artery and vein and external shunts, have been attempted, but do not provide adequate blood flow for effective hemofiltration. Patients with femoral artery bypass grafts or those with severe atherosclerotic vascular disease may be extremely poor candidates for arteriovenous techniques. Prior to femoral artery cannulation, dorsalis pedis pulses should be examined by doppler. If pulses are inaudible or if a bruit is present over the femoral artery, an alternative dialytic modality should be considered.

Peritoneal dialysis

Dialysates

Compared with the dialysates used for hemodialysis or hemofiltration, the composition of the dialysates used for peritoneal dialysis is relatively constant. The conventional dialysate sodium concentration is 132 meq/L, potassium concentration 0 meq/L, and lactate concentration 35 meq/L. Hypokalemia in peritoneal dialysis patients is usually managed by increasing the potassium intake. If oral therapy is either ineffective or not feasible, potassium can be added to the dialysate to attenuate its diffusive gradient. A typical potassium concentration in the dialysate is 0–4 meq/L. The dialysate calcium concentration varies from 2.5 to 3.5 meq/L; the choice of dialysate calcium depends on the propensity to develop hypercalcemia. Many peritoneal dialysis patients, who ingest calcium salts as phosphate binders, become hypercalcemic using the traditional 3.5 meq/L containing calcium dialysate.

Therefore, like hemodialysis, the trend has been to lower the calcium concentration in peritoneal dialysates. Magnesium is provided in the dialysate at 0.5 meq/L. The other electrolyte present in the dialysate is chloride, whose concentration is determined solely by the requirements to achieve electrical neutrality.

Ultrafiltration during PD is achieved by the infusion of a hyperosmolal dialysate. Dextrose in concentrations of 1.5, 2.5, or 4.25% are used to induce ultrafiltration. Because the osmotic gradient is less with a 1.5% dextrose-containing dialysate than with a 4.25% dialysate, the nadir in ultrafiltration develops relatively sooner using the 1.5% dextrose solution. Similarly, if the osmotic gradient is attenuated by the development of hyperglycemia, ultrafiltration will decline. Therefore, in PD patients with glucose intolerance, ultrafiltration with dialysates containing high levels of glucose may be compromised if glycemic control is not maintained.

Access into the peritoneal cavity

Access for peritoneal dialysis may be provided acutely by the percutaneous placement of a stylet-guided catheter connected to a closed-gravity, manual instillation drainage system or to an automated dialysate cycler.[279] Although simple to install and position in the peritoneal cavity, patients cannot be ambulatory, and the risk of infection is so great that the catheters must be removed after only 48 hours. If dialysis is required for more than 48–72 hours, a new site should be selected and the original catheter removed.[317]

An alternative means of establishing access into the peritoneal cavity with much greater permanency, and one that permits patient ambulation, is to place a soft Silastic catheter with one or two Dacron cuffs. The most frequently used dual-cuffed catheter is the Tenckhoff catheter, which has an open end and multiple holes in the distal 15 cm.[318] These cuffed catheters minimize bacterial migration down the catheter tract. Such catheters are highly desirable not only for ESRF patients on continuous PD but also in the ARF population if the expected duration of dialytic support by PD is more than 2 weeks. Although the placement of a chronic dialysis catheter can be performed in the ICU by experienced skilled personnel using a percutaneous technique, the method used in most hospitals is surgical placement under sterile conditions in the operating suite.

Placement of stylet-guided temporary catheters can be difficult and dangerous in patients who have intra-abdominal adhesions, which are usually secondary to prior major abdominal surgery. The most common catastrophes are vascular and viscus organ puncture. Even if successfully positioned, the resultant compartmentalization of the dialysate in the peritoneal cavity greatly decreases the surface area available for solute clearance and ultrafiltration. Similar limitations exist for the placement of surgically implanted Tenckhoff catheters. For this reason, PD is not generally offered to renal failure patients with previous major abdominal surgery and probable intra-abdominal adhesions.

Selected complications of dialysis

Conventional hemodialysis

The complications of hemodialysis are best managed conceptually in the same manner as those arising from ultrafiltration, solute clearance, access related, and from technical variances (Table 16.4).[319]

Table 16.4 Selected dialysis procedure–related complications

Manifestations	Causes
Hypotension ± arrythmia (factors—left ventricular dysfunction, autonomic dysfunction, sepsis, medications)	Excessive ultrafiltration Dialysate (acetate, low calcium, low sodium, potassium concentration) Membrane induced Bleeding Pyrogen reaction Air embolus
Hypoxemia (factors—pulmonary status, fluid status)	Acetate dialysate Membrane induced Air embolus
Dysequilibrium/cerebral edema (factors—liver failure, uremia)	Rapid solute removal with fluid and electrolyte shifts
Bleeding (factors—uremic platelet dysfunction, previous bleeding, medications)	Leak or disconnection Excessive anticoagulation, usually with heparin Access aneurysm rupture
Access dysfunction	Infection Clotting/hematoma formation
Miscellaneous	Hemolysis Electrolyte disorders Nutrient deficiency

Cardiovascular complications

A common complication is intradialytic hypotension, which is typically ascribed to excessive ultrafiltration (frank intravascular volume depletion resulting in diminished left ventricular filling pressure) or to an excessive rate of ultrafiltration (volume removal from the intravascular space at a rate that exceeds the capacity of interstitial fluid to migrate into this compartment).[205,320] Common additional contributory factors include left ventricular dysfunction (systolic or diastolic secondary to comorbid illness or medications),[3–5] autonomic dysfunction (secondary to disease processes or medications),[321] lack of pressor hormones stimulation,[322] inappropriate vasodilatation (secondary to sepsis, medications, nitric oxide),[319,323] disease of the pericardium or the pericardial space,[51] and bleeding.[88,149,285] It is important to appreciate that other critical components of the dialysis procedure may contribute to the development of hypotension. These include the choice of dialysate (buffer, sodium, and calcium concentrations)[205,227,229,230,251–253] and dialyzer membrane composition and porosity.[113,159,160]

Specific provocative issues are the (1) vasodilatory and cardiodepressant effects of acetate,[227,230] (2) impairment of vasoconstriction,[319,322,323] exacerbation of autonomic dysfunction,[321] and declining serum osmolality with a hyponatremic dialysate,[205,320] (3) vasodilatory and cardiodepressant effects of a lowered calcium dialysate,[251,253] (4) cellulosic membrane-induced complement activation,[160,170] (5) cellulosic membrane-induced and/or acetate-induced hypoxemia,[160,161,231] (6) complement and/or pyrogen-induced production of pro-inflammatory cytokines,[155,157,232] and (7) dialysis membrane immediate hypersensitivity mediated by kallikrein/bradykinin activation.[159,160,174]

Pre-emptive strategies should be taken to prevent hypotension in the setting of hemodialysis. The dialysate solution should have a higher concentration of sodium 140–145 meq/L and calcium 2.5–3.5 meq/L, and use bicarbonate as a buffer. In some cases the temperature of the dialysate can be lowered to 34–36°C;[324] cooler dialysate results in increased myocardial contractility[325] and peripheral vasoconstriction.[326] The ultrafiltration rate (as determine to achieve the estimated dry weight) should be closely regulated,[327] and a volumetric-controlled machine is preferable. The time on dialysis can be increased if large-volume ultrafiltration is desired (decreased rate of ultrafiltration) and sequential ultrafiltration/clearance can be instituted to give better cardiovascular tolerance. The use of a biocompatible membrane material may provide additional benefit as discussed.[158,170] Sodium ramping can be tried in some patients.[206–210] Recently, on-line monitoring systems have been tried in order to predict and/or prevent intradialytic symptoms. Measurement of ultrafiltrate and plasma conductivity with on-line monitoring (to modulate sodium removal to match sodium load),[328] non-invasive optical blood volume monitoring (to follow changes in hematocrit),[329] and bioimpedance spectroscopy (to delineate extracellular fluid and intracellular fluid volumes),[330] singly or in combination,[331] are being studied to guide dialysis therapy in real time. However, as in any new technology, larger studies are needed to validate these techniques.

Antihypertensive medications should be withheld if hypotension is known to occur during dialysis. Hypotension is managed acutely by intravenous infusion of saline, hypertonic saline, dextran, mannitol, packed red cells, or albumin. These therapies are all designed to improve intravascular volume and/or draw interstitial fluid into the vascular bed. Caution must be exercised in giving hyperosmolar substances (e.g. mannitol) which may leak into the interstitium or even into the pulmonary capillaries if not dialyzed out. Ultrafiltration should cease transiently with continuation of hemodialysis. In hemodynamically unstable patients, inotropic agents and supplemental oxygen may be required. Other potential causes of low blood pressure during hemodialysis should be considered, such as myocardial ischemia with left ventricular dysfunction, arrhythmias, and pericardial tamponade from hemorrhage and bleeding.

As stated earlier, dialysis-associated arrhythmias occur most often in patients with comorbid cardiovascular disease, cardiac glycoside administration, and/or a concurrent rapid decline in plasma potassium concentration.[219] In high-risk patients, the dialysate potassium concentration should be increased to 3–4 meq/L. Interdialytic hyperkalemia can be managed by more frequent dialysis treatments or the supplemental administration of kayexalate. Myocardial ischemia and hypoxemia must be ruled out and treated if present.

Hypoxemia

In some hemodialysis patients, a 5–35 mmHg decline in arterial oxygen tension is observed with hemodialysis. For most patients, this decline in arterial oxygen tension is usually of no clinical significance. However, in critically ill, non-ventilated patients with pre-existing respiratory and cardiac compromise, this small decline can result in overt respiratory failure, CNS hypoxemia, cardiac arrhythmias, and/or hypotension. Dialysis-associated hypoxemia appears to result from the interaction of the dialysate, dialysis membrane, lungs, and respiratory control center. Specifically, with acetate-based dialysates, carbon dioxide is cleared from the blood into the dialysate. The dialysance of carbon dioxide results in hypocapnia, which causes compensatory hypoventilation and hypoxemia (normocapnic hypoventilation).[231] Less contribution to the development of dialysis-associated hypoxemia is the interaction between blood complement and selected dialysis membrane materials.[160,161] Cellulosic membrane materials activate complement by the alternate pathway giving rise to anaphylatoxins that alter pulmonary regional ventilatory and perfusion patterns.[158] In addition, leukocyte interactions with the dialysis membrane enhance cell membrane expression of selected leukocyte adhesion molecules, causing leukocyte pulmonary sequestration.[155,158] Modifications of the hemodialysis procedure that minimize this complication include the use of a bicarbonate-based dialysate containing 30–35 meq/L and use of a non-complement activating dialysis membrane material. In addition, patients at high risk should have the inspired oxygen concentration empirically increased during the hemodialysis treatment.

Dialysis dysequilibrium

The dialysis dysequilibrium syndrome is an admixture of neurological symptoms and signs associated with the excessive removal of solute that occurs with the initiation of hemodialysis or in the setting of a dramatic increase in the amount of hemodialysis delivered to a chronically poorly dialyzed patient. The precise pathobiology of this disorder is undefined, but seems to be associated with increases in intracerebral pressure.[332] Although not uniformly supported experimentally, most evidence suggests that during rapid solute clearance with hemodialysis, urea departure from the CSF is delayed. The brain becomes relatively hyperosmolal and water shifts into the brain.[333] Because such adaptation is not prominent in ARF, dialysis dysequilibrium is uncommon with ARF.

Vascular access complications

The femoral site is also prone to infection, particularly in obese individuals. Meticulous local care is required to limit infection risk. The use of prophylactic antibiotics has not been demonstrated to be of benefit. Under optimal conditions, a femoral dialysis catheter may remain in place for up to 2–3 weeks, although the catheter should be changed after a week.[308] A patient with an indwelling femoral dialysis catheter should remain supine as much as possible to limit bending and kinking of the catheter. Unfortunately, this may delay rehabilitation and recovery. It is reasonable to perform same-day femoral vein catheterizations with hemodialysis, if the anticipated duration of therapy is limited or the risk of infection is especially great. Although laborious, this frequency of cannulation reduces the risks of thromboembolism, infection, and catheter malfunction.

With central venous catheters, early-occurring complications such as local bleeding, hemothorax, pneumothorax, hemopericardium, arrhythmia, and hemomediastinum are usually related to catheter placement.[334] Catheter placement under ultrasound guidance may make this procedure safer.[335] Late-occurring complications such as arteriovenous fistula formation, local catheter infection or sepsis, central vein thrombosis or stenosis, and catheter malfunction are particularly vexing. Infectious complications are a function of the duration of catheter usage. If the central catheter is left in place for less than 2 weeks, the incidence of infections is less than 5%. Longer periods of catheter placement *in situ* are associated with an increased incidence of infections ($\leq$25%).[336] The usual therapy is 10–14 days of systemic antibiotics and removal of the dialysis catheter. Suppurative thrombophlebitis requires prompt discontinuation of the catheter and 4–6 weeks of bacteriocidal antibiotics. This is particularly of great concern in the postoperative patient in the CT-ICU and portends poor outcome especially with multiorgan failure[23,29,31] Central venous thrombosis (which occurs more commonly with subclavian vein positioning) necessitates immediate removal of the catheter.[309]

Catheter malfunction with inadequate or absent blood flow is most often secondary to intraluminal thrombosis or catheter malposition.[308] Forced irrigation is usually of no benefit and may be detrimental. If the patient is postoperative and cannot be anticoagulated, the catheter can be threaded with a guide wire, removed, and a replacement catheter repositioned.[337] If the risk of bleeding is low, inadequate blood flow may be treated by the instillation of urokinase (5000 units per catheter port) in a volume sufficiently large to fill the catheter. After 15 minutes, the solution should be aspirated out of the catheter and dialysis reattempted. If unsuccessful, the procedure should be repeated. A single systemic dose of 250 000 units of urokinase or a low-dose systemic infusion of 5000 units/hour for 24 hours may be tried if low-dose urokinase is without benefit.[308] If thrombolytic therapy is of no benefit, catheter malposition should be considered.

Technical variances

As the monitoring techniques for the performance of hemodialysis have improved, technical errors such as air emboli, incorrect dialysates, and hemolysis, are now remarkably uncommon. As discussed earlier, pyrogen reactions are a persistent and vexing problem that result from the development of high-porosity dialysis membranes[155] and ultrafiltration controllers, combined with the greatly increased use of bicarbonate-based dialysates.[156] Arguably, strict adherence to prescribed guidelines for water and dialysate purity can minimize this occurrence.[157] In the case of a suspected pyrogen reaction, blood cultures should be obtained and the patient should be treated with systemic antibiotics until septicemia has been eliminated as the cause of the illness.

CRRT

Technical evolution and increased experience have made CRRT a well-tolerated therapy with a low complication rate. The most frequent complications are those related to the need for intensive anticoagulation and the establishment of vascular access, especially for CAVH. Unique to CAVH will be the maintenance of the arterial access with increased propensity for bleeding on insertion, but local thrombosis becomes the problem (in up to 3% of cases) later. Occasionally, this may critically affect perfusion of the leg, especially in those with severe arteriosclerosis, leading to urgent surgical intervention.[338] Less frequently, problems arise from incorrect matching of ultrafiltration and clearance needs.[339]

Bleeding is the most common and onerous problem encountered in CRRT techniques. Its risk is increased by the continuous need for anticoagulation during CRRT.[339] Bleeding may be visceral or localized to the catheter insertion site. Although not typically life-threatening, infection of a hematoma or distortion and compression of vascular anatomy can be problematic if protracted dialysis is needed. An infected hematoma may lead to sepsis in the critically ill patients in ICU.

Techniques like CRRT, that depend on convective clearance, obligate the formation of large volumes of ultrafiltrate and require the administration of a replacement fluid. This must be done with precision, in that errors can result in gross fluid imbalances of both extremes.[338] Changes in key parameters (central venous pressure, mean arterial pressure, pulmonary artery wedge pressure) should prompt reassessment and changes to the dialysis prescription. Because automated safeguards are fewer with CRRT, and replacement solutions are often needed, errors are more common. Hence, vigilant and experienced staff are mandatory.[271] A host of metabolic abnormalities may develop as a consequence of variations in the replacement solution or the dialysate. For example, if CRRT is performed in the absence of a bicarbonate-containing replacement solution, severe hyperchloremic metabolic acidosis develops.[272,279] Excessive solute replacement can result in hypernatremia, metabolic alkalosis, hyperkalemia, hypercalcemia, and hypermagnesemia. Inadequate solute replacement may cause hyponatremia, hyperchloremic metabolic acidosis, hypokalemia, hypocalcemia, and hypomagnesemia. The removal of phosphate is usually high in CRRT and can result in hypophosphatemia.[771]

Peritoneal dialysis

Peritoneal catheter malfunction, manifest by slow dialysate instillation and/or drainage, may be caused by catheter malpositioning (catheter tip migration, entrapment in adhesions, or kinking) or luminal obstruction (blood clot, fibrin, or incarcerated omentum). An initial approach to this problem is to obtain an abdominal X-ray to determine the position of the catheter tip.[279] If appropriately positioned, urokinase may be instilled into the catheter. After the liquid is aspirated, an exchange may be attempted. If catheter dysfunction continues, it should be replaced. Catheter exit-site infection, as evident by local redness and drainage, needs antibiotic treatment and usually does not mandate a change of catheter to a new exit location.[340] More extensive infections such as tunnel infection with or without peritonitis obligate removal of the catheter and transient substitution of PD with another dialytic modality.[279]

The most common complication of PD is peritonitis, which is reviewed in detail elsewhere.[341] Although peritonitis may occur as a consequence of bacteremia, it is usually a complication of introduction of bacteria through the catheter during an exchange or secondary to bacterial migration along the catheter tunnel. The incidence of peritonitis has declined, predominantly because of improvements in the connectors between the dialysis bag and the intraperitoneal catheter.[342] Typically, the diagnosis of bacterial peritonitis is not difficult. If a particular provocative event can be identified, symptoms and signs of fever, abdominal pain and tenderness, and a cloudy dialysate begin within 6–24 hours. The usual presentations in the ICU are pyrexia and turbid dialysate effluent, but it must be recognized that dialysate turbidity may not be apparent due to the rapid cycling with short dwell times typical of acute PD. The diagnosis of peritonitis is made if the leukocyte count is more than 100 cells/ml (or >50% polymorphonuclear leukocytes). Routine sentinel cell counts and cultures of dialysate fluid may help to detect early infections. Antibiotics should be initiated while awaiting definitive culture results. *Staphylococcus aureus* and *epidermidus* account for more than 50% of the cases of bacterial peritonitis, although polymicrobial[343] and fungal infections should not be discounted in the ICU. Appropriate antibiotics may be administered intraperitoneally.[344] In some cases of peritonitis, especially in the CT-ICU, discontinuation of PD should be considered and the patient converted to an alternative dialysis modality.

Common metabolic abnormalities associated with PD are hyperglycemia, hyper- and hyponatremia, hypokalemia, and hypercalcemia. Insulin may be required for adequate glycemic control, and hypokalemia can be corrected with addition of potassium into the dialysate. Less common, but with devastating ramifications, is the occurrence of a hydrothorax.[345] Present in about 5% of patients, it is due to tracking of dialysate into the pleural space through a defect in the diaphragm. The diagnosis is straightforward from thoracocentesis; the pleural fluid has a high glucose and urea content. Lastly, dialysate in the peritoneum can also contribute to respiratory compromise by inspiratory limiting lung volumes.

Patient outcomes and discontinuation of dialysis

Recovery from ARF usually occurs within 4 weeks, but may take at least 6–8 weeks if a severe renal insult has occurred and/or pre-existing renal insufficiency was present. It is imperative to periodically examine factors which may be associated with functional recovery. Generally, a urine output of <0.75 L/day is insufficient to provide obligate clearance of daily solute generation. However, the urine output alone cannot be used to gage the safety of discontinuing dialysis, particularly in critically ill patients. This aspect of care must be individualized, balancing the risks of holding renal replacement therapy against the benefit and risks of continued dialysis, which includes the reduced chance for recovery of renal function with continued therapy.[32]

Paradoxically, the BUN concentration may increase during recovery of renal function as tubular reabsorptive capacity improves. As the glomerular filtration rate improves, the serum creatinine concentration will plateau or the daily rate of rise slows. A stable or declining concentration of serum creatinine between dialysis treatments also heralds the recovery of renal function. If the patient is not threatened by volume overload or metabolic complications, dialysis should be withheld, and the patient followed carefully.

Discontinuing dialysis because of declining clinical status and the perception of medical futility is far more challenging. In most critically ill patients who develop ARF, the extent of comorbid disease, such as sepsis, cardiac failure, and surgical trauma, determines the patient's mortality.[23,29,31,122,187] The decision to withdraw dialysis may be appropriate when further aggressive care is futile, because it will not alter the patient's clinical outcome. Like most medico-ethical dilemmas encountered by ICU staff, the end-of-life issues for the dying patient must be individualized to reflect the wishes of the patient or their designated advocate. Therefore, it is critical that with inpatients with ARF, or those with ESRF, pre-emptive discussions be held to clarify the patient's wishes for the initiation or continuation of dialysis.[346] It is mandatory to fully inform the patient and/or their healthcare proxy of the potential risks and benefits of dialysis before it is initiated.

The initiation of dialysis does not mandate that this intervention be continued indefinitely. Many patients agree to a limited, short-term course of dialysis, but elect a priori to decline chronic dialysis based on perceived quality-of-life considerations. Therefore, in cases in which the patient, their health proxy, and the proximate care-givers are ambivalent because of an uncertain outcome, it may be helpful to recommend dialysis for a limited period. After the trial of dialysis is completed, the patient's clinical condition should be reassessed and discussed with the health proxy. Only then should the decision to proceed with additional dialysis treatments be made. A thoughtful, realistic, and compassionate approach to the patient with ARF should allow the patient, their family, and physicians to participate in shared decision-making.

For patients with CRF, especially those who have preoperative creatinine of >2.5 mg/dl, a quarter may develop ESRF.[347] On the other hand, chronic dialysis patients face an extremely high acute mortality rate (8–42%) compared with non-dialysis patients (1–2%).[24–27,348–352] Several studies report similar short- and long-term survival rates for ESRF patients post-CABG.[353–355] For example, one center reported a 9% short-term mortality and actuarial survival rates of 84 ± 8% in 1 year and 45 + 13% in 2 years.[353] Another center reported a 17% short-term mortality rate with a 5-year event-free rate of 70% among the surviving patients.[354] Lastly, a final center reported a short-term mortality rate of 5% with actuarial survival rates of 87, 78, and 59% at 1, 2, and 3 years, respectively.[355] Patient selection bias, publication bias, and only single institution outcomes among these reports compromise their general applicability. However, as long as patients benefit with improved quality of life in the context of shared clinical decision-making, dialytic management should be offered.

References

1. United States Renal Data System. USRDS *Annual Data Report* (1998). National Institutes of Health; National Institute of Diabetes and Digestive and Kidney Diseases, Bethesda, MD.
2. Bloembergen WE. (1997). Cardiac disease in chronic uremia: epidemiology. *Advances in Renal Replacement Therapy*, 4, 185–93.
3. Foley RN, Parfrey PS, Harnett JD, Kent GM, Martin CJ, Murray DC, *et al.* (1995). Clinical and echocardiographic disease in patients starting end-stage renal disease therapy. *Kidney International*, 47, 186–92.
4. Covic A, Goldsmith DJ, Georgescu G, Venning MC, Ackrill P. (1996). Echocardiographic findings in long-term, long-hour hemodialysis patients. *Clinical Nephrology*, 45, 104–10.
5. Dahan M, Siohan P, Viron B, Michel C, Paillole C, Gourgon R, *et al.* (1997). Relationship between LVH, myocardial contractility, and load conditions in hemodialysis patients: an echocardiographic study. *American Journal of Kidney Diseases*, 30, 780–5.
6. Parfrey PS, Foley RN, Harnett JD, Kent GM, Murray D, Barre P. (1996). Outcome and risk factors of ischemic heart disease in chronic uremia. *Kidney International*, 49, 1428–34.
7. Harnett JD, Foley RN, Kent GM, Barre P, Murray D, Parfrey PS. (1995). Congestive heart failure in dialysis patients: prevalence, incidence, prognosis, and risk factors. *Kidney International*, 47, 884–90.
8. Collins AJ, Hanson G, Umen A, Kjellstrand G, Keshaviah P. (1990). Changing risk factor demographics in end-stage renal disease patients entering hemodialysis and the impact on long term mortality. *American Journal of Kidney Diseases*, 15, 422–32.

9. Keane WF, Collins AJ. (1994). Influence of co-morbidity on mortality and morbidity in patients treated with hemodialysis. *American Journal of Kidney Diseases*, 24, 1010–18.

10. Herzog CA, Ma JZ, Collins AJ. (1998). Poor long term survival after myocardial infarction among patients on long term dialysis. *New England Journal of Medicine*, 339, 799–805.

11. Foley RN, Parfrey PS, Sarnak MJ. (1998). Clinical epidemiology of cardiovascular disease in chronic renal disease. *American Journal of Kidney Diseases*, 32, S112–19.

12. Tucker B, Fabbian F, Giles M, Thuraisingham RC, Raine AE, Baker LR. (1997). Left ventricular hypertrophy and ambulatory blood pressure monitoring in chronic renal failure. *Nephrology, Dialysis, Transplantation*, 12, 724–8.

13. Levin A, Singer J, Thompson CR, Ross H, Lewis M. (1996). Prevalent LVH in the pre-dialysis population: identifying opportunities for intervention. *American Journal of Kidney Diseases*, 27, 347–54.

14. Frost L, Pedersen RS, Lund O, Hansen OK, Hansen HE. (1991). Prognosis and risk factors in acute, dialysis-requiring renal failure after open-heart surgery. *Scandinavian Journal of Thoracic and Cardiovascular Surgery*, 25, 161–6.

15. Andersson LG, Ekroth R, Brattebe LE, Hallhagen S, Wesslen O. (1993). Acute renal failure after coronary surgery—A study of incidence and risk factors in 2009 consecutive patients. *Thoracic and Cardiovascular Surgeon*, 41, 237–41.

16. Zanardo G, Michielon P, Paccagnella A, Rosi P, Calo M, Salandin V, *et al.* (1994). Acute renal failure in the patient undergoing cardiac operation: prevalence, mortality rate, and main risk factors. *Journal of Thoracic and Cardiovascular Surgery*, 107, 1489–95.

17. Safi HJ, Harlin SA, Miller CC, Iliopoulos DC, Joshi A, Mohasci TG, *et al.* (1996). Predictive factors for acute renal failure in thoracic and thoracoabdominal aortic aneurysm surgery. *Journal of Vascular Surgery*, 24, 338–44.

18. Godet G, Fleron MH, Vicaut E, Zubicki A, Bertrand M, Riou B, *et al.* (1997). Risk factors for acute postoperative renal failure in thoracic or thoracoabdominal aortic surgery: a prospective study. *Anesthesia and Analgesia*, 85, 1227–32.

19. Swan RC, Merrill JP. (1953). The clinical course of acute renal failure. *Medicine*, 32, 215.

20. Rasmussen HH, Pitt EA, Ibels LS, McNeil DR. (1985). Prediction of outcome in acute renal failure by discriminant analysis of clinical variables. *Archives of Internal Medicine*, 145, 2015–18.

21. Chertow GM, Christiansen CL, Cleary PD, Munro C, Lazarus JM. (1995). Prognostic stratification in critically ill patients with acute renal failure requiring dialysis. *Archives of Internal Medicine*, 155, 1505–11.

22. McCarthy JT. (1996). Prognosis of patients with acute renal failure in the intensive care unit: a tale of two eras. *Mayo Clinic Proceedings*, 71, 117–26.

23. Chang TJ, Hung KY, Jung HK, Tsai TJ. (1999). Prognostic factors of postoperative acute renal failure. *Dialysis and Transplantation*, 28, 11–17.

24. Ko W, Krieger KH, Isom OW. (1993). Cardiopulmonary bypass procedures in dialysis patients. *Annals of Thoracic Surgery*, 55, 677–84.

25. Blum U, Skupin M, Wagner R, Matheis G, Oppermann F, Satter P. (1994). Early and long term results of cardiac surgery in dialysis patients. *Cardiovascular Surgery* 2, 97–100.

26. Galli R, Nicolini F, Napoleone CP, Longo M, Fiorani V, Cattabriga I, *et al.* (1996). Heart surgery with cardiopulmonary bypass in patients on chronic dialysis treatment: our experience. *Giornale Italiano di Cardiologia*, 26, 1025–30.

27. Shibuya M, Kitamura M, Koyanagi T, Hachida M, Nishida H, Endo M, *et al.* (1996). Cardiac surgery in patients on chronic hemodialysis. *Nippon Kyobu Geka Gakkai Zasshi*, 44, 1698–1703.

28. Grunenfelder J, von Segesser LK, Huyhn-Do U, Binswanger U, Turina MI. (1997). Is hemofiltration following acute kidney failure in elderly cardiovascular surgery patients justified? *Schweizerische Medizinische Wochenschrift*, 127, 53–9.

29. Llopart T, Lombardi R, Forselledo M, Andrade R. (1997). Acute renal failure in open heart surgery. *Renal Failure*, 19, 319–23.

30. Koning HM, Leusink JA, Nas AA, van Scheyen EJ, van Urk P, Haas PJ, *et al.* (1988). Renal function following open heart surgery: the influence of postoperative artificial ventilation. *Thoracic and Cardiovascular Surgeon*, 36, 1–4.

31. Lange HW, Aeppli DM, Brown DC. (1987). Survival of patients with acute renal failure requiring dialysis after open heart surgery: early prognostic indicators. *American Heart Journal*, 113, 1138–43.

32. Spurney RF, Fulkerson WJ, Schwab SJ. (1991). Acute renal failure in critically ill patients: prognosis for recovery of kidney function after prolonged dialysis support. *Critical Care Medicine*, 19, 8–11.

33. Jindal KK, McDougall J, Woods B, Nowakowski L, Goldstein MB. (1989). A study of the basic principles determining the performance of several high flux dialyzers. *American Journal of Kidney Diseases*, 14, 507–11.

34. Fernandez JM, Carbonell ME, Mazzuchi N, Petrucelli D. (1992). Simultaneous analysis of morbidity and mortality factors in chronic hemodialysis patients. *Kidney International*, 41, 1029–34.

35. Owen WF, Lew NL, Liu Y, Lowrie EG, Lazarus JM. (1993). The urea reduction ratio and serum albumin concentration as predictors of mortality in patients undergoing hemodialysis. *New England Journal of Medicine*, 329, 1001–6.

36. Collins AJ, Ma JZ, Umen A, Keshaviah P. (1994). Urea index and other predictors of hemodialysis patient survival. *American Journal of Kidney Diseases*, 23, 272–82.

37. Hakim RM, Breyer J, Ismail N, Schulman G. (1994). Effects of dose of dialysis on morbidity and mortality. *American Journal of Kidney Diseases*, 23, 661–9.

38. Held PJ, Port FK, Wolfe RA, Stannard DC, Carroll CE, Dagirdas JT, *et al.* (1996). The dose of hemodialysis and patient mortality. *Kidney International*, 50, 550–6.

39. National Kidney Foundation–Dialysis Outcome Quality Initiative. (1997). NKF–DOQI: clinical practice guidelines on hemodialysis adequacy. *American Journal of Kidney Diseases*, 30 (Suppl. 2), S15–66.

40. Paganini EP, Tapolyai M, Goormastic M, Halstenberg W, Kozlowski L, Leblanc M, *et al.* (1996). Establishing a dialysis therapy/patient outcome link in intensive care unit acute dialysis for patients with acute renal failure. *American Journal of Kidney Diseases*, 28 (Suppl. 3), S81–9.

41. Gotch FA, Sargent JA. (1985). A mechanistic analysis of the National Cooperative Dialysis Study (NCDS). *Kidney International*, 28, 526–34.

42. Lowrie E, Lew N. (1991). The urea reduction ratio (URR): a simple method for evaluating hemodialysis treatment. *Contemporary Dialysis and Nephrology*, 12, 11–20.

43. Ronco C, Bellomo R. (1998). Continuous renal replacement therapy: evolution in technology and current nomenclature. *Kidney International*, 53 (Suppl. 66), S160–4.

44. Maher JF. (1990). Physiology of the peritoneum: implications for peritoneal dialysis. *Medical Clinics of North America*, 74, 985–96.

45. Khanna R, Nolph KD, Oreopoulos DG. (1993). *The essentials of peritoneal dialysis*, pp. 35–44. Kluwer Academic, Dordrecht.

46. Dulaney JT, Hatch FE. (1984). Peritoneal dialysis and loss of proteins: a review. *Kidney International*, 26, 253–62.

47. Merrill JP. (1952). Medical progress: the artificial kidney. *New England Journal of Medicine*, 246, 17.

48. Locke S, Merrill JP, Tyler HR. (1961). Neurologic complications of acute uremia. *New England Journal of Medicine*, 108, 75.

49. Drueke T, Le Pailleur C, Zingraff J, Jungers P. (1980). Uremic cardiomyopathy and pericarditis. *Advances in Nephrology*, 9, 33–70.

50. De Broe M, Lins R, De Backer W. (1996). Pulmonary aspects of dialysis patients. In: Jacobs C, Kjellstrand C, Koch K, Winchester J, editors. *Replacement of renal function by dialysis*, p. 1034. Kluwer Academic.

51. Rostand SG, Rutsky EA. (1990). Pericarditis in end-stage renal disease. *Cardiology Clinics*, 8, 701–7.

52. Luke RG. (1981). Uremia and the BUN. *New England Journal of Medicine*, 305, 1213–15.
53. Kopple JD. (1996). The nutrition management of the patients with acute renal failure. *Journal of Parenteral and Enteral Nutrition*, 20, 3–12.
54. Kopple JD. (1998). Dietary protein and energy requirements in ESRD patients. *American Journal of Kidney Diseases*, 32 (Suppl. 4), S97–104.
55. Allon M. (1995). Hyperkalemia in end stage renal disease: mechanisms and management. *Journal of the American Society of Nephrology*, 6, 1134–42.
56. Brown RS. (1986). Extrarenal potassium homeostasis. *Kidney International*, 30, 116–27.
57. Simon GE, Bove JR. (1971). The potassium load from blood transfusion. *Postgraduate Medicine*, 49, 61–4.
58. Schlarmanr J, Schurek HJ, Neumann KH, Eckert G. (1984). Chloride-induced increase of plasma potassium after transfusion of erythrocytes in dialysis patients. *Nephron*, 37, 240–5.
59. Bastl C, Hayslett JP, Binder HJ. (1977). Increased large intestinal secretion of potassium in renal insufficiency. *Kidney International*, 12, 9–16.
60. Kunis CL, Lowenstein J. (1981). The emergency treatment of hyperkalemia. *Medical Clinics of North America*, 65, 165–76.
61. De Castro MC, De Freitas IF, Marcondes M, Sabbaga E. (1999). Prolonged β-adrenergic stimulation: a new way to reduce plasma potassium concentration in hemodialysis patients. *Dialysis and Transplantation*, 28, 125–7 and 154.
62. Allon M, Shanklin N. (1996). Effect of bicarbonate administration on plasma potassium in dialysis patients: interactions with insulin and albuterol. *American Journal of Kidney Diseases*, 28, 508–14.
63. Sun X, Iles M, Weissman C. (1993). Physiologic variables and fluid resuscitation in the postoperative intensive care unit patient. *Critical Care Medicine*, 21, 555–61.
64. Kellum JA. (1998). Use of diuretics in the acute care setting. *Kidney International*, 66, S67–70.
65. Brater DC. (1998). Diuretic therapy. *New England Journal of Medicine*, 339, 387–95.
66. Brater DC, Day B, Burdette A, Anderson S. (1984). Bumetanide and furosemide in heart failure. *Kidney International*, 26, 183–9.
67. Rudy DW, Voelker JR, Greene PK, Esparza FA, Brater DC. (1991). Loop diuretics for chronic renal failure: a continuous infusion is more efficacious than bolus therapy. *Annals of Internal Medicine*, 115, 360–6.
68. Inoue M, Okajima K, Itoh K, Ando Y, Watanabe N, Yasaka T, *et al.* (1987). Mechanism of furosemide resistance in analbuminemic rats and hypoalbuminemic patients. *Kidney International*, 32, 198–203.
69. Sica DA, Gehr TW. (1996). Diuretic combinations in refractory edema states: pharmacokinetic–pharmacodynamic relationships. *Clinical Pharmacokinetics*, 30, 229–49.
70. Anderson CC, Shahvari MB, Zimmerman JE. (1979). The treatment of pulmonary edema in the absence of renal function—a role for sorbitol and furosemide. *JAMA*, 241, 1008–10.
71. Brown RS. (1979). Renal dysfunction in the surgical patient: maintenance of high output state with furosemide. *Critical Care Medicine*, 7, 63–8.
72. Brown CB, Ogg CS, Cameron JS. (1981). High dose furosemide in acute renal failure: a controlled trial. *Clinical Nephrology*, 15, 90–6.
73. Conger JD, Schultz MF, Miller F, Robinette JB. (1994). Responses to hemorrhagic arterial pressure reduction in different ischemic renal failure models. *Kidney International*, 46, 318–23.
74. Gennari FJ, Rimmer JM. (1990). Acid–base disorders in end stage renal disease. Part I. *Seminars in Dialysis*, 3, 81–5.
75. Ypersele de Strihou CV, Frans A. (1970). The pattern of respiratory compensation in chronic uremic acidosis. The influence of dialysis. *Nephron*, 7, 37–50.
76. Walker JA. (1988). Aluminum and citrate: a cautionary note. *Seminars in Dialysis*, 1, 91–3.
77. Walker JA, Sherman RA, Cody RP. (1990). The effect of oral bases on enteral aluminum absorption. *Archives of Internal Medicine*, 150, 2037–9.

78. Levin T. (1983). What this patient didn't need: a dose of salts. *Hospital Practice*, 18, 95–8.
79. Graham K, Goodship T. (1997). Correction of acidosis in hemodialysis decreases whole body protein degradation. *Journal of the American Society of Nephrology*, 16, 632–7.
80. Ogata K. (1990). Clinicopathological study of kidneys from patients on chronic dialysis. *Kidney International*, 37, 1333–40.
81. Rottembourg J. (1993). Residual renal function and recovery of renal function in patients treated by CAPD. *Kidney International*, 40, S106–10.
82. Conger JD, Robinette JB, Schrier RW. (1988). Smooth muscle calcium and endothelial-derived relaxing factor in abnormal vascular responses of acute renal failure. *Journal of Clinical Investigation*, 82, 532–7.
83. Hakim RM, Wingard RL, Parker RA. (1994). Effect of the dialysis membrane in the treatment of patients with acute renal failure. *New England Journal of Medicine*, 331, 1338–42.
84. Lynn RI, Feinfeld DA. (1989). Importance of residual renal function in end-stage renal disease. *Seminars in Dialysis*, 2, 1–3.
85. Benabe JE, Martinez-Maldonado M. (1978). Hypercalcemic nephropathy. *Archives of Internal Medicine*, 138, 777–9.
86. Kjellstrand CM, Campbell DC, von Hartitizach B, Buselmeier TJ. (1974). Hyperuricemic acute renal failure. *Archives of Internal Medicine*, 133, 349–59.
87. Randall RE, Cohen MD, Spray CC. (1964). Hypermagnesemia in renal failure. *Annals of Internal Medicine*, 61, 73.
88. Remuzzi G. (1988). Bleeding in renal failure. *Lancet*, 1, 1205–8.
89. Livio M, Gotti E, Marchasi D, Remuzzi G, Mecca G, DeGaetano G. (1982). Uremic bleeding: role of anemia and beneficial effect of red cell transfusion. *Lancet*, 2, 1013–15.
90. Escolar G, Cases A, Bastida E, Garrido M, Lopez J, Revert L, *et al.* (1990). Uremic platelets have a functional defect affecting the interaction of von Willebrand factor with glycoprotein IIb–IIIa. *Blood*, 76, 1336–40.
91. Remuzzi G, Perico N, Zoja C, Corna D, Macconi D, Vigano G. (1990). Role of endothelium-derived nitric oxide in the bleeding tendency of uremia. *Journal of Clinical Investigation*, 86, 1768–71.
92. Lindsay RM, Friesen M, Koens F, Linton AL, Oreopoulos D, De Veber G. (1976). Platelet function in patients on long term peritoneal dialysis. *Clinical Nephrology*, 6, 335–9.
93. Di Minno G, Martinez J, McKean M, De la Rosa J, Burke JF, Murphy S. (1985). Platelet dysfunction in uremia: multifaceted defect partially corrected by dialysis. *American Journal of Medicine*, 79, 552–9.
94. Janson PA, Jubelirer SJ, Weinstein MJ, Deykin D. (1980). Treatment of the bleeding tendency in uremia with cryoprecipitate. *New England Journal of Medicine*, 303, 1318–21.
95. Mannuccci PM, Remuzzi G, Pusineri F, Lombardi R, Valsecchi C, Mecca G, *et al.* (1983). Deamino-8-D-arginine vasopressin shortens the bleeding time in uremia. *New England Journal of Medicine*, 308, 8–12.
96. Cases A, Escolar G, Reverter JC, Ordinas A, Lopez-Pedret J, Revert L, *et al.* (1992). Recombinant human erythropoietin treatment improves platelet function in uremic patients. *Kidney International*, 42, 668–72.
97. Livio M, Mannucci PM, Vigano G, Mingardi G, Lombardi R, Mecca G, *et al.* (1986). Conjugated estrogens for the management of bleeding associated with renal failure. *New England Journal of Medicine*, 315, 731–5.
98. Shemin D, Elnour M, Amarantes B, Abuelo JG, Chazan JA. (1990). Oral estrogens decrease bleeding time and improve clinical bleeding in patients with renal failure. *American Journal of Medicine*, 89, 436–40.
99. Sloand JA, Schiff MJ. (1995). Beneficial effect of low-dose transdermal estrogen on bleeding time and clinical bleeding in uremia. *American Journal of Kidney Diseases*, 26, 22–6.

100. Schetz MR. (1998). Classical and alternative indications for continuous renal replacement therapy. *Kidney International*, Suppl. 66, S129–32.

101. Bellomo R, Ronco C. (1998). Indications and criteria for initiating renal replacement therapy in the intensive care unit. *Kidney International*, Suppl. 66, S106–9.

102. Bellomo R, Kearly Y, Parkin G, Love J, Boyce N. (1991). The treatment of life threatening lithium toxicity with continuous arteriovenous hemodiafiltration. *Critical Care Medicine*, 19, 836–7.

103. Kroh, UF. (1995). Drug administration in critically ill patients with renal failure. *New Horizons* 3, 748–59.

104. Moonka R, Gentilello L. (1996). Hypothermia induced by continuous arteriovenous hemofiltration as a treatment for adult inflammatory distress syndrome: a case report. *Journal of Trauma*, 40, 1024–8.

105. Consentino F, Paganini E, Lockrem J, Stoler J. (1991). Continuous arteriovenous hemofiltration in the adult respiratory distress syndrome. A randomized trial. *Contributions to Nephrology*, 93, 94–7.

106. Berns JS, Cohen RM, Rudnick MR. (1991). Removal of myoglobin by CAVH-D in traumatic rhabdomyolysis. *American Journal of Medicine*, 11, 73–5.

107. Shigemoto T, Rinka H, Matsuo Y, Kaji A, Tsukioka K, Ukai T, *et al.* (1997). Blood purification for crush syndrome. *Renal Failure*, 19, 711–19.

108. Agostoni P, Marenzi G, Lauri G, Perego G, Schianni M, Sganzerla P, *et al.* (1994). Sustained improvement in functional capacity after removal of body fluid with isolated ultrafiltration in chronic cardiac insufficiency: failure of furosamide to provide the same result. *American Journal of Medicine*, 96, 191–9.

109. Davenport A, Will EJ, Davidson AM. (1993). Improved cardiovascular stability during continuous modes of renal replacement therapy in critically ill patients with acute hepatic and renal failure. *Critical Care Medicine*, 21, 328–8.

110. Bellomo R, Ronco C. (1996). Nutritional management of ARF in the critically ill patients. *American Journal of Kidney Diseases*, 28 (Suppl. 3), S58–61.

111. Misset B, Timsit JF, Chevret S, Renaud B, Tamion F, Carlet J. (1996). A randomized cross-over comparison of hemodynamic response to intermittent hemodialysis and continuous hemofiltration in ICU patients with acute renal failure. *Intensive Care Medicine*, 22, 742–6.

112. Bellomo R, Ronco C. (1996). Acute renal failure in the intensive care unit: adequacy of dialysis and the case for continuous therapies. *Nephrology, Dialysis, Transplantation*, 11, 424–8.

113. Clark WR, Mueller BA, Alaka KJ, Macias WL. (1994). A comparison of metabolic control by continuous and intermittent therapies in acute renal failure. *Journal of the American Society of Nephrology*, 4, 1413–20.

114. Davenport A, Will EJ, Davison AM. (1993). Effect of renal replacement therapy on patients with combined acute renal and fulminant hepatic failure. *Kidney International*, Suppl. 41, S245–51.

115. Liano F, Junco E, Pascual J, Madero R, Verde E, and the Madrid Acute Renal Failure Study Group. (1998). The spectrum of acute renal failure in the intensive care unit compared with that seen in other settings. *Kidney International*, Suppl. 66, S16–24.

116. Billiau A, Vandekerckhove F. (1991). Cytokines and their interactions with other inflammatory mediators in the pathogenesis of sepsis and septic shock. *European Journal of Clinical Investigation*, 21, 559–73.

117. Bellomo R, Tipping P, Boyce N. (1993). CVVH with dialysis removes cytokines from the circulation of septic patients. *Critical Care Medicine*, 21, 522–6.

118. Ronco C, Tetta C, Lupi H, Galloni E, Bettini MC, Sereni L, *et al.* (1995). Removal of platelet activating factors in experimental CAVH. *Critical Care Medicine*, 23, 99–107.

119. Sander A, Armbruster W, Sander B, Daul AE, Lange R, Peters J. (1997). Hemofiltration increases IL-6 clearance in early systemic inflammatory response syndrome but does not alter IL-6 and TNFα plasma concentrations. *Intensive Care Medicine*, 23, 878–84.

120. Journois D, Silvester W. (1996). Continuous hemofiltration in patients with sepsis or multiorgan failure. *Seminars in Dialysis*, 9, 175–8.

121. Jakob SM, Frey PJ, Uehlinger DE. (1996). Does CRRT favourably influence the outcome of the patients? *Nephrology, Dialysis, Transplantation*, 11, 1250–5.

122. Brivet FG, Kleinknecht DJ, Loirat P, Landais PJ. (1996). Acute renal failure in intensive care units—causes, outcome, and prognostic factors of hospital mortality; a prospective, multicenter study. *Critical Care Medicine*, 24, 192–8.

123. Mehta RL, McDonald B, Gabbai F, Pahl M, Farkas A, Pascual M, et al. (1996). Continuous versus intermittent dialysis for acute renal failure in the ICU: results from a randomized multicenter trial (abstract). *Journal of the American Society of Nephrology*, 7, 1456.

124. Lameire N, Van Biesen W, Vanholder R, Colardijn F. (1998). The place of intermittent hemodialysis in the treatment of acute renal failure in the ICU patient. *Kidney International*, Suppl. 66, S110–19.

125. Henrich WL. (1993). Arteriovenous or venovenous continuous therapies are not superior to standard hemodialysis in all patients with acute renal failure. *Seminars in Dialysis*, 6, 174–6.

126. Hoyt DB. (1997). CRRT in the area of cost containment: is it justified? *American Journal of Kidney Diseases*, 30 (Suppl. 4), S102–4.

127. Moreno L, Heyka RJ, Paganini EP. (1993). Continuous renal replacement therapy: cost considerations and reimbursement. *Seminars in Dialysis*, 9, 209–14.

128. Journois D. (1998). Hemofiltration during cardiopulmonary bypass. *Kidney International*, Suppl. 66, S174–7.

129. Elliott MJ. (1993). Ultrafiltration and modified ultrafiltration in pediatric open heart operations. *Annals of Thoracic Surgery*, 56, 1518–22.

130. Tanaka S, Watanabe S, Hayashi K, Ogawa M, Yamanishi H, Minami M, et al. (1997). Perioperative management of uremia and fluid balance in patients with compromised renal function undergoing open heart surgery. *Kyobu Geka*, 50, 286–91.

131. Chertow GM, Levy EM, Hammermeister KE, Grover F, Daley J. (1998). Independent association between acute renal failure and mortality following cardiac surgery. *American Journal of Medicine*, 104, 343–8.

132. Hong JJ, Lin JL, Huang CC, Lin PJ, Chang CH. (1993). Acute renal failure after open heart surgery: clinical experience with continuous arteriovenous hemodialysis. *Journal of the Formosa Medical Association*, 92, 519–23.

133. Alarabi A, Nystrom SO, Stahle E, Wikstrom B. (1997). Acute renal failure and outcome of continuous arteriovenous hemodialysis (CAVHD) and continuous hemofiltration (CAVH) in elderly patients following cardiovascular surgery. *Geriatric Nephrology and Urology*, 7, 45–9.

134. Caprioli R, Favilla G, Palmarini D, Comite C, Gemignani R, Rindi P, et al. (1993). Automatic continuous venovenous hemodiafiltration in cardiosurgical patients. *ASAIO Journal*, 39, M606–8.

135. Chen JM, Levin HR, Catanese KA, Sistino JJ, Landry DW, Rose EA, et al. (1995). Use of a pulsatile right ventricular assist device and continuous arteriovenous hemodialysis in a 57-year-old man with a pulsatile left ventricular assist device. *Journal of Heart and Lung Transplantation*, 14, 186–91.

136. Tsang GM, Khan I, Dar M, Clayton D, Waller D, Patel RL. (1996). Hemofiltration in a cardiac intensive care unit: time for a rational approach. *ASAIO Journal*, 42, M710–13.

137. Lazarus JM. (1992). Which dialysis therapy is best for the patient with an unstable cardiovascular system? Hemodialysis is the optimal therapy. *Seminars in Dialysis*, 5, 208–11.

138. Gailiunas P, Chawla R, Lazarus JM, Cohn L, Sanders J, Merrill JP. (1980). Acute renal failure following cardiac operations. *Journal of Thoracic and Cardiovascular Surgery*, 79, 241–3.

139. Stone HH, Fabian TC. (1980). Peritoneal dialysis in the treatment of acute alcoholic pancreatitis. *Surgery, Gynecology and Obstetrics*, 150, 878–82.

140. Lowrie EG, Lew NL. (1990). Death risk in hemodialysis patients: the predictive value of commonly measured variables and an evaluation of death rate differences between facilities. *American Journal of Kidney Diseases*, 15, 458–82.

141. Chima CS, Meyer L, Hummell AC, Bosworth C, Heyka R, Paganini EP, *et al.* (1993). Protein catabolic rate in patients with acute renal failure on continuous arteriovenous hemofiltration and total parenteral nutrition. *Journal of the American Society of Nephrology*, 3, 1516–21.

142. Ikizler TA, Flakoll PJ, Parker RA, Hakim RM. (1994). Amino acid and albumin losses in during hemodialysis. *Kidney International*, 46, 830–7.

143. Rocco MV, Makoff R. (1997). Appropriate vitamin therapy for dialysis patients. *Seminars in Dialysis*, 10, 272–7.

144. Gutierrez A. (1996). Protein catabolism in maintenance hemodialysis: the influence of the dialysis membrane. *Nephrology, Dialysis, Transplantation*, 11 (Suppl. 2), 108–11.

145. Fiaccadori E, Lombardi M, Leonardi S, Rotelli CF, Tortorella G, Borghetti A. (1999). Prevalence and clinical outcome associated with preexisting malnutrition in acute renal failure: a prospective cohort study. *Journal of the American Society of Nephrology*, 10, 581–93.

146. Hirschberg R, Maroni BJ. (1997). Protein and energy metabolism in acute renal failure. *Seminars in Dialysis*, 10, 74–81.

147. Wolfson M. (1998). Effectiveness of nutrition interventions in the pre-ESRD and the ESRD population. *American Journal of Kidney Diseases*, 32 (Suppl. 4), S126–30.

148. Kierdorf HP, Sieberth H. (1996). Continuous renal replacement therapies versus intermittent hemodialysis in acute renal failure: what do we know? *American Journal of Kidney Diseases*, 28 (Suppl. 5), S90–6.

149. Schwab S, Onorato J, Sharar L, Dennis P. (1987). Hemodialysis without anticoagulation: 1 year prospective trial in hospitalized patients at risk for bleeding. *American Journal of Medicine*, 83, 405–10.

150. Lysaght MJ. (1988). Hemodialysis membranes in transition. *Contributions to Nephrology*, 61, 1–17.

151. Cheung AK. (1990). Biocompatibility of hemodialysis membranes. *Journal of the American Society of Nephrology*, 1, 150–61.

152. Task Force on Reuse of Dialyzers, Council on Dialysis, National Kidney Foundation. (1997). National Kidney Foundation report on dialyzer reuse. *American Journal of Kidney Diseases*, 30, 859–71.

153. Vanholder R. (1994). Middle molecules as uremic toxins—still a viable hypothesis? *Seminars in Dialysis*, 7, 65–8.

154. McCarthy JT, Williams AW, Johnson WJ. (1994). Serum beta 2-microglobulin concentration in dialysis patients: importance of intrinsic renal function. *Journal of Laboratory and Clinical Medicine*, 123, 495–505.

155. Pereira BJ, Snodgrass BR, Hogan PJ, King AJ. (1995). Diffusive and convective transfer of cytokine inducing bacterial products across hemodialysis membranes. *Kidney International*, 47, 603–10.

156. Bland LA, Ridgeway MR, Aguero SM, Carson LA, Favero MS. (1987). Potential bacteriological and endotoxin hazards associated with liquid bicarbonate concentrate. *American Society of Artificial Internal Organs Transactions*, 33, 542–5.

157. Klein E, Pass T, Harding GB, Wright R, Million C. (1990). Microbial and endotoxin contamination in water and dialysate in the central United States. *Artificial Organs*, 14, 85–94.

158. Lazarus JM, Owen WF. (1994). Role of biocompatibility in dialysis morbidity and mortality. *American Journal of Kidney Diseases*, 24, 1019–32.

159. Henderson LW, Koch KM, Dinarello CA, Shaldon S. (1983). Hemodialysis hypotension: the interleukin hypothesis. *Blood Purification*, 1, 3–8.

160. Hakim RM, Breillatt J, Lazarus JM, Port FK. (1984). Complement activation and hypersensitivity reactions to dialysis membranes. *New England Journal of Medicine*, 311, 878–82.

161. Ross EA, Nissenson AR. (1988). Dialysis associated hypoxemia: insights into pathophysiology and prevention. *Seminars in Dialysis*, 1, 33–9.

162. Dinarello CA, Koch KM, Shaldon S. (1988). Interleukin-1 and its relevance in patients treated with hemodialysis. *Kidney International*, Suppl. 24, S21–6.

163. Roccatello D, Mazzucco G, Coppo R, Piccoli G, Rollino C, Scalzo B, *et al.* (1989). Functional changes of monocytes due to dialysis membranes. *Kidney International*, 35, 622–31.

164. Vanholder R, Ringoir S, Dhondt A, Hakim R. (1991). Phagocytosis in uremic and hemodialysis patients: a prospective and cross sectional study. *Kidney International*, 39, 320–7.

165. Vanholder R, Ringoir S. (1992). Polymorphonuclear cell function and infection in dialysis. *Kidney International*, Suppl. 38, S91–5.

166. Parker TF, Wingard RL, Husni L, Ikizler TA, Parker RA, Hakim RM. (1996). Effect of the membrane biocompatibility on nutritional parameters in chronic hemodialysis patients. *Kidney International*, 49, 551–6.

167. McCarthy JT, Jenson BM, Squillace DP, Williams AW. (1997). Improved preservation of residual renal function in chronic hemodialysis patients using polysulfone dialyzers. *American Journal of Kidney Diseases*, 29, 576–83.

168. Koch KM. (1992). Dialysis-related amyloidosis (clinical conference). *Kidney International*, 41, 1416–29.

169. Seres DS, Strain GW, Hashim SA, Goldberg IJ, Levin NW. (1993). Improvement of plasma lipoprotein profiles during high flux dialysis. *Journal of the American Society of Nephrology*, 3, 1409–15.

170. Hakim RM. (1995). Recent advances in the biocompatibility of hemodialysis membranes. *Nephrology, Dialysis, Transplantation*, 10 (Suppl. 10), 7–11.

171. Himmelfarb J, Zaoui P, Hakim R. (1992). Modulation of granulocyte LAM-1 and MAC-1 during dialysis—a prospective, randomized controlled trial. *Kidney International*, 41, 388–95.

172. Himmelfarb J, Ault KA, Holbrook D, Leeber DA, Hakim RM. (1993). Intradialytic granulocyte reactive oxygen species production: a prospective, cross-over trial. *Journal of the American Society of Nephrology*, 4, 178–86.

173. Ward RA. (1995). Effects of hemodialysis on coagulation and platelets: are we measuring membrane biocompatibility? *Nephrology, Dialysis, and Transplantation*, 10 (Suppl. 10), 12–17.

174. Schulman G, Hakim R, Arias R, Silverberg M, Kaplan AP, Arbeit L. (1993). Bradykinin generation by dialysis membranes: possible role in anaphylactic reaction. *Journal of the American Society of Nephrology*, 3, 1563–9.

175. Shaldon S, Lonnemann G, Koch KM. (1989). Cytokine relevance in biocompatibility. *Contributions to Nephrology*, 70, 227–36.

176. Pertosa G, Gesualdo L, Tarantino EA, Ranieri E, Bottalico D, Schena FP. (1993). Influence of hemodialysis on interleukin-6 production and gene expression by peripheral blood mononuclear cells. *Kidney International*, Suppl. 39, S149–53.

177. Zaoui P, Green W, Hakim RM. (1991). Hemodialysis with cuprophane membrane modulates interleukin-2 receptor expression. *Kidney International*, 39, 1020–6.

178. Zaoui P, Hakim RM. (1993). Natural killer-cell function in hemodialysis patients: effect of the dialysis membrane. *Kidney International*, 43, 1298–305.

179. Pascual M, Schifferli JA. (1993). Adsorption of complement factor D by polyacrylonitrile dialysis membranes. *Kidney International*, 43, 903–11.

180. Pascual M, Tolkoff-Rubin N, Schifferli JA. (1996). Is adsorption an important characteristic of dialysis membranes? *Kidney International*, 49, 309–13.

181. Hakim RM. (1998). Influence of the dialysis membrane on outcome of ESRD patients. *American Journal of Kidney Diseases*, 32 (Suppl. 4), S71–5.

182. Locatelli F. (1996). Influence of membranes on morbidity. *Nephrology, Dialysis, Transplantation*, 11 (Suppl. 2), 116–20.

183. Himmerfarb J, Hakim R. (1997). The use of biocompatible dialysis membranes in acute renal failure. *Advances in Renal Replacement Therapy*, 4 (Suppl. 1), 72–80.

184. Schulman G, Fogo A, Gung A, Badr K, Hakim R. (1991). Complement activation retards resolution of acute ischaemic renal failure in the rat. *Kidney International*, 40, 1069–74.

185. Schiffl LA, Lang SM, Konig A, Strasser T, Haider MC, Held E. (1994). Biocompatible membrane in ARF: prospective case control study. *Lancet*, 344, 570–2.
186. Alkhunaizi A, Schrier R. (1996). Management of acute renal failure: new perspectives. *American Journal of Kidney Diseases*, 28, 315–28.
187. Liano F, Pascual J. (1996). Epidemiology of acute renal failure: a prospective, multicenter, community-based study. Madrid Acute Renal Failure Study Group. *Kidney International*, 50, 811–18.
188. Consentino F, Chaff C, Piedmonte M. (1994). Risk factors influencing survival in ICU acute renal failure. *Nephrology, Dialysis, Transplantation*, 9 (Suppl. 4), 179–82.
189. Bergamo Collaborative Dialysis Study Group. (1991). Acute intradialytic well-being: results of a clinical trial comparing polysulfone with cuprophan. *Kidney International*, 40, 714–19.
190. Kranzlin B, Reuss A, Gretz N, Kirschfink M, Ryan CJ, Mujais SK. (1996). Recovery from ischemic renal failure: independence from dialysis membrane type. *Nephron*, 73, 644–51.
191. Jacobs C. (1997). The costs of dialysis treatments for patients with end-stage renal disease in France. *Nephrology, Dialysis, Transplantation*, 12 (Suppl. 1), 29–32.
192. Bloembergen WE, Hakim RM, Stannard DC, Held PJ, Wolfe RA, Agodoa LYC, *et al.* (1999). Relationship of dialysis membrane and cause-specific mortality. *American Journal of Kidney Diseases*, 33, 1–10.
193. Association for the Advancement of Medical Instrumentation. (1993). Reuse of hemodialyzers. In: *AAMI standards and recommended practices*, vol. 3, pp. 85–118. ANSI/AAMI-RD-47, Arlington, VA.
194. Rasborough DC, Van Stone JC. (1993). Dialysate glucose. *Seminars in Dialysis*, 6, 260–3.
195. Ward RA, Walthen RL, Williams TE, Harding GB. (1987). Hemodialysate composition and intradialytic metabolic, acid–base, and potassium changes. *Kidney International*, 32, 129–135.
196. Arem R. (1989). Hypoglycemia associated with renal failure. *Endocrinology and Metabolic Clinics of North America*, 18, 103–21.
197. Grajower MM, Walter L, Albin J. (1980). Hypoglycemia in chronic hemodialysis patients: association with propranolol use. *Nephron*, 26, 126–9.
198. Kopple JD, Swendseid ME, Shinaberger JH, Umezawa CY. (1973). The free and bound amino acids removed by hemodialysis. *Transactions of the American Society of Artificial Internal Organs*, 19, 309–13.
199. Ganda OP, Aoki TT, Soeldner JS, Morrison RS, Cahill GF. (1976). Hormone-fuel concentrations in anephric subjects: effects of hemodialysis (with special reference to amino acids). *Journal of Clinical Investigation*, 57, 1403–11.
200. Wilkinson R, Barber SG, Robson V. (1977). Cramps, thirst, and hypertension in hemodialysis patients—the influence of dialysate sodium concentration. *Clinical Nephrology*, 7, 101–5.
201. Ogden D. (1978). A double-blind crossover comparison of high and low sodium dialysis. *Proceedings from the Clinical Dialysis and Transplantation Forum*, 8, 157–65.
202. Henrich WL, Woodard TD, McPhaul JJ. (1982). The chronic efficacy and safety of high sodium dialysate: double-blind crossover study. *American Journal of Kidney Diseases*, 2, 349–53.
203. Cybulsky AV, Matni A, Hollomby DJ. (1985). Effects of high sodium dialysate during maintenance hemodialysis. *Nephron*, 41, 57–61.
204. Port FK, Johnson WJ, Klass DW. (1973). Prevention of dialysis disequilibrium syndrome by use of high sodium concentration in the dialysate. *Kidney International*, 3, 327–33.
205. Van Stone JC, Bauer J, Carey J. (1980). The effect of dialysate sodium concentration on body fluid distribution during hemodialysis. *Transactions of the American Society of Artificial Internal Organs*, 26, 383–6.
206. Raja RM. (1996). Sodium profiling in the elderly hemodialysis patients. *Nephrology, Dialysis, Transplantation*, 11 (Suppl. 8), 42–5.
207. Palmer BF. (1992). The effect of dialysate composition on systemic hemodynamics. *Seminars in Dialysis*, 5, 54–9.

208. Sang GL, Kovithavongs C, Ulan R, Kjellstrand CM. (1997). Sodium ramping in hemodialysis: a study of beneficial and adverse effects. *American Journal of Kidney Diseases*, 29, 669–77.

209. Sadowski RH, Allred EN, Jabs K. (1993). Sodium modelling ameliorates and interdialytic symptoms in young hemodialysis patients. *Journal of the American Society of Nephrology*, 4, 1192–8.

210. Paganini EP, Sandy D, Moreno L, Kozlowski L, Sakai K. (1996). The effect of sodium and ultrafiltration modelling on plasma volume changes and hemodynamic stability in intensive care patients receiving hemodialysis for acute renal failure: a prospective, stratified, randomized, cross-over study. *Nephrology, Dialysis, Transplantation*, 11 (Suppl. 8), 32–7.

211. William M, Epstein FH. (1989). Internal exchanges of potassium. In: Seldin DW, Giebisch G, editors. *The regulation of potassium balance*, p. 3. Raven Press, New York.

212. Ketchersid TL, Van Stone JC. (1991). Dialysate potassium. *Seminars in Dialysis*, 4, 46–51.

213. Sherman RA, Hwang ER, Bernholc AS, Eisinger RP. (1986). Variability in potassium removal by hemodialysis. *American Journal of Nephrology*, 6, 284–8.

214. Fcig PU, Shook A, Sterns RH. (1981). Effect of potassium removal during hemodialysis on the plasma potassium concentration. *Nephron*, 27, 25–30.

215. Hou S, McElroy PA, Nooters S, Beach M. (1989). Safety and efficacy of low potassium dialysate. *American Journal of Kidney Diseases*, 13, 137–43.

216. Papadakis MA, Wexman MP, Fraser C, Sedlacek SM. (1985). Hyperkalemia complicating digoxin toxicity in a patient with renal failure. *American Journal of Kidney Diseases*, 5, 64–6.

217. Williams AJ, Barnes JN, Cunningham J, Goodwin FJ, Marsh FP. (1985). Effect of dialysate buffer on potassium removal during haemodialysis. *Proceedings of the European Dialysis and Transplant Association/European Renal Association*, 21, 209–14.

218. Redaelli B, Sforzini B, Bonoldi L, Limido D, Princella G, Vigano MR, et al. (1982). Potassium removal as a factor limiting the correction of acidosis during dialysis. *Proceedings of the European Dialysis and Transplant Association/European Renal Association*, 19, 366–71.

219. Morrison G, Michelson FI, Brown S, Morganroth J. (1980). Mechanism and prevention of cardiac arrhythmias in chronic hemodialysis patients. *Kidney International*, 17, 811–19.

220. Redaelli B, Locatelli F, Limido D, Andrulli S, Signorini MG, Sforzini S, et al. (1996). Effect of a new model of hemodialysis potassium removal on the control of ventricular arrythmias. *Kidney International*, 50, 690–717.

221. Wiegand CF, Davin TD, Raij L, Kjellstrand CM. (1981). Severe hypokalemia induced by hemodialysis. *Archives of Internal Medicine*, 141, 167–70.

222. Ebel H, Saure B, Laage C, Dittmar A, Keuchel M, Stellwaag M, et al. (1990). Influence of computer-modulated profile haemodialysis on cardiac arrhythmias. *Nephrology, Dialysis, Transplantation*, 5 (Suppl. 1), 165–6.

223. Kveim M, Nesbakken R. (19??). Utilization of exogenous acetate during hemodialysis. *Transactions of the American Society for Artificial Internal Organs*, 21, 138–43.

224. Vinay P, Prud'homme M, Vinet B, Cournoyer G, Degoulet P, Leville M, et al. (1987). Acetate metabolism and bicarbonate generation during hemodialysis: 10 years of observation. *Kidney International*, 31, 1194–204.

225. Mastrangelo F, Rizzelli S, Corliano C, Montinaro AM, De Blasi V, Alfonso L, et al. (1985). Benefits of bicarbonate dialysis. *Kidney International*, 28 (Suppl. 17), S188–93.

226. Henrich WL. (1986). Hemodynamic instability during hemodialysis. *Kidney International*, 30, 605–12.

227. Wolff J, Pedersen T, Rossen M, Cleeman-Rasmussen K. (1986). Effects of acetate and bicarbonate dialysis on cardiac performance, transmural myocardial perfusion and acid–base balance. *International Journal of Artificial Organs*, 9, 105–10.

228. Daugirdas JT. (1991). Dialysis hypotension: a hemodynamic analysis. *Kidney International*, 39, 233–46.

229. Wehle B, Asaba H, Castenfors J, Furst P, Grahn A, Gunnarson B, *et al.* (1978). The influence of dialysis fluid composition on the blood pressure response during dialysis. *Clinical Nephrology*, 10, 62–6.

230. Borges HF, Fryd DS, Rosa AA, Kjellstrand CM. (1981). Hypotension during acetate and bicarbonate dialysis in patients with acute renal failure. *American Journal of Nephrology*, 1, 24–30.

231. Garella S, Chang BS. (1984). Hemodialysis associated hypoxemia. *American Journal of Nephrology*, 4, 273–9.

232. Ward RA, Luehmann DA, Klein E. (19??). Are current standards for the microbiological purity of hemodialysate adequate? *Seminars in Dialysis*, 2, 69.

233. Pegues DA, Oettinger CW, Bland LA, Oliver JC, Arduino MJ, Aguero SM, *et al.* (1992). A prospective study of pyrogenic reactions in hemodialysis patients using bicarbonate dialysis fluids filtered to remove bacteria and endotoxin. *Journal of the American Society of Nephrology*, 3, 1002–7.

234. Sherman RA. (1988). On lowering dialysate calcium. *Seminars in Dialysis*, 1, 78–9.

235. Goodman WG, Coburn JW. (1992). The use of 1,25-dihydroxyvitamin D3 in early renal failure. *Annual Review in Medicine*, 43, 227–37.

236. Sutton RA, Cameron EC. (1992). Renal osteodystrophy: pathophysiology. *Seminars in Nephrology*, 12, 91–100.

237. Wing AJ. (1968). Optimum calcium concentration of dialysis fluid for maintenance hemodialysis. *British Medical Journal*, 4, 145–9.

238. Raman A, Chong YK, Sreenevasan GA. (1976). Effects of varying dialysate calcium concentrations on the plasma calcium fractions in patients on dialysis. *Nephron*, 16, 181–7.

239. Bouillon R, Verberckmoes R, Moor PD. (1975). Influence of dialysate calcium concentration and vitamin D on serum parathyroid hormone during repetitive dialysis. *Kidney International*, 7, 422–32.

240. Salusky IB, Foley J, Nelson P, Goodman WG. (1991). Aluminum accumulation during treatment with aluminum hydroxide and dialysis in children and young adults with chronic renal disease. *New England Journal of Medicine*, 324, 527–31.

241. Touam M, Martinez F, Lacour B, Bourdon R, Zingraff J, Di Giulio S, *et al.* (1983). Aluminum-induced, reversible microcytic anemia in chronic renal failure: clinical and experimental studies. *Clinical Nephrology*, 19, 295–8.

242. Alfrey AC, Le Gendre GR, Kaehny WD. (1976). The dialysis encephalopathy syndrome. Possible aluminum intoxication. *New England Journal of Medicine*, 294, 184–8.

243. Slatopolsky E, Weerts C, Lopez-Hilker S, Norwood K, Zink M, Windus D, *et al.* (1986). Calcium carbonate as a phosphate binder in patients with chronic renal failure undergoing dialysis. *New England Journal of Medicine* 315:157–61.

244. Mai ML, Emmett M, Sheikh MS, Santa Ana CA, Schiller L, Fordtran JS. (1989). Calcium acetate, an effective phosphorus binder in patients with renal failure. *Kidney International*, 36, 690–5.

245. Fernandez E, Montoliu J. (1994). Successful treatment of massive uremic tumoral calcinosis with daily hemodialysis and very low calcium dialysate. *Nephrology, Dialysis Transplantation*, 9, 1207–9.

246. Chertow GM, Burke SK, Lazarus JM, Stenzel KH, Wombolt D, Goldberg D, *et al.* (1997). Poly[allylamine hydrochloride] (RenaGel): a noncalcemic phosphate binder for the treatment of hyperphosphatemia in chronic renal failure. *American Journal of Kidney Diseases*, 29, 66–71.

247. Kurokawa K, Akizawa T, Suzuki M, Akiba T, Ogata E, Slatopolsky E. (1996). Effect of 22-oxa-calcitriol on hyperparathyroidism of dialysis patients: results of a preliminary study. *Nephrology, Dialysis Transplantation*, 11, 121–4.

248. Tan AU, Levine BS, Mazess RB, Kyllo DM, Bishop CW, Knutson JC, *et al.* (1997). Effective suppression of parathyroid hormone by 1α-hydroxy-vitamin D2 in hemodialysis patients with moderate to severe secondary hyperparathyroidism. *Kidney International*, 51, 317–23.

249. Martin KJ, Gonzales EA, Gellens M, Hamm LL, Abboud H, Lindberg J. (1998). 19-nor-1-α-25-dihydroxyvitamin D2 (Paricalcitol) safely and effectively reduces the levels of intact parathyroid hormone in patients on hemodialysis. *Journal of the American Society of Nephrology*, 9, 1427–32.
250. Antonsen JE, Sherrard DJ, Andress DL. (1998). A calcimimetic agent acutely suppresses parathyroid hormone levels in patients with chronic renal failure. *Kidney International*, 53, 223–7.
251. Sherman RA, Bialy GB, Gazinski B, Bernhole AS, Eisinger RP. (1986). The effect of dialysate calcium levels on blood pressure during hemodialysis. *American Journal of Kidney Diseases*, 8, 244–7.
252. Maynard JC, Cruz C, Kleerekoper M, Levin NW. (1986). Blood pressure response to changes in serum ionized calcium during hemodialysis. *Annals of Internal Medicine*, 104, 358–61.
253. Fellner SK, Lang RM, Neumann A, Spencer KT, Bushinsky DA, Borow KM. (1989). Physiological mechanisms for calcium-induced changes in systemic arterial pressure in stable dialysis patients. *Hypertension*, 13, 213–18.
254. Vaporean ML, Van Stone JC. (1993). Dialysate magnesium. *Seminars in Dialysis*, 6, 46–51.
255. Breuer J, Moniz C, Baldwin D, Parsons V. (1987). The effects of zero magnesium dialysate and magnesium supplements on ionized calcium concentration in patients on regular dialysis treatment. *Nephrology, Dialysis Transplantation*, 2, 347–50.
256. Gonella M, Ballanti P, Della Rocca C, Calabrese G, Pratesi G, Vagelli G, et al. (1988). Improved bone morphology by normalizing serum magnesium in chronically hemodialyzed patients. *Mineral and Electrolyte Metabolism*, 14, 240–5.
257. Gonella M, Calabrese G. (1989) Magnesium status in chronically haemodialyzed patients: the role of dialysate magnesium concentration. *Magnesium Research*, 2, 259–65.
258. Navarro-Gonzalez JF. (1998). Magnesium in dialysis patients: serum levels and clinical implications. *Clinical Nephrology*, 49, 373–8.
259. Zehender M, Meinertz T, Faber T, Caspary A, Jeron A, Bremm K, et al. (1997). Antiarrhythmic effects of increasing the daily intake of magnesium and potassium in patients with frequent ventricular arrythmias. Magnesium in Cardiac Arrythmias (MAGICA) Investigators. *Journal of the American College of Cardiology*, 29, 1028–34.
260. Specter MJ, Schweizer E, Goldman RH. (1975). Studies on magnesium's mechanism of action in digitalis-induced arrythmias. *Circulation*, 52, 1001–5.
261. Prielipp RC, Butterworth JF, Roberts PR, Black KW, Zaloga GP. (1995). Magnesium antagonizes the actions of lysophosphatidyl choline (LPC) in myocardial cells: a possible mechanism for its antiarrhythmic effect. *Anesthesia and Analgesia*, 80, 1083–7.
262. Pearson PJ, Evora PR, Seccombe JF, Schaff HV. (1998). Hypomagnesemia inhibits nitric oxide release from coronary endothelium: protective role of magnesium infusion after cardiac operations. *Annals of Thoracic Surgery*, 65, 967–72.
263. Aglio LS, Stanford GG, Maddi R, Boyd JL, Nussbaum S, Chernow B. (1991). Hypomagnesemia is common following cardiac surgery. *Journal of Cardiothoracic and Vascular Anesthesia*, 5, 201–8.
264. Yurvati AH, Sanders SP, Dullye LJ, Carney MP, Archer RL, Karo PP. (1992). Antiarrhythmic response to intravenously administered magnesium after cardiac surgery. *Southern Medical Journal*, 85, 714–17.
265. Colquhoun IW, Berg GA, el-Fiky M, Hurle A, Fell GS, Wheatley DJ. (1993). Arrhythmia prophylaxis after coronary artery surgery: a randomised controlled trial of intravenous magnesium chloride. *European Journal of Cardiothoracic Surgery*, 7, 520–3.
266. Casthely PA, Yoganathan T, Komer C, Kelly M. (1994). Magnesium and arrhythmias after coronary artery bypass surgery. *Journal of Cardiothoracic and Vascular Anesthesia*, 8, 188–91.
267. Vyvyan HA, Mayne PN, Cutfield GR. (1994). Magnesium flux and cardiac surgery: a study of the relationship between magnesium exchange, serum magnesium levels, and postoperative arrhythmias. *Anaesthesia*, 49, 245–9.
268. Steinberger HA, Hanson CW. (1998). Outcome-based justification for implementing new point-of-care tests: there is no difference between magnesium replacement based on ionized magnesium

and total magnesium as a predictor of development of arrhythmias in the postoperative cardiac surgical patient. *Clinical Laboratory Management Review*, 12, 87–90.

269. Takayasu H, Sato S, Yanadori H, Hirata T. (1962). Serum magnesium level in acute renal failure. *Acta Medica et Biologica*, 10, 117–25.

270. Coburn JW, Popovtzer MM, Massry SG, Kleeman CR. (1969). The physico-chemical state and renal handling of divalent cations in CRF. *Archives of Internal Medicine*, 124, 302–11.

271. Locatelli F, Pontoriero G, Di Filippo S. (1998). Electrolyte disorders and substitution fluid in continuous renal replacement therapy. *Kidney International*, 53 (Suppl.66), S151–55.

272. Macias WL. (1996). Choice of replacement fluid/dialysate anion in continuous renal replacement therapy. *American Journal of Kidney Diseases*, 28 (Suppl. 3), S15–20.

273. Davenport A, Will EJ, Davison AM. (1991). Hyperlactatemia and metabolic acidosis during hemofiltration using lactate-buffered fluids. *Nephron*, 59, 461–5.

274. Leblanc M, Moreno L, Paganini E, Robinson OP, Tapolyai M. (1995). Bicarbonate dialysate for continuous renal replacement therapy in intensive care unit patients with acute renal failure. *American Journal of Kidney Diseases*, 26, 910–17.

275. Story DA, Ronco C, Bellomo R. (1999). Trace element and vitamin concentrations and losses in critically ill patients treated with continuous venovenous hemofiltration. *Critical Care Medicine*, 27, 220–3.

276. Bistrian BR. (1999). To replace or not to replace vitamins and minerals in CVVH: this is the question (Editorial). *Critical Care Medicine*, 27, 36.

277. Cazenave JP, Mulvihill J. (1988). Interactions of blood with surfaces: hemocompatibility and thromboresistance of biomaterials. *Contributions to Nephrology*, 62, 118–27.

278. Grant ME, Lovell HB, Wiegmann TB. (1991). Current use of anticoagulation in hemodialysis. *Seminars in Dialysis*, 4, 168–73.

279. Owen WF, Lazarus JM. (1993). Dialytic management of acute renal failure. In: Lazarus JM, Brenner BM, editors. *Acute renal failure*, pp. 487–525. Churchill Livingstone, New York.

280. Eiswirth G, Walch S, Bommer J. (1998). New bedside test for monitoring anticoagulation during hemodialysis. *Artificial Organs*, 22, 346–8.

281. Flanigan MJ, Pillsbury L, Sadewasser G, Lim VS. (1996). Regional hemodialysis anticoagulation: hypertonic tri-sodium citrate or anticoagulant citrate dextrose-A. *American Journal of Kidney Diseases*, 27, 519–24.

282. Pinnick RV, Wiegmann TB, Diederich DA. (1983). Regional citrate anticoagulation for hemodialysis in the patient at high risk for bleeding. *New England Journal of Medicine*, 308, 258–61.

283. von Brecht JH, Flannigan MJ, Freeman RM, Lim VS. (1986). Regional anticoagulation: hemodialysis with hypertonic trisodium citrate. *American Journal of Kidney Diseases*, 8, 196–201.

284. Kelleher SP, Schulman G. (1987). Severe metabolic alkalosis complicating regional citrate hemodialysis. *American Journal of Kidney Diseases*, 9, 235–6.

285. Caruana R, Raja R, Bush J, Kramer MS, Goldstein SJ. (1987). Heparin free dialysis: comparative data and results in high risk patients. *Kidney International*, 31, 1351–5.

286. Jastrzebski J, Sykes MK, Woods JB. (1974). Cardiorespiratory effects of protamine after cardiopulmonary bypass in man. *Thorax*, 29, 534–8.

287. Hampers CL, Balufox MD, Merrill JP. (1966). Anticoagulation rebound after hemodialysis. *New England Journal of Medicine*, 275, 766–8.

288. Ljungberg B, Jacobson SH, Lins LE, Pejler G. (1992). Effective anticoagulation by a low molecular weight heparin (Fragmin) in hemodialysis with a highly permeable polysulfone membrane. *Clinical Nephrology*, 38, 97–100.

289. Boccardo P, Melacini D, Rota S, Mecca G, Boletta A, Casiraghi F, *et al.* (1997). Individualized anticoagulation with dermatan sulphate for haemodialysis in chronic renal failure. *Nephrology, Dialysis, Transplantation*, 12, 2349–54.

290. Nowak G, Bucha E, Brauns I, Czerwinski R. (1997). Anticoagulation with r-hirudin in regular haemodialysis with heparin induced thrombocytopenia (HIT II): the first long-term application of r-hirudin in a haemodialysis patient. *Wiener Klinische Wochenschrift*, 109, 354–8.

291. van Wyk V, Badenhorst PN, Luus HG, Kotze HF. (1995). A comparison between the use of recombinant hirudin and heparin during hemodialysis. *Kidney International*, 48, 1338–43.

292. Mehta R. (1996). Anticoagulation strategies for continuous renal replacement therapies: what works? *American Journal of Kidney Diseases*, 38 (Suppl. 3), S8–14.

293. Mehta RL, McDonald BR, Aguilar MM, Ward DM. (1990). Regional citrate anticoagulation for continuous arteriovenous hemodialysis in critically ill patients. *Kidney International*, 38, 976–81.

294. Davenport A, Will EJ, Davison AM. (1994). Comparison of the use of standard heparin and prostacyclin anticoagulation in spontaneous and pump driven extracorporeal circuits in patients with combined acute renal and hepatic failure. *Nephron*, 66, 431–7.

295. Jeffrey RF, Khan AA, Douglas JT, Will EJ, Davison AM. (1993). Anticoagulation with low molecular weight heparin (Fragmin) during continuous hemodialysis in the intensive care unit. *Artificial Organs*, 17, 717–20.

296. Favre H, Martin PY, Stoerman C. (1996). Anticoagulation in continuous renal replacement therapy. *Seminars in Dialysis*, 9, 112–18.

297. Falkenhain ME, Bou-Khalil PK, Hernandez RA, Naman NS, Bay WH. (1993). Anticoagulation with low dose citrate or heparin prolongs hemofilter survival in continuous arteriovenous hemodialysis (CAVHD). *Journal of the American Society of Nephrology*, 4, 344. [Abstract].

298. Hsu CY, Palsson R, Niles JL. (1997). Continuous hemofiltration (letter). *New England Journal of Medicine*, 337, 713.

299. Apsner R, Druml W. (1998). More on anticoagulation for continuous hemofiltration (letter). *New England Journal of Medicine*, 338, 131–2.

300. Palsson R, Niles JL. (1999). Regional citrate anticoagulation in continuous venovenous hemofiltration (CVVH) in critically ill patients with high risk of bleeding. *Kidney International*, 55, 1991–7.

301. Kirschbaum B, Galishoff M, Reines HD. (1992). Lactic acidosis treated with continuous hemodiafiltration and regional citrate anticoagulation. *Critical Care Medicine*, 20, 349–53.

302. Paganini EP. (1988). Slow continuous hemofiltration and slow continuous ultrafiltration. *American Society of Artificial Internal Organ Transactions*, 34, 63–6.

303. Schwab SJ, Raymond JR, Saeed M, Newman GE, Dennis PA, Bollinger RR. (1989). Prevention of hemodialysis fistula thrombosis: early detection of venous stenoses. *Kidney International*, 36, 707–11.

304. Windus DW, Audrain J, Vanderson R, Jendrisak M, Picus D, Delmez JA. (1990). Optimization of high-efficiency hemodialysis by detection and correction of fistula dysfunction. *Kidney International*, 38, 337–41.

305. Storck M, Hartl WH, Zimmerer E, Inthorn D. (1991). Comparison of pump-driven and spontaneous continuous hemofiltration in postoperative acute renal failure. *Lancet*, 337, 452–5.

306. Kelber J, Delmez JA, Windus DW. (1993). Factors affecting delivery of high efficiency dialysis using temporary vascular access. *American Journal of Kidney Diseases*, 22, 24–9.

307. Goldstein MB. (1992). Prevention of sepsis from central vein dialysis catheters. *Seminars in Dialysis*, 5, 106–7.

308. Besarab A, Al-Ejel F. (1996). Creating and maintaining acute access for hemodialysis. *Seminars in Dialysis*, 9 (Suppl. 1), S2–6.

309. Cimochowski GE, Worley E, Rutherford WE, Sartain J, Blondin J, Harter H. (1990). Superiority of the internal jugular over the subclavian access for temporary dialysis. *Nephron*, 54, 154–61.

310. Schwab SJ, Buller GL, McCann RL, Bollinger RR, Stickel DL. (1988). Prospective evaluation of a Dacron cuffed hemodialysis catheter for prolonged use. *American Journal of Kidney Diseases*, 11, 166–9.

311. Moss AH, Vasilakis C, Holley JL, Foulks CJ, Pillai K, McDowell DE. (1990). Use of a silicone dual lumen catheter with a Dacron cuff as long-term vascular access for hemodialysis. *American Journal of Kidney Diseases*, 16, 211–15.
312. Uldall R, DeBruyne M, Besley M, Mcmillan J, Simons M, Francoeur R. (1993). A new vascular access catheter for hemodialysis. *American Journal of Kidney Diseases*, 21, 270–7.
313. National Kidney Foundation–Dialysis Outcome Quality Initiative. (1997). NKF–DOQI: clinical practice guidelines for vascular access. *American Journal of Kidney Diseases*, 30 (Suppl. 3), S150–91.
314. Agraharkar M, Isaacson S, Mendelssohn D, Muralidharan J, Mustafa S, Zevallos G, *et al.* (1995). Percutaneously inserted silastic jugular hemodialysis catheters seldom cause jugular vein thrombosis. *American Society of Artificial Internal Organ Transactions*, 41, 169–72.
315. Kramer P, Wigger W, Reiger J, Matthaei D, Scheler F. (1977). Arteriovenous haemofiltration: a new and simple method for treatment of over-hydrated patients resistant to diuretics. *Klinische Wochenschrift*, 55, 1121–2.
316. Quinton WE, Dillard DH, Scribner BH. (1960). Cannulation of blood vessels for prolonged hemodialysis. *American Society for Artificial Internal Organs Transactions*, 6, 106–8.
317. Ash SR. (1993). Peritoneal access devices and placement techniques. In: Nissenson AR, Fine RN, editors. *Dialysis therapy*, vol. 3, 2nd edn, pp. 23–8. Hanley and Belfus, Philadelphia.
318. Tenckhoff H, Schechter H. (1968). A bacteriologically shaped peritoneal access device. *Transactions of the American Society for Artificial Internal Organs*, 14, 181–7.
319. Anonymous. (1980). Complications in hemodialysis. An overview. *Kidney International*, 18, 783–96.
320. Henrich WL, Woodard TD, Blachley JD, Gomez-Sanchez C, Pettinger W, Cronin RE. (1980). Role of osmolality in blood pressure stability after dialysis and ultrafiltration. *Kidney International*, 18, 480–8.
321. Travis M, Henrich WL. (1989). Autonomic nervous system and hemodialysis hypotension. *Seminars in Dialysis*, 2,158–62.
322. Moore TJ, Lazarus JM, Hakim RM. (1989). Reduced angiotensin receptors and pressor responses in hypotensive hemodialysis patients. *Kidney International*, 36, 696–701.
323. Beasley D, Brenner BM. (1992). Role of nitric oxide in hemodialysis hypotension. *Kidney International*, 42 (Suppl. 38), S96–100.
324. Kaufman AM, Morris AT, Lavarias VA, Wang Y, Leung JF, Glabman MB, *et al.* (1998). Effects of controlled blood cooling on hemodynamic stability and urea kinetics during high efficiency hemodialysis. *Journal of the American Society of Nephrology*, 9, 877–83.
325. Levy FL, Grayburn PA, Foulks CJ, Brickner ME, Henrich WL. (1992). Improved left ventricular contractility with cool temperature hemodialysis. *Kidney International*, 41, 961–5.
326. Jost C, Agarwal R, Khair-El-Din T, Grayburn P, Henrich WL. (1993). Effects of cooler temperature dialysate on hemodynamic stability in 'problem' dialysis patients. *Kidney International*, 44, 606–12.
327. Jaeger JQ, Mehta RL. (1999). Assessment of dry weight in hemodialysis: an overview. *Journal of the American Society of Nephrology*, 10, 392–403.
328. Locatelli F, Andrulli S, Di Filippo S, Redaelli B, Mangano S, Navino C, *et al.* (1998). Effect of on-line conductivity plasma ultrafiltrate kinetic modelling on cardiovascular stability of hemodialysis patients. *Kidney International*, 53, 1052–60.
329. Steuer RR, Leypoldt JK, Cheung AK, Harris DH, Conis JM. (1994). Hematocrit as an indicator of blood volume and a predictor of intradialytic morbid events. *American Society for Artificial Internal Organs Journal*, 40, M691–6.
330. Fisch BJ, Spiegel DM. (1996). Assessment of excess fluid distribution in chronic hemodialysis patients using bioimpedance spectroscopy. *Kidney International*, 49, 1105–9.
331. Jabara A, Mehta RL. (1995). Determination of fluid shifts during chronic hemodialysis using bioimpedance spectroscopy and an in-line hematocrit monitor. *ASAIO Journal*, 41, M682–7.

332. Silver SM, Sterns RH, Halperin ML. (1996). Brain swelling after dialysis: old urea or new osmoles? *American Journal of Kidney Diseases*, 28, 1–13.
333. Silver SM, DeSimone JA Jr, Smith DA, Sterns RH. (1992). Dialysis dysequilibrium syndrome (DDS) in the rat: role of the 'reverse urea effect.' *Kidney International*, 42, 161–6.
334. Bander SJ, Schwab SJ. (1992). Central venous angioaccess for hemodialysis and its complications. *Seminars in Dialysis*, 5, 121–8.
335. Mallory DL, McGee WT, Shawker TH, Brenner M, Bailey KR, Ecans RG, et al. (1990). Ultrasound guidance improves the success rate of internal jugular vein cannulations. A prospective randomized trial. *Chest*, 98, 157–60.
336. Hung KY, Tsai TJ, Yen CJ, Yen TS. (1995). Infection associated with double lumen catheterization for temporary haemodialysis: experience of 168 cases. *Nephrology, Dialysis Transplantation*, 10, 247–51.
337. Suhocki P, Conlon P, Knelson M, Harland RC, Schwab SJ. (1996). Silastic cuffed catheters for hemodialysis vascular access: thrombolytic and mechanical correction of malfunction. *American Journal of Kidney Diseases*, 28, 379–86.
338. Ronco C, Bellomo R. (1996). Complications with continuous renal replacement therapy. *American Journal of Kidney Diseases*, 28 (Suppl. 5), S100–4.
339. Ward DM, Mehta RL. (1993). Extracorporeal management of acute renal failure patients at high risk of bleeding. *Kidney International*, 43 (Suppl. 41), S237–44.
340. Twardowski ZJ. (1992). Peritoneal dialysis catheter exit site infections: prevention, diagnosis, treatment, and future directions. *Seminars in Dialysis*, 5, 305–15.
341. Tzamaloukas AH. (1996). Peritonitis in peritoneal dialysis patients: an overview. *Advances in Renal Replacement Therapy*, 3, 232–6.
342. Port FK, Held PJ, Nolph KD, Turenne MN, Wolfe RA. (1992). Risk of peritonitis and technique failure by CAPD connection technique: a national study. *Kidney International*, 42, 967–74.
343. Holley JL, Bernardini J, Piraino B. (1992). Polymicrobial peritonitis on continuous peritoneal dialysis. *American Journal of Kidney Diseases*, 19, 162–6.
344. Keane WF, Alexander SR, Bailie GR, Boeschoten E, Gokal R, Golper TA, et al. (1996). Peritoneal dialysis-related peritonitis treatment recommendations: 1996 update. *Peritoneal Dialysis International*, 16, 557–73.
345. Saillen P, Mosimann F, Wauters JP. (1991). Hydrothorax and end-stage renal failure. *Chest*, 99, 1010–11.
346. Sehgal AR, Weisheit C, Miura Y, Butzlaff M, Kielstein R, Taguchi Y. (1996). Advance directives and withdrawal of dialysis in the United States, Germany, and Japan. *Journal of the American Medical Association*, 276, 1652–6.
347. Samuels LE, Sharma S, Morris RJ, Kuretu ML, Grunewald KE, Strong MD, et al. (1996). Coronary artery bypass grafting in patients with chronic renal failure: a reappraisal. *Journal of Cardiac Surgery*, 11, 128–33 (discussion on 134–5).
348. Rutsky EA, Rostand SG. (1994). Coronary artery bypass graft surgery in end-stage renal disease: indications, contraindications, and uncertainties. *Seminars in Dialysis*, 7, 91–5.
349. Rostand SG, Kirk K, Rutsky EA, Pacifico A. (1988). Results of coronary artery bypass grafting in end-stage renal disease. *American Journal of Kidney Diseases*, 12, 266–70.
350. Opsahl J, Husebyc D, Helseth H, Collins A. (1988). Coronary artery bypass surgery in patients on maintenance hemodialysis: long term survival. *American Journal of Kidney Diseases*, 271–4.
351. Deutsch E, Bernstein R, Addonizio V, Kussmaul W. (1989). Coronary artery bypass surgery in patients on chronic hemodialysis: a case control study. *Annals of Internal Medicine*, 110, 369–72.
352. Batiuk T, Kurtz S, Oh J, Orszulak T. (1991). Coronary artery bypass operation in dialysis patients. *Mayo Clinic Proceedings*, 66, 45–53.

353. Owen CH, Cummings RG, Sell TL, Schwab SJ, Jones RH, Glower DD. (1994). Coronary artery bypass grafting in patients with dialysis-dependent renal failure. *Annals of Thoracic Surgery*, 58, 1729–33.

354. Koyanagi T, Nishida H, Kitamura M, Endo M, Koyanagi H, Kawaguchi M, *et al.* (1996). Comparison of clinical outcomes of coronary artery bypass grafting and percutaneous transluminal coronary angioplasty in renal dialysis patients. *Annals of Thoracic Surgery*, 61, 1793–6.

355. Jahangiri M, Wright J, Edmondson S, Magee P. (1997). Coronary artery bypass graft surgery in dialysis patients. *Heart*, 78, 343–5.

17

Management of peripheral arterial disease among end-stage renal failure patients

Fabien Koskas, Philippe Cluzel, Gilbert Deray, Thierry Petitclerc, Benoît Barrou, Marc-Olivier Bitker, and Edouard Kieffer

Introduction

Overview

Peripheral arterial complications of end-stage renal failure (ESRF) are the non-coronary arterial lesions that occur because of ESRF or are worsened by its presence. The attribution of peripheral arterial lesions to ESRF alone is questionable compared with their representing the complication of well-defined vascular risk factors commonly present in ESRF patients, including diabetes mellitus and hypertension (HT). Although ESRF alone is able to induce arterial lesions, hints towards arterial lesions existing before the development of uremia should evolve more rapidly than among non-ESRF patients. This explains the importance of a steady arterial surveillance among ESRF patients using non-invasive methods. Preventive detection of arterial lesions through complete clinical examination, duplex scanning, and computed tomography (CT) scanning in selected cases offers a unique opportunity for earlier management of such lesions. Such a work-up should take place the earliest as possible in the course of ESRF and before any attempt at transplantation. Even asymptomatic patients must at least undergo duplex of all arteries accessible to transcutaneous ultrasound. Moreover, these non-invasive studies should be repeated annually if 'mild' lesions were formerly detected, given the tendency of such lesions to evolve rapidly. ESRF patients may present with occlusive disease, aneurysmal disease, or both. The risk of these arterial lesions is generally considered more important than in the non-ESRF population. They are accessible to the same therapeutic interventions as in non-ESRF patients with a tolerable but clearly higher operative risk than in the latter group. Dialysis and transplantation have transformed the prognosis of ESRF without significantly improving the life expectancy of these patients. Indications for arterial intervention must, therefore, take into account the spontaneous and therapeutic risks, and not only the life expectancy but also quality of survival. In the current context of shortage of renal allografts, the fact that these grafts are offered to recipients with the longest life expectancy is logical. However, the presence of an arterial lesion alone, which is amenable to treatment, should not deter from renal transplantation when indicated.

Pathological patterns of arterial lesions

The atherosclerotic plaque

Atherosclerotic disease is by far the most frequent lesion in the peripheral vasculature. Among ESRF patients, it is often diffuse, long, and circumferential, and may produce stenoses or complete occlusions whose hemodynamic consequences depend on the development of collateral arterial circulation. Even if often calcified in ESRF patients, atherosclerotic plaques must be distinguished from medial calcinosis. The structure of plaques varies a great deal. Fibrous plaques with a smooth surface are most stable but may be the starting point of occlusive thrombosis if the degree of stenosis is high enough. Calcified coral-like burgeoning plaques are frequent among ESRF patients, and the surfaces of these plaques may host a thrombus. Frequent sites of hemorrhage, local thrombosis, or necrosis, soft plaques are most unstable, and manifest a strong thromboembolic or atheroembolic potential.

Atherosclerosis has grossly the same topography in ESRF patients as that found in the general population. Most frequent locations include the cerebral arteries and particulary the carotid bifurcation, and the aortoiliac, mesenteric, and peripheral arteries. Atherosclerotic renal arterial occlusive disease may have participated in the genesis of ESRF through a thromboembolic or hemodynamic mechanism.

Aneurysms

Aneurysms are increasingly reported in the general population, as well as among ESRF patients. Their most frequent locations are the aortic bifurcation, the thoracoabdominal aorta, and the iliac and femoropopliteal arteries. Less common are those of arteries feeding an older arteriovenous fistula. Thoracoabdominal aneurysms, as well as atherothrombotic occlusive disease, may have participated in the genesis of ESRF through a thromboembolic mechanism.

Defined as a loss of parallelism of arterial walls, aneurysms are self-aggravating disorders. A vicious circle augments tensile stress applied on the aneurysmal wall as a consequence of the radial distance from the axis of the vessel (Laplace's law), and this distance is itself a direct consequence of transmural pressure. An aneurysm is said to exist when the diameter of the involved artery reaches 1.5 times that of the healthy immediately proximal vessel. When this ratio reaches 2, the aneurysm may be considered large. Growth of aneurysms, although non-isotropic, may be observed in all directions, including radial and longitudinal dimensions with lengthening and tortuosity. In addition, growth is associated with a thinning of the arterial wall. This thinning explains the diphasic pattern of the growth curve: the rate of growth remains constant until the ratio of diameters reaches two. Beyond this level, growth accelerates.

The best-known complication of aneurysms is rupture. Although possible at any arterial level, such rupture is the main complication of aortoiliac aneurysms. Turbulence in the aneurysm explains shear stress anomalies responsible for thrombosis. The presence of thrombus in the aneurysmal sac must always be viewed as indicating the clinical significance of the lesion. Dynamic equilibrium between thrombosis and thrombolysis leads to a complex, stratified coating of the native arterial wall, which becomes host to various types of lesion due to necrosis, inflammation, and infection. Up to 15% of aneurysmal thrombi contain bacteria; in particular, *Staphylococcus epidermidis*. These lesions probably provide initiation sites for rupture. Aneurysmal thrombus sometimes molds the aneurysmal cavity to the point that, at first glance, arteriograms may be considered normal. However, it is now clearly demonstrated that the thrombus does not offer any protection against rupture because it transmits pressure like a fluid rather than a solid. Aneurysmal thrombi may lead to embolic events and total occlusion. Such thromboembolic complications are most common for femoropopliteal aneurysms. These femoropopliteal aneurysms may remain silent for years, during which arteries of the leg are occluded by embolic phenomena. Only after the embolic occlusion of the last patent artery or the blocking of the aneurysm itself does the patient present with an acute ischemic limb.

Other lesions

Other lesions are less frequently observed among ESRF patients but can occur. Aortic or arterial dissection, fibromuscular dysplasia, and arterial inflammatory diseases are seen sufficiently frequently among ESRF patients that they or their etiological determinants may participate in the genesis of ESRF.

Management

General principles and medical management

The clinical presentation of these arterial lesions varies a great deal. The most frequent clinical entities deserve to be specifically described herein. A common medical treatment applies to all patients including the control of all risk factors and the use of antithrombotic drugs. As ESRF alone constitutes a major risk factor, it must be clearly explained to the patient that there is no place for any other risk factor. Tobacco abuse must be ruled out using all available methods. Most claudicants enjoy a benefit from stopping smoking within 2 weeks. Diabetes and hyperlipemia must be controlled using diet, drugs, or both. Low doses of aspirin (100 mg per day) offer primary and secondary protection against many thromboembolic events. The control of HT deserves a special place among ESRF patients, given the frequency of this risk factor. Of course, HT must be controlled if the vascular tree of the patient is to be preserved from rapid degeneration. However, a subtle equilibrium between hypertension and fluid overload, on one hand, and an overzealous control, on the other, may be difficult to attain. Many mildly ischemic states will be destabilized by a too vigorous attempt at controlling hypertension or fluid overload. Frequent examples are transient ischemic attacks (TIAs) or strokes, foot ischemic tissue loss, and intestinal angina. Such barodependent or volodependent hemodynamic ischemic events or lesions are known to occur from the brain to the foot. On the other hand, even if a temporary relief of such lesions may be obtained with a higher blood pressure or volemia, the limits and dangers of such a 'therapy' are well known, including cardiac failure and pulmonary edema. It is precisely in those situations where the optimal therapeutic window proves too hard to find that revascularization is the only solution. HT cannot be safely treated among ESRF patients without an exhaustive non-invasive investigation of the whole vascular tree.

Cerebrovascular lesions

As in the general population, cerebrovascular lesions, especially atherosclerotic plaques and stenoses at the level of carotid bifurcations, may cause strokes or TIAs through a thromboembolic or hemodynamic mechanism (Fig. 17.1). Moreover, this latter mechanism, which is less common among non-ESRF patients, is not rare among ESRF patients given the often tight and multivessel character of lesions. This diffuse atherosclerotic process may serve as the basis for cerebral ischemia or infarction, especially if too vigorous an attempt at controlling HT has been undertaken.

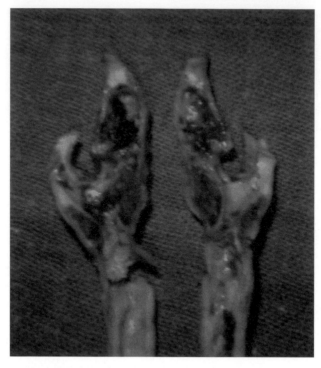

Fig. 17.1 Bilateral carotid endarterectomy specimen in an ESRF patient. Note the necrotic structure of the plaque.

Stenoses of the carotid bifurcation

As in the non-ESRF population, lesions are most frequent at the level of the carotid bifurcation, and ocular or hemispheric TIAs or minor strokes are the most frequent clinical presentations. Given the multivessel distribution of arterial disease, the occurrence of less characteristic clinical presentations, such as seizures or non-hemispheric symptoms, during hemodialysis is not rare and must be considered as typical (Fig. 17.2). More and more frequently, asymptomatic cases with sufficiently threatening lesions are considered good candidates for surgery, especially if silent brain infarcts are seen on CT.

Diagnosis of arterial lesions is currently straightforward using duplex-scanning and CT. As in the general population, tightly (>70%) stenotic, symptomatic or long and irregular lesions are the best candidates for revascularization. Frequently, patients are operated upon without preoperative arteriography, given the accuracy of less-invasive investigations like duplex studies, angio–CT or magnetic resonance (MR)-angiography. However, we continue to use preoperative arteriography in multivessel diseased patients or cases with non-hemispheric symptoms in order to define the best strategic approach to those frequently multiple-staged revascularization procedures.

Carotid endarterectomy (CE) is currently the gold standard among the various techniques available for the revascularization of the carotid bifurcation. Its ratio of benefit to invasiveness is one of the most favorable among vascular operations. The choice of technical details like saphenous or prosthetic patch closure versus direct closure or eversion endarterectomy

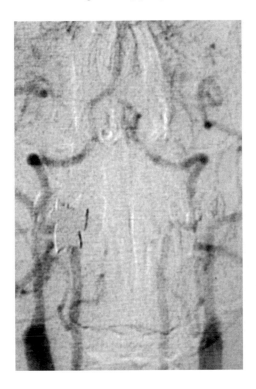

Fig. 17.2 Bilateral total occlusion of both internal carotids in an ESRF patient with seizures during hemodialysis.

and the type of anesthesia, cerebral monitoring, or protection and shunting remain a matter of personal preference for surgeons, given the inconsistencies in a large literature and limited published data on ESRF patients in particular.

As shown in well-known randomized trials, CE has definitely improved the neurological prognosis of carotid stenoses among the general population. This is also true in the ESRF population, but with morbidity slightly higher than that observed among non-ESRF patients.[1] Good selection of patients and surgeons provides rates of death or stroke lower than 5% in our experience. Cases amenable to transluminal angioplasty with comparable rates must remain anecdotal until endoluminal techniques mature.

Lesions of the mediastinal supra-aortic trunks

Lesions of the mediastinal supra-aortic trunks (SAT) increase the risk of cerebral ischemia through a mechanism similar to that described for lesions of the carotid bifurcation. Moreover, subclavian lesions may threaten not only the hind-brain but also the superior limb, especially ipsilateral to angioaccess. It is noteworthy that angioaccess is frequently established on the left side among right-handed patients and that stenoses and complete occlusions of the mediastinal left subclavian artery are among the most frequent atherosclerotic lesions. These findings stresses the importance of checking the adequacy of the arterial inflow of the chosen limb before the installation of angioaccess. Even moderate proximal lesions can behave like tight stenoses or worsen after the placement of an arteriovenous fistula (AVF) on the same limb.

Non-invasive investigation methods offer sufficient accuracy for a positive diagnosis, but for the purpose of planning revascularization we continue to rely on aortography in this field. Also, given the frequency of cardiac comorbidity among these patients, all of them are preoperatively explored with echocardiography, while coronary angiography is performed in selected cases.

Direct open-chest surgical revascularization procedures using endarterectomy or prosthetic transposition into the ascending aorta offer the best long-term results but necessitate a sternotomy or, less frequently, a left thoracotomy. Hence, these procedures are reserved for low-risk patients with multivessel disease involving both common carotids or the innominate artery or for patients undergoing simultaneous coronary artery bypass. Single-vessel disease is most frequently amenable to revascularization through a cervical or remote approach of lesser invasiveness. The best benefit-to-invasiveness ratio is provided by the direct or prosthetic transposition of the cervical part of the diseased artery into the adjacent patent artery. Examples of such a strategy include the direct transposition of the cervical subclavian or vertebral arteries into the ipsilateral common carotid, transposition of the cervical common carotid into the ipsilateral subclavian artery or the contralateral common carotid (Fig. 17.3), or the crossed carotid-to-carotid bypass. These extra-anatomic cervical procedures offer excellent hemodynamics and good long-term results, and only necessitate a generally well-tolerated cervicotomy. Very high risk patients may also be treated using transluminal angioplasty with or without stenting, when lesions are short and uncomplicated. A percutaneous transfemoral route is reserved for cases where the anticipated embolic risk to the brain is considered reasonably low. In all other cases, a cervical or a brachial cut-down is preferred, especially if a CE is performed on the same artery (Fig. 17.4).

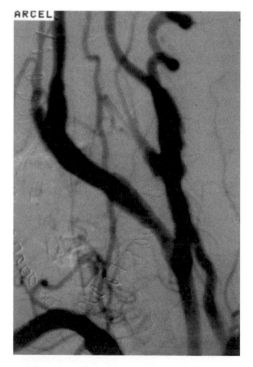

Fig. 17.3 Direct transposition of the right common carotid into the left common carotid and simultaneous bilateral endarterectomy of the carotid bifurcations in a case including a tight stenosis of the innominate and a stenosis of both carotid bifurcations. Such multilevel revascularizations can be performed using a well-tolerated bilateral cervicotomy.

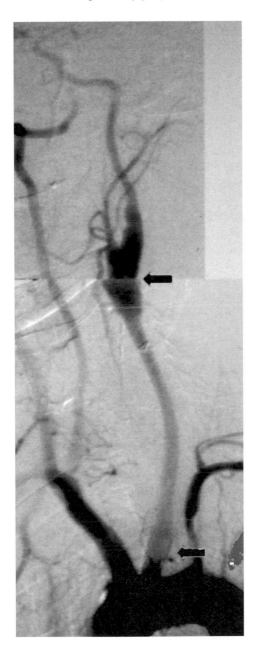

Fig. 17.4   Simultaneous reconstruction of a stenosis of the ostium of the left common carotid using transluminal angioplasty with stenting through the arteriotomy of a simultaneous endarterectomy of the carotid bifurcation.

Aneurysms

The natural history of aortoiliac aneurysms (AIAs) is well known in the general population, causing the patient complications among which the best known is rupture. Other complications such as embolic events leading to blue toe or 'trash foot syndrome', thrombotic occlusion, compression of the adjacent thoracic or abdominal structures, inflammation, and infection account for significant morbidity. Even though the definite etiology of AIAs remains to be discovered, the mechanisms of worsening are now known. Among all predictors of rupture, the best is the maximal transverse diameter of the aneurysmal section of the aorta. When this diameter is larger than two times the diameter of the healthy proximal aorta, the risk of rupture must be considered high. Among ESRF patients, the frequency of HT accounts for a more rapid evolution. Among transplant recipients, this evolution is accelerated even more by corticosteroid therapy.

Aneurysms of the infrarenal aorta

Aneurysms of the infrarenal aorta (AAAs) are the most frequent AIAs. It is becoming less frequent that a pre-existing AAA escapes the initial work-up in a patient with ESRF. Even the most basic ultrasonographic assessment of the kidneys shows the state of the adjacent large vessels. This accounts, at least in part, for the increase of ESRF cases reported initially as having AAAs (Fig. 17.5). Whatever the progress made in the domain of elective surgery, results of surgery for rupture remain dismal, with mortality rates of at least 50%.[2] In comparison, rates around 4% are reported in the general population after elective surgery.[3] Cardiovascular comorbidity factors increase operative risk. Their incidence among ESRF patients accounts for higher mortality rates after elective surgery at approximately 8%. However, in the absence of unstable coronary disease, congestive heart failure, or severe respiratory disease, reported surgical results are good.[4,5] Given this background, our strategy is to offer surgery to all patients with AAAs of sufficient size, unless the surgical risk is considered prohibitive.

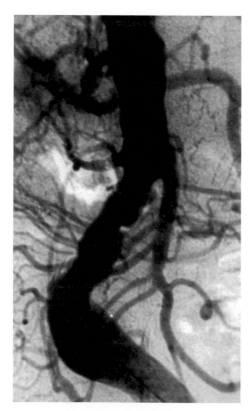

Fig. 17.5 Aneurysm of the infrarenal aorta discovered in a candidate for kidney transplant. Even medium-sized aortic aneurysms must be treated before any attempt at transplantation if difficult management problems are to be avoided after the kidney transplant.

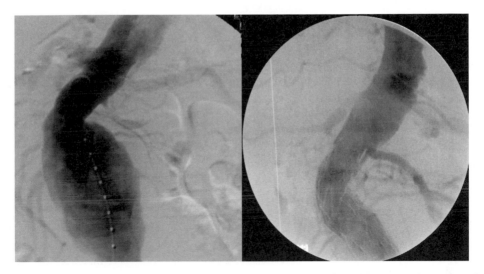

Fig. 17.6 Treatment of an aneurysm of the infrarenal aorta (left) using a custom-made stent-graft in a high-risk patient. The lack of effect of covering the ostia of the renal arteries on renal perfusion extends the feasibility of this method among ESRF patients (right).

Even if conventional surgery offers good short- and long-term results in the general population, it requires some form of laparotomy and aortic cross-clamping. Those maneuvers represent an ordeal for patients with cardiac or respiratory disease. When a kidney transplant is connected to the outflow of the AAA, it is exposed to warm ischemia during the repair of the AAA if specific measures are not taken. In view of the widespread use of renal allografts, the discovery of an aortic aneurysm above a functional renal allograft is not unusual. The aneurysm is, however, accessible to surgical treatment using a modified technique including perfusion of the transplant through the collaterals or a specific temporary circuit if the collaterals are not sufficient.

Despite unanswered questions regarding long-term performance, the transfemoral or iliac endovascular treatment of AAAs using stent-grafts is an appealing solution when dealing with low-risk ESRF patients. The lesser invasiveness of this technique, owing to the absence of laparotomy and aortic cross-clamping, has the disadvantage of requiring very restrictive anatomical conditions to be feasible. Using standard-sized stent-grafts, only 15–20% of AAAs can be treated. We, therefore, turned to custom-made stent-grafts, and this approach has increased the percentage of patients who can be treated in this manner to 80%. With stent-grafts made to measure, the only remaining limitation for the endovascular treatment of an AAA is the length of the proximal neck. One must point out that among many ESRF patients, the ostia of the renal arteries may be safely covered by the stent-graft, thus extending the length of the proximal neck and the indications of endovascular treatment (Fig. 17.6).

Given the armamentarium currently available for the treatment of AAA, every AAA with a maximal transverse diameter greater than two times the diameter of the proximal healthy aorta should be considered for surgery and studied with angio-CT, graduated aortography, and respiratory and cardiac evaluation. Low-risk patients are best candidates for open surgery, and high-risk patients are probably better candidates for a custom-made stent-graft. Among future recipients of renal allografts, even smaller AAAs must preferably be treated before any attempt at transplantation in order to avoid more technically difficult procedures after the transplantation with a risk for the health of the transplant.

Thoracic and thoracoabdominal aneurysms

Although the same strategic schemes apply to thoracic and thoracoabdominal aneurysms (TTAAs) as those described for AAAs, the higher invasiveness of the surgery has deterred its broad application among ESRF patients. Only very low-risk patients can withstand the extensive surgical approaches, including cardiopulmonary bypass and often hypothermic circulatory arrest, necessary for the conventional surgical treatment of such lesions. Nevertheless, TTAAs are more frequent among ESRF patients than the rest of the population, and especially among vascular ESRF patients in whom they may have contributed to the development of ESRF (Fig. 17.7). Using custom-made stent-grafts in combination with extra-anatomic cervical surgery of the SAT, an increasing number of those TTAAs are amenable to a lesser invasive curative procedure than has been the case with conventional surgical approaches (Fig. 17.8).

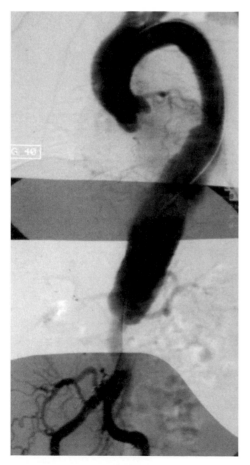

Fig. 17.7 Type III thoracoabdominal aneurysm above a functional renal transplant. This aneurysm has probably contributed to the genesis of ESRF. Distal perfusion is required during the surgical repair of such an aneurysm if loss of the kidney transplant is to be avoided.

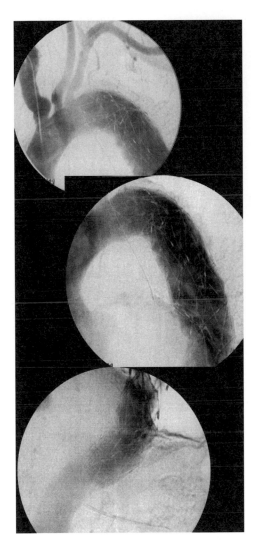

Fig. 17.8 Aneurysm of the descending aorta responsible for ESRF through repeated embolic events treated with a long, custom-made stent-graft through a femoral access.

Femoropopliteal aneurysms

Femoropopliteal aneurysms may be detected at two different stages of their evolution among ESRF patients. The first stage is asymptomatic. The patient or the physician detects a pulsatile, expansile mass identified as an aneurysm at non-invasive investigations. Large, thrombosed or silent complicated aneurysms should be preventively operated upon. Femoral aneurysms are easier to deal with since they are of easy access and the caliber of the arteries involved permits the use of prosthetic conduits with excellent long-term results. The outcome is very different for popliteal aneurysms where the reconstructions that are necessary are basically similar to those described for occlusive infrainguinal disease, and need an autologous saphenous graft and acceptable arterial outflow for a good long-term result. The work-up of such asymptomatic popliteal aneurysms must be performed carefully and include arteriography to check for embolic occlusion of the distal arteries of the leg or the foot,

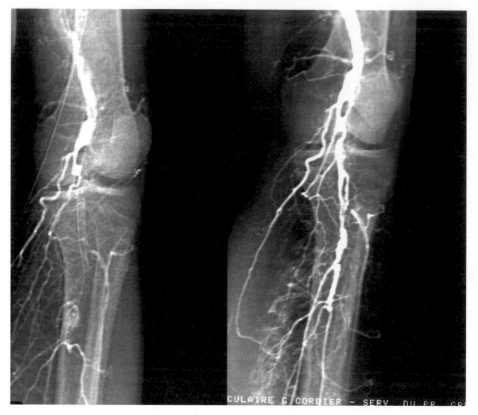

Fig. 17.9 Acute ischemia due to the complete occlusion of a popliteal aneurysm. The initial angiogram (left) shows no outflow arteries. The angiogram after local thrombolysis (right) shows the outflow arteries. Bypass surgery must follow rapidly to avoid rethrombosis.

which would increase the risk of a reconstruction. Duplex ultrasonography of the saphenous veins is also required to check their usability.

The second stage is acute ischemia after thrombotic occlusion of the aneurysm. Silent, progressive embolic destruction of the arterial outflow of arteries of the leg and the foot during the months or years preceding the acute event explains the high rate of failure and secondary amputation after surgery for acute ischemia following occlusion of a popliteal aneurysm. The best solution currently available involves local thrombolysis to restore the immediately prethrombotic status, followed by definitive surgical reconstruction (Fig. 17.9).

Aortoiliac occlusive disease

Most often, patients are seen for claudication. Owing to the extensiveness of lesions, claudication may be severe or progress to rest pain or gangrene, even if aortoiliac disease is isolated. However, the severity of symptoms is most frequently the consequence of concomitant infrainguinal occlusive disease. The distribution of atherosclerosis along the aortoiliac tree varies, but frequent sites for plaques are the dorsal wall of the aorta (Fig. 17.10), particularly around the ostia of intercostal and lumbar arteries, the ostium of the celiac, mesenteric, and

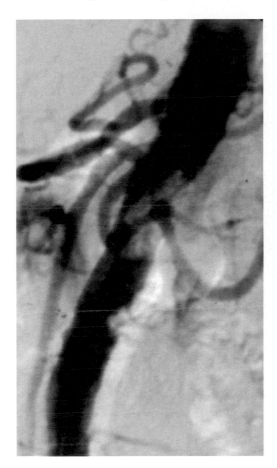

Fig. 17.10 Aortography showing a calcified plaque of the dorsal aortic wall responsible for ESRF and claudication of the thighs.

renal arteries, the ostia of iliac arteries, and the dorso-medial wall of common, external, and internal iliac arteries. Depending on this distribution, other symptoms may add to those affecting the lower extremities. Embolic events through the intercostal arteries are rare but can induce paraplegia or paraparesis if the intercostal artery involved gives rise to spinal arteries such as the artery of Adamkiewicz. Lesions at the origin of celiac or mesenteric arteries may induce visceral ischemia. Embolic events arising from such lesions lead typically to diffuse or localized intestinal infarcts. The management of such infarcts falls beyond the scope of this chapter but typically requires intestinal resection. More frequently, lesions at the origin of celiac or mesenteric arteries provoke intestinal angina. Abdominal pain or diarrhea occurring 30–60 minutes after meals and especially during hemodialysis is particularly characteristic (Fig. 17.11).

As already mentioned, lesions at the origin of the renal arteries may have participated in the genesis of ESRF. Lesions of the aortic bifurcation and of the iliac arteries are by far the most frequent. It is generally through a hemodynamic mechanism that these lesions provoke symptoms in the lower limbs, especially as far as claudication is concerned. However, embolic events from these lesions are not rare, although less than that observed with AAAs. Severe lesions of the hypogastric arteries, like those of the profunda femoris, impair the col-

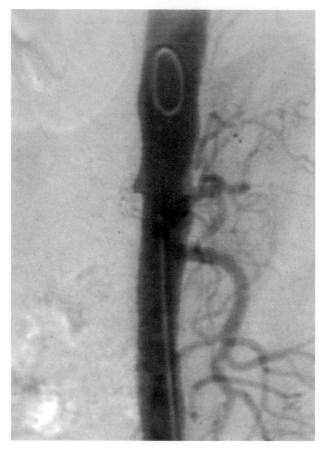

Fig. 17.11 Aortography showing total occlusion of the celiac and mesenteric arteries in a patient with abdominal pain after meals and during dialysis.

lateral circulation and lessen the tolerance for a given lesion of the common or external iliac arteries. If bilateral, hypogastric lesions can lead to sexual impotence.

Lesions of conduit arteries, like the common and external iliac and the common and superficial femoral arteries, are the most frequent among non-diabetic ESRF patients. Disease at these levels must be seen as segmental, even if focal lesions prevail, and may worsen with time. The segmental character of disease is particularly important to understand for the external iliac arteries and explains many failures of transluminal angioplasty at this level. In addition, the external iliac artery is the most widely used for the vascular anastomosis of a renal allograft. A frequent mistake is the use of a mildly diseased external iliac artery for such a connection. Transplant surgeons must bear in mind that after trauma due to handling and cross-clamping of a diseased external iliac artery, intimal hyperplasia and spontaneous worsening of the iliac lesions may develop with time, threatening the allograft and provoking ischemia of the lower limb (Fig. 17.12). Only perfect external iliac arteries should be used for the anastomosis of a renal allograft. In the absence of healthy external iliac arteries, we recommend the use of other donor native arterial sites or, on occasion, anastomosing the renal allograft to a prosthetic aortofemoral bypass (Fig. 17.13). Otherwise, the

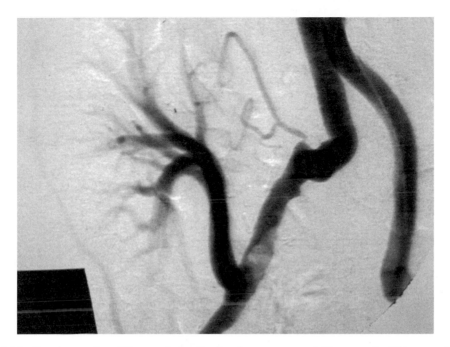

Fig. 17.12 Renal transplant failure and claudication from an external iliac stenosis. This stenosis was mild at the time of kidney transplant but evolved rapidly after transplantation.

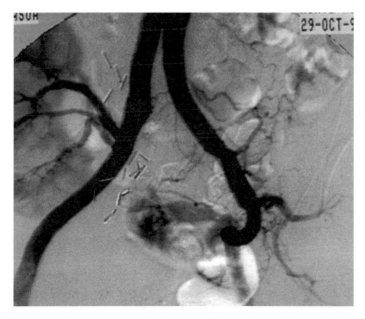

Fig. 17.13 Kidney transplant anastomosed to an aortobifemoral prosthetic graft. Such an approach is necessary when the donor aortoiliac arteries of the recipient are less than perfect to avoid problems shown Fig. 17.12.

conjunction of a failing renal allograft and ischemia of the lower limb may cause problems. Unaffected hypogastrics and profunda femoris arteries permit the development of a collateral circuit. In diabetics, muscular arteries of distribution, like the hypogastric and the profunda femoris, are impaired at an early phase of the disease, leaving fewer sites for a development of collateral circuits. Even in the absence of diabetes, the presence of lesions of the hypogastric arteries is indicative of the severity of atherosclerotic disease.

Clinical diagnosis of aortoiliac occlusive disease is generally made with the absence or the diminution of one or both femoral pulses and the presence of an iliofemoral bruit. However, excellent femoral pulses may be present at rest. Even if MR-angiography gives more promising results, duplex scanning is the best non-invasive investigation technique available if carried out by an experienced operator. Only cases of marked obesity prevent obtaining a good investigation using duplex scanning. However, in most cases, aortography remains necessary for the planning of revascularization.

An increasingly extensive therapeutic armamentarium allows for individualized approaches for each patient. Direct open surgical revascularization is the most invasive procedure but gives the most complete and durable results. Given the segmental characteristics of aortoiliac occlusive disease, aorto(bi)femoral prosthetic bypass is the best choice for low-risk patients, even though selected cases may benefit from unilateral iliac or iliofemoral bypass or endarterectomy. Use of the proximal infrarenal aorta as a donor artery requires excellent and durable inflow. If the patient is to be a renal allograft recipient, the prosthetic graft offers an excellent donor site for anastomosing the transplanted kidney with better long-term results than those had a diseased native iliac artery been used. Visceral arterial or hypogastric occlusive disease is easily treated using the same incision (Fig. 17.14). However, direct open surgery necessitates deep general anesthesia, laparotomy, and aortic cross-clamping. It is, therefore, reserved for low-risk ESRF patients.

Preoperative work-up is of a paramount importance among ESRF patients having to undergo open surgery. The cardiac status must be precisely evaluated with echocardiography and coronary angiography if doubt persists. Irreversible coronary insufficiency must deter from direct open surgery. Significant silent coronary disease is more and more frequently identified during the preoperative work-up of candidates for open surgical aortoiliac reconstruction. Multidisciplinary discussion of the choice between a less invasive technique of revascularization of the lower limbs or the combination of open direct surgery with coronary artery bypass or angioplasty must take place in those cases. In this discussion, which falls outside the scope of the present chapter, not only the immediate cardiac tolerance of aortoiliac direct surgery must be taken into account but also the fact that the preoperative work-up offers an opportunity for an attempt at extending life expectancy of these patients. Respiratory insufficiency must also be taken into account in the preoperative work-up. Severe chronic obstructive pulmonary disease patients are best treated using limited retroperitoneal incisions or with less invasive techniques. An assessment of all general metabolic functions is necessary before open direct aortoiliac reconstruction. The evaluation of hepatic and hemostatic liver function is most important if severe intraoperative or postoperative hemorrhage is to be avoided. Severe concomitant cerebrovascular occlusive disease is frequent and easily treated preoperatively.

For higher risk patients, endovascular methods of revascularization and extra-anatomic bypass are available and permit limb salvage and treatment of severe claudication in selected cases.[6] Transluminal angioplasty, once the only endovascular method available, remains the core tool of less invasive revascularization. Technological and technical improvements, better

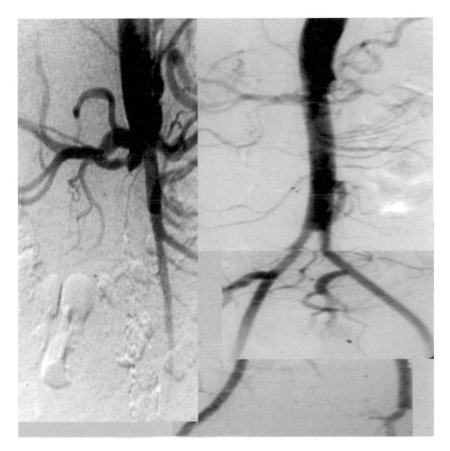

Fig. 17.14 Leriche syndrome with claudication of both legs and sexual impotence in an ESRF patient. Preoperative aortogram (left). Postoperative aortogram (right) showing a good result and revascularization of both hypogastrics, both femoral arteries, and the inferior mesenteric artery using a prosthetic aortic graft.

knowledge of indications, and the addition of new techniques like stenting, thrombolysis, clot aspiration, and instrumental closed recanalization continue to extend the potential of endovascular surgery. However, to obtain not only an immediate result but also long-term success, indications must be carefully observed. The best indications for the endovascular techniques are very short lesions, ideally concentric and non-calcified, of the common iliac, especially if they are located at a distance from bifurcations (Fig. 17.15). Other lesions that are amenable to endovascular revascularization are short occlusions or longer stenoses of the infrarenal aorta or the external or internal iliac arteries, stenoses at the bifurcations, and lesions of the visceral arteries. However, one must bear in mind that the more remote the indication from the ideal case, the higher the risk of immediate or long-term failure. Once the only solution when direct open surgery is contraindicated, extra-anatomic bypass has a very limited place owing to the development of endovascular surgery. Axillofemoral bypass must, however, be distinguished from crossed femoral bypass as the former is really only used when nothing else is possible, given its poor long-term results, and the latter offers sufficient hemodynamics for long-term results.

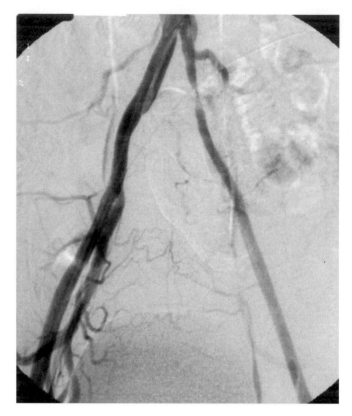

Fig. 17.15 Good indication for a transluminal angioplasty of a stenosis of the left common iliac artery.

Femoral and infrainguinal occlusive disease

Occlusive disease of the iliofemoral junction and the femoral bifurcation is frequent among ESRF patients where the most prominent pattern is the calcified plaque arising from the dorsal arterial wall or the ostia of the superficial femoral artery or the profunda femoris arteries. Given the place of the femoral bifurcation as the main site in the anastomotic net of the root of the inferior limb, the hemodynamic and, thus, clinical consequences of its occlusive disease are significant, and include claudication and rest pain or tissue loss if infrainguinal disease is also present. The femoral bifurcation is of very easy surgical access, even under local anesthesia, rendering direct open revascularization using endarterectomy, patch angioplasty, or bypass the method of choice at this level, even for high-risk ESRF patients.

Infrainguinal occlusive disease is the most frequent cause of critical limb ischemia among ESRF patients. It is almost constant after some years in ESRF, but may also remain asymptomatic for years or only cause claudication. In this context, control of risk factors and especially tobacco use is, in general, sufficient to obtain good clinical results, rendering surgical or endovascular indications limited at this level for claudication. Endovascular or surgical infrainguinal revascularization has limited expectancy of patency. The result of distal bypass depends highly on the availability of limited autologous venous grafts. Infrainguinal revascularization must be seen principally as an instrument of limb salvage. Rest pain, acute ischemia, and tissue loss constitute its indication. These conditions are generally considered as the end-stage of arterial disease and are often precipitated by a local or a general factor. Trauma, especially that caused by ill-adapted footwear and infection, is the best known local triggering factor, particularly among diabetics. Cutaneous complications of immunosuppressive drugs are often seen as local initiators of tissue loss. General factors include congestive heart failure and edema. Such general factors can doom revascularization to failure and must, therefore, be controlled before it. The existence of such general factors must be suspected particularly when perfusion of the ischemic limb appears to be dependent on blood volume or pressure.

There are three simple steps in approaching infrainguinal arterial occlusive disease: (1) impute tissue loss to ischemia; (2) identify culprit arterial lesions and a patent outflow; and (3) revascularize. The first step is based on clinical examination of tissue loss, analysis of symptoms, the absence of pulses, and duplex-scanning, and seldom necessitates more sophisticated methods. The gold standard for the second stage remains the arteriogram. The technique of this investigative method must be irreproachable and provide excellent images. In practice, and in the absence of aortoiliac occlusive disease, conventional arteriograms using direct femoral punction provide the best results. Most frequently, the addition of femoral, popliteal, and infrapopliteal stenoses is responsible for tissue loss, which explains why treatment most frequently is best achieved through a distal bypass using a saphenous autograft. However, in selected cases where an isolated and short culprit arterial lesion is identified, transluminal angioplasty or recanalization may offer good results as well.

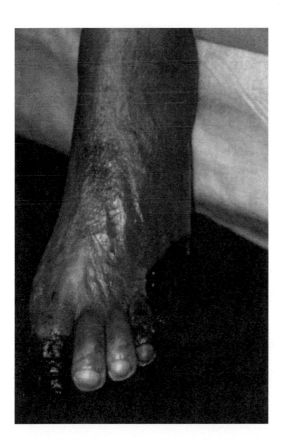

Fig. 17.16 Gangrene of the foot in an ESRF patient.

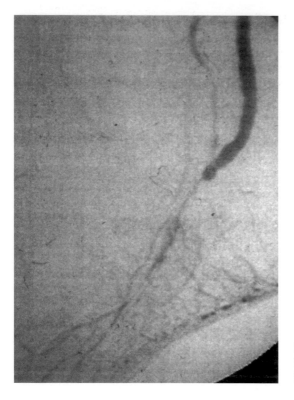

Fig. 17.17   A distal posterior tibial saphenous bypass achieves limb salvage in the case shown in Fig. 17.16.

It is increasingly rare that revascularization is not feasible. Even distal diseased arteries of the foot may provide a sufficient run-off for a bypass (Figs 17.16 and 17.7). However, the odds of success in the short term and especially the long term remain very dependent on the availability of a suitable venous autograft, the other materials giving poor results in this setting. The development of reversed or *in situ* saphenous bypass has reduced the rate of primary major amputation. The technical choice between reversed or *in situ* bypass remains a question of personal preference for surgeons, even if *in situ* bypass is technically easier to perform. The most difficult problem is how to perform a distal bypass in the absence of a suitable saphenous graft of sufficient length. Saphenous veins are sufficiently easy to visualize at duplex scanning to recommend this investigation in the preoperative work-up of distal bypass. Alternative autologous veins are the contralateral greater saphenous vein, the lesser saphenous veins, and the veins of the arms. However, none of these alternative solutions is ideal as there is frequent contralateral occlusive infrainguinal disease, the lesser saphenous vein is often too thin and too short for use, and the veins of superior limbs are a precious capital for angioaccess. Since prostheses give poor results when used in long segments, composite bypass using the available length of venous graft and with a prosthetic complement to optimize length may represent a solution. Other solutions await validation, including the use of endarterectomized segments of occluded autogenous arteries such as the superficial femoral artery, arterial or venous allografts, and prostheses with venous cuffs or distal AVF. Such low-flow revascularizations require long-term anticoagulation, in our experience. Distal minor amputations and debridement of infected lesions are often necessary, even after successful revascularization, and extend the duration of the hospital stay. In this setting, the development of multidisciplinary centers of foot-care is highly desirable. Efficiency of distal bypass has as its principal cost the duration of the operation. Even under locoregional anesthesia, this duration may constitute an ordeal for very high-risk cardiac ESRF patients. It is in these situations that primary amputation below or above the knee is still considered reasonable.

Reported results of limb salvage surgery are less favorable among ESRF patients than among non-ESRF patients, especially in cases of diabetes. Operative mortality rates average 9% (2–15%), depending essentially on the type of recruitment and selection of patients. The reported rates of limb salvage at 2 years vary from 70 to 90%. A certain number of amputations remain necessary for the control of infection despite successful revascularization.[7–11]

Arterial disease of the upper extremities

Apart from their unquestioned functional interest, the upper extremities of ESRF patients host angioaccess settings of a vital importance. Years of ESRF and associated diseases like diabetes mellitus, on the one hand, and the proper consequences of AVF, on the other, contribute to damage to the arterial bed of the superior limb. As any artery with a distal AVF, arteries of the upper extremity anastomosed to the angioaccess site enlarge moderately. Over years, this enlargement may become aneurysmal and expose the patient to the same complications as any aneurysm, namely thromboembolism and rupture (Fig. 17.18). For this reason, the donor artery of an angioaccess must be regularly surveyed with duplex-scanning. Aneurysms are easily treated by segmental replacement using saphenous autografts or even prostheses if suitable autografts are not available.

Much more frequent is the deterioration of the arterial bed distal to the AVF. The AVF adds hemodynamic steal to the effects of arterial occlusive disease with important consequences like digital rest pain or gangrene. Classically, such cases are treated with suppression of the AVF, establishment of angioaccess on another limb, and cervicodorsal sympathectomy. It is, indeed, becoming more and more frequent that endovascular or surgical arterial repair permits the conservation of the angioaccess along with limb salvage.

Conclusion

Peripheral arterial disease that may threaten the life expectancy and the quality of life of ESRF patients is more often amenable to revascularization than generally thought. All ESRF and kidney transplanted patients must be considered vasculopaths and surveyed for peripheral vascular disease.

References

1. Plecha EJ, King TA, Pitluk HC, Rubin JR (1993). Risk assessment in patients undergoing carotid endarterectomy. *Cardiovasc Surg*; 1:30–2.
2. Koskas F, Kieffer E, AURC (1997). Long-term survival after elective repair of intrarenal abdominal aortic aneurysm: results of a prospective multicentric study. *Ann Vasc Surg*; 11:473–81.
3. Koskas F, Kieffer E, AURC (1997). Surgery for ruptured abdominal aortic aneurysm: early and late results of a prospective study by the AURC in 1989. *Ann Vasc Surg*; 11:90–9.
4. Cohen JR, Mannick JA, Couch NP, Wittemore AD (1986). Abdominal aortic aneurysm repair in patients with preoperative renal failure. *J Vasc Surg*; 3:867–70.
5. Johnston KW (1989). Multicenter prospective study of nonruptured abdominal aortic aneurysm. Part II. Variables predicting morbidity and mortality. *J Vasc Surg*; 9:437–47.

(18 years and over), were included in that year. Blood pressure was measured by a nurse or doctor using a standard mercury sphygmomanometer. Blood tests were performed when abnormal urinalysis, hypertension, or any other significant problems were encountered, or upon the participant's request. Because the cost of the blood test was not paid for by the government, it was not mandatory.

The OKIDS registry defined patients with ESRF as follows: people who (1) are resident in Okinawa, (2) have chronic renal failure, and (3) have survived at least 1 month on scheduled dialysis therapy. The prognoses of ESRF patients were traced by reviewing medical records and/or by interviewing physicians and paramedical staff.[3] Strokes were diagnosed by both clinical symptoms and computed tomography (CT) of the head, which was performed within 48 hours of the initial symptoms and repeated if necessary. A CT scan of the head was also performed in almost all patients with clinical disorders related to strokes.[10] We registered only definite cases of stroke as determined by both clinical symptoms and CT scan, so patients who had suffered asymptomatic stroke were not included. Both first-ever and subsequent strokes were registered.

The cumulative incidence of stroke was calculated to be the ratio of the number of cases of stroke to the number of patients at risk, expressed per 1000 patient-years. The observation period was the sum of the duration of dialysis during the study period in each gender- and age-class, expressed in patient-years. The latter was calculated from the start of the study or the beginning of dialysis (whichever came later) until death, renal transplantation, transfer to another part of Japan, or the end of the study period (whichever came earlier). Multiple logistic analysis was performed on age and other variables simultaneously. The dependent variable in this model was binary: the presence or absence of a stroke in the subject. Statistical analysis was performed using an SAS statistical package.

Epidemiology of stroke in ESRF patients

We prospectively examined the incidence of stroke in both dialysis patients and the general population over a 3-year period from 1 April 1988 to 31 March 1991.[11] A total of 1609 dialysis patients (674 female and 935 male) were observed for a total observation period of 3576 patient-years (1533 among females and 2043 among males). We observed a total of 41 strokes, which were distributed as 8 thrombo(embolic) cerebral infarctions, 31 cerebral hemorrhages, and 2 subarachnoid hemorrhages. The incidence per 1000 patient-years of stroke, thrombo(embolic) cerebral infarction, cerebral hemorrhage, and subarachnoid hemorrhage was 11.5, 2.2, 8.7, and 0.6, respectively. The relative incidence (observed/expected ratio), when compared with the general population, was 5.2 for stroke, 2.0 for thrombo(embolic) cerebral infarction, 10.7 for cerebral hemorrhage, and 4.0 for subarachnoid hemorrhage. Cerebral hemorrhages occurred an average of 10 years earlier in ESRF patients (mean age 52.6 ± 2.4 years) than in the general population (63.4 ± SD 15.0 years). Mean (SD) age at the onset of cerebral infarction was 63.0 (9.6) years in the ESRF patients and 69.9 (12.8) years in the general population. The ratio of thrombo(embolic) cerebral infarction to cerebral hemorrhage was 1.4:1.0 (1.5:1.0 for males and 1.4:1.0 for females) in the general population, whereas it was 0.26:1.0 (0.3:1.0 in males and 0.18:1.0 in females) in ESRF patients.

Figure 18.1 shows the cumulative incidence of stroke by age and gender in the general population and in the dialysis patients. Dialysis patients have a higher incidence of stroke irrespective of age and gender. It is noteworthy that stroke, and cerebral hemorrhagic stroke in particular, occurred at significantly higher rates in the ESRF patients than in the general population.[11] Accordingly, the life expectancy of ESRF patients is obviously shorter than

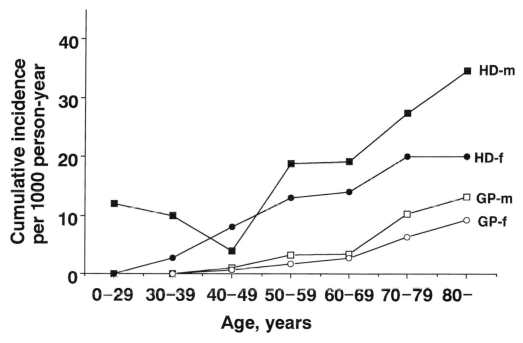

Fig. 18.1 Cumulative incidence of stroke per 1000 person-years. HD, hemodialysis patients; GP, general population; m, male; f, female. Data were derived from reference 11 for the ESRF patients and from reference 6 for the general population.

that of the general population, and considerably so in younger patients (Fig. 18.2). The life expectancy was 42.9 years (women) and 37.6 years (men) in the general population, but 27.7 years (women) and 24.3 years (men) in the dialysis patients at age 40. This is partly explained by the high incidence of stroke. The difference in life expectancy between the general population and ESRF patients is less in older people, demonstrating the benefits of dialysis treatment for prolonging life in this group. This benefit may be a consequence of a 'catch-up' phenomenon for non-dialysis patients, or it may be a consequence of better medical care and observation, as dialysis patients are under frequent medical supervision. However, the decision to undergo this treatment depends on many socio-economic factors in both the family and the community. For example, all patients must consider the possibility that uremic or hypertensive encephalopathy, which can be reversed after only a few dialysis treatments, may be replaced by senile dementia, which cannot be cured.

Our observation is similar to reports from France[4] and other parts of Japan.[12] However, the stroke-related mortality rate is different between Japan (12.7%)[13] and the USA (4.8%).[14] This could be explained by the difference in renal transplantation. In Okinawa, the stroke mortality rate, per 1000 patient-years, was 1.5 for renal transplant recipient and 10.9 for dialysis patients.[15] One possible explanation for this different rate could be the difference in renal transplantation between countries.

Risk factors for stroke in ESRF patients

To identify the risk factors for stroke in dialysis patients, we conducted a prospective study, from 1991 to 1995, of 1243 chronic hemodialysis patients (524 female and 719 male).[16] The

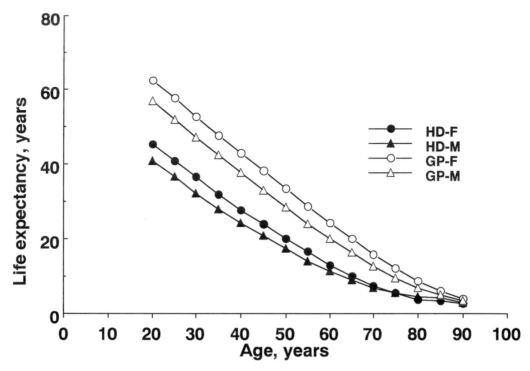

Fig. 18.2 Comparison between the life expectancy of the ESRF patients and the general population in Okinawa (1990). HD, hemodialysis patients; GP, general population; F, female; M, male.

mean age and duration of hemodialysis at the start of the study was 52.2 years and 61.9 months, respectively. Two hundred and eleven subjects (17.0%) were diabetic. In most of the patients (N = 1041, 83.7%), hemodialysis was performed three times a week. In 708 patients (57.0%), hemodialysis lasted 3.5–4.0 hours per session. Hypertensive patients were defined as those having a diastolic blood pressure of 90 mmHg or higher, those having a systolic blood pressure of 140 mmHg or higher, or those for whom treatment of hypertension had been implemented. Patients with dyslipidemia were defined as having a serum cholesterol level greater than 220 mg/dl or less than 150 mg/dl, or having a serum triglyceride level greater than 180 mg/dl or less than 40 mg/dl.

Of the 1243 patients studied, 342 (27.5%) died, 45 (3.6%) underwent renal transplantation, and 12 (1.0%) were transferred outside Okinawa by the end of 1995. Seventy-eight (22.8%) of the deaths were cardiac in nature, 62 (18.1%) were due to infection, 56 (16.4%) followed withdrawal from dialysis treatment, 26 (7.6%) were sudden, 67 (19.6%) were a consequence of vascular problems including strokes, and 53 (15.5%) were due to other causes.[5]

During the 5-year period, we observed 90 strokes distributed as 63 cerebral hemorrhages, 20 thrombo(embolic) cerebral infarctions, and 7 subarachnoid hemorrhages. The incidence per 1000 patient-years of stroke, cerebral hemorrhage, thrombo(embolic) cerebral infarction, and subarachnoid hemorrhage was 17.6, 12.3, 3.9, and 1.4, respectively. The cumulative incidence of stroke increased linearly with the duration of dialysis, reaching approximately 8.6% after 5 years (Fig. 18.3).

Multiple logistic analysis identified hypertension as an independent predictor of stroke, with an odds ratio of 2.38 and a 95% confidence interval ranging from 1.26 to 4.50. This

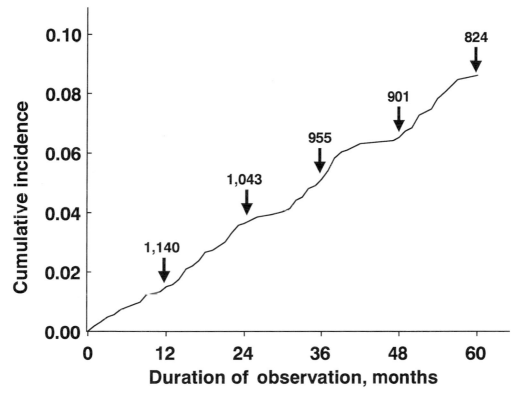

Fig. 18.3 Cumulative incidence of stroke, calculated by the Kaplan–Meier method. Numbers above the line are the number of dialysis patients at risk. The observation period was from 1 January 1991 to 31 December 1995. Reproduced from reference 16, with permission.

study confirmed a previous report showing the high prevalence of hypertension in dialysis patients who sustain strokes.[11] However, other possible risk factors for stroke (for example, dyslipidemia, diabetes mellitus, smoking, and the duration of dialysis) were not identified as significant predictors of stroke (Table 18.1).

From 1971 to 1997 we observed significant changes in patient demographics. The study group was divided into six subgroups according to comorbid predialysis conditions. These subgroups, consisting of patients who suffered from atherosclerotic heart disease, chronic obstructive pulmonary disease, peripheral vascular disease, malignancy, cerebrovascular disease, or other miscellaneous conditions, were registered after a review of their medical charts.[3,17] Such comorbid conditions were found to have a significant impact on survival in ESRF patients.[18] The frequency of positive comorbid conditions increased with each decade, from 5.6% in 1971–1980 to 15.5% in 1981–1990[3] to 20.0% in 1991–1997. There was a significant, linear relationship between the annual entry rate into the registry, the prevalence rate, and age at the start of dialysis, and the year dialysis treatment began.[3] It is still uncertain whether the higher entry rate can be explained by the increasing incidence of renal disease or of the referral rate of ESRF patients.

We have observed a gradual increase in stroke incidence with the introduction of erythropoietin in 1990.[19] The annual incidence of stroke was 12.5 (1988), 10.5 (1989), 12.7 (1990), 14.0 (1991), and 17.5 (1992), per 1000 patient-years, respectively. However, it is unknown

Table 18.1   Multiple logistic analysis of clinical predictors of stroke in chronic hemodialysis patients[a]

Predictor	Odds ratio (95% confidence interval) Unadjusted	Adjusted[b]
Male (vs. female)	1.42 (0.91–2.23)	1.22 (0.75–1.99)
Age (vs. <35 years)	1.10 (0.94–1.30)	1.16 (0.97–1.38)
Hypertension (vs. normotension)	2.41 (1.30–4.49)	2.38 (1.26–4.50)
Diabetes mellitus (vs. non-DM)	1.24 (0.72–2.12)	1.14 (0.63–2.06)
Smoker (vs. non-smoker)	1.46 (0.91–2.34)	1.35 (0.81–2.24)
Dyslipidemia (vs. normal)	1.01 (0.64–1.58)	0.96 (0.61–1.52)
Duration of dialysis (vs. <60 months)	1.13 (0.86–1.50)	1.24 (0.93–1.67)

[a]Reproduced from reference 16, with permission.
[b]Adjusted for other predictors.
DM is diabetes mellitus. Hypertension is defined as diastolic blood pressure ≥ 90 mmHg, systolic blood pressure is ≥ 140 mmHg, or treatment of hypertension already implemented. Dyslipidemia is defined as serum cholesterol >220 mg/dl or <150 mg/dl, or serum triglyceride >180 mg/dl or <40 mg/dl. Duration of dialysis is categorized as <60 months, 60–119 months, and 120 months.

whether erythropoietin use was the cause of this increase, given the rapid changes in patient demographics. A higher incidence of women, aged patients, and diabetic patients are erythropoietin users compared with erythropoietin non-users. Currently, the annual number of stroke cases is approximately 30 per 1000 patient-years. The hematocrit level achieved with erythropoietin therapy is variable. In our registry, the target hematocrit has been set empirically at approximately 30–35% before the hemodialysis session. Recently, it has been shown that mortality rate is higher in patients with a hemoglobin concentration below 10 g/dl, but that there is no benefit associated with values exceeding 11 g/dl.[20] One of the possible confounding factors would be an increase of blood pressure in response to erythropoietin therapy, in association with the correction of anemia. Such an increase occurs more frequently in the case of a rapid rise of hematocrit. Since rapid correction of anemia by erythropoietin can cause hypertensive encephalopathy,[21] and therefore should be avoided.

Malnutrition and hypoalbuminemia are common in ESRF patients and are significant predictors of mortality.[5,22,23] Patients with a low diastolic blood pressure also have a high mortality rate.[24] Such patients may have severe heart failure, infection, cachexia, and withdrawal of dialysis before sustaining a stroke. Neither a J-shaped nor a U-shaped relationship was observed between the incidence of stroke and blood pressure, as shown by the stroke recurrence rate in the non-ESRF population.[25]

Comparison of risk factors for stroke between ESRF patients and the general population

To learn more about the risk of stroke in dialysis patients, we analyzed data from OGHMA and COSMO[26] or OGHMA and OKIDS registries simultaneously.[9,27] By using names, genders, birth dates, and ZIP codes, candidates were identified in both registries. If needed, further confirmation was provided by chart review.

Among the OGHMA participants, a total of 38 053 participants (17 859 men and 20 194 women) had data on serum cholesterol. The median serum cholesterol level was 180–

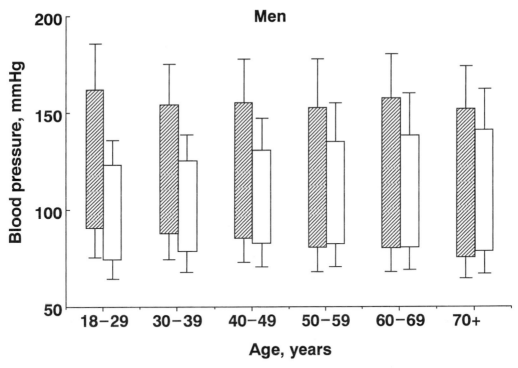

Fig. 18.4 Comparison of the mean (SD) levels of systolic and diastolic blood pressure in the general population[8,9] (□) and ESRF patients[5,16] (▨) for men.

189 mg/dl in both genders. Serum cholesterol levels varied widely, with a minimum level of 66 mg/dl and a maximum level of 748 mg/dl. The screened subjects were grouped into quartiles according to their basal serum cholesterol level: 167 mg/dl, 168–191 mg/dl, 192–217 mg/dl, and 218 mg/dl. The mean (SD) serum cholesterol level in each quartile was 149.3 (14.1), 179.8 (6.8), 203.7 (7.4), and 245.3 (26.9), respectively.[26]

At the time of this report, we have determined the following:

1. Mean levels of blood pressure in dialysis patients were higher than those of the general population, and in particular those of both younger men (Fig. 18.4) and women (Fig. 18.5).

2. The cumulative incidence of stroke increased with blood pressure both in the general population and in the ESRF patients. Dialysis patients had a higher incidence of stroke even in the normal range of blood pressure (Fig. 18.6).

3. The cumulative incidence of cerebral hemorrhage was inversely correlated with serum cholesterol levels in the general population. The mean levels of serum cholesterol were approximately 20 mg/dl lower in dialysis patients than in the general population. The mean (SD) serum cholesterol was 163.8 (41.1) mg/dl ($N = 114$), ranging from 99 to 281 mg/dl.

4. The role of cholesterol may be different among the various subtypes of stroke, such as cerebral hemorrhage and thrombo(embolic) cerebral infarction. Whereas, dyslipidemia itself is not a significant predictor of stroke in general,[16] several lines of evidence have

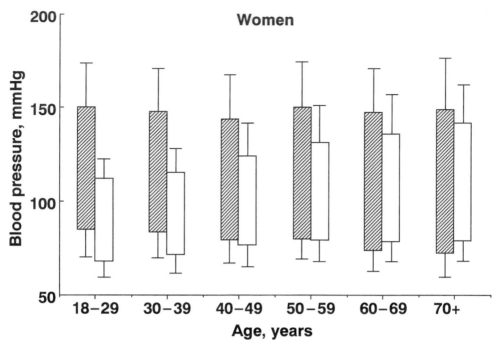

Fig. 18.5 Comparison of the mean (SD) levels of systolic and diastolic blood pressure in the general population[8,9] (□) and ESRF[5,16] patients (▨) for women.

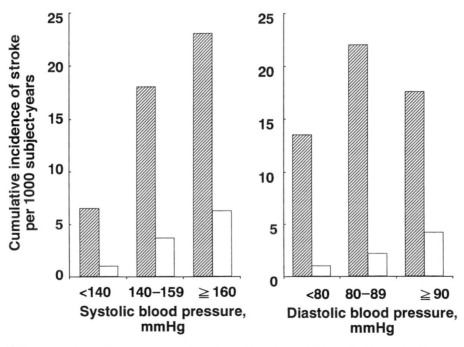

Fig. 18.6 Comparison of the cumulative incidence of stroke at different levels of blood pressure in the general population (□) and in ESRF patients (▨).

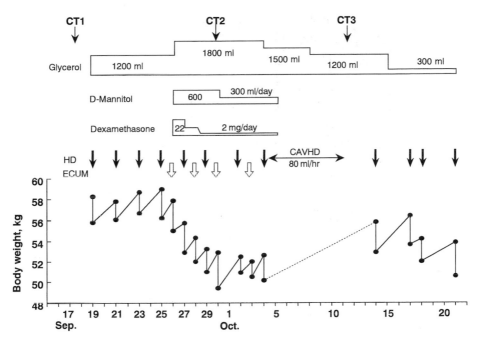

Fig. 18.7 Clinical course of a hemodialysis patient with cerebral hemorrhage. CT, computed tomography head scan; HD, hemodialysis; ECUM, extracorporeal ultrafiltration method; CAVHD, continuous arteriovenous hemodiafiltration.

shown that the incidence of cerebral hemorrhage is inversely correlated with serum cholesterol.[28,29]

Treatment of stroke in patients on dialysis treatment

Case presentation

A 53-year-old man was referred to us because of right hemiplegia and dysphagia 36 hours after his most recent hemodialysis session. He had been on intermittent hemodialysis for 5 hours, three times per week since 1977. The blood pressure was 196/100 mmHg, body temperature 39.1°C, plasma glucose 113 mg/dl, blood urea nitrogen (BUN) 57 mg/dl, plasma creatinine 10.8 mg/dl, sodium 138 meq/l, potassium 4.5 meq/l, chloride 107 meq/l, arterial pH 7.39, pCO_2 33.4 mmHg, and pO_2 98.9 mmHg. The clinical course is summarized in Fig. 18.7.

A CT scan of the head showed hemorrhage in the left hemisphere, 5.0 cm in size, with some surrounding edema (Fig. 18.8, CT1). In addition to standard hemodialysis, 1200–1800 ml of glycerol was infused per day to reduce cerebral edema, but this was not effective. The patient lost consciousness and there were signs of increased intracranial pressure. A second CT scan (Fig. 18.9, CT2) revealed an increase in cerebral edema. To remove excess fluid from the brain, isolated ultrafiltration and continuous arteriovenous hemodiafiltration (CAVHD) were initiated. The patient's body weight decreased to 50 kg, 6 kg lower than before the hemorrhagic event. The cerebral edema disappeared following this procedure and the patient's clinical condition gradually improved, as shown by a third CT scan (Fig. 18.10, CT3). The patient is now rehabilitated.

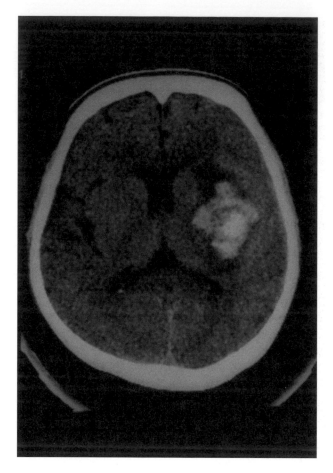

Fig. 18.8 The computed tomography head scan (CT1) taken on the day of the onset of cerebral hemorrhage.

Comments

The prognosis following cerebral hemorrhage is very poor in hemodialysis patients. The acute mortality rate (within 30 days after the onset of the event) is 74.4% in the these patients,[11] in contrast only 12.3% in the general population.[6] The size of the hemorrhage tends to be larger in hemodialysis patients than in the general population,[11,30] which may account for the higher acute mortality. Even in the general population, the prognosis is very poor in patients with a large bleed (>6 cm diameter).[6]

The relationship between the use of heparin and the size of the hemorrhage is not clear. The mean length of time between the most recent hemodialysis and the onset of cerebral hemorrhage was 35.5 hours,[11] by which time the effects of heparin had already disappeared. It is advisable to avoid the use of heparin within 24 hours after the onset of bleeding. However, the clinical significance of heparin use remains to be determined. If the patient has been prescribed warfarin as an anticoagulant, its effect should be reversed quickly with vitamin K and fresh frozen plasma.[31] Recently, Kawamura *et al.*[12] reported that there was no difference in the dose of heparin, the size of hematomas, or the frequency of intraventricular

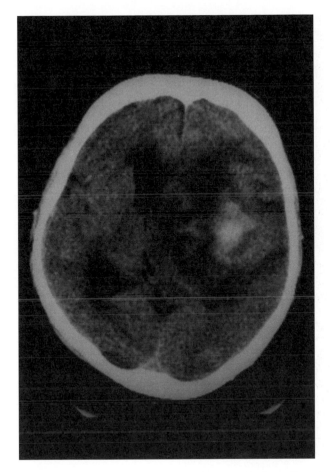

Fig. 18.9 The computed tomography head scan (CT2) taken 13 days after the onset of cerebral hemorrhage.

hemorrhage between patients with respectively early and late onset of cerebral hemorrhage after a previous hemodialysis session.

During the acute phase of stroke, lean body mass may be significantly reduced by factors such as low caloric intake and infection. Dry-weight should be monitored weekly. The serum potassium level may be increased or decreased.

Excessive bleeding tendency can be reduced by controlling uremia. However, choosing between hemodialysis and peritoneal dialysis can be difficult. Some prefer using peritoneal dialysis, to eliminate the risk of bleeding from heparin use. In the case presented above, we chose to perform hemodialysis with judicious use of nafamostat mesylate for two reasons. First, the patient had a good blood flow in his arteriovenous fistula. Second, we needed a high rate of ultrafiltration to reduce the cerebral edema.

This case suggests that an efficient reduction in cerebral edema can be achieved with a significant weight reduction. For this purpose, slow diffusion-dialysis, such as CAVHD, may be superior to regular hemodialysis because it can prevent dialysis dysequilibrium syndrome.[32,33] To assess the adequacy of cerebral perfusion, frequent monitoring of the state of alertness and other neurological signs is better than measuring blood pressure.[31]

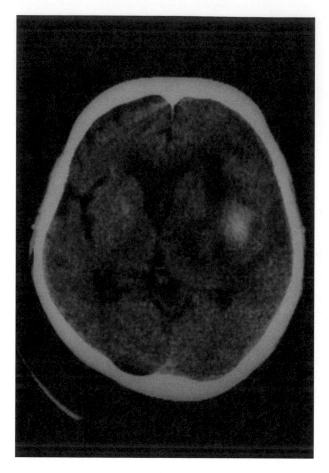

Fig. 18.10 The computed tomography head scan (CT3) taken 26 days after the onset cerebral hemorrhage.

Strategy for the prevention of stroke in ESRF patients

Strokes are a heavier burden for ESRF patients than for the general population. Therefore, every possible means of stroke prevention should be applied to ESRF patients. Table 18.2 summarizes the causes of a high incidence of stroke in ESRF patients.

Better control of uremia should lead to better control of hypertension and a lower mortality rate.[34] Platelet dysfunction due to uremia[35] is probably the underlying cause of the larger hemorrhagic lesions seen in dialysis patients. However, it is not realistic to prescribe a lengthy hemodialysis (such as Tassin[34]) in Japan, where the national average hemodialysis time has decreased from 4.12 hours in 1993 to 4.05 hours in 1996 for patients dialyzed three times a week.[36] In the general population, serum creatinine is a marker for increased risk of stroke even when within normal range.[37]

As shown in Figs 18.4 and 18.5, the mean blood pressure values in ESRF patients was higher than that of the general population. Antihypertensive drugs are commonly used, but

Table 18.2 Mechanistic basis for the high incidence of stroke in ESRF patients

1. Uremia
2. Hypertension
3. Predialysis comorbid conditions
4. Conditions associated with long-term dialysis
   Heparin use
   Malnutrition
   Vascular calcification
   Atherosclerosis
   Bioincompatible membrane
   Homocysteine
   C-reactive protein
   Bleeding diathesis of uremia

blood pressure is often inadequately controlled. In our survey, patients who were prescribed antihypertensives had a mean systolic (diastolic) blood pressure of 160.9 (84.6) mmHg, whereas those who were not prescribed antihypertensives had a mean systolic (diastolic) blood pressure of 141.3 (77.0) mmHg.[38] These data may, however, be misleading. Hypertensive patients can develop symptomatic hypotension during hemodialysis if they take antihypertensives, so they often refuse to take medications on the day of hemodialysis. Blood pressure is often volume-sensitive among hemodialysis patients. It is quite variable, and easily decreases by removing excess fluid. On the other hand, cross-sectional values of blood pressure (calculated from one pre-dialysis value) are quite similar to the mean levels calculated over 1 year (more than 150 dialysis sessions) (Fig. 18.11). The goal of blood pressure control should be approximately 130/85 mmHg in ESRF patients and not lower[39] since they all have target organ damage (even those without comorbid conditions other than ESRF). According to this target, our patients had uncontrolled systolic hypertension, even those who had not been prescribed antihypertensives.

Six hundred and forty-six patients in our study group (52.0%) were prescribed at least one antihypertensive drug.[38] Calcium channel blockers were used most frequently ($N = 552$, 80.8%), followed by angiotensin-converting enzyme (ACE) inhibitors ($N = 216$, 33.4%), beta blockers ($N = 159$, 24.6%), centrally acting agents ($N = 77$, 11.9%), alpha blockers ($N = 45$, 7.0%), and vasodilators ($N = 22$, 3.4%). ACE inhibitors may cause a decrease in hematocrit[40] as well as lead to an anaphylactoid reaction if used together with PAN AN-69 membrane dialyzers.[41] Both non-compliance[42] and the use of shortened hemodialysis times in adult patients may further increase the incidence of hypertension and lead to deterioration of nutritional status. It has been reported that more cardiovascular events are experienced by patients with salt-sensitive hypertension than patients with non-salt-sensitive hypertension.[43] ESRF patients commonly display salt-sensitive hypertension, as well as insulin-resistance, and 'non-dipping' while asleep (i.e. their blood pressure does not decrease overnight). The reason why such patients also have a high incidence of stroke remains unknown, but sodium sensitivity may provide a better estimate of blood pressure risk in these patients.[43]

An increasing number of aged and sick patients are currently accepted into the ESRF program.[3,44] These patients often suffer from cerebrovascular disease and autonomic nerve dysfunction.[45] In such patients, precise determination of dry-weight is very difficult as dry-weight was originally defined using young patients without comorbid conditions.[46]

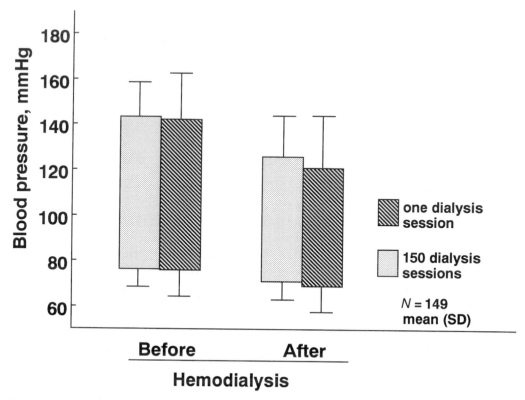

Fig. 18.11 Comparison of mean (SD) blood pressures measured at one dialysis session and over the course of 1 year (more than 150 dialysis sessions).

Occasional severe atherosclerotic changes in ESRF patients may make renal transplantation impossible.[47] In hemodialysis patients, vessel wall distensibility of the common carotid artery was shown to be lower than that of age-matched healthy subjects.[48] Asymptomatic cerebral infarction is frequently detected by head CT scan and magnetic resonance imaging. Decreased cerebral blood flow has been detected by positron emission tomography in long-term hemodialysis patients.[49] Thus, greater arterial stiffness may also contribute to the higher incidence of stroke. Whether dialysis therapy *per se* can accelerate atherosclerosis is still debatable.[50–52] Impaired cardiac function, which significantly correlates with the incidence of stroke and atheroembolic cerebral infarction, may be a prior condition that contributes to the acceleration of atherosclerosis and eventually to stroke. Atrial fibrillation, in particular, is a common precursor of stroke, especially embolic stroke in the general population.[53]

The role of nutrition in stroke, as measured by serum albumin and cholesterol, has not yet been clearly defined in our study. However, protein malnutrition has been linked to a higher incidence of cerebral hemorrhage among both the general population[54,55] and hemodialysis patients.[4] Although the mechanisms are not clear, hypoalbuminemia is associated with a hypercoagulable state and is related to the development of ischemic heart disease,[56] vascular access thrombosis,[57] and possibly ischemic stroke. Hypoalbuminemia directly affects red cell deformability and possibly endothelial function, and therefore would be an additional component of the risk factors that are associated with hypoalbuminemia.[58,58a]

During the past three decades, the stroke mortality rate decreased dramatically in Japan from 175.8 in 1965 to 99.4 per 100 000 people in 1992.[59] The precise reasons for this decrease are not clear.[60] On the other hand, in dialysis patients, the calculated gross stroke mortality rate was more than 800 per 100 000 patients.

Currently, the average life expectancy in Japan is the highest in the world. However, the incidence of stroke is higher than that for ischemic heart disease.[6] Serum C-reactive protein (CRP) is a good predictor of ischemic stroke.[61,62] Therefore, it is advisable to prevent any sort of tissue damage, such as infection or trauma, and to use biocompatible dialysis membranes to keep CRP levels low. Regarding the former, it has been shown that both bacterial and viral infection are risk factors for cerebrovascular ischemia.[63] CRP reflects the depletion of body protein, not inflammation.[64]

It was reported that hypoalbuminemia predisposes patients to hyperhomocysteinemia.[65] This observation became significant when prospectively obtained data confirmed that ESRF patients with increased homocysteine concentrations were more likely to develop fatal or non-fatal thrombotic or atherosclerotic complications.[66] Hyperhomocysteinemia can be partially corrected with the administration of folic acid, either alone or combined with vitamin B6 or B12.[67] In cases of clinically evident malnutrition in dialysis patients, administration of intradialytic-parenteral nutrition may be effective for reducing the risk of death and of stroke.[68]

Patients with polycystic kidney disease are at increased risk of subarachnoid hemorrhage from the rupture of intracranial aneurysms. Optional cerebral arteriography may be beneficial for young adults (less than 25 years old).[69] This procedure should precede the average age at which dialysis is initiated in patients with polycystic kidney disease (49.9 years in our study).[18] The benefits of non-invasive screening tests, such as CT scans, are not clear, and these cannot be routinely recommended.

An association between physical inactivity and an increased incidence of coronary heart disease is well known. However, no increased frequency of stroke was observed in patients with sedentary as opposed to active lifestyles.[53]

In summary, our study and other reports[70–72] have shown that blood pressure control is inadequate with current strategies of chronic hemodialysis, despite universal recognition of the role of hypertension in stroke. On the other hand, opinions may vary about the relative importance of hypertension in ESRF patients. We consider the average predialysis blood pressure levels of ESRF patients conventionally considered to be acceptable to be too high. Restriction of salt intake, maintenance of dry-weight, and use of antihypertensive drugs are good means of lowering blood pressure in ESRF patients. However, because of the rapid increase in the number of dialysis patients, these procedures may be neglected as they are time-consuming. Every dialysis patient should be informed about their risk of stroke and its poor prognosis. In this regard, we may need advance directives,[73] concerning the possibility of stopping long-term dialysis in all ESRF patients.[74]

Conclusions

We present clinico-epidemiological data collected since 1971 as part of the Okinawa Dialysis Study (OKIDS) of patients undergoing chronic dialysis due to end-stage renal failure (ESRF). OKIDS focused on a comparison of stroke incidence and risk factors in the general population (hospital-based) stroke registries in Okinawa, Japan. Strokes, in particular cerebral hemorrhage, were found to occur at a significantly higher rate in dialysis patients than in the general population. By logistic analysis, hypertension was demonstrated to be the single most reliable predictor of strokes; however, the risk was still elevated in dialysis patients with normal blood pressure. Therefore, the effects of uremia *per se* and malnutrition were thought to be the underlying causes of stroke. We suggest that strict blood pressure control, along with good nutritional support, should be effective in decreasing the incidence of stroke, particularly cerebral hemorrhages, in patients with ESRF. The shorter life expectancy of these patients, due in part to the high incidence of stroke, leads us to suggest further that current strategies of dialysis should be modified to place more emphasis on lowering blood pressure.

Acknowledgments

We thank the staff of the Okinawa Dialysis Study group and the Okinawa General Health Maintenance Association, and M. Itokazu in particular for retrieving data files from a 1983 health check. A complete list of physicians participating in OKIDS appears in reference 9. We are also grateful to Dr O. Morita from the Department of Physics, Kyushu University, Fukuoka, Japan, who wrote our computer program and made other technical suggestions. We thank Mrs C. Iseki for data processing and secretarial work, and Professor K. Fukiyama for his encouragement and valuable suggestions.

References

1. Hull AR, Parker III. (1990). Introduction and Summary. Proceedings from the Morbidity, Mortality and Prescription of Dialysis Symposium, Dallas, 15–17 September 1989. *American Journal of Kidney Diseases* 15, 375–85.
2. Held PJ, Brunner F, Odaka M, Garcia JR, Port FK, Gaylin DS. (1990). Five-year survival for end-stage renal disease patients in the United States, Europe, and Japan, 1982 to 1987. *American Journal of Kidney Diseases* 15, 397–401.
3. Iseki K, Kawazoe N, Osawa A, Fukiyama K. (1993). Survival analysis of dialysis patients in Okinawa, Japan (1971–1990). *Kidney International* 43, 404–9.
4. Degoulet P, Legrain M, Reach I, Aime F, Devries C, Rojas P, *et al.* (1982). Mortality risk factors in patients treated by chronic hemodialysis. Reports of the Diaphane Collaborative Study. *Nephron* 31, 103–10.
5. Iseki K, Kawazoe N, Fukiyama K. (1993). Serum albumin is a strong predictor of death in chronic dialysis patients. *Kidney International* 44, 115–19.
6. Kinjo K, Kimura Y, Shinzato Y, Kawazoe N, Takishita S, Fukiyama K, and COSMO Group. (1992). An epidemiological analysis of cardiovascular diseases in Okinawa, Japan. *Hypertension Research* 15, 111–19.
7. Iseki K, Miyasato F, Oura T, Uehara H, Nishime K, Fukiyama K. (1994). An epidemiologic analysis of end-stage lupus nephritis. *American Journal of Kidney Diseases* 23, 547–54.
8. Iseki K, Ikemiya Y, Fukiyama K. (1996). Blood pressure and risk of end-stage renal disease in a screened cohort. *Kidney International* 49, Suppl. 55, S69–71.
9. Iseki K, Iseki C, Ikemiya Y, Fukiyama K. (1996). Risk of developing end-stage renal disease in a cohort of mass screening. *Kidney International* 49, 800–5.
10. Special report from the National Institute of Neurological Disorders and Stroke: classification of cerebrovascular disorders III. (1990). *Stroke* 21, 637–76.
11. Iseki K, Kinjo K, Kimura Y, Osawa A, Fukiyama K. (1993). Evidence for high risk of cerebral hemorrahge in chronic dialysis patients. *Kidney International* 44, 1086–90.

12. Kawamura M, Fujimoto S, Hisanaga S, Yamamoto Y, Eto T. (1998). Incidence, outcome, and risk factors of cerebrovascular events in patients undergoing maintenance hemodialysis. *American Journal of Kidney Diseases* 31, 991–6.
13. Japanese Society for Dialysis Therapy. (1998). *Annual report on dialysis in Japan* (as of 31 December 1997). (In Japanese.)
14. United States Renal Data System: USRDS (1994). Annual data report. *American Journal of Kidney Diseases* 24, (Suppl. 2), 88–95.
15. Shiohira Y, Iseki K, Kowatari T, Uehara H, Yoshihara K, Nishime K, *et al.* (1996). A community-based evaluation of the effect of renal transplantation on survival in patients with renal replacement therapy. *Nippon Jinzo Gakkai Shi* 38, 449–54.
16. Iseki K, Fukiyama K. (1996). Predictors of stroke in patients receiving chronic hemodialysis. *Kidney International* 50, 1672–5.
17. Mailloux LU, Bellucci AG, Wilkes BM, Napolitano B, Mossey RT, Lesser M, *et al.* (1991). Mortality in dialysis patients: analysis of the causes of death. *American Journal of Kidney Diseases* 18, S326–35.
18. Iseki K, Nishime K, Uehara H, Osawa A, Fukiyama K. (1994). Effect of renal diseases and comorbid conditions on survival in chronic dialysis patients. *Nephron* 68, 80–6.
19. Iseki K, Nishime K, Uehara H, Tokuyama K, Toma S, Yoshihara K, *et al.* (1996). Increased risk of cardiovascular disease with erythropoietin in chronic dialysis patients. *Nephron* 72, 30–6.
20. Madore F, Lowrie EG, Brugnara C, Lew NL, Lazarus JM, Bridges K, *et al.* (1997). Anemia in hemodialysis patients: variables affecting this outcome predictor. *Journal of the American Society of Nephrology* 8, 1921–9.
21. Eschbach JW, Egrie J, Downing M, Browne J, Adamson J. (1987). Correction of anemia of end-stage renal disease with recombinant human erythropoietin. Results of a combined phase I and II clinical trial. *New England Journal of Medicine* 316, 73–8.
22. Acchiardo SR, Moore LW, Latour PA. (1983). Malnutrition as the main factor in morbidity and mortality of hemodialysis patients. *Kidney International* 24, S199–203.
23. Lowrie EG, Lew NL. (1990). Death risk in hemodialysis patients: the predictive value of commonly measured variables and an evaluation of death rate differences between facilities. *American Journal of Kidney Diseases* 15, 458–82.
24. Iseki K, Miyasato F, Tokuyama K, Nishime K, Uehara H, Shiohira Y, *et al.* (1997). Low diastolic blood pressure, hypoalbuminemia, and risk of death in a cohort of chronic hemodialysis patients. *Kidney International* 51, 1212–17.
25. Irie K, Yamaguchi T, Minematsu K, Omae T. (1993). The J-curve phenomenon in stroke recurrence. *Stroke* 24, 1844–9.
26. Wakugami K, Iseki K, Kimura Y, Okumura K, Ikemiya Y, Muratani H, *et al.* (1998). Relationship between serum cholesterol and the risk of acute myocardial infarction in a screened cohort in Okinawa, Japan. *Japanese Circulation Journal* 62, 7–14.
27. Iseki K, Ikemiya Y, Fukiyama K. (1998). Serum cholesterol and risk of end-stage renal disease in a cohort of mass screening. *Clinical Experiments in Nephrology* 2, 18–24.
28. Iso H, Jacob DR, Wentworth D, Neaton JD, Cohen JD, for the MRFIT Research Group. (1989). Serum cholesterol levels and six-year mortality from stroke in 350,977 men screened for The Multiple Risk Factor Intervention Trial. *New England Journal of Medicine* 320, 904–10.
29. Tanaka H, Ueda Y, Hayashi M, Date C, Baba T, Yamashita H, *et al.* (1982). Risk factor for cerebral hemorrhage and cerebral infarction in a Japanese rural community. *Stroke* 13, 62–73.
30. Onoyama K, Ibayashi S, Nanishi F, Okuda S, Oh Y, Hirakata H, *et al.* (1987). Cerebral hemorrhage in patients on maintenance hemodialysis. CT analysis of 25 cases. *European Neurology* 26, 171–5.
31. Caplan LR. (1992). Intracerebral haemorrhage. *Lancet* 339, 656–8.
32. Arieff AI, Massry SG, Barrientos A, Kleeman XCR. (1973). Brain water and electrolyte metabolism in uremia: effects of slow and rapid hemodialysis. *Kidney International* 4, 177–87.

33. Silver SM, DeSimone JA Jr, Smith DA Jr, Sterns RH. (1992). Dialysis disequilibrium syndrome (DDS) in the rat: role of the 'reverse urea effect'. *Kidney International* 42, 161–6.
34. Charra B, Calemard E, Chazot C, Terrat JC, Vanel T, Laurent G. (1992). Survival as an index of adequacy of dialysis. *Kidney International* 41, 1286–91.
35. Lindsay RM, Dennis BN, Bergstrom J, Johnsson C, Furst P. (1980). Platelet function as an assay for uremic toxin. *Artificial Organs* 4, (Suppl. 1), 82–9.
36. Japanese Society for Dialysis Therapy. (1996). *An overview of regular dialysis treatment in Japan* (as of 31 December 1995).
37. Wannamethee SG, Shaper AG, Perry IJ. (1997). Serum creatinine concentration and risk of cardiovascular disease: a possible marker for increased risk of stroke. *Stroke* 28, 557–63.
38. Tozawa M, Iseki K, Fukiyama K. (1996). Hypertension in dialysis patients: a cross-sectional analysis. *Japanese Journal of Nephrology* 38, 129–35.
39. The Sixth Report of the Joint National Committee on Prevention, Detection, Evaluation, and Treatment of High Blood Pressure. (1997). *Archives of Internal Medicine* 157, 2413–46.
40. Hirakata H, Onoyama K, Iseki K, Kumagai H, Fujimi S, Omae T. (1984). Worsening of anemia induced by long-term use of captopril in hemodialysis patients. *American Journal of Nephrology* 4, 355–60.
41. Brunet PH, Jaber K, Berland Y, Baz M. (1992). Anaphylactoid reactions during hemodialysis and hemofiltration: role of associating AN 69 membrane and angiotensin 1-converting enzyme inhibitors. *American Journal of Kidney Diseases* 19, 444–7.
42. Wolcott DL, Maida CA, Diamond R, Nissenson AR. (1986). Treatment compliance in end-stage renal disease patients on dialysis. *American Journal of Nephrology* 6, 329–38.
43. Morimoto A, Uzu T, Fujii T, Nishimura M, Kuroda S, Nakamura S, *et al.* (1997). Sodium sensitivity and cardiovascular events in patients with essential hypertension. *Lancet* 350, 1734–7.
44. Collins AJ, Hanson G, Umen A, Kjellstrand C, Keshaviah P. (1990). Changing risk factor demographics in end-stage renal disease patients entering hemodialysis and the impact on long-term mortality. *American Journal of Kidney Diseases* 15, 422–32.
45. Campese VM, Romoff MS, Levitan D, Lane K, Massry SG. (1981). Mechanisms of autonomic nervous dysfunction in uremia. *Kidney International* 20, 246–53.
46. Thomson GE, Waterhouse K, McDonald HP Jr, Friedman EA. (1967). Hemodialysis for chronic renal failure. Clinical observations. *Archives of Internal Medicine* 120, 153–67.
47. Vincenti F, Amend WJ, Abele J, Feduska NJ, Salvatierra O. (1980). The role of hypertension in hemodialysis-associated atherosclerosis. *American Journal of Medicine* 68, 363–9.
48. Barenbrock M, Spieker C, Laske V, Heidenreich S, Hohage H, Bachmann J, *et al.* (1994). Studies of the vessel wall properties in hemodialysis patients. *Kidney International* 45, 1397–400.
49. Hirakata H, Yano H, Osato S, Ibayashi S, Onoyama K, Otsuka M, *et al.* (1992). CBF and oxygen metabolism in hemodialysis patients: effects of anemia correction with recombinant human EPO. *American Journal of Physiology* 262, 737–43.
50. Lindner A, Charra B, Sherrard D, Scribner B. (1974). Accelerated atherosclerosis in prolonged maintenance hemodialysis. *New England Journal of Medicine* 290, 697–701.
51. Burke JF, Francos GC, Moore LL, Cho SY, Lasker N. (1978). Accelerated atherosclerosis in chronic-dialysis patients—another look. *Nephron* 21, 181–5.
52. Lundin AP, Friedman GA. (1978). Vascular consequences of maintenance hemodialysis—an unproved case. *Nephron* 21, 177–80.
53. Wolf PA, Kannel WB, Verter J. (1983). Current status of risk factors for stroke. *Neurologic Clinics* 1, 317–43.
54. Kagan A, Popper JR, Rhoads GG. (1980). Factors related to stroke incidence in Hawaii Japanese men. The Honolulu Heart Study. *Stroke* 11, 14–21.
55. Kimura N, Toshima Y, Nakayama Y, Takayama K, Tasiro H, Takagi M. (1979). Fifteen-year follow-up population survey on stroke: a multivariate analysis of the risk of stroke in farmers of Tanushimaru and fisherman of Ushibuka. In: Yamori Y, editor. *Prophylactic approach to hypertensive diseases*, pp. 505–51. Raven Press, New York.

56. Parfrey PS, Foley RN, Harnett JD, Kent GM, Murray D, Barre PE. (1996). Outcome and risk factors of ischemic heart disease in chronic uremia. *Kidney International* 49, 1428–34.

57. Churchill DN, Taylor DW, Cook RJ, La Plante P, Barre P, Cartier P, *et al.* (1992). Canadian hemodialysis morbidity study. *American Journal of Kidney Diseases* 19, 214–34.

58. Joles JA, Willekes-Koolschijn N, Koomans HA. (1997). Hypoalbuminemia causes high blood viscosity by increasing red cell lysophosphatidylcholine. *Kidney International* 52, 761–70.

58a. Stenvinkel P, Heimburger O, Paultre F, Diczfalusy U, Wang T, Berglund L, *et al.* (1999). Strong association between malnutrition, inflammation, and atherosclerosis in chronic renal failure. *Kidney International* 55, 1899–1911.

59. *Vital Statistics of Japan.* (1990). Statistics and Information Department. Minister's Secretariat. Ministry of Health and Welfare.

60. Marmot MG, Smith GD. (1989). Why are the Japanese living longer? *British Medical Journal* 299, 1547–51.

61. Bergstrom J, Heimburger O, Indholm B, Qureshi AR. (1995). Elevated serum C-reactive protein is a strong predictor of increased mortality and low serum albumin in hemodialysis (HD) patients. *Journal of the American Society of Nephrology* 6, 573 (Abstract).

62. Ridker PM, Cushman M, Stampfer MJ, Tracy RP, Hennekens CH. (1997). Inflammation, aspirin, and the risk of cardiovascular disease in apparently healthy men. *New England Journal of Medicine* 336, 973–9.

63. Grau AJ, Buggle F, Becher H, Zimmermann E, Spiel M, Fent T, *et al.* (1998). Recent bacterial and viral infection is a risk factor for cerebrovascular ischemia. Clinical and biochemical studies. *Neurology* 50, 196–203.

64. Owen WF, Lowrie EG. (1998). C-reactive protein as an outcome predictor for maintenance hemodialysis patients. *Kidney International* 54, 627–36.

65. Selhub J, Jacques PF, Wilson PW, Rush D, Rosenberg IH. (1993). Vitamin status and intake as primary determinants of homocysteinemia in an elderly population. *Journal of the American Medical Association* 270, 2693–8.

66. Moustapha A, Naso A, Nahlawi M, Gupta A, Arheart KL, *et al.* (1998). Prospective study of hyperhomocysteinemia as an adverse cardiovascular risk factor in end-stage renal disease. *Circulation* 97, 138–41.

67. Bostom AG, Shemin D, Lapane KL, Hume AL, Yoburn D, Nadeau MR, *et al.* (1996). High dose B-vitamin treatment of hyperhomocysteinemia in dialysis patients. *Kidney International* 49, 147–52.

68. Chertow GM, Ling J, Lew NL, Lazarus JM, Lowrie EG. (1994). The association of intradialytic parenteral nutrition administration with survival in hemodialysis patients. *American Journal of Kidney Diseases* 24, 912–20.

69. Levey AS, Pauker SG, Kassirer JP. (1983). Occult intracranial aneurysms in polycystic kidney disease. When is cerebral arteriography indicated? *New England Journal of Medicine* 308, 986–94.

70. Salem MM. (1995). Hypertension in the hemodialysis population: a survey of 649 patients. *American Journal of Kidney Diseases* 26, 461–8.

71. Cheigh JS, Milite C, Sullivan JF, Rubin AL, Stenzel KH. (1992). Hypertension is not adequately controlled in hemodialysis patients. *American Journal of Kidney Diseases* 19, 453–9.

72. Mansoor GA, White WB. (1997). Ambulatory blood pressure monitoring is a useful clinical tool in nephrology. *American Journal of Kidney Diseases* 30, 591–605.

73. Sehgal AR, Weisheit C, Miura Y, Butzlaff M, Kielstein R, Taguchi Y. (1996). Advance directives and withdrawal of dialysis in the United States, Germany, and Japan. *Journal of the American Medical Association* 276, 1652–6.

74. Neu S, Kjellstrand CM. (1986). Stopping long-term dialysis. An empirical study of withdrawal of life-supporting treatment. *New England Journal of Medicine* 314, 14–20.

19

Prevention of cardiovascular complications in chronic renal disease

Z.A. Massy and B.L. Kasiske

Introduction

Cardiovascular disease (CVD) is common in patients with renal failure. Indeed, data from both the United States and Europe suggest that CVD is the most common cause of death in patients with end-stage renal failure (ESRF).[1,2] In addition, risk factors for CVD may also be risk factors for renal disease and its rate of progression. In 1997 the National Kidney Foundation (NKF) convened a Task Force on CVD.[3] The Task Force examined CVD and its risk factors in four groups: (1) patients with renal insufficiency, further divided into those with and without nephrotic syndrome (NS); (2) patients treated with hemodialysis (HD); (3) peritoneal dialysis (PD) patients, and (4) renal transplant recipients (RTRs). The NKF Task Force concluded that patients in each of these four categories were at very high risk for CVD, and that the excess risk could be explained, in part, by risk factors for CVD in the general population. These include age, hypertension, hyperlipidemia, diabetes, and physical inactivity. In addition, hemodynamic and metabolic factors that are characteristically found in patients with renal disease may also play a role. These include proteinuria, increased extracellular volume, electrolyte abnormalities, anemia, thrombogenic factors, and homocysteine. The Task Force recommended that strategies for risk factor reduction should target both traditional CVD risk factors and those specific to patients with renal disease.

In this chapter we focus on the major, modifiable risk factors for CVD in patients with renal disease: hypertension, diabetes, cigarette smoking, hyperlipidemia, hyperhomocyst(e)inemia, anemia, and hyperparathyroidism. Since there are few randomized, controlled, clinical trials in renal disease patients to establish the basis for the therapy of these risk factors, in each case we will first review the evidence and strategies for intervention based on studies in the general population. We will then review factors unique to patients with renal disease that may affect the decision to treat or the approach to therapy.

Treating hypertension

Evidence from the general population, guidelines

A substantial amount of data suggests that hypertension contributes to CVD in the general population. These data come not only from large observational trials, but also from intervention trials that have been carried out using a number of different therapies in diverse populations. As a result of the strength of evidence suggesting that treatment of hypertension reduces CVD, several clinical practice guidelines for hypertension have emerged in recent years.[4–7]

Evidence supporting the treatment of hypertension in the general population has recently been summarized in the Sixth Report of the Joint National Committee (JNC VI) on Prevention, Detection, Evaluation, and Treatment of High Blood Pressure.[7] Some aspects of the JNC guidelines have been controversial. It is generally agreed that hypertension is a major risk factor for CVD and few would dispute that hypertension should be treated. More controversial, however, have been the JNC recommendations on the prioritization of specific therapies used to treat hypertension. A strictly evidence-based approach would suggest that emphasis should be placed on therapies proven to be effective in reducing CVD in large, multicenter, randomized, controlled trials. However, newer antihypertensive agents may more effectively lower blood pressure, and may have a more favorable effect on a number of 'surrogate endpoints' such as hyperglycemia and hyperlipidemia. The controversy has centered on the question of how much emphasis should placed on these surrogate endpoints and how much should remain on the results of the older, gold-standard, randomized trials.

The controversy was recently brought into focus by reports that immediate-release and short-acting nifedipine may cause an increase in mortality in patients with CVD.[8,9] More recently, the Appropriate Blood Pressure Control in Diabetes (ABCD) Trial of patients with non–insulin-dependent diabetes compared nisoldipine with enalapril for the prevention and progression of complications of diabetes. Analysis of 470 patients who had baseline diastolic blood pressure <90 mmHg showed a higher incidence of fatal and non-fatal myocardial infarctions in the nisoldipine group ($n = 237$) compared to the enalapril group ($n = 233$).[10] This finding in the ABCD Trials was in a secondary endpoint and other trials have failed to confirm adverse effects of calcium antagonists. Therefore, the matter is yet to be completely resolved. Nevertheless, the possibility that adverse effects of agents such as nifedipine may negate otherwise beneficial effects on blood pressure and other endpoints demonstrates the usefulness of large-scale clinical trials in proving the efficacy and toxicity of specific therapies for reducing CVD and all-cause mortality. Blood pressure reduction alone may not be a suitable surrogate endpoint to evaluate the usefulness of a new therapy.

Special considerations for patients with renal disease

Many observational studies have shown that blood pressure treatment slows the rate of progression of renal disease. In the Modification of Diet in Renal Disease (MDRD) Study, for example, blood pressure reduction slowed the rate of progression of renal disease, and the benefits from blood pressure reduction were greatest in patients with proteinuria. In fact, the greater the degree of proteinuria, the more effective was the blood pressure treatment in slowing the rate of renal function decline.[11] A substantial proportion of the patients that benefited from blood pressure reduction in the MDRD trial were treated with converting enzyme inhibitors. It is now recognized that converting enzyme inhibitors may be particularly beneficial in both diabetic and non-diabetic renal disease. The uniquely beneficial effect of converting enzyme inhibitors in slowing the rate of renal disease progression also appears to be proportional to the amount of proteinuria.[12] This has given rise to the concept that proteinuria *per se* contributes to renal disease progression, and that at least some of the beneficial effects of antihypertensive agents in general, and converting enzyme inhibitors in particular, may stem from their ability to reduce proteinuria. JNC VI acknowledges the unique role of converting enzyme inhibitors in the treatment of hypertension in patients with renal insufficiency.[7]

In general, hypertension is not adequately controlled in patients with renal insufficiency. In the MDRD study, for example, only 54% had blood pressure less than 140/90 mmHg.[11] There are few studies documenting the role of hypertension in CVD in patients with renal insufficiency.[13,14] However, several studies have shown that proteinuria is a risk factor for CVD. It is interesting to speculate, therefore, that the measures which reduce proteinuria might not only slow the rate of renal disease progression, but might also reduce the incidence of CVD events. In any case, it is reasonable to conclude, in the absence of solid data, that the treatment of hypertension will be at least as effective in reducing CVD in patients with renal insufficiency as it is in the general population.

The prevalence of hypertension in HD patients is approximately 80%, i.e. far higher than in the general population.[15] Hypertension is probably poorly controlled in HD patients.[15] Although there are no controlled trials proving that hypertension causes CVD in HD patients, a number of observational studies have linked blood pressure to left ventricular hypertrophy, congestive heart failure, and coronary artery disease,[15] which are, in turn, associated with increased mortality in HD patients. Nevertheless, it has been difficult to establish whether hypertension is directly linked to mortality in HD patients. This might be explained by the U-shaped curvilinear relationship between blood pressure and mortality. HD patients with either high or low blood pressure have an increased risk of dying. A similar U-shaped curvilinear relationship between blood pressure and mortality has also been observed in the general population. In both cases the association between low blood pressure and mortality can be explained by severe CVD causing reduced blood pressure and increased mortality. Intervention trials in the general population have generally failed to show any increased mortality from overzealous treatment of blood pressure. In the absence of randomized, controlled, intervention trials in HD, it is reasonable to assume that treating hypertension in HD patients will help to reduce the high incidence of CVD.

The prevalence of hypertension in PD patients is approximately 50%, which appears to be higher than in the general population, but lower than in HD patients.[15] The relationship between blood pressure and CVD appears to be similar in PD patients to that in hemodialysis patients.[15] Therefore, it is also reasonable to recommend treatment of blood pressure in this population in order to reduce CVD.

The prevalence of hypertension in RTRs is probably around 80%.[15] Possible causes of hypertension in RTRs include (1) essential hypertension, (2) graft dysfunction from chronic rejection, (3) diseased native kidneys, (4) renal artery stenosis in the transplanted kidney, and (5) immunosuppressive drugs such as cyclosporin, tacrolimus, and corticosteroids. Hypertension has been linked to renal allograft failure, counting as graft failures patients who return to dialysis and those who die with a functioning kidney.[16] Hypertension has also been associated with CVD in RTRs.[2] However, not all have been able to detect a relationship between hypertension and CVD, possibly reflecting effective intervention in some populations, or inadequate sample size.[17] In any case, it is reasonable to expect that the benefit from hypertension treatment observed in the general population should also be seen in RTRs. It is also possible that aggressive blood pressure treatment may prolong allograft survival, although this remains to be tested in clinical trials.

The NKF Task Force on CVD concluded that hypertension is common and not optimally treated in patients with ESRF.[3] The Task Force also concluded that hypertension is associated with CVD in all chronic renal disease populations, and that target blood pressure should be <140/90 mmHg in patients with ESRF. However, in patients with renal insufficiency, especially those with proteinuria, target blood pressure should be lower, i.e. <125/75 mmHg. Although clinical trials are warranted in patients with ESRF, it seems reasonable to treat blood pressure in the absence of trial data, given the high incidence of both hypertension and CVD in this population.

Diabetes control

Evidence from the general population, guidelines

Whether or not intensive blood-glucose management reduces the incidence of CVD complications in diabetics has been controversial. Many observational studies have demonstrated that individuals with poor glycemic control are at greater risk for developing CVD events. However, it cannot be inferred from this that intensive treatment will reduce this increased incidence of CVD. Only well-designed, randomized, controlled trials can establish the role of intensive insulin therapy in reducing CVD risk.

The Diabetes Control and Complications Trial (DCCT) was a multicenter, randomized, controlled trial that demonstrated that intensive insulin therapy delayed the onset and slowed the progression of retinopathy, nephropathy, and neuropathy in patients with type 1 diabetes.[18] A subgroup analysis of the DCCT examined whether intensive insulin therapy also reduced the incidence of CVD events.[19] In this study, 1441 patients aged 13–39 years, who were free of CVD at baseline, were randomly assigned to intensive insulin or conventional therapy. Patients with hypertension, hypercholesterolemia, or obesity were excluded. The number of combined macrovascular disease events was 23 in the intensive therapy group compared to 40 in the conventional treatment group, i.e. almost a 50% reduction. However, this difference was not statistically significant ($p = 0.08$). Mean cholesterol, low-density lipoprotein cholesterol, and triglycerides were each significantly lower in the intensive treatment group; however, weight gain was higher. There were no differences in other CVD risk factors between the two treatment groups.

In the Stockholm Diabetes Intervention Study 102 insulin-dependent diabetic patients were randomly allocated to intensive glucose control or usual management.[20] In a 10-year follow-up, carotid doppler study, 28 patients from the original control group had increased intima–media thickening compared to 31 from the original intensive treatment group.[21] Similarly, control patients had reduced flow-mediated dilatation of brachial arteries compared to the intensive treatment group. Mean hemoglobin A1C values were also significantly higher in the control patients (8.2 ± 0.2%) compared to the intensive treatment group (7.1 ± 0.1%, $p < 0.0001$). Unfortunately, the small sample size and post hoc nature of this analysis make it difficult to draw firm conclusions based on this study.

The results of the United Kingdom Prospective Diabetes Study (UKPDS) were reported recently.[22] This study examined the effect of intensive blood-glucose control in 3867 newly diagnosed patients with type 2 diabetes. These patients were randomly allocated to intensive therapy with a sulfonylurea or insulin versus conventional therapy with diet alone. Over 10 years the median glycated hemoglobin level was 7.0% in the intensive group and 7.9% in the conventional group. Intensive insulin therapy reduced the risk of any diabetes-related endpoint (micro- and macrovascular disease) by 12% ($p = 0.029$). However, diabetes-related deaths (death from myocardial infarction, stroke, peripheral vascular disease, renal disease, hypoglycemia, hyperglycemia, or sudden death) were not different between the two groups ($p = 0.44$). The investigators concluded that intensive blood-glucose control with either sulfonylureas or insulin decreased microvascular complications, but had no effect on macrovascular disease endpoints in patients with type 2 diabetes.[22].

The UKPDS also examined whether intensive glucose therapy with the biguanide metformin had any particular advantage.[23] In this portion of the study 753 of the 1704 obese patients with type 2 diabetes were randomly allocated to intensive blood-glucose control with metformin ($n = 342$) or to conventional treatment with diet alone ($n = 411$). In patients from the metformin group, the median glycated hemogobin level was 7.4% compared to 8.0% in the conventional group. Patients allocated to intensive blood-glucose control with metformin had a 42% ($p = 0.011$) risk reduction for diabetes-related deaths (death from myocardial infarction, stroke, peripheral vascular disease, renal disease, hypoglycemia, hyperglycemia, or sudden death) compared to conventional treatment. The metformin group also had a 39% ($p = 0.010$) lower risk for myocardial infarction (a secondary endpoint) compared to the conventional group. For all macrovascular diseases combined (myocardial infarction, sudden death, angina, stroke, and peripheral vascular disease) metformin reduced the risk by 30% ($p = 0.020$) compared to the conventional group. The authors concluded that first-line therapy with metformin appeared to be advantageous compared to diet alone in obese type 2 diabetic patients.

Thus, whether or not intensive blood-glucose management with insulin in type 1 diabetes prevents CVD remains unproven. In type 2 diabetes, intensive management with either insulin or sulfonylureas does not appear to reduce macrovascular disease events. More promising are the data from the UKPDS showing that metformin, used as first-line, intensive therapy in obese type 2 diabetic patients, reduces macrovascular disease. However, the UKPDS also demonstrated that the same results may not be obtained when metformin is added to sulfonylurea.[23]

Some data suggest that secondary intervention with intensive blood-glucose control may be beneficial in diabetic patients with myocardial infarction. Mortality from myocardial infarction is increased in patients with diabetes.[24,25] A recent trial randomly allocated 620 patients admitted to a coronary care unit with myocardial infarction and blood-glucose > 11 mmol/l (with or without previous diagnosed diabetes) to insulin–glucose infusion followed by multidose insulin treatment or conventional management.[26] The group assigned to receive intensive insulin treatment had fewer deaths during follow-up (relative risk and 95% confidence interval 0.72 (0.55–0.92), $p = 0.011$). Patients who had not been previously treated with insulin benefited the most. The mechanism for the beneficial effect of intensive insulin therapy is unknown. Whether the effect is the result of acute or chronic changes is also unclear. Suggested mechanisms include a reduction in acute ischemic injury, the restoration of altered platelet function, a decrease in plasma activity of plasminogen activator inhibitor, or a chronic reduction in risk factors such as hyperlipidemia.

Intensive control of diabetes comes with a price. That price is an increase in hypoglycemic episodes. In the DCCT trial, patients in the intensive treatment group had coma and seizures three times more frequently than patients in the control group.[18] Hypoglycemia and its consequences may be even worse in patients with renal disease who typically have had diabetes for a longer time than the mean duration of diabetes in patients enrolled in trials such as the DCCT. Similarly, in the UKPDS, major hypoglycemic episodes were significantly more frequent in intensively managed type 2 diabetics compared to patients managed with diet alone.[22] Thus, it is clear that intensive blood-glucose management increases the frequency of major hypoglycemic episodes in both type 1 and type 2 diabetes.

Special considerations for patients with renal disease

Clearly, diabetic patients with chronic renal failure (CRF) have a higher incidence of CVD compared to patients without renal insufficiency. Even patients in early stages of diabetic nephropathy manifest by microalbuminuria have an increased risk of death.[27,28] Other studies have also shown that proteinuria in patients with diabetes is associated with an increased risk of CVD.[29–31]

In theory, diabetic patients with CRF could have the added benefit from intensive blood-glucose therapy of a delay in the progression of nephropathy. Several studies have shown that glycemic control helps to prevent the development of microalbuminuria in normoalbuminuric, diabetic patients. The DCCT results, for example, demonstrated that intensive insulin therapy in type 1 diabetics delayed the onset of nephropathy.[18] Less clear is whether intensive glucose control affects the rate of progression of established diabetic nephropathy. The best evidence for this comes from studies in type 1 diabetic patients with microalbuminuria.[32–34] However, others have been unable to show that strict glycemic control slows the rate of progression of diabetic nephropathy.[35] In the DCCT there was a trend toward reduced transition from microalbuminuria to clinical proteinuria among 73 patients, but the difference was not statistically significant.[18] Perhaps the most convincing evidence that strict diabetes control can slow the rate of progression of nephropathy in type 1 diabetes comes from a study of pancreatic transplant recipients.[36] In this study the progression of diabetic morphological changes during the first 5 years of follow-up improved during the subsequent 5–10-year follow-up period.

There are no large, randomized, controlled trials examining whether strict glycemic control slows the rate of progression of type 1 diabetic nephropathy in patients with clinical proteinuria with or without decreased renal function. There are also few data examining whether intensive blood-glucose control affects the progression of renal disease in type 2 diabetic patients.[37] Thus, the attractive theory that strict glycemic control will slow the rate of progression of established diabetic nephropathy still needs rigorous testing in controlled clinical trials. Similarly, it remains unproven that strict glycemic control will reduce the incidence of cardiovascular disease in diabetic patients with renal insufficiency.

The incidence of CVD is extremely high in diabetic patients with ESRF. However, there are no observational studies examining whether the degree of glycemic control correlates with the incidence of CVD in HD patients, PD patients, or RTRs. Similarly, there are no controlled trials examining whether intensive glucose management in patients with ESRF reduces the risk of CVD.

Intensive insulin therapy for type 1 diabetes is more problematic in patients with renal disease than in the general population. Patients with diabetic nephropathy more often have long-standing diabetes, and as a result more often have autonomic neuropathy that makes it difficult to detect hypoglycemia. Similarly, gastroparesis is common in patients with long-term diabetes and nephropathy, and erratic gastric emptying makes it more difficult to regulate insulin and blood-glucose levels. Insulin metabolism is also delayed in patients with renal failure, necessitating modification of usual dosing regimens. Finally, patients with renal disease and long-standing diabetes may be more prone to severe complications of hypoglycemia, e.g. myocardial infarction or stroke, as a result of pre-existing CVD. For all of these reasons, the risk to benefit ratio of intensive insulin therapy for type 1 diabetes may not be as advantageous for patients with renal disease as it is for patients in the general population.

In patients with type 2 diabetes, as discussed above, there is no good evidence from studies in the general population that intensive management with sulfonylureas or insulin reduces the incidence of macrovascular disease complications. On the other hand, intensive therapies clearly increase the risk of hypoglycemic episodes, and the risk of adverse events could well be increased in type 2 diabetics with renal disease. Unfortunately, the encouraging results with metformin as first-line therapy in obese patients with type 2 diabetes cannot be extrapolated to type 2 diabetic patients with renal disease. Indeed, metformin is considered contraindicated in patients with renal failure.[38]

Pancreatic transplantation offers a unique opportunity to normalize blood-glucose. Pancreatic transplantation is generally limited to diabetic patients who have already undergone, or patients who undergo, simultaneous renal transplantation. Unfortunately, the number of such patients is still relatively small and it is difficult to ascertain what influence pancreatic transplantation may have on CVD. To date there have been no randomized, controlled trials to compare any aspects of pancreatic transplantation with other management strategies for diabetes.

In summary, the incidence of CVD is much higher in diabetic patients with, compared to diabetic patients without, renal disease. As a result, the potential benefit of therapies that reduce the risk of CVD could be greater in diabetics with renal disease. On the other hand, the risks of therapies to achieve strict glycemic control are greater in diabetic patients with renal disease compared to diabetics in the general population. Unfortunately, there are no large, randomized, controlled trials that define the risk to benefit ratio of intensive glucose management in diabetic patients with renal disease. Thus, the role of intensive therapy in reducing CVD in this population remains unclear.

Smoking cessation

Evidence from the general population, guidelines

The evidence that cigarette smoking causes CVD in the general population is very compelling. Indeed, in the United States smoking cessation has become a matter of public policy.[39] Comprehensive clinical practice guidelines for smoking cessation have been developed.[40,41] Guidelines were developed under the auspices of the Agency for Health Care Policy and Research by an independent panel of scientists, clinicians, consumers, and methodologists. These guidelines recommend that five major steps be taken by clinicians: (1) systematically identify all tobacco users at every visit; (2) strongly urge a smoker to quit; (3) identify smokers willing to make an effort to quit; (4) aid the patient in quitting through multiple means, including the use of nicotine patches or gum; and (5) schedule follow-up contact. A number of studies, and a meta-analysis of these studies, have confirmed the usefulness of nicotine replacement therapies in smoking cessation.[42] Finally, data suggest that smoking cessation reduces the risk of CVD.[43,44] In the Nurses' Health Study, one-third of the excess risk of coronary artery disease was eliminated within 2 years of smoking cessation.[44]

Special considerations for patients with renal disease

Recent data have suggested that smoking may contribute to renal disease and its rate of progression. In patients with insulin-dependent diabetes, for example, smoking was associated with a higher incidence of microalbuminuria and proteinuria.[45] Ravid and co-workers[46] demonstrated that cigarette smoking was a risk factor for both nephropathy and CVD in a cohort of 574 patients with type 2 diabetes. Yokoyama and co-workers[47] also found that smoking was an independent risk factor for the progression of renal disease in 182 patients with type 2 diabetic nephropathy. In a retrospective study of 160 patients with systemic lupus erythematosus, the median time to ESRF was shorter in smokers compared to non-smokers.[48] Thus, accumulating evidence suggests that smoking may contribute to renal disease and its progression.

How cigarette smoking contributes to renal disease is unclear. Ritz and co-workers[49] recently demonstrated that cigarette smoking causes acute renal hemodynamic changes and albuminuria. These acute effects of smoking were reproduced by nicotine gum. Interestingly, plasma levels of nicotine from smoking are inversely proportional to the degree of renal insufficiency.[50]

It has long been appreciated that smoking is associated with increased CVD risk in HD patients.[51] Recent data from the United States Renal Data System (USRDS) Case Mix Severity Study demonstrated that mortality in smokers was 1.26 times greater than that of non-smokers ($p < 0.002$).[52] In the USRDS Dialysis Morbidity and Mortality Study (Wave 2), the relative risk of myocardial infarction was more than twofold greater in smokers compared to non-smokers.[53] Few studies have examined the effects of cigarette smoking on CVD in RTRs or in CRF patients.[14,17] In multivariate analysis we found that cigarette smoking was an independent risk factor for CVD in a large cohort of RTRs.[17]

There are no controlled trials to prove that smoking cessation will reduce the incidence of CVD in patients with renal disease. Nevertheless, it is reasonable to conclude, based on the substantial amount of data demonstrating an adverse effect of smoking on CVD in the general population, and the limited data showing correlation between cigarette smoking and CVD in renal patients, that smoking cessation may reduce the risk of CVD in patients with renal disease. In addition, it is possible that smoking cessation may reduce the incidence and slow the rate of progression of renal disease. The lack of any risk to smoking cessation makes this intervention attractive, even if the data proving its effectiveness are incomplete. Since combining CVD risk factors results in a greater risk than can be explained by their additive effects, smoking cessation is likely to be particularly beneficial in smokers with additional CVD risk factors. Indeed, the NKF Task Force on CVD concluded that the prevalence of tobacco use in patients with renal disease is similar to that seen in the general population, and that tobacco use is associated with an increased risk for CVD.[3,54] The NKF Task Force also concluded that smoking may be linked to a greater risk of renal disease, and that it is reasonable to use general population guidelines regarding smoking cessation strategies.

Treating hyperlipidemia

Evidence from the general population, guidelines

The National Cholesterol Education Program (NCEP)–Adult Treatment Panel II guidelines continue to identify low-density lipoprotein (LDL) as the primary target of lipid-lowering therapy to reduce the incidence of CVD.[55] However, more attention to high-density lipoprotein (HDL) as a negative CVD risk factor is emphasized.[55] The role of hypertriglyceridemia, as surrogate for very low-density lipoprotein (VLDL) remnants, in the absence of elevated total or LDL cholesterol levels has not been yet documented with certainty by clinical trials.[55] Consequently, only two major treatment categories are recognized: elevated LDL cholesterol with triglycerides <2.2 mM (200 mg/dl), and elevated LDL cholesterol with triglyccrides >2.2 mM. The treatment goals based on LDL cholesterol levels and a different degree of CVD risk are divided into the following categories: in subjects without CVD and with fewer than two risk factors, LDL cholesterol should be <4.1 mM (<160 mg/dl); with two or more risk factors, <3.4 mM (<130 mg/dl). In the subjects with CVD, LDL cholesterol should be <2.6 mM (<100 mg/dl).[55] The initial approach to treatment of hyperlipidemia should be by dietary means (restriction of saturated fat and cholesterol), increase of physical activity, and, if appropriate, weight reduction.[55] If treatment goals are not achieved by this conservative approach, drug therapy should be introduced. The statins are considered as first choice to treat hypercholesterolemia, and nicotinic acid followed by fibrates to treat hypercholesterolemia associated with hypertriglyceridemia.[55] Recently, reduction of CVD morbidity and mortality has been obtained using lipid lowering therapies in both primary and secondary prevention.[56–59]

Special considerations for patients with renal disease

Hyperlipidemia (also referred to as dyslipidemia) is common in patients with renal disease;[60,61] however, lipoprotein abnormalities are different in the NS, CRF without NS, HD patients, and PD patients, as well as RTRs.[60,61] Hypertriglycerdimia secondary to triglyceride-enriched apolipoprotein-B particles and reduced HDL cholesterol are features of CRF and HD.[60,62] In addition, NS and PD patients and RTRs usually have an increase in LDL cholesterol levels.[60,62,63] There are few observational studies examining the relationship between hyperlipidemia and CVD in renal disease.[14,64,65] However, whether lipid-lowering therapies reduce the incidence of CVD events in renal disease patients remains to be determined. In a recent meta-analysis, we compared and contrasted the relative efficacy of different lipid-lowering strategies in various clinical settings of renal disease.[60] We found that antilipemic therapies had similar effects on lipoprotein abnormalities in different renal disease settings; however, only 3-hydroxy-3-methylglutaryl–coenzyme A (HMG–CoA) reductase inhibitors and fibric acid analogs had a consistent and substantial effect on lipoprotein abnormalities.[60] The effect of diet and other therapies were less consistent.[60] However, lipid-lowering therapies do not appear to be sufficient to obtain treatment goals for lipid levels in patients with renal disease as recommended by NECP guidelines for high-risk patients.[55] Of note, lipid-lowering therapies in patients with renal disease had no harmful consequences when the doses were reduced and concomitant therapy with other drugs known to cause rhabdomyolysis was avoided,[60] although long-term safety of lipid-lowering therapies in such patients is unknown.

Meanwhile it is reasonable, we believe, to follow in general the recent recommendations of the NKF Task Force on CVD.[61] In patients with NS, efforts should be made to induce a remission of NS. If this is not possible, efforts should be made to reduce proteinuria with angiotensin-converting enzyme inhibitors or by other means. If these efforts are unsuccessful, diet and subsequently lipid-lowering therapies should be added. HMG–CoA reductase inhibitors are the most effective in reducing total and LDL cholesterol levels in NS, and should generally be the first choice among pharmacological agents.[60,61]

In CRF without NS and dialysis (PD and HD), diet and lipid-lowering therapies are effective in improving lipid abnormalities.[60,61] Adjusted doses according to the level of renal function of fibric acid analogs should be the first choice in CRF and dialysis patients with both hypercholesterolemia and hypertriglyceridemia. Similar adjusted doses of HMG–CoA reductase inhibitors should generally be useful among pharmacological agents in such patients with hypercholesterolemia. The NCEP guidelines do not recommend the treatment of borderline-high triglycerides (2.2–4.4 mM, 200–400 mg/dl) without increased LDL levels except in the presence of established CVD as secondary prevention.[55] Therefore, it is reasonable to treat CRF and dialysis patients who have CVD and borderline-high triglycerides, but it is difficult to make general recommendations for primary prevention in such patients, and individual judgment should be used.

In RTRs, diet followed by the use of HMG–CoA reductase inhibitors should generally be the first choice.[60,61] Since blood levels of HMG–CoA reductase inhibitors have been shown to be high under cyclosporin and tacrolimus treatment,[66] it is necessary to reduce the doses of HMG–CoA reductase inhibitors by half in RTRs receiving such treatment. In some cases with combined hyperlipidemia, adjusted doses for reduced renal function of fibric acid analogs, particularly gemfibrozil, could be used.[67,68]

Treating hyperhomocyst(e)inemia

Evidence from the general population, guidelines

An elevated level of total homocyst(e)ine (tHcy) in blood, denoted hyperhomocyst(e)inemia, appears to be emerging as a prevalent and graded risk factor (with no threshold) for CVD in the general population.[69,70] Genetic and acquired factors, including deficiencies of folate and vitamin B12, are involved in the elevation of circulating tHcy levels.[70] In typical Western populations, supplementation with both 0.5–5 mg daily folic acid and about 0.5 mg daily vitamin B12 should reduce blood tHcy concentrations by about a quarter to a third (for example, from about 12 mM to 8–9 mM).[71] In a recent randomized and controlled trial, Malinow and colleagues[72] showed that consuming breakfast cereal fortified with 400 or 600 mg of folic acid for 5 weeks reduced plasma tHcy concentrations. Intake of this level of folic acid has been shown to reduce the incidence of neural tube birth defects,[73] and it was recommended that flour and cereal products be fortified with folic acid beginning in January 1998 in the United States to prevent such defects.[74] It is also argued that fortification of food with folic acid will significantly reduce the incidence of CVD attributable to moderate hyperhomocyst(e)inemia observed in the general population.[75] Whether this therapy effectively reduces the incidence of CVD in the general population remains to be determined.

Special considerations for patients with renal disease

Moderate elevation of plasma tHcy concentrations is present in the early stage of CRF and increases in parallel with the degree of reduction in renal function.[76] Moderate elevation of plasma tHcy concentrations is also present in HD and PD patients, and in RTRs as well.[76] Several recent prospective studies, but not all, show an association between high tHcy concentrations and CVD or events in renal disease patients.[14,65,77–79] In view of the atherogenic role of hyperhomocyst(e)inemia, attempts have been made to lower plasma tHcy concentrations in renal disease patients, although the optimum protocol has not yet been determined. Oral folic acid supplementation at 5 mg thrice weekly together with pyridoxine (250 mg twice weekly) and vitamin B12 (1 mg twice weekly) allowed a substantial (40%) and sustained (up to 6 years) reduction of plasma tHcy concentrations in pre-dialysis CRF patients.[80] Several studies in dialysis patients have shown that the supplementation with a higher pharmacological dose of folic acid (2.5–15 mg/day) than used in pre-dialysis CRF patients, either alone or combined with other B vitamins, reduced plasma tHcy levels by about 30–40%.[81–83] Recently, the use of 5-methyltetrahydrofolate, the circulating form of folate, at a dose of 15 mg/day *per os* for 2 months has led to better decrease of plasma tHcy levels (70%) than observed with folic acid supplementation in HD patients.[84] It should be noted that neither serine nor betaine effectively lowers tHcy levels in dialysis patients.[85,86] In RTRs, folic acid supplementation at 5 mg/day in combination with 50 mg/day vitamin B6 and 0.4 mg/day vitamin B12 resulted in a decrease in plasma tHcy concentrations of about 25%.[87] Of note, folate supplementation in patients with renal disease had no harmful consequences (particularly gastrointestinal distress), although data concerning long-term evaluation in such patients are limited.[80,83] Whether this therapy also reduces the incidence of CVD events in renal disease patients remains to be determined and requires controlled trials. Meanwhile it is reasonable, we believe, to prescribe a combination of high-dose folic acid (5 mg/day), vitamin B12 (0.4 mg/day), and vitamin B6 (50 mg/day) as recommended recently by the NKF Task Force on CVD,[54] which is sufficient to restore normal tHcy levels in patients with moderate CRF or in RTRs, but not in patients with severe CRF or in dialysis patients. However, the use of high-flux membrane, erythropoietin therapy, and the growing number of elderly patients may increase the need for vitamin B12 supplementation, and the use of 1 mg/day may be necessary in dialysis patients.[88] Moreover, the use of 5-methyltetrahydrofolate appears to be preferable in such patients.[84]

Treating risk factors for arteriosclerosis

Anemia

Anemia, which is present in the majority of dialysis and severe pre-dialysis CRF patients, has been found to be associated with an elevated risk of developing CVD morbidity, particularly left ventricular (LV) hypertrophy or LV dilatation in such patients.[89–92] An association between anemia and overall mortality has been also reported in dialysis patients.[90,93,94] The impact of anemia on specific CVD mortality in dialysis patients has been evaluated in only two studies with conflicting results.[95,96] In the first study, the decline in overall mortality seems to be exclusively attributable to a decline in cardiovascular deaths.[95] In the second study, the authors failed to demonstrate any statistical association between anemia and CVD mortality, although such association was present for overall mortality in dialysis patients.[96] Of note, the results of both studies were not adjusted for other confounding mortality risk factors in such patients. Thus, the role of anemia correction by recombinant human erythropoietin (r-HuEPO) in reducing CVD morbidity and mortality in this population remains unclear. There is still no demonstration to date that anemia, when present, is associated with CVD morbidity and mortality in RTRs.

In numerous studies the high efficacy of r-HuEPO in the treatment of renal anemia has been documented.[97,98] Partial correction of anemia with r-HuEPO results in reduction in LV hypertrophy or LV dilatation, although these do not return to normal in dialysis and pre-dialysis CRF patients.[99–103] However, none of these studies has demonstrated that improvement of LV abnormalities could reduce CVD morbidity and mortality in CRF patients treated with r-HuEPO. Moreover, although there is evidence that partial correction of anemia with r-HuEPO is accompanied by some CVD benefits, the issue of hemoglobin targets remains unresolved. Recently, the administration of r-HuEPO in dialysis patients with clinically evident CVD to normalize hematocrit (i.e. 42%) has been shown to be associated with an elevated number of all causes of mortality.[98] Taking into consideration the economic issue and long-term adverse events (e.g. vascular access failure and hypertension), it is reasonable, we believe, to target the hematocrit value between 33 and 36% as recommended recently by the NKF guidelines,[104] which appears to be a reasonable cost-effective level to improve cardiovascular abnormalities in ESRF patients.

Hyperparathyroidism

Secondary hyperparathyroidism is a common complication of CRF, evident with rather modest reductions in glomerular filtration rate and frequently present among dialysis patients.[105] Untreated, secondary hyperparathyroidism has been associated with LV hypertrophy and impaired cardiac function in dialysis patients,[106–109] although not in all studies.[89] There is no demonstration to date that secondary hyperparathyroidism is associated with CVD mortality in dialysis patients, although it has been observed that elevated Ca × PO$_4$ product (>72) and serum phosphorus concentration (>6.5 mg/dl) significantly increased the risk of mortality in such patients.[110] The use of phosphate binders, vitamin D metabolites and analogs, calcimimetic agents, and/or parathyroidectomy could correct secondary hyperparathyroidism in dialysis patients.[111] However, correction of secondary hyperparathyroidism, principally by parathyroidectomy, is not consistently associated with reduction of LV hypertrophy or improvement in cardiac function.[109,112–115] Until clarification of this issue, it is reasonable, we believe, to target an intact plasma parathyroid hormone concentration 2–3 times the upper limit of normal (i.e. normal range for a uremic patient),[105] which appears to be a reasonable level to improve secondary hyperparathyroidism morbidity, including cardiovascular abnormalities, in ESRF patients.

Conclusions

Despite many therapeutic advances in renal patient care, CVD morbidity and mortality remain high. A number of modifiable CVD risk factors, either traditional or specific to

Table 19.1 Recommended target of cardiovascular risk factors in patients with renal disease

Risk factor	Optimal target
Hypertension	Blood pressure level <140/90 mmHg[a]
Diabetes	ND
Smoking	Complete cessation
Hyperlipidemia	LDL cholesterol concentration <3.4 mM (for primary prevention)
	LDL cholesterol concentration <2.6 mM (for secondary prevention)
Hyperhomocyst(e)inemia	Total homocyst(e)ine concentration <14 μM
Anemia	Hematocrit value between 33 and 36%
Intact parathyroid hormone	Parathyroid hormone concentration 2–3 times the upper limit of normal range

[a]<125/75 mmHg for patients with renal insufficiency and proteinuria.
LDL, low-density lipoprotein; ND, not defined.

patients with renal disease, seem to contribute. These patients are most likely to be exposed to CVD risk factors for a long period of time, starting when they had their renal disease. It is therefore of capital importance to provide adequate intervention(s) as soon as possible in order to obtain effective cardiovascular prevention. Such preventive treatment is most likely to be multifactorial (Table 19.1). Although there are few randomized, controlled intervention trials examining whether preventive therapies are beneficial in the prevention of CVD in renal patients, it is reasonable to assume that the risks associated with CVD and the benefits of correcting such factors in renal patients are at least comparable with those in the general population. The recent recommendations of the NKF Task Force on CVD seem to be a reasonable choice to approach such therapy.[3] However, it is clear that such an approach is not sufficient, and further clinical trials are warranted in order to optimize cardiovascular prevention in patients with renal disease.

References

1. Raine, A.E., Margreiter, R., Brunner, F.P., Ehrich, J.H., Geerlings, W., Landais, P., *et al.* (1992). Report on management of renal failure in Europe, XXII, 1991. *Nephrology Dialysis Transplantation*, **7**, 7–35.
2. United States Renal Data System (1998). The USRDS and its products. *American Journal of Kidney Diseases*, **32**, S20–37.
3. Levey, A.S., Beto, J.A., Coronado, B.E., Eknoyan, G., Foley, R.N., Kasiske, B.L., *et al.* (1998). Controlling the epidemic of cardiovascular disease in chronic renal disease—what do we know—what do we need to learn—where do we go from here. *American Journal of Kidney Diseases*, **32**, 853–906.
4. Guidelines for the management of mild hypertension (1993). Memorandum from a WHO/ISH meeting. *Bulletin of the World Health Organization*, **71**, 503–17.
5. Ogilvie, R.I., Burgess, E.D., Cusson, J.R., Feldman, R.D., Leiter, L.A., Myers, M.G. (1993). Report of the Canadian Hypertension Society Consensus Conference: 3. Pharmacologic treatment of essential hypertension. *Canadian Medical Association Journal*, **149**, 575–84.
6. Sever, P., Beevers, G., Bulpitt, C., Lever, A., Ramsay, L., Reid, J., *et al.* (1993). Management guidelines in essential hypertension: report of the second working party of the British Hypertension Society. *British Medical Journal*, **306**, 983–7.
7. JNC VI (1997). The sixth report of the Joint National Committee on prevention, detection, evaluation, and treatment of high blood pressure. *Archives of Internal Medicine*, **157**, 2413–46.
8. Furberg, C.D., Psaty, B.M., Meyer, J.V. (1995). Nifedipine. Dose-related increase in mortality in patients with coronary heart disease. *Circulation*, **92**, 1326–31.
9. Grossman, E., Messerli, F.H., Grodzicki, T., Kowey, P. (1996). Should a moratorium be placed on sublingual nifedipine capsules given for hypertensive emergencies and pseudoemergencies? *Journal of the American Medical Association*, **276**, 1328–31.
10. Estacio, R.O., Jeffers, B.W., Hiatt, W.R., Biggerstaff, S.L., Gifford, N., Schrier, R.W. (1998). The effect of nisoldipine as compared with enalapril on cardiovascular outcomes in patients with non-insulin-dependent diabetes and hypertension. *New England Journal of Medicine*, **338**, 645–52.
11. Peterson, J.C., Adler, S., Burkart, J.M., Greene, T., Hebert, L.A., Hunsicker, L.G., *et al.* (1995). Blood pressure control, proteinuria, and the progression of renal disease. The Modification of Diet in Renal Disease Study. *Annals of Internal Medicine*, **123**, 754–62.
12. The GISEN (Gruppo Italiano di Studi Epidemiologici in Nefrologia) group (1997). Randomised placebo-controlled trial of effect of ramipril on decline in glomerular filtration rate and risk of terminal renal failure in proteinuric, non-diabetic nephropathy. *Lancet*, **349**, 1857–63.
13. London, G.M., Guerin, A., Pannier, B., Marchais, S., Benetos, A., Safar, M. (1992). Increased systolic pressure in chronic uremia. Role of arterial wave reflections. *Hypertension*, **20**, 10–19.

14. Jungers, P., Massy, Z.A., Khao, T., Fumeron, C., Labrunie, M., Lacour, B., *et al.* (1997). Incidence and risk factors of atherosclerotic cardiovascular accidents in predialysis chronic renal failure patients: a prospective study. *Nephrology Dialysis Transplantation*, **12**, 2597–602.

15. Mailloux, L.U., Levey, A.S. (1998). Hypertension in patients with chronic renal disease. *American Journal of Kidney Diseases*, **32**, S120–41.

16. Opelz, G., Wujciak, T., Ritz, E. (1998). Association of chronic kidney graft failure with recipient blood pressure. Collaborative Transplant Study. *Kidney International*, **53**, 217–22.

17. Kasiske, B.L., Guijarro, C., Massy, Z.A., Wiederkehr, M.R., Ma, J.Z. (1996). Cardiovascular disease after renal transplantation. *Journal of the American Journal of Nephrology*, **7**, 158–65.

18. The Diabetes Control and Complications Trial (DCCT) Research Group (1993). The effect of intensive treatment of diabetes on the development and progression of long-term complications in insulin-dependent diabetes mellitus. *New England Journal of Medicine*, **329**, 977–86.

19. The Diabetes Control and Complications Trial (DCCT) Research Group (1995). Effect of intensive diabetes management on macrovascular events and risk factors. *American Journal of Cardiology*, **75**, 894–903.

20. Reichard, P., Nilsson, B.Y., Rosenqvist, U. (1993). The effect of long-term intensified insulin treatment on the development of microvascular complications of diabetes mellitus. *New England Journal of Medicine*, **329**, 304–9.

21. Jensen-Urstad, K.J., Reichard, P.G., Rosfors, J.S., Lindblad, L.E., Jensen-Urstad, M.T. (1996). Early atherosclerosis is retarded by improved long-term blood glucose control in patients with IDDM. *Diabetes*, **45**, 1253–8.

22. UK Prospective Diabetes Study (UKPDS) Group (1998). Intensive blood-glucose control with sulphonylureas or insulin compared with conventional treatment and risk of complications in patients with type 2 diabetes (UKPDS 33). *Lancet*, **352**, 837–53.

23. UK Prospective Diabetes Study (UKPDS) Group (1998). Effect of intensive blood-glucose control with metformin on complications in overweight patients with type 2 diabetes (UKPDS 34). *Lancet*, **352**, 854–65.

24. Malmberg, K., Ryden, L. (1988). Myocardial infarction in patients with diabetes mellitus. *European Heart Journal*, **9**, 259–64.

25. Abbud, Z.A., Shindler, D.M., Wilson, A.C., Kostis, J.B. (1995). Effect of diabetes mellitus on short- and long-term mortality rates of patients with acute myocardial infarction: a statewide study. Myocardial Infarction Data Acquisition System Study Group. *American Heart Journal*, **130**, 51–8.

26. Malmberg, K. (1997). Prospective randomised study of intensive insulin treatment on long term survival after acute myocardial infarction in patients with diabetes mellitus. DIGAMI (Diabetes Mellitus, Insulin Glucose Infusion in Acute Myocardial Infarction) Study Group. *British Medical Journal*, **314**, 1512–15.

27. Mogensen, C.E. (1984). Microalbuminuria predicts clinical proteinuria and early mortality in maturity-onset diabetes. *New England Journal of Medicine*, **310**, 356–60.

28. Mattock, M.B., Morrish, N.J., Viberti, G., Keen, H., Fitzgerald, A.P., Jackson, G. (1992). Prospective study of microalbuminuria as predictor of mortality in NIDDM. *Diabetes*, **41**, 736–41.

29. Borch-Johnsen, K., Kreiner, S. (1987). Proteinuria: value as predictor of cardiovascular mortality in insulin dependent diabetes mellitus. *British Medical Journal*, **294**, 1651–4.

30. Jensen, T., Borch-Johnsen, K., Kofoed-Enevoldsen, A., Deckert, T. (1987). Coronary heart disease in young type 1 (insulin-dependent) diabetic patients with and without diabetic nephropathy: incidence and risk factors. *Diabetologia*, **30**, 144–8.

31. Nelson, R.G., Pettitt, D.J., Carraher, M.J., Baird, H.R., Knowler, W.C. (1988). Effect of proteinuria on mortality in NIDDM. *Diabetes*, **37**, 1499–504.

32. Feldt-Rasmussen, B., Mathiesen, E.R., Jensen, T., Lauritzen, T., Deckert, T. (1991). Effect of improved metabolic control on loss of kidney function in type 1 (insulin-dependent) diabetic patients: an update of the Steno studies. *Diabetologia*, **34**, 164–70.

33. Dahl-Jorgensen, K., Bjoro, T., Kierulf, P., Sandvik, L., Bangstad, H.J., Hanssen, K.F. (1992). Long-term glycemic control and kidney function in insulin-dependent diabetes mellitus. *Kidney International*, **41**, 920–3.
34. Bangstad, H.J., Osterby, R., Dahl-Jorgensen, K., Berg, K.J., Hartmann, A., Hanssen, K.F. (1994). Improvement of blood glucose control in IDDM patients retards the progression of morphological changes in early diabetic nephropathy. *Diabetologia*, **37**, 483–90.
35. Microalbuminuria Collaborative Study Group, United Kingdom (1995). Intensive therapy and progression to clinical albuminuria in patients with insulin dependent diabetes mellitus and microalbuminuria. *British Medical Journal*, **311**, 973–7.
36. Fioretto, P., Steffes, M.W., Sutherland, D.E., Goetz, F.C., Mauer, M. (1998). Reversal of lesions of diabetic nephropathy after pancreas transplantation. *New England Journal of Medicine*, **339**, 69–75.
37. Ohkubo, Y., Kishikawa, H., Araki, E., Miyata, T., Isami, S., Motoyoshi, S., *et al.* (1995). Intensive insulin therapy prevents the progression of diabetic microvascular complications in Japanese patients with non-insulin-dependent diabetes mellitus: a randomized prospective 6-year study. *Diabetes Research and Clinical Practice*, **28**, 103–17.
38. Bailey, C.J., Turner, R.C. (1996). Metformin. *New England Journal of Medicine*, **334**, 574–9.
39. Manley, A.F. (1997). Cardiovascular implications of smoking: the surgeon general's point of view. *Journal of Health Care Poor Underserved*, **8**, 303–10.
40. American Psychiatric Association (1996). Practice guideline for the treatment of patients with nicotine dependence. *American Journal of Psychiatry*, **153**, 1–31.
41. The Agency for Health Care Policy and Research Smoking Cessation Clinical Practice Guideline (1996). *Journal of the American Medical Association*, **275**, 1270–80.
42. Silagy, C., Mant, D., Fowler, G., Lodge, M. (1994). Meta-analysis on efficacy of nicotine replacement therapies in smoking cessation. *Lancet*, **343**, 139–42.
43. Hermanson, B., Omenn, G.S., Kronmal, R.A., Gersh, B.J. (1988). Beneficial six-year outcome of smoking cessation in older men and women with coronary artery disease. Results from the CASS registry. *New England Journal of Medicine*, **319**, 21, 1365–9.
44. Kawachi, I., Colditz, G.A., Stampfer, M.J., Willett, W.C., Manson, J.E., Rosner, B., *et al.* (1994). Smoking cessation and time course of decreased risks of coronary heart disease in middle-aged women. *Archives of Internal Medicine*, **154**, 169–75.
45. Microalbuminuria Collaborative Study Group, United Kingdom (1993). Risk factors for development of microalbuminuria in insulin dependent diabetic patients: a cohort study. *British Medical Journal*, **306**, 1235–9.
46. Ravid, M., Brosh, D., Ravid-Safran, D., Levy, Z., Rachmani, R. (1998). Main risk factors for nephropathy in type 2 diabetes mellitus are plasma cholesterol levels, mean blood pressure, and hyperglycemia. *Archives of Internal Medicine*, **158**, 998–1004.
47. Yokoyama, H., Tomonaga, O., Hirayama, M., Ishii, A., Takeda, M., Babazono, T., *et al.* (1997). Predictors of the progression of diabetic nephropathy and the beneficial effect of angiotensin-converting enzyme inhibitors in NIDDM patients. *Diabetologia*, **40**, 405–11.
48. Ward, M.M., Studenski, S. (1992). Clinical prognostic factors in lupus nephritis. The importance of hypertension and smoking. *Archives of Internal Medicine*, **152**, 2082–8.
49. Ritz, E., Benck, U., Franek, E., Keller, C., Seyfarth, M., Clorius, J. (1998). Effects of smoking on renal hemodynamics in healthy volunteers and in patients with glomerular disease. *Journal of the American Journal of Nephrology*, **9**, 1798–804.
50. Orth, S.R., Ritz, E., Schrier, R.W. (1997). The renal risks of smoking. *Kidney International*, **51**, 1669–77.
51. Haire, H.H., Sherrard, D.J., Scardapane, D., Curtis, F.K., Brunzell, J.D. (1978). Smoking, hypertension, and mortality in a maintenance dialysis population. *Cardiovascular Medicine*, **3**, 1163–8.

52. Anonymous. (1992). Comorbid conditions and correlations with mortality risk among 3,399 incident hemodialysis patients. *American Journal of Kidney Diseases*, **20**, 32–8.
53. United States Renal Data System (1997). The USRDS Dialysis Morbidity and Mortality Study: Wave 2. *American Journal of Kidney Diseases*, **30**, S67–85.
54. Beto, J.A., Bansal, V.K. (1998). Interventions for other risk factors—tobacco use, physical inactivity, menopause, and homocysteine. *American Journal of Kidney Diseases*, **32**, S172–83.
55. Expert Panel on Detection Evaluation and Treatment of High Blood Cholesterol in Adults (1994). Summary of the second report of the National Cholesterol Education Program (NCEP) Expert Panel on detection, evaluation, and treatment of high blood cholesterol in adults (Adult Treatment Panel II). *Circulation*, **89**, 1336–445.
56. Scandinavian Simvastatin Survival Study Group (1994). Randomized trial of cholesterol lowering in 4444 patients with coronary heart disease: the Scandinavian Simvastatin Survival Study (4S). *Lancet*, **344**, 1383–9.
57. Shepherd, J., Cobbe, S.M., Ford, I., Isles, C.G., Lorimer, A.R., Macfarlane, P.W., et al. (1995). Prevention of coronary heart disease with pravastatin in men with hypercholesterolemia. *New England Journal of Medicine*, **333**, 1301–7.
58. Sacks, F.M., Pfeffer, M.A., Moye, L.A., Rouleau, J.L., Rutherford, J.D., Cole, T.G., et al. (1996). The effect of pravastatin on coronary events after myocardial infarction in patients with average cholesterol and recurrent events. *New England Journal of Medicine*, **335**, 1001–9.
59. The Long-term Intervention with Pravastatin in Ischaemic Disease (LIPID) Study Group (1998). Prevention of cardiovascular events and death with pravastatin in patients with coronary heart disease and a broad range of initial cholesterol levels. *New England Journal of Medicine*, **339**, 1349–57.
60. Massy, Z.A., Ma, J.Z., Louis, T.A., Kasiske, B.L. (1995). Lipid-lowering therapy in patients with renal disease. *Kidney International*, **48**, 188–98.
61. Kasiske, B.L. (1998). Hyperlipidemia in patients with chronic renal disease. *American Journal of Kidney Diseases*, **32**, S142–56.
62. Attman, P.O., Samuelsson, O., Alaupovic, P. (1993). Lipoprotein metabolism and renal failure. *American Journal of Kidney Diseases*, **21**, 573–92.
63. Keane, W.F., Kasiske, B.L. (1990). Hyperlipidemia in the nephrotic syndrome. *New England Journal of Medicine*, **323**, 603–4.
64. Massy, Z.A., Kasiske, B.L. (1996). Hyperlipidemia and its management in renal disease. *Current Opinion in Nephrology and Hypertension*, **5**, 141–6.
65. Massy, Z.A., Mamzer-Bruneel, M.F., Chevalier, A., Millet, P., Helenon, O., Chadefaux-Vekemans, B., et al. (1998). Carotid atherosclerosis in renal transplant recipients. *Nephrology Dialysis Transplantation*, **13**, 1792–8.
66. Christians, U., Jacobsen, W., Floren, L.C. (1998). Metabolism and drug interactions of 3-hydroxy-3-methylglutaryl coenzyme A reductase inhibitors in transplant patients: are the statins mechanistically similar? *Pharmacology and Therapy*, **80**, 1–34.
67. Chan, T.M., Cheng, I.K.P., Tam, S.C.F. (1994). Hyperlipidemia after renal transplantation: treatment with gemfibrozil. *Nephron*, **67**, 317–21.
68. Fuhrer, J.A., Montandon, A., Descoeudres, C., Jaeger, P., Horber, F.F. (1993). Impact of time-interval after transplantation and therapy with fibrates on serum cholesterol levels in renal transplant patients. *Clinical Nephrology*, **39**, 265–71.
69. Boushey, C.J., Beresford, S.A.A., Omenn, G.S., Motulsky, A.G. (1995). A quantitative assessment of plasma homocysteine as a risk factor for vascular disease—probable benefits of increasing folic acid intakes. *Journal of the American Medical Association*, **274**, 1049–57.
70. Refsum, H., Ueland, P.M., Nygard, O., Vollset, S.E. (1998). Homocysteine and cardiovascular disease. *Annual Review of Medicine*, **49**, 31–62.

71. Anonymous. (1998). Lowering blood homocysteine with folic acid based supplements: meta-analysis of randomised trials. Homocysteine Lowering Trialists' Collaboration. *British Medical Journal*, 3, 894–8.

72. Malinow, M.R., Duell, P.B., Hess, D.L., Anderson, P.H., Kruger, W.D., Phillipson, B.E., *et al.* (1998). Reduction of plasma homocyst(e)ine levels by breakfast cereal fortified with folic acid in patients with coronary heart disease. *New England Journal of Medicine*, 338, 1009–15.

73. Pietrzik, K., Brönstrup, A. (1997). Folate in preventive medicine: a new role in cardiovascular disease, neural tube defects, and cancer. *Annals of Nutrition and Metabolism*, 41, 331–43.

74. Center for Disease Control and Prevention (1993). Recommendations for use of folic acid to reduce number of spina bifida cases and other neural tube defects. *Journal of the American Medical Association*, **269**, 1233–8.

75. Oakley, G.P.J. (1998). Eat right and take a multivitamin. *New England Journal of Medicine*, 338, 1060–1.

76. Massy, Z.A. (1996). Hyperhomocyst(e)inemia in renal failure—what are the implications? *Nephrology Dialysis Transplantation*, 11, 2392–3.

77. Massy, Z.A., Chadefaux-Vekemans, B., Chevalier, A., Bader, C.A., Drüeke, T.B., Legendre, C., *et al.* (1994). Hyperhomocysteinaemia: a significant risk factor for cardiovascular disease in renal transplant recipients. *Nephrology Dialysis Transplantation*, 9, 1103–8.

78. Bostom, A.G., Shemin, D., Verhoef, P., Nadeau, M.R., Jacques, P.F., Selhub, J., *et al.* (1997). Elevated fasting total plasma homocysteine levels and cardiovascular disease outcomes in maintenance dialysis patients—a prospective study. *Arteriosclerosis Thrombosis and Vascular Biology*, 17, 2554–8.

79. Moustapha, A., Naso, A., Nahlawi, M., Gupta, A., Arheart, K., Jacobsen, D.W., *et al.* (1998). Prospective study of hyperhomocysteinemia as an adverse cardiovascular risk factor in end-stage renal disease. *Circulation*, 97, 138–41.

80. Jungers, P., Joly, D., Massy, Z.A., Nguyen, A.T., Chabli, A., Aupetit, J., *et al.* (1998). Sustained reduction of hyperhomocysteinemia in predialysis chronic renal failure (CRF) patients by long-term folic acid supplementation. *Journal of the American Journal of Nephrology*, 9, 613 (Abstract).

81. Bostom, A.G., Shemin, D., Lapane, K.L., Hume, A.L., Yoburn, D., Nadeau, M.R., *et al.* (1996). High dose B-vitamin treatment of hyperhomocysteinemia in dialysis patients. *Kidney International*, 49, 147–52.

82. Janssen, M.J., van Guldener, C., de Jong, G.M., van den Berg, M., Stehouver, C.D., Donker, A.J. (1996). Folic acid treatment of hyperhomocysteinemia in dialysis patients. *Mineral and Electrolyte Metabolism*, 22, 110–14.

83. van Guldener, C., Janssen, M.J., Lambert, J., ter Wee, P.M., Jakobs, C., Donker, A.J., *et al.* (1998). No change in impaired endothelial function after long-term folic acid therapy of hyperhomocysteinemia in hemodialysis patients. *Nephrology Dialysis Transplantation*, 13, 106–12.

84. Perna, A., Ingrosso, D., De Santo, N.G., Galletti, P., Brunone, M., Zappia, V. (1997). Metabolic consequences of folate-induced reduction of hyperhomocysteinemia in uremia. *Journal of the American Journal of Nephrology*, 8, 1899–905.

85. Bostom, A.G., Shemin, D., Yoburn, D., Fisher, D.H., Nadeau, M., Selhub, J. (1996). Lack of effect of oral N-acetylcysteine on the acute dialysis-related lowering of total plasma homocysteine in hemodialysis patients. *Atherosclerosis*, 120, 241–4.

86. Bostom, A.G., Shemin, D., Nadeau, M.R., Shih, V., Stabler, S.P., Allen, R.H., *et al.* (1995). Short term betaine therapy fails to lower elevated fasting total plasma homocysteine concentrations in hemodialysis patients maintained in chronic folic acid supplementation. *Atherosclerosis*, 113, 129–32.

87. Bostom, A.G., Gohh, R.Y., Beaulieu, A.J., Nadeau, M.R., Hume, L., Jacques, P.F., *et al.* (1997). Treatment of hyperhomocysteinemia in renal transplant recipients. A randomized, placebo-controlled trial. *Annals of Internal Medicine*, 127, 1089–92.

88. Chandna, S.M., Tattersall, J.E., Nevett, G., Tew, C.J., O'Sullivan, J., Greenwood, R.N., *et al.* (1997). Low serum vitamin B12 levels in chronic high-flux haemodialysis patients. *Nephron*, **75**, 259–63.

89. Silberberg, J.S., Rahal, D.P., Patton, D.R., Sniderman, A.D. (1989). Role of anemia in the pathogenesis of left ventricular hypertrophy in end-stage renal disease. *American Journal of Cardiology*, **64**, 222–4.

90. Foley, R.N., Parfrey, P.S., Harnett, J.D., Kent, G.M., Murray, D.C., Barre, P.E. (1996). The impact of anemia on cardiomyopathy, morbidity, and mortality in end-stage renal disease. *American Journal of Kidney Diseases*, **28**, 53–61.

91. Levin, A., Singer, J., Thompson, C.R., Ross, H., Lewis, M. (1996). Prevalent left ventricular hypertrophy in the predialysis population: identifying opportunities for prevention. *American Journal of Kidney Diseases*, **27**, 347–54.

92. Washio, M., Okuda, S., Mizoue, T., Kiyama, S., Ando, T., Sanai, T., *et al.* (1997). Risk factors for left ventricular hypertrophy in chronic hemodialysis patients. *Clinical Nephrology*, **47**, 362–6.

93. Yang, C.S., Chen, S.W., Chiang, C.H., Wang, M., Peng, S.J., Kan, Y.T. (1996). Effects of increasing dialysis dose on serum albumin and mortality in hemodialysis patients. *American Journal of Kidney Diseases*, **27**, 380–6.

94. Madore, F., Lowrie, E.G., Brugnara, C., Lew, N.L., Lazarus, J.M., Bridges, K., *et al.* (1997). Anemia in hemodialysis patients: variables affecting this outcome predictor. *Journal of the American Journal of Nephrology*, **8**, 1921–9.

95. Mocks, J., Franke, W., Ehmer, B., Scigalla, P., Quarder, O. (1997). Analysis of safety database for long-term epoetin-beta treatment. A meta-analysis covering 3697 patients. In: Koch, K.M., Stein, G., editors. *Pathogenetic and therapeutic aspects of chronic renal failure*, pp. 163–79. Marcel Dekker, New York.

96. Locatelli, F., Conte, F., Marcelli, D. (1998). The impact of hematocrit levels and erythropoietin treatment on overall and cardiovascular mortality and morbidity—the experience of the Lombardy Dialysis Registry. *Nephrology Dialysis Transplantation*, **13**, 1642–4.

97. Eschbach, J.W. (1991). Erythropoietin 1991—an overview. *American Journal of Kidney Diseases*, **18**, 3–9.

98. Besarab, A., Bolton, W.K., Browne, J.K., Egrie, J.C., Nissenson, A.R., Okamoto, D.M., *et al.* (1998). The effects of normal as compared with low hematocrit values in patients with cardiac disease who are receiving hemodialysis and epoetin. *New England Journal of Medicine*, **339**, 584–90.

99. Macdougall, I.C., Lewis, N., Saunders, M.J., Cochlin, D.L., Davies, M.E., Hutton, R.D., *et al.* (1990). Long-term cardiorespiratory effects of amelioration of renal anaemia by erythropoietin. *Lancet*, **335**, 489–93.

100. Pascual, J., Teruel, J.L., Moya, J.L., Liaño, F., Jiménez-Mena, M., Ortuño, J. (1991). Regression of left ventricular hypertrophy after partial correction of anemia with erythropoietin in patients on hemodialysis: a prospective study. *Clinical Nephrology*, **35**, 280–7.

101. Wizemann, V., Schafer, R., Kramer, W. (1993). Follow-up of cardiac changes induced by anemia compensation in normotensive hemodialysis patients with left-ventricular hypertrophy. *Nephron*, **64**, 202–6.

102. Portoles, J., Torralbo, A., Martin, P., Rodrigo, J., Herrero, J.A., Barrientos, A. (1997). Cardiovascular effects of recombinant human erythropoietin in predialysis patients. *American Journal of Kidney Diseases*, **29**, 541–8.

103. London, G.M., Zins, B., Pannier, B., Naret, C., Berthelot, J.M., Jacquot, C., *et al.* (1989). Vascular changes in hemodialysis patients in response to recombinant human erythropoietin. *Kidney International*, **36**, 878–82.

104. Anemia Work Group for National Kidney Foundation (1997). National Kidney Foundation–Dialysis Outcomes Quality Initiative (NFK–DOQI): Clinical practice guidelines for the treatment of anemia of chronic renal failure. *American Journal of Kidney Diseases*, **12**, 192–240.

105. Fournier, A., Oprisiu, R., Hottelart, C., Yverneau, P.H., Ghazali, A., Atik, A., *et al.* (1998). Renal osteodystrophy in dialysis patients: diagnosis and treatment. *Artificial Organs*, **22**, 530–57.

106. London, G.M., De Vernejoul, M.C., Fabiani, F., Marchais, S., Guerin, A.P., Metvier, F., *et al.* (1987). Secondary hyperparathyroidism and cardiac hypertrophy in hemodialysis patients. *Kidney International*, **32**, 900–7.

107. Harnett, J.D., Parfrey, P.S., Griffiths, S.M., Gault, M.H., Barre, P., Guttmann, R.D. (1988). Left ventricular hypertrophy in end-stage renal disease. *Nephron*, **48**, 107–15.

108. Rostand, S.G., Sanders, C., Kirk, K.A., Rutsky, E.A., Fraser, R.G. (1988). Myocardial calcification and cardiac dysfunction in chronic renal failure. *American Journal of Medicine*, **85**, 651–6.

109. Rostand, S.G., Sanders, P.C., Rutsky, E.A. (1994). Cardiac calcification in uremia. *Contributions to Nephrology*, **106**, 26–9.

110. Block, G.A., Hulbert-Shearon, T.E., Levin, N.W., Port, F.K. (1998). Association of serum phosphorus and calcium x phosphate product with mortality risk in chronic hemodialysis patients: a national study. *American Journal of Kidney Diseases*, **31**, 607–17.

111. Chertow, G., Martin, K.J. (1998). Current and future therapies for the medical management of secondary hyperparathyroidism. *Seminars in Dialysis*, **11**, 267–70.

112. Drüeke, T., Fauchet, M., Fleury, I., Lesourd, P., Toure, Y., Le Pailleur, C., *et al.* (1980). Effect of parathyroidectomy on left ventricular function in hemodialysis patients. *Lancet*, **I**, 112–14.

113. Gafter, U., Battler, A., Eldar, M., Zevin, D., Neufeld, H.N., Levi, J. (1985). Effect of hyperparathyroidism on cardiac function in patients with end-stage renal disease. *Nephron*, **41**, 30–3.

114. Fellner, S.K., Lang, R.M., Neumann, A., Bushinsky, D.A., Borow, K.M. (1991). Parathyroid hormone and myocardial performance in dialysis patients. *American Journal of Kidney Diseases*, **18**, 320–5.

115. Lemmilä, S., Saha, H., Virtanen, V., Ala-Houhala, I., Pasternack, A. (1998). Effect of intravenous calcitriol on cardiac systolic and diastolic function in patients on hemodialysis. *American Journal of Nephrology*, **18**, 404–10.

Index